PLATE 2-1

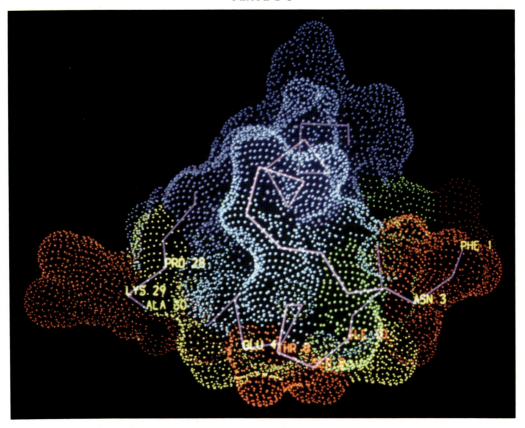

View of Insulin This computer-generated image shows that antigenic determinants cluster at highly flexible regions. The α-carbon backbone is shown
with purple lines. The molecular surface is indicate with dots, color-coded
from most mobile to most rigid in the order red, yellow, green, deep blue,
light blue. Residues forming antigenic determinants are labeled in orange
(contiguous) and yellow (discontiguous) and can be seen to correspond with
the more mobile regions. [Computer image by J. A. Tainer and E. D. Getzoff,
Research Institute of Scripps Clinic; used with permission]

PLATE 3-1

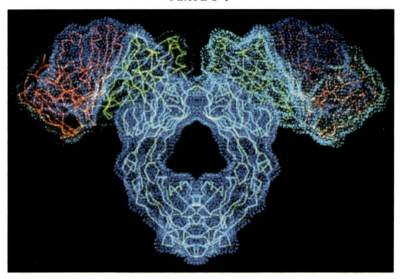

An Antibody Molecule The four-chain antibody molecule is depicted in this computer graphic. The heavy chains are shown as dark blue surfaces and the light chains as green surfaces. The constant regions are shown as light blue (heavy chain) and yellow (light chain) skeletons. The variable regions are shown as red skeletons. [Computer image by A.J. Olson; used with permission]

PLATE 4-1

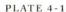

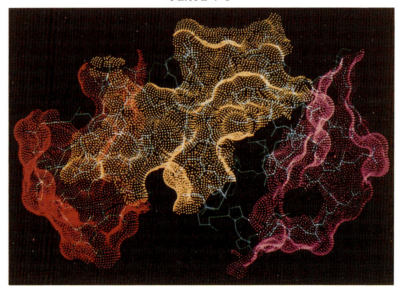

Epitopes of Lysozyme The three epitopes of lysozyme are shown from X-ray crystallographic data and computer-generated images. Each of the three epitopes is shown in a different color. From this depiction it is clear that the epitopes comprise large areas of the surface.

PLATE 4-2

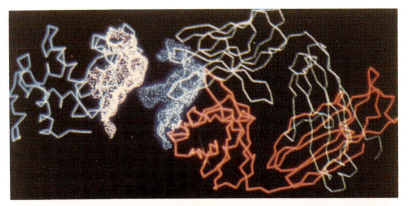

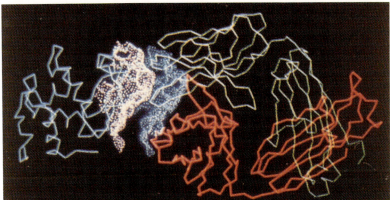

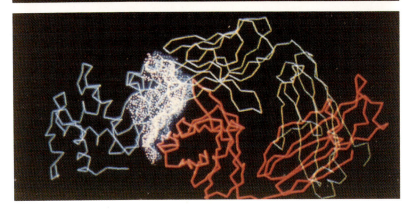

Interaction of Lysozyme and Anti-Lysozyme The α-carbon representation of lysozyme is on the left in blue, with the interacting surface shown in pink. The anti-lysozyme Fab is on the right with the L chain shown in yellow, the H chain in red and its interacting surface in blue. (Top image) The molecules are 15 Å apart. (Middle image) The molecules are 7.5 Å apart. (Bottom image) The molecules as they interact and are found in the crystal. [From Davies, Sheriff, and Padlan, 1988. *J. Biol. Chem.* 263: 10541. Used with permission]

PLATE 4-3

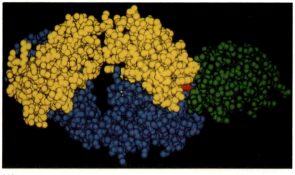

(A)

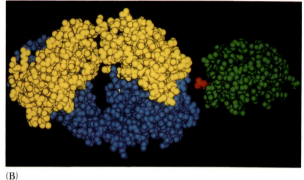

(B)

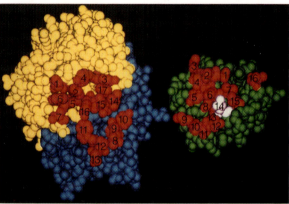

(C)

Space-Filling Representation of Anti-Lysozyme Fab and Lysozyme Interaction (A) The antigen-antibody interaction between HEL (hen egg lysozyme) and a Fab of anti-HEL. (B) The Fab and HEL models have been pulled apart to indicate that the protuberances and depressions of each fit in the complementary surface features of the other. (C) End-on views of the antibody-combining site (left) and the epitopes of the antigen. This view is obtained by rotating each of the molecules approximately 90 degrees around a vertical axis. Contacting residues on the antigen and antibody are shown in red. The antibody H chain is shown in blue, and the L chain is in yellow. Lysozyme is shown in green. (Gln 121 of HEL is shown in red for reasons we have not discussed.) [From Amit, Mariuzza, Philips and Poljak, 1986. *Science* 233: 747. Used with permission]

PLATE 7-1

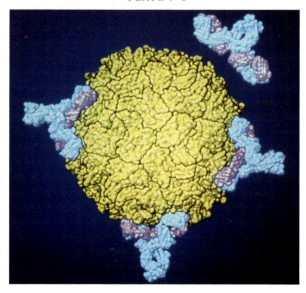

Neutralization of Poliovirus by Antibody Antibodies against sites on the virus involved in binding to cells interfere with viral infection. This computer graphic model is of four Ig molecules interacting with a poliovirus particle (gold). The H chains of each Ig are light blue; the L chains are purple. Although the interaction depicted is hypothetical, it shows the relationship of size and symmetry between Ig and virus in a model that uses X-ray crystallographic coordinates for the independently solved structures of both. A. J. Olson developed the model by using the independently solved structures of an intact Ig (D. R. Davies, NIH) and polio virus (W. Hogle, Scripps). [Courtesy of A. J. Olson]

PLATE 9-1

Model of CDR-Grafted Antibody Molecular model of V region of humanized mouse anti-Tac antibody. Amino acids of a human Ig molecule are shown in light blue. The amino acids in the CDRs are shown in red, and amino acids from a mouse molecule that potentially interact with the CDRs are shown in deep blue. Some other mouse amino acids that were incorporated into the human molecule are shown in yellow. [From Queen et al., 1989. *Proc. Natl. Acad. Sci. U.S.A.* 86: 1029. Illustration courtesy of C. Queen]

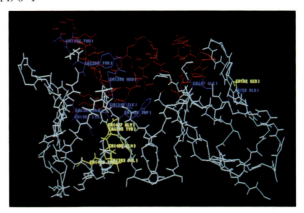

PLATE 20-1

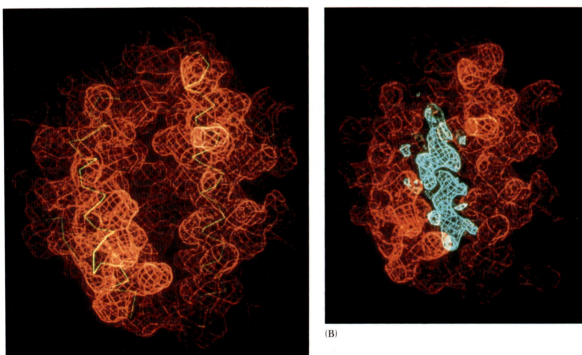

(A)

(B)

The Class I Molecule "Groove" An X-ray crystallographic view of the class I MHC molecule "groove," which probably contains processed antigen fragments. (A) View looking "down" on the HLA-A2 MHC molecule, as discussed in Chapter 15. (B) The groove is filled with an electron density that probably represents a number of different antigenic fragments bound to the MHC molecules in the crystal. [Courtesy of P. Bjorkman]

PLATE 22-1

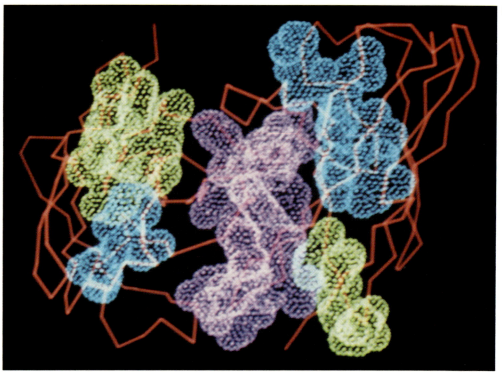

(A)

The T-Cell Receptor, the MHC–Peptide Complex, and the Possible Interaction Between Them (A) Immunoglobulin-like binding sites (CDRs) on the T-cell receptor. The van der Waals surfaces of the three CDRs are shown for both the V_H and V_L. CDR1 is blue, CDR2 is purple, and CDR3 is yellow. (B) Model for the T-cell receptor interaction with the peptide–MHC complex. This view is a side view of one that would be obtained by rotating the views seen (A) so that it would fit on top of the hypothetical peptide in the groove on the top of the MHC molecule (see PLATE 20-1B). [For details of the representations see Davis and Bjorkman, 1988. *Nature* 334: 395. Courtesy of P. Bjorkman]

PLATE 22-1

(B)

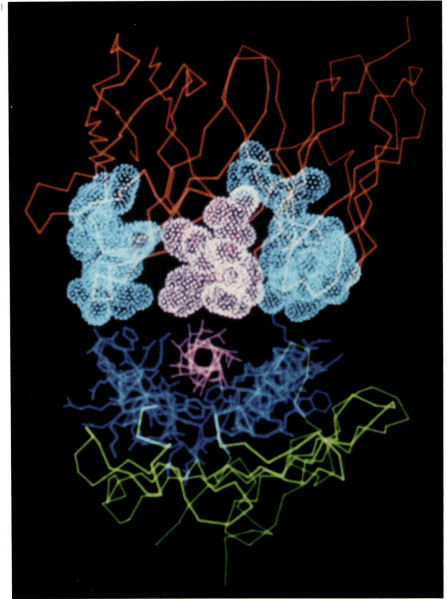

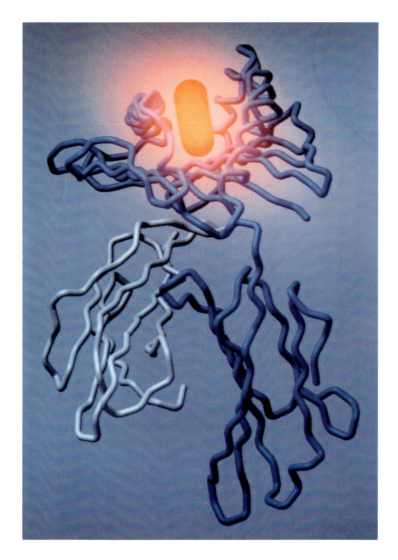

Computer graphic model of the human class I histocompatibility antigen HLA-A2, created by Arthur J. Olson, Research Institute of Scripps Clinic. This model uses the X-ray crystallographic coordinates from the structure reported by Bjorkman et al., 1987 (*Nature* 329: 506). The α-carbon backbone of the HLA structure is shown in two shades, with the heavy chain in deep blue and the β_2-microglobulin in light blue. The glowing orange shape, representing a peptide, sits in the proposed antigen-binding groove of the heavy chain, which is formed by two α helices lying on a large β sheet. The molecular models were rendered using the program MCS, written by Michael Connolly. The glowing effect surrounding the antigen was created on a Sun Microsystems TAAC-1 by compositing a low-pass Fourier filtered image of the peptide tube with the original image, using software developed by Michael Pique of Scripps Clinic.

IMMUNOLOGY
A SYNTHESIS
Second Edition

EDWARD S. GOLUB

R. W. Johnson Pharmaceutical Research Institute
Scripps Clinic and Research Foundation

DOUGLAS R. GREEN

La Jolla Institute of Allergy and Immunology and
The University of Alberta

SINAUER ASSOCIATES, INC. • PUBLISHERS
Sunderland, Massachusetts

PART-OPENING ELECTRON MICROGRAPHS

Part 1 (page 19): Antibody–hapten complex (purified rabbit anti-2,4-dinitro-phenyl antibody and a bivalent hapten). [From Valentine and Green, 1967. *J. Mol. Biol.* 27: 615]

Part 2 (page 191): A resting lymphocyte, probably a T cell (×21,800). [Courtesy of D. Zucker-Franklin, New York University Medical Center]

Part 3 (page 543): Immune complexes, seen as electron-dense, hump-shaped deposits in the upper third of the photo, along a capillary wall in a glomerulus following streptococcal glomerulonephritis (×17,250). [Courtesy of M. N. Yum, Indiana University Medical Center]

IMMUNOLOGY: A SYNTHESIS
Second Edition

Library of Congress Cataloging-in-Publication Data

Golub, Edward S., 1934–
    Immunology, a synthesis / Edward S. Golub, Douglas R. Green. —
2nd ed.
        p.   cm.
    Includes bibliographical references.
    Includes index.
    ISBN 0-87893-263-1 (cloth)
    1. Immunology.   I. Green, Douglas R.   II. Title.
    [DNLM: 1. Immunity.   2. Immunologic Diseases.   QW 504 G629i]
    QR181.G66   1991
    616.07′9—dc20
    DNLM/DLC
    for Library of Congress   91-4617
                                                                                            CIP

Printed in U.S.A.

5   4   3   2

This book is for our wives, Constance Jordan and Rona Mogil, both of whom we know always wanted a book like this.

*The **next** edition will be dedicated to our parents.*

Brief Contents

Contents

PART 2: CELLULAR IMMUNOLOGY   191

Section I: Origin and Organization of Lymphoid Tissue   192

Section V: Regulation of the Immune Response 480

PART 3: IMMUNITY AND IMMUNOPATHOLOGY 543

Preface

This book was written by the two of us. One of us (ESG) has been writing textbooks of immunology since the mid-1970s, a time when the complexity and beauty of the immune system was first being glimpsed. He has seen the repeated application of new approaches and technologies to old problems, sometimes resulting in solutions and sometimes opening up whole new areas of investigation. He thus brings what we hope is a mature perspective to the book and a healthy skepticism towards current fashions in the field. (This is a kind way of saying that he is becoming a skeptical curmudgeon.) The second author (DRG) is beginning now where the first author began all those years ago—caught up in the excitement of recent developments and looking forward to the new directions these developments will bring. (This is a kind way of saying that what he lacks in age he makes up for in enthusiasm.) There have been a great many intellectual arguments along the way (and of course none of the other kind); several bets have been duly registered; and both of us feel we have written a book that neither of us could have written alone.

In the past two decades, immunology has metamorphosed from a field that was tolerated by the scientific community only because of its practical applications into a major area of biological research. The reader, however, should not fall into the trap of thinking the research that preceded this "emergence" is only of historical interest. Science builds on what has gone before, and we have attempted to develop our current ideas about the immune system from the early observations. We will see how nearly every major advance in immunology was presaged by prior experiments, and how even "wrong turns" on the path to our present understanding have been important. But there is an even more important effect of laying these foundations. It is a fact of science that our views are in a state of flux; interpretations change regularly, and without knowing *how* we know what we know, these changes can render an earlier view of the field worthless. However, one who is versed in the development of the current viewpoint will experience the excitement of incorporating new findings into this perspective.

Acknowledgments

We would like to thank the following colleagues for the time they have spent with us in discussions and for providing selected literature for our education: Pam Bjorkman, Lee Hood, Charlie Janeway, Tak Mak, Gordon Mills, John Monroe, Carey Queen, Eli Sercarz, Liz Simpson, Hung-Sia Teh, and Irv Weissman.

We would especially like to thank our colleagues in Edmonton and La Jolla, many of whom had to put up with the mood swings and absences engendered by this project. In Edmonton: Mike Belosovic, Chris Bleackley, Erwin Diener, Mike Longnecker, Bhagi Singh, Tim Mosmann, Tom Wegman, and the medical school classes of 1985–1989. In La Jolla: Amnon Altman, Dennis Burton, Dick Dutton, Carol Forsyth, Arun Fotedar, Howie Grey, Steve Hedrick, Kimi and Teri Ishizaka, Norman Klinman, Rich Lerner, Art Olson, Jonas Salk, John Sprent, Susie Swain, Barry Toyonaga, Bill Weigle, Ian Wilson, and Maurizio Zanetti.

For artwork we thank Jana Lauzon, Art Olson, and John Woolsey. Critical reviews of various sections of the manuscript by Dennis Burton, Tommy Douglas, Pat Jones, Roberta Pollock, Susie Swain, and Maurizio Zanetti were very helpful. We are especially indebted to Judith Owen and Jeffrey Sich for their very thorough critiques of the entire manuscript. Our wonderful copyeditor, Gretchen Becker, saved us from some embarassing errors. The good-natured crowd at Sinauer Associates were pushed to the limits of congeniality by this time having to deal with two mad immunologists. It must be more than money that keeps them coming back for more.

Finally, readers must get bored with all of the thanks writers give to their families, but anyone who has had the misfortune to write a whole book knows that the price paid by those who are near and dear is much greater than that paid by the authors. Our wives Constance and Rona have put up with so much that it seems too cruel to tell them we will be starting work on the next edition soon.

Edward S. Golub
Douglas R. Green
La Jolla, California

A Note to the Reader

It has struck us in our teaching that textbooks are almost always dull but science is almost always fun. As in the earlier incarnations of this book, we have attempted to make immunology as exciting and enjoyable to the beginner as it is to us and to our colleagues. This note tells you what we plan to do and how the book can be used. Perhaps most important, it tells what the book is *not* going to do. We urge you to read it, because it may save you a lot of work if you find this isn't your cup of tea.

What this book is not

Immunology has become a growth industry. It is impossible for any one person to follow all of the literature in the scientific journals, and it is rapidly becoming a full-time job to follow stories about immunology in the popular press. In a field in which information is accumulating so rapidly, only a fool would attempt to write a full book that claimed to have all the very latest data. In fact, during the time it will take you to read this book, it is safe to assume that there will be at least four articles published that radically change at least one of the areas in this field.

Therefore, this book is not a review of the latest advances in immunology. It is a synthesis of the field in general that attempts to prepare the reader to follow the scientific literature and be a critical reader of the popular writing about immunology.

Who this book is not for

Since the sole purpose of this book is to prepare the reader to be an intelligent reader of the immunological literature, if you are already able to do this, then this book is not for you. After working through this book you may want to keep up with the field by reading review journals such as *Immunology Today, Annual Review of Immunology, Immunological Reviews*, or *Advances in Immunol-*

ogy. If you are at the stage where you can do that now, Stop! Do Not Pass Go! Give the book to someone who needs it to get to your exalted state. He or she will thank you for it.

How to use this book if it is for you

As you go through this book you will see that we have written it with the idea in mind that *science is a process*, not a series of facts. Obviously one needs facts in order to have a process, and you will get plenty of facts in this book. But remember, the facts come from experiments, and these experimental facts must be put into a conceptual framework to make sense. Knowing that there are approximately 10^{12} lymphocytes in a human being is of little value. Using that fact in attempting to determine how large the immune repertoire of the human can be is science. Whenever it is reasonable to do so, we will lead you to experimental facts by guiding you through experimental designs. This means that you will understand the question that was being asked, how the experiment was designed to answer that question, how it was carried out, and how the results were interpreted.

The data that emerge from a good experiment last forever, but their interpretation can change often. That is the essence of scientific progress; not that the old facts are wrong, only that because of the emergence of new facts they are seen in a different light. We will give you what we feel are the current interpretations of the experimental facts in the sections marked *Synthesis* (hence the title of the book). Remember, these syntheses are opinion; the experiments are fact. In the next edition we will use many of the same experiments and facts, but because of new experiments, we will change some of the syntheses.

We hope you will find immunology as intellectually rewarding and as much fun as we do.

BUILDING AN IMMUNE SYSTEM
Clonal Selection and the Nature of the Immune Response

Overview Immunology is the study of the immune system. Unlike many systems in the body (or in nature), the existence of the immune system was not recognized until the end of the nineteenth century, making this a relatively new field of study. The principles of immunity to disease had been recognized for millenia and may have been applied to preventing disease for the same period of time. Yet the idea that a specialized system in the body performs this service required fundamental changes in the understanding of the basis of disease. Once this idea was grasped, it became apparent that the body has the capability of responding in a specific way to nearly any foreign substance that enters, resulting in the destruction, removal, or neutralization of a threat to health. Finding ways to enhance this effect ushered in the Golden Age of immunization, when many widespread diseases were brought under control through vaccination. Even then, however, the immune system did not reveal itself; instead, researchers slowly had to build an increasingly complex scaffold onto which they could hang their findings.

Today, the underlying assumption of modern immunology is that the cells that carry out the reactions leading to specific immune responses are preprogrammed to respond to the substance (called antigen) that induces the response. An antigen does not instruct the immune system in what specificity to generate; rather, it selects those cells displaying a receptor of the appropriate specificity and induces them to proliferate and differentiate, resulting in the expansion of specific clones of reactive cells. This process is called CLONAL SELECTION. A solid comprehension of clonal selection is the first step in understanding how the immune system is built, and further, how the immune system changes to respond to any foreign substance through interactions with the environment. Throughout this book we will assume the validity of

CHAPTER

1

The moral is that although the "ordinary processes of scientific discovery" are culpably wasteful and inefficient, and are looked upon with contemptuous disfavour by people who have never made a discovery of any importance in their lives, we cannot do better; *scientific discovery cannot be premeditated.*

P. B. Medawar
The Uniqueness of the Individual, Introduction to the Second Edition

clonal selection and follow its development from the origin of immunology in folk medicine to the modern era of molecular biology. And although this chapter does not convey many scientific "facts" in the manner usual in textbooks, the reader is urged to read it because of the importance of the idea of clonal selection to the understanding of immunology.

Before Immunology: The Phenomenon of Immunity

The study of immunology is to a great extent the study of the cell biology of lymphocytes. Immunology is a discipline that, using the tools of cell and molecular biology, asks questions about self–nonself discrimination, cellular recognition, and genetic organization. As the reader will soon learn, it requires an interest in and a knowledge of many aspects of modern biology and biochemistry. Yet the beginnings of immunology are to be found in the ancient folk observation that people, having once recovered from a disease, do not get the disease again.[1]

> Yet still the ones who felt most pity for the sick and the dying were those who had had the plague themselves and had recovered from it. They knew what it was like and at the same time felt themselves to be safe, *for no one caught the disease twice,* or, if he did, the second attack was never fatal. Such people were congratulated on all sides, and they themselves were so elated at the time of their recovery that *they fondly imagined that they could never die of any other disease in the future.* [Thucydides, *The Peloponnesian War* (italics added)]

The fortunate few who recovered from the plague conceived of this *immunitas* as a boon from the gods. If a benevolent deity spared you from one plague, they reasoned, it was only natural to assume that you were to be spared from *all* diseases. Of course, people learned, over a period of time, that this is not the case. Immunity from one disease does not grant you immunity to another; the immunity is *specific*, whatever (or whoever) was responsible for it.

Because the concept of specific immunity came to be firmly

---

[1] Even the name immunology comes from this experience. The Latin words *immunitas* and *immunis* derive from the Roman notion of being exempt from service (usually military) to the state. Arthur Silverstein, who has arguably become the foremost historian of immunology, points out that the word was probably first used in the context in which we use it today by the Roman Marcus Annaeus Lucanus (A.D. 39–65) in his poem *Pharsalia* to describe the resistance to snakebite of the Psylli tribe of North Africa. [Silverstein, A. M. and A. A. Bialasiewicz. 1980. *Cell. Immunol.* 51: 151]

implanted in folklore, it is not surprising that eventually it was given a practical application in some societies. (It is interesting to ask why it was *not* put into practice in others.) It is not known who first intentionally immunized healthy individuals in order to prevent subsequent disease. Several African peoples had the long-standing practice of mixing the dried and pulverized poison glands from different venomous snakes and placing them under the skin to produce resistance to snakebite. Similarly, resistance to some poisons can be produced by taking very small doses of the poison and gradually increasing the dose, a practice ascribed to Mithridates VI, King of Pontus from 120 to 63 B.C.

At least as early as 1000 A.D. (and probably much earlier) the Chinese inoculated healthy people with material removed from a pustule of a person suffering from smallpox. According to a letter from an English trader of the East India Company in 1700, the method involved "opening the pustules of one who has the Small Pox ripe upon them and drying up the Matter with a little Cotton, . . . and afterwards put it up the nostrils of those they would infect." The letter was communicated to the Royal Society that same year; but the members of this august body failed to follow the suggestion of their compatriot even though smallpox was then a scourge in England.

It is likely that the Chinese introduced this practice into Turkey, where it gained popularity as a way to ensure the fair complexions of young girls bound for harems. Lady Mary Montagu, the wife of the British ambassador to Constantinople (now Istanbul) in the early 1700s, is usually credited with introducing the practice of inoculation against smallpox into European society. In a much-quoted letter to her friend Sarah Chiswell in 1717, she wrote: "I am going to tell you a thing that I am sure will make you wish yourself here. The small-pox, so fatal, and so general amongst us, is here entirely harmless by the invention of *ingrafting*. . . . I am patriot enough to take pains to bring this useful invention into fashion in England and I should not fail to write to some of our doctors very particularly about it, if I knew any one of them that I thought had virtue enough to destroy such a considerable branch of their revenue for the good of mankind!" In 1718, while still in Constantinople, the six-year-old Montagu son was inoculated by Charles Maitland, the surgeon to the embassy. Upon her return to London, Lady Montagu attempted to get the same Dr. Maitland, now retired and also returned to England, to inoculate her three-year-old daughter with pustules from people afflicted in the smallpox epidemic of 1721. But Maitland consented to perform the deed, which he had done in the East with no apparent reservations, only if outside physicians were present as witnesses. (Perhaps we see here not only the origins of vaccination but also an incident in the early history of malpractice suits.) Witnesses were found, and the child was successfully inoculated; in fact, one witness was so impressed that he had the only one of his children who had not died of the pox similarly inoculated. But the practice of inoculating healthy individuals with pustules from infected ones did not gain favor in England despite further testing.[2] Edward Jenner introduced a safer (and esthetically more pleasing) method of vaccination in 1798. It is part of medical lore that Jenner had noted that milkmaids had the scars of the pox on their hands and not on their faces. Milkmaids themselves knew that because they were infected with cowpox they did not get smallpox; and Jenner, reasoning from this experience, intentionally induced a mild case of cowpox in his patients in order to protect them from smallpox.

Jenner's methods of immunization against smallpox (and the twentieth century efforts of the World Health Organization) led eventually to the worldwide elimination of this disease in the 1980s. As important as Jenner's contribution is, he did not envision any further application of his work. It took nearly 100 years, and a new theory of disease, to realize that vaccination is a general approach to preventing disease. With that realization came the beginnings of the science of immunology.

The Invention of Immunization

Louis Pasteur and the Golden Age

The middle of the nineteenth century was a time of political and scientific ferment. The career of Louis Pasteur (1822–1895) exemplified the times. Trained as a chemist, he made important contributions to structural chemistry before turning to the nature of fermentation in 1857. Fermentation was then a loosely applied term referring to the "spontaneous" changes seen in the making of wine or beer (alcoholic fermentation) and the souring of milk (lactic fermentation). These were thought to be caused by chemical agents that catalyzed chemical reactions. Even though Schwann and others had shown in 1837 that yeasts were living entities, the great chemists and their followers did not see any value in micro-

[2] The complex reasons for this are discussed in Silverstein and Miller, 1981 [*Cell. Immunol.* 61: 437].

scopic evidence. The idea that living agents were involved was relegated to "vitalism," which was anathema to scientists like Leibig, Berzelius, Helmholz, and Wohler. The yeasts seen in fermentation were considered by them to be chemical precipitates.[3]

By 1860, Pasteur had moved from the views of the chemist to that of the biologist and had formalized the theory that different kinds of fermentations are produced by different kinds of organisms. The extension of this idea is that "disease" is a fermentation also due to a living agent. Ultimately, this was to lead Pasteur and the world to the germ theory of disease, that is, the crucial idea that each infectious disease is caused by a specific microbe.

It is important to realize the tenor of the times. Charles Darwin had published *On the Origin of Species* in 1859. The hold of the church and the past on the European mind was changing rapidly. In France a great (and final) debate on the subject of the spontaneous origin of life was raging, and Pasteur, who never avoided a conflict, was at the center of it. The now famous swan-necked flask experiment is still used as the final argument against the idea that microbial life arises spontaneously. Thus by 1860 the ideas that specific diseases are caused by specific microbial agents and that these do not arise spontaneously had been formulated and were on their way to being accepted.

In 1879 Pasteur made a chance discovery that began the field of modern immunology. In the spring of the year he had begun experiments on chicken cholera. After the summer vacation it was found that the cultures of chicken cholera bacillus that had been kept during the summer did not produce disease when inoculated into healthy chickens. A new, virulent culture was obtained from a natural outbreak and was injected into new chickens. However, when this culture was injected into the animals that had not succumbed to the old cultures, the animals remained free of disease. Pasteur immediately recognized the analogy between his results and Jenner's cowpox protection against smallpox. In homage to Jenner he called the phenomenon he had found VACCINATION, thus forever enlarging the meaning of the word. With this, Pasteur established the *general* principle that an organism can be altered (ATTENUATED) so that it does not cause disease but still retains the property of inducing immunity. What had been a brilliant but

---

[3] The great Liebig summed up the chemist's view of a vitalistic nature of ferments: "As to the opinion which explains the putrefaction of animal substances by the presence of microscopic animicula, it may be compared to that of a child who would explain the rapidity of the Rhine current by attributing it to the violent movement of the many millwheels at Mainz."

apparently anecdotal clinical insight for Jenner was given a scientific basis and raised to the level of a scientific principle by Pasteur.

In one of the most famous (and widely publicized) experiments of the era, Pasteur immunized sheep, goats, and cows with an attenuated anthrax bacillus and then exposed them to a virulent anthrax. What made this experiment so unusual was that it was public: crowds of doctors, veterinarians, farmers, and, of course, reporters gathered in the small village of Pouilly le Fort to watch the outcome. Pasteur's experiment turned out a brilliant success, and, in the account of his co-worker, Emile Roux, "In the multitude at Pouilly le Fort, that day, there were no longer any skeptics but only admirers."[4]

There followed two decades of competition between the French and German schools of immunologists, headed by Pasteur in Paris and Robert Koch in Berlin, that had important implications both in the history of immunology and in international relations. This was a time of extreme nationalism, and both Pasteur and Koch saw themselves (and were seen by their compatriots) as defenders of national honor. It is rare in the history of nations that chauvinism bears socially useful results, but this was the case. In the attempt to be the first to identify the organisms responsible for every disease and to develop procedures to immunize against them, the French and the Germans tried to outdo each other. While neither France nor Germany was ennobled, as their fervid citizenry hoped, the world acquired, along with war, hardship, and hatred, the means of inducing specific immunity to many diseases and the beginnings of the understanding of the mechanisms of immunity.

For the purposes of the present narrative, one fact that became very important was the realization that the mechanism of the immune response toward any innocuous substance was the same as that against a deadly bacillus. Thus, it became possible to study immunology using SURROGATE PATHOGENS. If this were not true and if it had not been realized early in the history of the science, the enormous progress that has been made in the understanding of the mechanisms of immunity might not have been possible.

---

[4] The public trial of Pasteur's methods did not go off without a hitch. On the day after the virulent challenge, Pasteur was informed that some of the immunized animals were sick. He lost heart and accused Roux of spoiling the test and insisted that Roux face the humiliation alone, as it was his fault. During the night, however, Pasteur received a telegram saying that all was well, and next morning he arrived at the train station, stood in his carriage, and announced to the crowds "Well then! Men of little faith!" [quoted in Dubos, R., 1950. *Louis Pasteur: Free Lance of Science*]

The use of surrogate pathogens in immunologic studies required that a new word be coined to describe the substances being employed to analyze the immune response. An ANTIGEN is any substance recognized in a specific way by the immune system. The word can refer to something harmful, like a toxin, or something completely innocuous, like egg albumen. The substance becomes an antigen when it can be recognized in an immunologic assay (that is, the definition is a functional one). If this is a new word for you, learn it! We use it repeatedly throughout the book. Two immunologists having a conversation will mention antigens at least once a minute (unless they're talking about baseball, when the rate drops to once every 10 minutes). The next chapter discusses antigens in some detail.

The Study of the Immune System

Characteristics of the Vertebrate Immune System

The turn of the century is considered the Golden Era of microbiology. Through the work of Pasteur, Koch, and their schools, the germ theory of disease became firmly established and the causative agents of many diseases were isolated. It was also the Golden Era of immunizations: these same people found that specific immunity to most of the organisms that cause disease could be developed in humans and animals.

Once the phenomenon of immunity was established and put into practice in the form of vaccination, the burning question became: How does immunity work? From the observations, several features of the immune response were apparent. These features apply to the immune systems of most vertebrate species.

The first feature is that the immune response is INDUCIBLE. When an antigen enters the body, the system responds to the presence of that antigen. This response is SPECIFIC for the antigen; that is, immunity induced by one antigen does not usually have any effect on a different antigen; this is the second feature of the immune system. When an individual is reexposed to an antigen it has experienced before, the subsequent immune response is usually faster and more vigorous; this third feature is called IMMUNO-LOGIC MEMORY.

The fourth feature of the immune response is obvious by hindsight. If the system responds to nearly any foreign substance that enters the body, why doesn't it respond to those substances that make up our bodies? The fact is, it usually doesn't, and this tells us that the immune response diplays SELF–NONSELF DISCRIMINATION.

These four features refer to the types of immune responses responsible for the effects of vaccination. We refer to these as SPECIFIC or ADAPTIVE IMMUNITY. The immune system also has a component that displays neither specificity (or only partial specificity) nor memory. This is called NATURAL IMMUNITY. Natural immunity is inducible, displays self–nonself discrimination, and plays important roles in resistance to disease (discussed in Part Three). Most of this book, however, is concerned with the mysteries of adaptive immune responses.

Humoral and Cellular Immunity

The above features of the immune response cried out for explanations, and after nearly a century of research, some of those explanations are now available. Early on, however, it was unclear how immunity happens. One school of thought insisted that immunity is HUMORAL, that is, that the mechanism resides in the serum and other fluids (humors) of the body. Another school argued that immunity is CELLULAR. We now know that there are several mechanisms of immunity that have cellular and/or humoral components.

The most important (from our point of view) component of humoral immunity is a protein called ANTIBODY. Antibodies, induced by the presence of an antigen, bind specifically to that antigen and not to others. Emil von Behring and Shibasaburo Kitasato recognized the existence of antibodies, for which von Behring was awarded the first Nobel prize.[5] This discovery focused attention on antibodies and raised the intriguing question: How can a protein show the properties of specificity and memory for each of a huge number of antigens?

Instructive Versus Selective Theories of Antibody Formation

Paul Ehrlich and the Side-Chain Theory

Because immunology was originally concerned with the prevention of disease, it is not surprising that the first theory to explain the phenomenon of specific antibody formation was fashioned

---

[5] Investigators in the field of immunology have received more than their share of Nobel prizes in medicine. For every one of these prizes, however, there are many outstanding researchers who have made extremely valuable contributions but who were not recognized in this way. In this book, we are not at all diligent in pointing out Nobel prize–winning work and prefer to let elegant research speak for itself.

with immunity to disease in mind. Paul Ehrlich (1854–1915), who was one of the great thinkers in all of biomedicine, presented the first theory of antibody formation in the Croonian Lecture of 1900. Ehrlich realized that the antibodies in the serum must come from cells and postulated the SIDE-CHAIN THEORY as an explanation. According to the side-chain theory, every cell capable of synthesizing antibody (the exact cells were not known at the time) has on its surface an array of "side chains," each of which is able to react with a different specific antigen (Figure 1). No doubt Ehrlich devel-

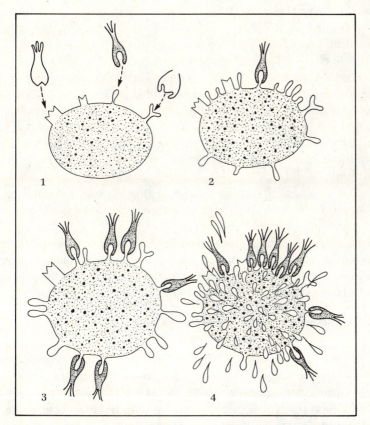

1 Side-Chain Theory. Paul Ehrlich's side-chain theory for antibody production. In this model, cells bear a large number of different receptors for antigen. If a particular antigen binds to one of the receptors, it directs the cell to secrete that receptor (i.e., the specific antibody). This model is distinct from clonal selection, but has some similarities, in that the various antibodies are preformed and are then selected through interaction with antigen (see Figure 3). [From Ehrlich, 1900. *Proc. R. Soc. London* 66: 424]

oped this theory with infectious microbes in mind. He assumed that each cell has a side chain for each of the microbial antigens to which the individual can produce antibody: for example, tetanus toxin, and the organisms that cause whooping cough, syphilis, and tuberculosis. When the specific agent (antigen) infects the body, it reacts with its specific side chain on the cell. This interaction between side chain and infectious agent (which in modern terms would be described as an interaction between a receptor and a ligand) somehow causes the cell to cease producing all the other side chains and initiate production of only the specific side chain with which the agent has interacted. Eventually, however, the cell overproduces this side chain and the excess appears in the serum as antibody.

Note, first of all, that the essential part of the theory is that all the side chains the cell can produce are PREDETERMINED. The infectious agent SELECTS the specific side chain; it has no role in instructing the cell how to make that side chain. Obviously, this theory requires that all the agents to which the organism can make antibody have complementary side chains on the surface of each antibody-producing cell. This theory is tenable if there are a reasonably small number of agents to which the animal makes antibody.

But at about the same time that Ehrlich was formulating his theory, others were showing that animals make perfectly fine antibody responses to nonpathogenic substances such as foreign red blood cells. In fact, it was soon learned that the easiest way to study the immune response was with these innocuous agents, because they could be used with no harm to investigator or animal and provided a perfect surrogate for the infectious agents.

Karl Landsteiner and Artificial Antigens

The side-chain theory was the dominant (and virtually the only) theory for many years. It fell out of favor for many reasons, but in retrospect the work of Karl Landsteiner ought to have been the most significant. Landsteiner (1868–1943) was a pathologist–chemist who won the Nobel prize for his work on red blood cell antigens. In Chapter 2 we will discuss his work with haptens—small molecules that can initiate an immune response when they are attached to carrier molecules. Landsteiner was able to raise antibodies against simple compounds such as nitrophenol. But he found that an alteration in the position of the nitro group resulted in unique antibodies. Thus he could get specific antibodies to *ortho-, meta-,* or *para-*nitrophenol. Moreover, he could get anti-bodies to arsenate, as well as to a vast array of other groups conjugated to carriers. If one can go into the laboratory and synthesize almost any compound, conjugate it to a carrier protein, and get antibodies against it, at some point one must realize that there will not be enough side chains to react with all possible antigens.

Felix Haurowitz and the Template Theory

In 1931 a new theory appeared on the scene. Its authors were Friedrich Breinl and Felix Haurowitz, both working in Prague. Breinl was a young virologist who had spent a few years at the Rockefeller Institute in New York, where he became fascinated with Landsteiner's work. Haurowitz was a protein chemist who worked on hemoglobin. When Breinl returned to Prague, he interested Haurowitz in the antibody problem.[6]

Breinl and Haurowitz immunized rabbits with hemoglobin and attempted to analyze the amino acid composition of the antibodies that were produced. In 1930 this was a tedious and inexact procedure, but they concluded that there is no difference between the amino acid composition of the protein molecules in serum before or after immunization. They reasoned that the difference between a normal molecule and an antibody molecule must be in the arrangement of the amino acids or in the shape of the molecule. They reasoned further that because the difference between a molecule with antibody activity and one without it is the fact that antigen has been introduced into the animal with the antibody molecules, antigen must *instruct* the cell about the specificity of the antibody.

Breinl and Haurowitz postulated that the antigen acts as a TEMPLATE; for example, each acidic amino acid in the antigen will be reflected as a basic group in the antibody molecule, and vice versa. This theory is fundamentally different from the selective theory, because in it, the cell that synthesizes the antibody mole-

---

[6] In an interview that one of us (E.S.G.) conducted with Haurowitz on his eighty-first birthday in 1976, he described the start of the short collaboration. "His [Breinl's] enthusiasm was infectious and, well, he declared he would introduce me to immunological matters. He would immunize animals . . . inject some of the antigens which I would supply him. He would bleed the animals, send me serum and I would try to isolate the antibodies. I remember he said, 'Haurowitz, we *must* find out what antibodies are!' Well, I said, I will try my best." Breinl died a few years later in a laboratory accident, and Haurowitz went on to devote his entire career to the study of antibody molecules. At 91 he still came to his laboratory every day to ponder the nature of the mechanism of antibody formation. He died in 1988.

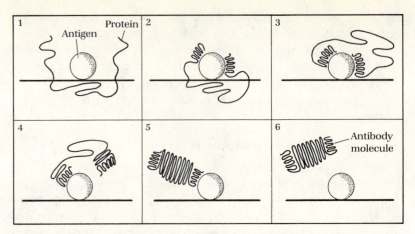

2   Direct Template Theory. Linus Pauling's direct template theory. In this model, all antibody molecules are identical before interaction with an antigen. Once a molecule interacts with protein, it folds into a specific antibody and subsequently can only react with the specific antigen. This clever idea is now known to be wrong, and has been replaced by clonal selection (see Figure 3). [From Pauling, 1940. *J. Am. Chem. Soc.* 62: 2643]

cule is not preprogrammed to make the antibody; rather, it makes "blank" molecules whose specificity is imposed by the antigen. Rather than a selective theory, the template theory is an INSTRUCTIVE THEORY of antibody formation.

The publication in German of the paper of Breinl and Haurowitz coincided with the formulation of a very similar theory by two Americans, Alexander and Mudd. The great chemist Linus Pauling also became interested in the problem and made the theory more accessible to a wider scientific audience (Figure 2). It quickly supplanted the side-chain theory and even influenced the development of early theories that attempted to explain regulatory phenomena in microbial systems. It was only when modern molecular biology began, with the understanding of the "trinity" (DNA, RNA, peptide), that the instructive theories had to be abandoned.

Niels Jerne, David Talmage, and Macfarlane Burnet: Clonal Selection

With the realization that the amino acid sequence and shape of proteins were the result of the nucleotide sequence of the genes in which they were encoded, the instructive model of antibody formation became difficult to defend. Niels Jerne, probably as a result of the influence of Max Delbrück and the Phage Group, evolved a new incarnation of the selective theory, which he called the NATURAL SELECTION THEORY. Here is Jerne's reminiscence about his insight:

"Can the truth [*the capacity to synthesize antibody*] be learned? If so, it must be assumed not to pre-exist; to be learned, it must be acquired. We are thus confronted with the difficulty to which Socrates calls attention in *Meno* (Socrates, 375 B.C.), namely that it makes as little sense to search for what one does not know as to search for what one knows; what one knows one cannot search for, since one knows it already, and what one does not know one cannot search for since one does not even know what to search for. Socrates resolves this difficulty by postulating that learning is nothing but recollection. The truth [*the capability to synthesize an antibody*] cannot be brought in, but was already inherent."

The above paragraph is a translation of the first lines of Soren Kierkegaard's "Philosophical Bits or a Bit of Philosophy" (Kierkegaard, 1844). By replacing the word "truth" by the italicized words, the statement can be made to present the logical basis of the selective theories of antibody formation. Or, in the parlance of Molecular Biology: synthetic potentialities cannot be imposed upon nucleic acid, but must pre-exist.

I do not know whether reverberations of Kierkegaard contributed to the idea of a selective mechanism of antibody formation that occurred to me one evening in March 1954, as I was walking home in Copenhagen from the Danish State Serum Institute to Amaliegade. The train of thought went like this: the only property that all antigens share is that they can attach to the combining site of an appropriate antibody molecule; this attachment must, therefore, be a crucial step in the sequence of events by which the introduction of an antigen into an animal leads to antibody formation; a million structurally different antibody-combining sites would suffice to explain structural specificity; if all 10^{17} gammaglobulin molecules per ml of blood are antibodies, they must include a vast number of different combining sites, because otherwise normal serum would show a high titer against all usual antigens; three mechanisms must be assumed: (1) a random mechanism for ensuring the limited synthesis of antibody molecules possessing all possible combining sites, in the absence of antigen, (2) a purging mechanism for repressing the synthesis of such antibody molecules that happen to fit to auto-antigens, and (3) a selective mechanism for promoting the synthesis of those antibody molecules that make the best fit to any antigen entering the animal. The framework of the theory was complete before I had crossed Knippelsbridge. I decided to let it mature and to preserve it for a first discussion with Max Delbrück on our freighter trip to the U.S.A., planned for that summer. [Niels K. Jerne, 1966. The natural selection theory of antibody formation: ten years later. In *Phage and the Origin of Molecular Biology*, Cold Spring Harbor Laboratory, New York, p. 301.]

The natural selection theory Jerne devised was based upon the fact that all animals have detectable levels of antibody to a wide array of antigens in their serum despite the fact that they have not been intentionally immunized to these antigens. Jerne postulated that antigen enters the system and reacts with one of these "natural antibody" molecules in the serum. The complex of antigen and antibody is then tranported to a cell, and this cell is induced to produce more of the antibody. The important point here is that Jerne has returned to a selective theory: antigen is the selective agent.[7]

In Denver in 1957, David Talmage pointed out that Jerne's theory was a modification of the side-chain theory and suggested that it would be improved if the selective elements were cellular. In Melbourne, F. M. Burnet, who had been at work on a similar theory at the time, then introduced what he called the CLONAL SELECTION THEORY. He found that the "major objection [to the Jerne theory] is the absence of any precedent for, and the intrinsic unlikelihood of the suggestion, that a molecule of partially denatured antibody could stimulate a cell, into which it had been taken, to produce a series of replicas of the molecule." He modified the natural selection theory by having the selection occur between the antigen and the cell that produces the antibody. The role of antigen was to select the proper clone of lymphocytes. In his theory, a given lymphocyte has the ability to produce antibodies of one (or at most a few) specificity. In addition, it expresses on its surface antibody that acts as a receptor so that the reaction between the antigen and the surface antibody causes the cell to proliferate. In this way a "clone" of the cells is generated and produces more antibodies of that specificity.

The Premises of Clonal Selection

The clonal selection theory is the central paradigm (see next section) of modern immunology and, for that reason, is central to this

---

[7] "The crucial point of the natural-selection theory is the postulate that the introduction of antibody molecules into appropriate cells can be the signal for the production of more of their kind. This notion is unfamiliar" [Jerne, N. K., 1955. *Proc. Natl. Acad. Sci. U.S.A.* 41:849]. Even though the theory is a return to *selection* explanations, Jerne apparently didn't know of the Ehrlich theory because it is not quoted in his paper.

book. From time to time, therefore, we will return to this theory to see how we're doing. Burnet laid out the basic premises behind this theory, which we've paraphrased below. As we'll see, a great deal of modern immunology has centered on confirming and understanding these premises as they apply to cells of the immune system. The premises are as follows:[8]

1. There exist in the body populations of cells differentiated for immune function by their ability to react to contact with specific antigen.

2. The specificity of antibody is determined by the genetic endowment of the cell that produces it.

3. The range of immune reactivity of any lymphocyte is sharply limited by a process of phenotypic restriction. It may be subject to limited extension by subsequent somatic mutation.

4. The origin of the diversity of immune specificity is to be sought at the genetic level.

5. Antigen acts essentially only as a signal or stimulus to such cells as are competent by possession of specific receptors for the antigen.

As we'll see as we explore the design of the immune system and its components in this book, the premises of clonal selection are met by the mechanisms underlying the immune response. The principles of clonal selection are sketched in Figure 3. You may find it worthwhile, at this early stage, to examine the process of clonal selection carefully and to think about what a system capable of clonal selection can do. Later, as we get into the real "nuts and bolts" of the immune system, you might want to come back to this section to see how the clonal selection theory holds up.

The Notion of the Paradigm

With only slight modification, clonal selection has passed from the status of theory to that of paradigm. According to Thomas Kuhn in *The Structure of Scientific Revolutions*, a paradigm is a commonly held belief among scientists of a given discipline. It need not be correct, only accepted. Scientific progress, according to Kuhn, comes from the changing of the paradigm. Paradigms are not changed lightly, but when they do change there is a revolution—hence the title of his book. Kuhn also argues that because the paradigm is assumed to be correct, all experiments

[8] Paraphrased slightly from Burnet, M., 1969. *Self and Not-Self*, Cambridge University Press, pp. 29–30.

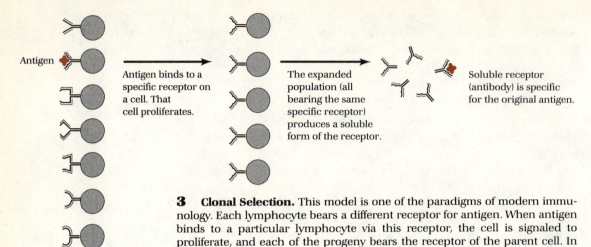

Antigen

Antigen binds to a specific receptor on a cell. That cell proliferates.

The expanded population (all bearing the same specific receptor) produces a soluble form of the receptor.

Soluble receptor (antibody) is specific for the original antigen.

3   Clonal Selection. This model is one of the paradigms of modern immunology. Each lymphocyte bears a different receptor for antigen. When antigen binds to a particular lymphocyte via this receptor, the cell is signaled to proliferate, and each of the progeny bears the receptor of the parent cell. In the case of antibody-producing cells, the activated clones produce antibodies that, being a soluble form of the surface receptor, specifically recognize the antigen.

are carried out within the confines of the paradigm. In this book we will be assuming the correctness of clonal selection, and the reader will see that the explanations of the immune response are all fashioned around this paradigm.

The Modern Era

The acceptance of clonal selection as the underlying paradigm of immunology allowed the phenomena observed by generations of immunologists to be put into a framework that had the promise of giving it coherence. It was fortunate that this new paradigm came at a time when technical and conceptual advances in biochemistry and cell biology allowed the generations of immunologists who followed to begin to solve the problems of the immune response.

In the following chapters we will examine the fascinating story of the attempt to determine what cells are involved in the immune response; the way they interact with each other; the nature of the antibody molecule; and the organization of the genes responsible for the generation of the great diversity in the immune response. We will also see the first successful attempts at the application of what we know in designing new vaccines, using immunologic techniques in diagnosis, and modulating the immune response.

The picture is complex and the solutions have not come easily. Embarking on an attempt to understand the immune system is a bit like starting to work your way through a labyrinth. In this case, by following the flow of the experiments the reader will emerge at the other end with an understanding of the picture as a whole.

"How do you know that? Are you an expert on labyrinths?"
"No, I am citing an ancient text I once read."
"And by observing this rule you get out?"
"Almost never, as far as I know. But we will try it, all the same."

Umberto Eco, *The Name of the Rose*

Additional Readings

Breinl, F. and F. Haurowitz. 1930. Chemical investigation of the precipitate from hemoglobin and anti-hemoglobin serum and remarks on the nature of antibodies. *Z. Physiol. Chem.* 192: 45 (in German).

Burnet, F. M. 1957. A modification of Jerne's theory of antibody production using the concept of clonal selection. *Aust. J. Sci.* 20:67.

Burnet, F. M. 1959. *The Clonal Selection Theory of Immunity*. Vanderbilt University Press, Nashville, Tenn.

Ehrlich, P. 1900. The Croonian lecture: On immunity. *Proc. R. Soc. London* 66:424.

Golub, E. S. 1980. Paradigms lost. *Immunol. Today* 1:v.

Golub, E. S. 1981. Shadows, stepping stones and the nature of scientific truth. *Immunol. Today* 2:v.

Golub, E. S. 1982. Paradigms regained. *Immunol. Today* 3:v.

Jerne, N. K. 1955. The natural selection theory of antibody formation. *Proc. Natl. Acad. Sci. U.S.A.* 41:849.

Landsteiner, K. 1936. *The Specificity of Serological Reactions*. Thomas, Springfield, Ill.

Lederberg, J. 1959. Genes and antibodies. *Science* 129:1669.

Pauling, L. 1940. A theory of the structure and process formation of antibodies. *J. Am. Chem. Soc.* 62:2643.

Silverstein, A. M. 1989. *A History of Immunology*. Academic Press, San Diego.

Talmage, D. W. 1957. Allergy and immunology. *Annu. Rev. Med.* 8:239.

IMMUNOCHEMISTRY

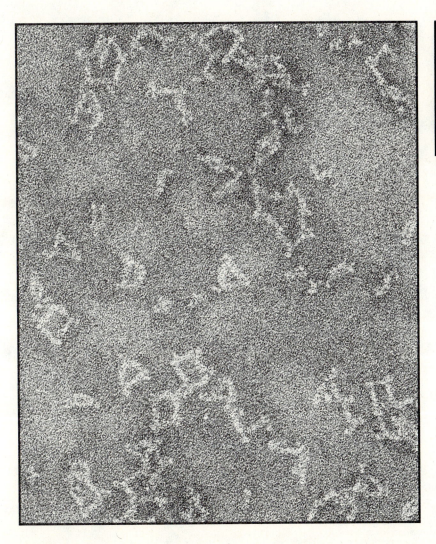

ANTIGENS, ANTIBODIES, AND COMPLEMENT

SECTION

I

There *is* a magic in the blood, but what does it consist of? [Emil von] Behring thinks it's a mysterious power in the blood. But if it can be augmented. . .

Edward G. Robinson as Ehrlich in
*Dr. Ehrlich's Magic Bullet**

In these chapters we will examine the nature of antigens and antibodies. The purpose of the chapters is to give the reader the theoretical basis for understanding modern developments such as monoclonal antibodies and new methods of vaccine production. In addition, the solution to one of the great problems of immunology—the organization of antibody genes—will be described so that the reader can participate vicariously in one of the great events of modern biology.

*Warner Brothers Studios, 1940.

THE NATURE OF ANTIGENS

CHAPTER

2

Overview The immune response begins with the introduction of antigen into the system, so we will begin by examining the nature of antigens. The properties of a molecule that enable it to induce a response are called immunogenicity; and the properties that allow it to react with antibodies are called antigenicity. Even though the factors that make a molecule immunogenic or antigenic are not yet clearly defined, advances in protein chemistry, computer-generated graphics, and monoclonal antibody techniques have allowed the nature of these properties to be addressed at molecular and even atomic levels. We will see that any stretch of amino acids can be antigenic if it is in the proper conformation. Even small stretches of peptides that have been synthesized and added to a proper carrier can in some cases induce the production of antibodies that react with the whole molecule. This technique has brought us to the threshold of constructing vaccines from synthetic peptides that have been synthesized on the basis of either the protein sequence as analyzed or the sequence deduced from the DNA code.

Antigenicity and Immunogenicity

The introduction of antigen into an animal initiates a series of events culminating in both cellular and humoral immunity. In this chapter we will deal only with humoral immunity: antibody formation and the reaction of antibodies with antigen. By convention, the property of a molecule that allows it to *induce* an immune response is called IMMUNOGENICITY. The property of being able to *react* with an antibody that has been induced is called ANTIGENICITY. Of course, in most cases an antigen molecule has both properties—immunogenicity and antigenicity. The hapten–carrier systems to be described in this chapter enable us to make a clear distinction between these two properties.

Studies with Haptens

Haptens and Carriers

The theme of specificity runs through the study of the immune response. Resistance to disease was known to be specific long before immunity and the immune system were studied scientifically. Karl Landsteiner was the first to systematically study specificity using a chemically defined system. Landsteiner studied the reaction of antibodies directed against HAPTENS, which are traditionally defined as small molecules that of themselves do not *induce* the production of antibody but are capable of *reacting* with antibodies. At first glance the last statement appears to be a contradiction—after all, how can something react with antibody but not induce its formation? The critical phrase in the statement is "of themselves." Haptens injected by themselves into an animal do not induce the production of antibody (Figure 1). But when the hapten is conjugated to a CARRIER (a large immunogenic molecule such as a protein), the animal responds by producing antibodies both to the hapten and to the carrier. Anti-hapten antibody, once it is induced by the hapten–carrier conjugate, is able to react with

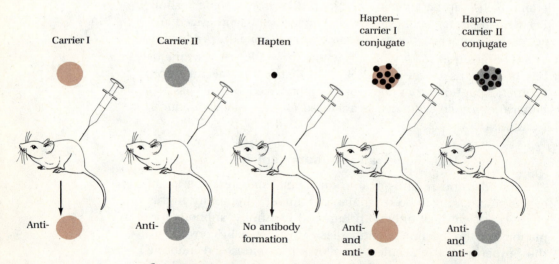

1   Antibody Responses to Haptens and Carriers The injection of immunogenic carrier alone (*large* gray and *large* brown *circles*) results in a carrier-specific antibody response. The injection of hapten alone (*small circle*) does not result in the formation of anti-hapten antibody. When hapten is conjugated to either carrier, the result is anti-hapten antibody as well as antibody specific to the carrier.

free hapten. In general, carriers are molecules that are of themselves immunogenic. Hence we may think of the hapten as an added determinant on an already immunogenic molecule. The study of hapten–carrier systems has given us much information about the nature of antigens and the antigen–antibody interaction, but it has also been one of the keys to understanding the cellular events in the immune response (see Chapter 17).

The Specificity of Serological Reactions

Landsteiner studied haptens and carriers in an attempt to work out the rules that govern antigenicity. The compilation of these studies appeared in his classic treatise, *The Specificity of Serological Reactions*. As we will see, no universal rules governing antigenicity came out of this work, but what did emerge was the realization that the chemical properties of the antigen molecule determine the specificity of the immune system. SPECIFICITY is defined as the ability of antibodies produced in response to an antigen to react with that antigen and not with others. The thoroughness of Landsteiner's approach and the elegance of his thought make browsing in this volume, which is available in paperback, a worthwhile experience for any scientist.

Landsteiner immunized a rabbit with a hapten–carrier conjugate. This injection resulted in antiserum with both anti-hapten and anti-carrier activity. He then conjugated the hapten to a different carrier and reacted the conjugate with the same antiserum to test for the presence of *anti-hapten* antibodies. Because he had changed carrier molecules for the test, there was no anti-carrier reaction; the reaction observed was between the anti-hapten antibodies and the hapten. He then varied the properties of the hapten in order to study, for example, the effect of acidic or ionic groups on the ability of the antibody raised against the original hapten to react with the modified hapten. Although no general rules emerged, it is instructive to look at some of Landsteiner's conclusions (Landsteiner, 1962):

> The principal results of numerous precipitin tests with azoproteins were the following . . .
> 1. First of all, the nature of the acidic groups was of decisive influence. [p. 163]

Data from Landsteiner's experiments are shown in Tables 1–4. Antibody is raised against aminobenzene or aminobenzene with

Table 1   Acidic groups and specificity.[a]

Antiserum against	Reactivity with			
	Aminobenzene (aniline)	p-Aminobenzoic acid	p-Aminobenzene sulfonic acid	p-Aminobenzene arsenic acid
Aminobenzene	+ + +	0	0	0
p-Aminobenzoic acid	0	+ + + ±	0	0
p-Aminobenzene sulfonic acid	0	0	+ + + ±	0
p-Aminobenzene arsenic acid	0	0	0	+ + + ±

Source: From Landsteiner, 1962. Modified by Klein.

[a]When an acidic group is substituted in the para position, the antibody raised against one of the haptens reacts only with that hapten.

acidic groups substituted at the para position (Table 1). In each case the antibody induced by one of the haptens reacts with *only* that hapten and none of the others.

2. In contrast to acid groups, substitution of the aromatic nucleus by methyl, halogen, methoxyl and nitro groups was of less influence on the specificity. [p. 163]

Antibody raised against any of these haptens is likely to react with all the haptens (Table 2). From this we see that the nature of the added group is critical in determining the ability to react.

3. Another rule, seen from the very distinctive reactions of the three isomeric aminobenzoic acids and aminocinnamic acids, is that the relative position of the acid radical to the azo group has a pronounced effect on specificity and the occurrence of cross reactions. [p. 167]

Moving the carboxyl group from ortho to meta to para results in different specificities (Table 3).

Another example deals with subtle differences between two molecules, such as the interchange of H and OH on one carbon atom. These data (which are actually from the work of Avery and

Table 2   Non-ionic groups and specificity.[a]

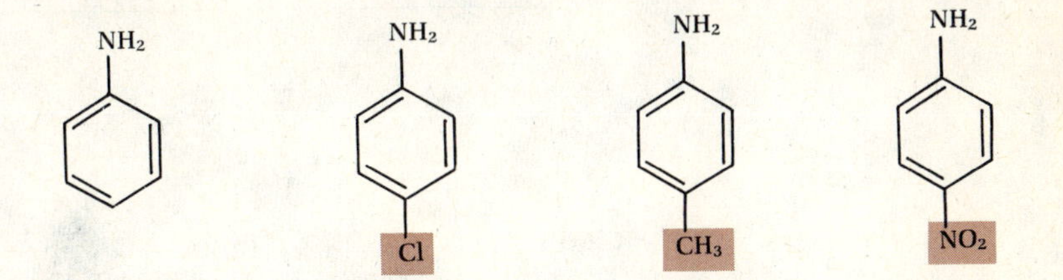

Reactivity with

Antiserum against	Aminobenzene (aniline)	p-Chloroamino-benzene	p-Toluidine	p-Nitroamino-benzene
Aminobenzene	+ + ±	+	+ ±	+
p-Chloroaminobenzene	± + + + ±	+ +	+ +	+ ±
p-Toluidine	+ ±	+ +	+ +	+
p-Nitroaminobenzene	+	+ +	+ ±	+

Source: From Landsteiner, 1962. Modified by Klein.
[a]Substituting nonionic groups has little influence on the specificity.

Table 3   Group position and specificity.[a]

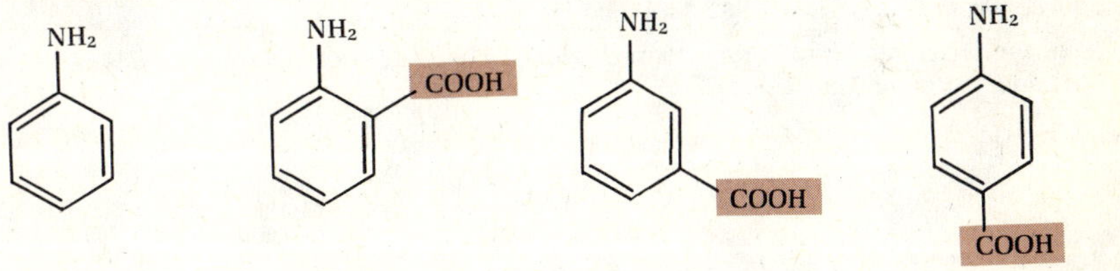

Reactivity with

Antiserum against	Aminobenzene (aniline)	o-Aminobenzoic acid	m-Aminobenzoic acid	p-Aminobenzoic acid
Aminobenzene	+ + +	0	0	0
o-Aminobenzoic acid	0	+ + +	0	0
m-Aminobenzoic acid	0	0	+ + + +	0
p-Aminobenzoic acid	0	0	0	+ + + ±

Source: From Landsteiner, 1962. Modified by Klein.
[a]The position of a group (in this case a carboxyl) has great influence on specificity.

Table 4   Glycoside bonds and specificity.[a]

Reactivity with

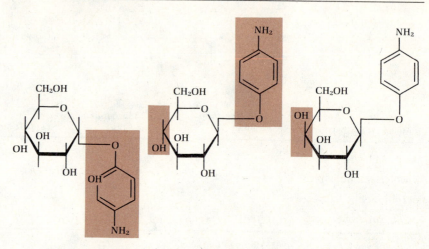

Antiserum against	p-Aminophenyl-α-glucoside	p-Aminophenyl-β-glucoside	p-Aminophenyl-β-galactoside
p-Aminophenyl-α-glucoside	+++	+	0
p-Aminophenyl-β-glucoside	++	++++	0
p-Aminophenyl-β-galactoside	0	0	+++

Source: From Landsteiner, 1962. Modified by Klein.

[a]Slight changes may have large or small effects. The α or β configuration does not have a large effect, but the rotation of H and OH on carbon 4 does.

Goebel and are quoted by Landsteiner) are shown in Table 4. The presentation of the aminophenyl group in either the α or β configuration from glucose has a slight effect on the reaction. However, rotation of the H and OH on the sugar to form galactose has a profound effect.

These experiments clearly demonstrate that subtle changes in the molecule have profound effects on the ability of the molecule to react with an antibody directed against a similar molecule, a fact that must be kept in mind throughout the text when the nature of specificity of the immune response is discussed.

Cross Reactivity

Antibody molecules can exhibit great specificity, but there are CROSS REACTIONS—cases in which antibody to antigen A also reacts with antigen B. This can be due to the presence of the same molecular configuration, or ANTIGENIC DETERMINANT, on the two antigens, or to properties of a determinant that allow it to be recognized as though it were another group. Antigenic determinants are also called *epitopes*. As we move through the book we will use these terms almost interchangeably. We can conceive of molecules that have similar but not identical structures and appear in closely related species. These molecules may have enough similarity to allow antibodies against one to react with the other.[1]

Table 5 shows the percentage of cross reactivity between albumins of different species. Antibody was made against bovine serum albumin (BSA), and the extent of the ability of albumins from other species to react with the anti-BSA was then determined. This cross reactivity is probably due to the presence of common determinants on the different albumins. To determine this, however, each of the determinants must be isolated and studied chemically. Even then, as we will see later in this chapter, we cannot be quite certain of

[1] The neurobiologist A. K. Hall has suggested the term IMMUNOFREQUENT for such determinants.

Table 5 Cross reaction between BSA and other albumins.[a]

Albumin source	Percentage of cross reactivity with BSA	Albumin source	Percentage of cross reactivity with BSA
Human	15	Mouse	10
Pig	32	Rat	13
Sheep	75	Hamster	13
Horse	13	Cat	25
Guinea pig	5	Vallaroo	6
Dog	13		

Source: Data from Weigle, 1961. *J. Immunol.* 87: 599.

[a]Rabbit anti-BSA was absorbed with each of the albumins listed and then tested for its ability to react with BSA. This ability is expressed as a percentage *cross reactivity*. The data show that sheep BSA has the highest amount of cross reactivity and guinea pig and vallaroo the least.

the causes of the cross reactivity because factors such as conformation are also involved.

Studies with Proteins

As elegant and informative as the hapten–carrier studies were, they were meant to be the groundwork for the study of the more complex protein and carbohydrate antigens found in nature. Landsteiner, in contemplating the vast array of natural antigens in the world, concluded that an antigenic determinant in a naturally occurring molecule would not be a simple structure.

> Clearly the highly selective action of the immune sera precludes specificity being determined by simple structures as single amino acids, and even reacting groups composed of di- or tripeptides could not furnish a sufficient number of combinations ... the specificity of proteins must be referable to complicated structures—possibly multiple, like groups in one molecule—or to several groupings whose affinities have to be satisfied before a visible reaction can occur, in which event the spatial arrangement of the reacting groups may be significant. [Landsteiner, quoted in Lerner, 1984. *Adv. Immunol.* 36:4]

The Roles of Conformation and Amino Acid Sequence in Antigenicity

True to Landsteiner's prediction, early studies on proteins did show that the *conformation* of a molecule could be important to its antigenicity. For example, when antibody was raised against a native protein, the antibody would not react with the protein after the protein had been denatured. In studies of controlled denaturation, for example, antibody against ribonuclease did not react with ribonuclease after its four disulfide bonds had been oxidized and the *shape* of the ribonuclease molecule changed.

Ruth Arnon, Michael Sela, and their colleagues in Israel carried out a particularly lovely series of experiments in the 1970s to examine the role of conformation in the antigenicity of lysozyme. In the lysozyme molecule (Figure 2A), residues 64–80 form a loop

2 **Effect of Conformation on Antigenicity.** (A) Amino acid sequence of hen egg-white lysozyme. The shaded area forms the "loop." (B) Diagram of the synthetic open and closed loops. (C) Reacting the anti-loop antiserum with lysozyme, natural loop, or synthetic loop inhibits the reaction between loop–anti-loop. However, reaction with open loop does not. These results show that the specificity of the anti-loop is for the conformation of the loop. [After Arnon and Sela, 1969. *Proc. Natl. Acad. Sci. U.S.A.* 62: 164; Arnon et al., 1971. *Proc. Natl. Acad. Sci. U.S.A.* 68: 1450]

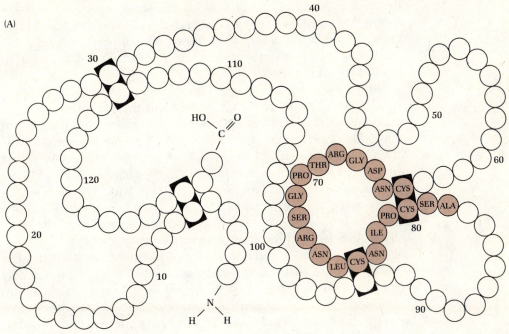

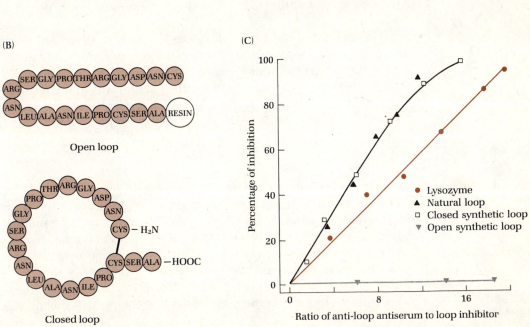

through the formation of a disulfide bond between Cys-64 and Cys-80. These investigators synthesized the amino acids that constitute the loop (Figure 2B) and found that antibodies against either the intact molecule or the isolated but still-closed loop and the synthetic closed loop reacted with both the whole molecule and the closed loop. However, when the synthetic open loop was used, there was a dramatic reduction in the ability of the antibody to bind to the intact molecule (Figure 2C).

Studies of this kind showed that the conformation of the protein is crucial for its antigenicity. At about the same time that the experiments showing the importance of conformation were being done, however, other studies showed that the requirement for complex structure is not absolute. These experiments showed that *amino acid sequence* is important to antigenicity. Results with the protein of the tobacco mosaic virus (TMV) provide a good example.

Tobacco mosaic virus is a large virus composed of a spiral series of protein subunits around a nucleic acid core. In the early 1960s, Anderer and his coworkers in Germany produced antibody against TMV and tested the ability of fragments of TMV protein (TMVP), produced by enzymatic digestion, to inhibit the reaction of anti-TMV with TMVP. They found that several peptides efficiently inhibited the reaction. Some of these peptides were very short and did not have significant three-dimensional conformation; thus the dependence of antigenicity on conformation was shown not to be absolute.

Eli Benjamini and his colleagues in California pursued these findings and demonstrated that the antibody to TMVP that reacted with the intact molecule was directed against one of the TMVP tryptic peptides. The specificity of the reaction was in the terminal five amino acids of the peptide, further demonstrating that a small stretch of amino acids with no apparent complex structure can serve as an antigen.

The Role of Segmental Mobility

Recent work from the laboratory of Aaron Klug in England has shown that the *mobility* of the segment of an antigen molecule influences whether it will be antigenic. Klug and van Regenmortel have identified in TMV seven antigenic determinants, each of which consists of between 5 and 10 amino acids. Because TMV can be crystallized and analyzed by X-ray diffraction, they were able to show that six of the seven determinants have high temperature factors along the polypeptide backbone. This means that the determinants had high SEGMENTAL MOBILITY (that is, they can move about 1 Å from the mean backbone position).

John Tainer and Elizabeth Getzoff in La Jolla have analyzed several proteins and found that mobile peptide segments are more likely to be antigenic than nonmobile segments. Figure 3A shows a computer-generated "glowing coal" model of insulin; the lighter areas have greater mobility than the dark ones. Figure 3B is a computer-generated view, in which the labeled amino acids are the antigenic determinants. It can be seen that the antigenic determinants are clustered in the more mobile segments. This is seen very dramatically in Plate 2-1.

Obviously, the flexibility or segmental mobility of a stretch of amino acids cannot be the sole factor in antigenicity. The *accessibility* of an epitope to the surface must be important, because the antibody molecule cannot reach a buried epitope. Eduardo Padlan at the National Institutes of Health (NIH) has pointed out that the amino acid residues in the interior of the protein can have an indirect effect on residues at the surface by causing them to

(A)   (B)

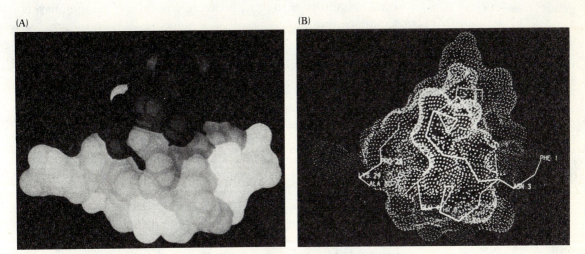

3   **Computer Graphic Views of Insulin.** Computer graphics show that the antigenic determinants cluster at flexible regions. (A) The "glowing coal" model illustrates the more mobile regions of insulin, which are highlighted with the lightest colors. (B) In this view (which is shown in color in Plate 2-1), the α-carbon backbone (lines) and the molecular surface (dots) are displayed with residue labels indicating the contiguous and discontiguous antigenic determinants. [Adapted from Tainer et al., 1985. *Annu. Rev. Immunol.* 3: 501, with permission]

assume certain configurations. Thus it seems prudent to conclude that a combination of factors, including segmental mobility and accessibility, determine if a stretch of amino acids will be antigenic.

SYNTHESIS
What Makes Something Antigenic?

We have seen so far that both amino acid sequence and conformation are important to the antigenicity of a molecule and that the segmental mobility of the determinant is crucial. These observations have led to the hypothesis that the surface of a protein is a continuum of *potential* antigenic sites. Or, in other words, almost any sequence of amino acids can be antigenic if it is accessible and is located in the larger molecule in such a manner that it has a conformation allowing segmental mobility. The antibody recognizes this structure based on its amino acid sequence, conformation, and shape. This notion has been called the MULTIDETERMINANT HYPOTHESIS. The reader should keep in mind that we have not discussed the factors that are responsible for *immunogenicity* (the ability to induce an antibody response). The complications involved in approaching this problem will be seen in the chapters on cellular immunology.

Blood Group Antigens

There are a very large number of blood groups in humans (over 300 serologically determined specificities), and many have been well studied. Of these, the ABO system and the Rh group are of the most general importance. The ABO system was discovered in 1901 by Landsteiner, who noted that serum from some individuals agglutinated the red blood cells from some other individuals. We now know that type A individuals have antibody to type B red cells in their serum. Because the blood group antigens are oligosaccharides that occur commonly in nature, type A people become immunized to type B antigen present in the environment, although they remain tolerant to A antigens. The reverse is true for type B individuals.

The A and B antigenic determinants of the red-cell surface molecule are not gene products. Rather, the genes encode *glycosyl transferases* that transfer specific monosaccharides to an acceptor molecule. These antigens are a good example of how a small change in *chemical structure* results in a unique *antigenic structure*. Blood group A individuals have an *N*-acetylgalactosamine transferase that attaches an *N*-acetylgalactosamine to the "stem" (Figure 4). Blood group B individuals have a galactose transferase and they transfer a galactose to the stem.

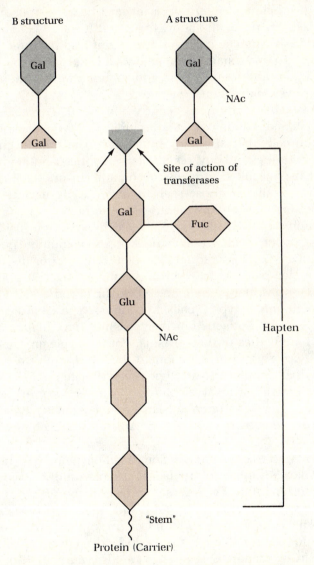

4 Blood Group Antigens. Blood group antigens are oligosaccharides. Groups A and B differ only in the terminal sugar on the "stem." Group A has an *N*-acetylgalactosamine and group B has a galactosamine. The genes that determine groups A and B do not encode the sugars but encode the proper transferase. These blood group antigens are haptens; the carrier is a protein on the red blood cell.

Transfusion Reactions and Rh Compatibility
(A Brief Clinical Interlude)

We have clearly embarked on a discussion of immunologic data. The reader may be wondering at this stage where this is leading. This brief clinical interlude is to give heart to those who have reached this point and show them that the study of antigens can not only be intellectually rewarding but also has practical implications. To understand what follows, it is necessary to understand that antibodies not only bind antigen but that this interaction can have physiological consequences.

TRANSFUSION REACTIONS occur when blood is transfused into a mismatched recipient, that is, an individual who has antibodies to the red cells that are being transfused. The transfused red cells react with the antibody, resulting in an antigen–antibody complex (see Chapter 10). The results of the antigen–antibody reaction in vivo are similar to those seen in vitro, that is, agglutination and the activation of complement leading to hemolysis. The resulting symptoms of this reaction are fever, hypotension, back pains, a feeling of chest compression, nausea, and vomiting. The red blood cells of a type O individual have neither the A nor the B antigens. His or her plasma, however, has antibody against both. Thus a type O individual is the UNIVERSAL DONOR of red cells but can be a recipient only of type O cells. In contrast, type AB individuals have both A and B antigens on their cells but have neither anti-A nor anti-B antibodies in their plasma. These people are therefore UNIVERSAL RECIPIENTS but can donate their cells only to another AB individual. People who are type A can donate red cells to another type A or to a universal recipient and can receive transfusions from another type A or from a universal donor. Similarly, type B individuals can donate only to type B or AB and can receive from another B or an O.

To avoid transfusion reactions a simple blood type test is done that takes advantage of the fact that type A individuals have antibody to type B and vice versa. To test for the presence of A or B antigens on the surface of red blood cells, the investigator takes two small drops of blood by finger prick, places them on a slide, and adds a drop of anti-A to one and a drop of anti-B to the other. A positive reaction is seen by a rapid agglutination of the cells. Agglutination in both drops indicates that the blood is type AB; no agglutination indicates that the person is type O.

The RH SYSTEM is very complex, but the only antigen in the system that is of clinical importance is the D antigen because of its involvement in HEMOLYTIC DISEASE OF THE NEWBORN, or *erythro-blastosis fetalis*. An Rh-negative mother carrying an Rh-positive child takes the risk of being immunized by the Rh antigens of the fetus during pregnancy and delivery, that is, she will make an anti-Rh response. This will have no effect on the child she is carrying because the sensitization process is slow (requiring many weeks or months) and the first antibody that is made is of a type that does not cross the placenta. However, it can have a very serious effect on the next child that she bears if that child is also Rh-positive. The maternal anti-Rh antibodies will by now be of another type that can cross the placenta and react with the red cells of the Rh-positive fetus. This results in hemolytic disease of the new-born, which is characterized by hemolytic anemia, hyperbilirubi-nemia (high blood levels of breakdown products of hemoglobin), enlarged spleen and liver, and severe neonatal jaundice and brain damage. Death can result in as many as 24 to 30% of the infants.

Because it is the antibody response only to the D antigen that is responsible, it is a simple task to determine if there is a possible problem with Rh compatibility between the parents. Obviously the group at risk is an Rh-negative mother whose fetus has an Rh-positive father (Table 6).

To prevent the sensitization of the Rh-negative mother by the Rh-positive red cells of her fetus, she is injected with *anti-Rh antibody* either before she develops a primary response to the Rh positive red cells or after delivery. This antibody binds to any Rh-positive fetal cells that get into her circulation during pregnancy and delivery and these cells are destroyed. In this manner there are no cells available to sensitize her, she will not make an anti-Rh antibody response of her own, and the fetus at the next pregnancy will not be in danger.

Molecular Mapping of Antigenic Determinants

It would be interesting and useful to understand the nature of antigenicity and to determine which parts of molecules are anti-genic. Indeed, these determinations have been made by using antibodies alone and in conjunction with X-ray crystallography. Before the advent of monoclonal antibodies, it was very difficult to map the antigenic determinants of a molecule because the antisera that were used had antibodies to all the determinants. But because monoclonal antibodies react with a single determinant on an anti-gen, they can be used in conjunction with sequence studies, com-

Table 6   Rh genotypes, phenotypes, and hemolytic disease of the newborn[a]

		Father		
		Rh+		Rh−
		DD	Dd	dd
Rh−	dd	Dd Rh+	Dd dd Rh+ & Rh−	dd Rh−
Rh+	Dd	DD Dd Rh+	DD Dd dd Rh+ & Rh−	Dd dd Rh+ & Rh−
	DD	DD Rh+	DD Dd Rh+	Dd Rh+

(left axis label: **Mother**)

[a]The D antigen of Rh is involved in hemolytic disease of the newborn (erythroblastosis fetalis). The chart above shows the possible genotypes and phenotypes of offspring with the indicated parental genotypes. The danger of the disease comes when an Rh− mother carries an Rh+ child. Both homozygous (DD) and heterozygous (Dd) individuals are Rh+. Shaded area indicates the combinations in which the infant is in danger.

puter-generated graphics, and crystallography to determine the fine structure of determinants.[2]

A very instructive example of the combined use of these methods can be seen in the work that determined the antigenic sites on the human rhinovirus (HRV; the virus that causes the common cold). Roland Rueckert and his colleagues in Madison studied this virus by producing monoclonal antibodies against it and selecting variants of the virus that were not neutralized by a given antibody. By comparing the nonbinding variants to the wild type viruses they were able to identify four antigenic groups, which they called

[2] Conventional antibodies from the serum are a mixture of antibodies of many specificities. Monoclonal antibodies are composed of antibody molecules all of which are identical and therefore have the same specificity (see Chapter 9).

NIm (for neutralizing immunogen) IA, IB, II, and III. The RNA of the variants was sequenced so that the positions of the amino acids responsible for each of the variants could be identified. Some of these data appeared to be anomalous, however, because some of the variants seemed to have substitutions that were located far from the clusters that were thought to be the antigenic determinants. This anomaly was cleared up when Michael Rossmann and his colleagues at Purdue and James Hogle and his colleagues in La Jolla worked out the three-dimensional structures of HRV and polio virus by X-ray crystallography. They found that picornaviruses, of which HRV and poliovirus are examples, have the same basic structure: several "β barrels." The individual strands of these barrels are connected by chains of peptides (Figure 5), which

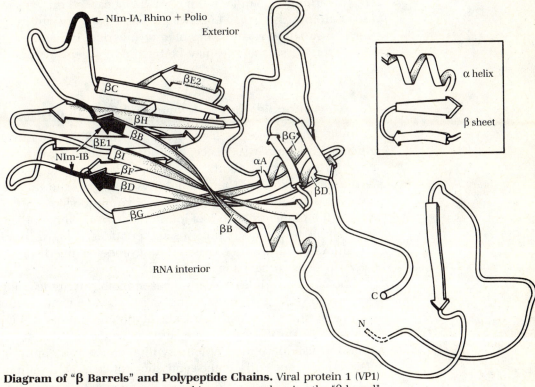

5   Diagram of "β Barrels" and Polypeptide Chains. Viral protein 1 (VP1) of human rhinovirus (HRV) is represented in a manner showing the "β barrel" structure. The barrel-like structure is composed of β-*sheets* (see inset) connected by polypeptide chains. The antigenic determinant NIm-IB is seen to be on two strands of the polypeptide chains, but the determinant NIm-IA is contiguous. [Diagram of HRV from Rossmann et al., 1985. *Nature* 317: 145. Similar structural data for poliovirus can be seen in Hogle et al., 1985. *Science* 229: 1358]

protrude from the virus surface and are likely candidate structures for antigenic determinants because they are accessible to antibody and have relatively high flexibility. When the three-dimensional structure of HRV was compared with its amino acid sequences, it was found that the antigenic determinants (NIm) were in fact located on the protruding peptides that connect the strands of β sheets (which compose the barrels) and that the anomalous data now made sense because some of the antigenic determinants were made up of amino acids that are distant from each other on a *linear* representation of the amino acid sequence but are adjacent to each other in the three-dimensional structure. In other words, the determinant can be formed by amino acids that are in close association by virtue of spatial orientation of the viral peptides. This finding is shown in Figure 5A; the black areas form the antigenic determinant. Similar studies are being carried out by several groups around the world and will give us greater insight into the structure–function relationship of antigenic determinants in their natural setting so that we may better modify them for our own purposes.

Antibodies of Predetermined Specificities

A protein immunogen[3] is usually composed of a large number of antigenic determinants. Hence, immunizing with a protein results in the formation of antibody molecules with different specificities, the number of different antibodies depending on the number of antigenic determinants and their inherent immunogenicity. On the basis of the pioneering work of immunochemists who studied the responses to fragments of proteins and peptides, a new technology that allows us to produce antibodies of predetermined specificity against protein antigens is developing.

One of the revolutionary advances in biology was the ability to sequence DNA. In fact, it is often easier to clone a gene, sequence it, and infer the amino acid sequence of the protein that it encodes than it is to purify the protein and sequence it. Consequently, immunologists have been able to synthesize the protein from the inferred sequence and use the synthetic protein as an immunogen.

Antibodies to Products of Nucleotide Sequence

The power of this technology is evident in the following example. In examining the nucleotide sequence of the Moloney leukemia

---

[3] IMMUNOGEN is the term used when the immunogenic properties of an antigen are discussed.

virus, Richard Lerner and his colleagues in La Jolla found that there was a stretch of nucleotides that could not be explained. This reading frame was part of the envelope gene and predicted a protein that was not known to exist in the virus. The predicted protein was synthesized, conjugated to a carrier, and used to immunize rabbits. The resulting antibody precipitated two previously unidentified proteins from infected and transformed cells. The proteins had not been isolated earlier because during the process of viral budding from the cell, the COOH termini of these two proteins are cleaved. The antibody had detected the cleaved portions of the proteins, which were parts of previously unknown precursor proteins. Their discovery allowed the synthesis and assembly of the virus to be studied in more detail.

Another example of the use of antigens synthesized from nucleotide sequences is seen in the work of Gregor Sutcliffe, Floyd Bloom, and their colleagues in La Jolla. There is a large amount of messenger RNA (mRNA) in the brain that is not accounted for in known brain proteins. These workers approached the problem of identifying the proteins by producing complementary DNA (cDNA) from mRNA of the whole brain. The cDNA was then hybridized to mRNA from different regions of the brain, and when a message coding for a product unique to an area of the brain was found, the corresponding cDNA was sequenced and the amino acid sequence of the protein inferred. Several regions of the predicted peptide were then synthesized and injected into animals to produce antibodies. The antibodies were used to search for the predicted protein in brain slices. Using this technique a protein was found that may be a precursor to a new neurotransmitter.

From these two examples it is clear that the application of antigens and antibodies goes far beyond the study of immunology. Other applications in cell biology, developmental biology, and clinical medicine are becoming increasingly common.

Antibodies to Predetermined Amino Acid Sequences

The amino acid sequences of many antigens, including those on pathogens (disease-causing organisms) that may be of importance in immunization strategies, have been determined since their genes have been sequenced. This advance should facilitate the production of vaccines because the immunogenic portion of the agents can be synthesized and used for immunization. One strategy for doing this has recently been worked out. Monoclonal antibodies to a feline leukemia virus protect cats from infection with the virus. To determine which of the viral antigens are responsible for the protection, advantage has been taken of the techniques of molecular biology. The gene for the immunogenic protein was cloned and then cut at random by DNase I. These fragments were then inserted individually into a phage so that they could be expressed in infected host bacteria. Colonies of bacteria that contained the gene for the antigen were plated and identified by treating the colonies with the monoclonal antibody. In this way, the fragment actually containing the antigenic determinant was identified. Because the DNA sequence of each fragment can be easily determined in the laboratory, the amino acid sequence was deduced and synthesized and the synthetic peptide used as immunogen. This elegant strategy can be used, in principle, for almost any pathogen.

Another interesting advance in immunization has also come about through the use of the methods of molecular biology. It is possible to put the DNA sequence for a desired antigenic determinant into the vaccinia virus genome so that when an individual is immunized with vaccinia they are also immunized with the desired antigen. One can foresee the construction of genomes containing DNA sequences for several antigenic determinants of several pathogens and the expression of these determinants in a single organism, which is then used for immunization.

Summary

1. Immunogenicity is the property of a molecule that allows it to induce an immune response. Antigenicity is the ability of a molecule to react with antibody.
2. Haptens are structures that are not immunogenic unless conjugated to a carrier but that are able to react with anti-hapten antibody. The distinction between hapten and hapten–carrier complexes is the distinction between antigenicity and immunogenicity.
3. Cross reactivity occurs when the same molecular conformation occurs in more than one molecule. In those cases, an antibody raised against one antigen will react with another.
4. The antigenicity of a protein is determined by its sequence of amino acids as well as by its conformation and accessibility. Peptide sequences with high segmental mobility are frequently antigenic.
5. The combined use of monoclonal antibody, computer-generated graphics, and X-ray crystallography is making molecular–antigenic mapping of complex structures possible.
6. Antibodies of predetermined specificity can be made by immunizing an animal with synthetic peptides. In this manner vaccines of desired specificity should be able to be made in the future.

Additional Readings

Benjamini, D. C., J. A. Berzofsky, I. J. East, F. R. N. Gurd, C. Hannum, S. J. Leach, E. Margoliash, J. G. Michael, A. Miller, E. M. Prager, M. Reichlin, E. E. Sercarz, S. J. Smith-Gill, P. E. Todd and A. C. Wilson. 1984. The antigenic structure of proteins: A reappraisal. *Annu. Rev. Immunol.* 2:67.

Landsteiner, K. 1962. *The Specificity of Serological Reactions*, rev. ed. Dover, New York.

Lerner, R. A. 1984. Antibodies to predetermined specificity in biology and medicine. *Adv. Immunol.* 36:1.

Novotny, J., M. Handschumacher and R. E. Bruccoleri. 1987. Protein antigenicity: A static surface property. *Immunol. Today* 8:26.

Padlan, E. H. 1985. Quantitation of the immunogenic potential of protein antigens. *Mol. Immunol.* 22:1243.

Silverstein, A. M. 1982. Development of the concept of immunological specificity. *Cell. Immunol.* 67:396.

Sutcliffe, J. G., R. J. Milner, T. N. Shennick and F. E. Bloom. 1983. Identifying the protein products of brain-specific genes with antibodies to chemically synthesized peptides. *Cell* 33:671.

Tainer, J. A., E. D. Getzoff, Y. Paterson, A. J. Olson and R. A. Lerner. 1985. The atomic mobility component of protein antigenicity. *Annu. Rev. Immunol.* 3:501.

Williams, W., E. Beutler, H. J. Erslev and M. H. Lichtman. 1983. *Hematology*, 3rd ed. McGraw-Hill, New York.

THE STRUCTURE OF IMMUNOGLOBULINS

CHAPTER

3

Overview The body can produce antibodies to what may be a limitless array of antigens, each antibody reacting specifically with the antigen that initiated the immune response leading to its appearance in the serum. Determining the structure of the molecule that can impart so much diversity and the structural basis for the specificity has been one of the profound problems of biology. During the past two decades, however, this problem has come very close to being solved, and the solution is one of the more thrilling episodes in modern biology—one that reads almost like a detective story. At each stage the problem was defined through an advance in immunology, although the solution required advances in other areas such as protein chemistry and molecular biology.

The antibody molecule should be thought of as a monomer composed of four chains: two identical heavy chains and two identical light chains held together by disulfide bonds. There are several classes of immunoglobulin molecules, and they differ in size and number of monomers. In the next chapter we will address the question of how such an apparently simple molecule can be varied to allow the enormous array of antigen reactivity that the system requires. But the reader must keep in mind through all of this that a given antibody is specific for a given antigen.

Antibodies and Immunoglobulins

It has been known from the earliest days of immunology that antibody activity is found in the SERUM, the fluid portion of blood that is left after the blood has been allowed to clot.[1] Serum contains many proteins, but antibodies are found almost exclusively in the

---

[1] Plasma is the fluid portion containing unreacted clotting factors.

globulin fraction. In a classic experiment, Tiselius and Kabat in 1939 showed that after reacting serum from an immune animal (called ANTISERUM) with specific antigen and collecting the immune precipitate, the γ-globulin fraction of the serum was diminished, indicating that the γ-globulins contained the antibody activity (Figure 1).

Later it appeared that the only function of the γ-globulins was antibody activity, and this group of molecules was called IMMUNO-GLOBULINS (IGS). An immense amount of work has been done to determine the chemical structure of Igs in order to understand how these molecules can bind specifically to antigen.

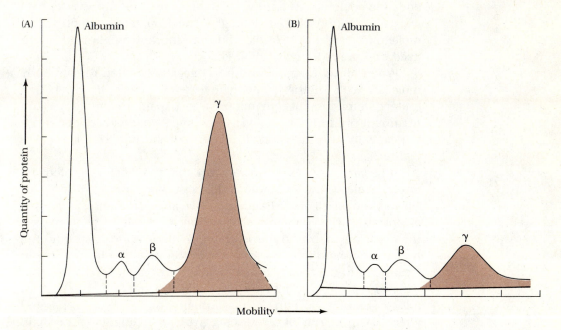

1   Antibodies are Found in the γ-Globulin Fraction of Serum. The classic experiment of Tiselius and Kabat showing that the serum from a rabbit hyperimmunized to egg albumin shows a reduction in the γ-globulin peak when the serum is analyzed by electrophoresis. (A) The electrophoretic pattern before the serum was treated with the antigen, egg albumin. (B) The pattern after the addition of the antigen and the removal of the antigen–antibody complexes that formed. [Redrawn from Tiselius and Kabat, 1939. *J. Exp. Med.* 69: 119]

The Chain Structure of Ig

Early Studies Using Antiserum:
Treatment with Proteolytic Enzymes

The early research into the structure of Igs showed that they are multichained proteins that are found in the serum as either monomers or polymers. The experiments leading to our understanding of the *chain structure* of the basic Ig monomer earned Nobel prizes for the two prime movers in the field, R. R. Porter and G. M. Edelman. Porter, working in England, treated rabbit antibody with the proteolytic enzyme papain and separated the products on a carboxymethyl cellulose column. This treatment produced three fragments. Two of the fragments were of equal molecular weight (~50,000) and could bind antigen. These two were called F$_{AB}$ fragments (**F**ragment with **a**ntigen **b**inding). It had been known from physicochemical studies done a very long time ago that the antibody molecule has two antigen-binding sites, and this was a physical confirmation of that data. The third fragment, which had a molecular weight of ~80,000, did not bind antigen, but it crystallized and therefore was called Fc.

When Alfred Nisonoff and his colleagues treated the antibody molecule with another proteolytic enzyme, pepsin, they obtained quite different results. In contrast to papain treatment, pepsin treatment produced a single large fragment that had antigen-binding capacity and many small pieces that did not. This is seen in Figure 2.

It became clear after further work that the different proteolytic enzymes cleave the molecule at different sites, thus accounting for the different sizes of the fragments. Two antigen-binding fragments are produced by papain treatment because this enzyme cleaves the molecule "above" the interchain disulfide bonds that hold the two antigen-binding sites together in the intact molecule. Pepsin treatment, in contrast, cleaves "below" this disulfide bond so that the two antigen-binding sites remain associated. In short, the two antigen-binding portions of the antibody molecule are separated after papain treatment (producing two Fab fragments) but remain united by a disulfide bond after pepsin treatment [producing a (Fab)$_2$ fragment]. This is seen in Figure 2.

The Use of Myeloma Proteins

The antibodies in serum (antiserum) are extremely heterogeneous. This is because they have a variety of molecular weights and reflect

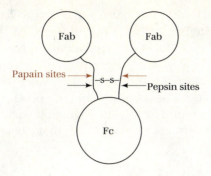

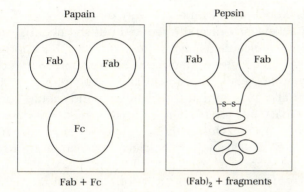

2   **The Generation of Fab and Fc Fragments by Enzymatic Cleavage.**
Treatment of Ig with papain results in two fragments with antigen-binding
activity (Fab) and a fragment that crystallizes (Fc). Treatment with pepsin
results in a single fragment that binds antigen [(Fab)$_2$] and fragments.

antibody specificities to every antigen the individual has recently
come in contact with. This heterogeneity was one of the stumbling
blocks in the study of the chemistry of antibodies. The use of
myeloma protein, however, overcame this difficulty. (The basis of
antibody heterogeneity will be covered in detail in Chapter 4.)

Multiple myeloma is a disease in which there is a malignant
transformation in a single cell that normally produces antibody.
The transformed cell, now a cancer cell (in this case a myeloma
cell), multiplies in an uncontrolled manner while continuing to
secrete its Ig product into the serum. The result is a very high
concentration of only one kind of Ig (the MYELOMA PROTEIN) in the
serum of the patient. The myeloma protein molecules are physically homogeneous, being the products of the progeny of a single

clone of cells. This unfortunate "experiment of nature," however, gave access to high concentrations of identical Ig molecules.

Henry Kunkel at Rockefeller University in New York introduced the use of homogeneous myeloma proteins for studying the structure of normal antibody molecules. His was a very creative move because he made the assumption that the product of the myeloma cell was normal even though the cell itself was abnormal, having lost its growth control. We will see that this assumption was correct.

Chain Dissociation Studies

The other Nobel prize winner for work on Ig structure, G. M. Edelman of Rockefeller University, worked out the chain structure of the antibody molecule using myeloma proteins. His approach was to allow the molecule to unfold in $6\,M$ urea and then reduce the disulfide bonds with mercaptoethanol. The reduced disulfides were then alkylated so that the disulfide bonds could not reform. He found that there are two kinds of reduced and alkylated chains in each Ig molecule. One of the chains has a molecular weight of approximately 20,000 and one a molecular weight of approximately 50,000. They were named LIGHT CHAINS and HEAVY CHAINS (L and H chains). From the relative concentrations of each it was determined that the monomeric Ig molecule contains four chains, two H and two L, held together by disulfide bonds. This is seen in Figure 3.

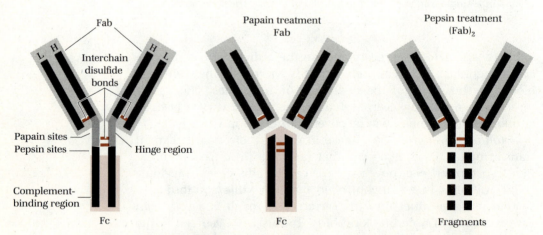

3 **The Chain Structure of Ig.** The monomeric Ig molecule is composed of two H and two L chains (H_2L_2). The diagram also shows the pepsin and papain sites within the chain structure.

4   The Relationship Between the Chain Structure and the Fab and Fc Parts of the Ig Molecule. The H chains contribute to both the Fab and the Fc but the L chains are found in only the Fab.

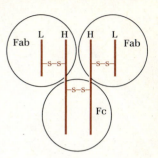

When the data from the proteolytic cleavage and the chain dissociation studies were combined, it became clear that the L chains and part of the H chains are located in the Fab portion of the molecule. The remainder of the H chains are contained in the Fc portion. The picture that emerged from this pioneering work is seen in Figure 4.

The basic Ig monomer thus consists of two H and two L chains. To avoid confusion, the reader should firmly establish in his or her mind that for any given antibody molecule, the two H chains will be identical to each other and the two L chains will be identical to each other. Another antibody molecule will also have the formula H_2L_2 and its H chains will be identical to each other as will its L chains. *But* (and this is perhaps the biggest *but* in the book) its H chains and the L chains will be different from the H and L chains of another antibody. It is this difference that confers the antigen-binding specificity upon the molecule.

The Hinge Region and Interchain Disulfide Bonds

The region of the Ig molecule between which papain and pepsin cleavages occur is called the HINGE REGION. This region, which is rich in cysteines and prolines, probably serves several functions: the cysteines contribute to the INTERCHAIN DISULFIDE BRIDGES. The prolines may keep the two combining sites of the molecule separated in space and contribute to the molecular mobility of the various parts of the Ig. This will be discussed in greater detail in Chapter 6.

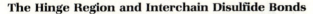

SYNTHESIS
The Basic Monomeric Structure of the Ig Molecule: The Theme from which Variations Occur

All Igs are composed of the four-chain structure described so far that serves as the basic monomeric form from which variations occur. We will see in the next several chapters that some Igs are composed of polymers of the H_2L_2 basic monomeric form and that there are slight differences in both H and L chains in different classes. But all the Ig molecules that we will be discussing are composed of monomers of two identical H and two identical L chains.

Domains of the Ig Molecule

Intrachain Disulfide Bonds and Structural Domains

In the discussion of the studies on enzymatic cleavage of the Ig molecule we noted that papain gives two antigen-binding fragments (Fab) and pepsin gives one fragment that has two antigen-binding sites [(Fab)$_2$]. We said this is because of the site at which the enzymes attack the molecule. This was the first indication that interchain disulfide bonds are involved in the structure of the Ig molecule. Further analysis of the disulfide bonds in the basic Ig molecule revealed that there are regularly spaced cysteines that result in INTRACHAIN DISULFIDE BONDS (intra = within, inside). The intrachain disulfide bonds are not to be confused with the interchain disulfide bonds discussed above (inter = among, between).[2]

The intrachain disulfide bonds are important in giving the molecule its unique shape and result in clear STRUCTURAL DOMAINS. Domains are conserved units of molecular structure within the protein that confer a unique motif (see below). Figure 5 depicts an Ig molecule and shows the intrachain disulfide bonds and the structural domains.

The Ig Superfamily

The distinct loop formed by the intrachain disulfide bond is a motif that defines a large family of molecules called the IMMUNO-GLOBULIN SUPERFAMILY. As seen in Figure 6, the loop motif appears in molecules other than antibodies, but many of them are associated with the immune system. This association will become apparent as we work our way through the molecules of the immune system and the reader may want to refer back to this section from time to time.

As the name implies, the Ig superfamily is a very large (and a growing) family. Table 1 lists the current members of the superfamily. It can be seen that the two major functional divisions of cells that use members of the superfamily are the immune system and the nervous system. This may be because the motif that characterizes the family allows domain–domain interaction.

Functional Domains

We will see in Chapter 5 that these structural domains reflect exon–intron relationships at the DNA level and are in fact also *functional*

---

[2] A device to avoid confusion is to think of *inter*collegiate athletics (Purdue vs. UCLA) as compared with *intra*mural athletics (Biology Bombers vs. ΠΚΓ).

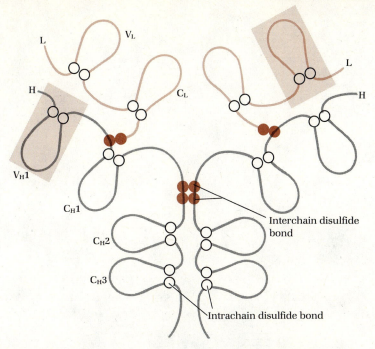

5   The Domain Structure of Igs. This diagram shows the structural motif imposed upon the molecule by the intrachain disulfide bonds (open circles). The L chain has two such domains and the H chain has four. The H and L chains are joined by interchain disulfide bonds (color circles). Note that each domain has one intrachain disulfide bond. Single domains in H and L are indicated in light color. In this diagram there are 4 H and 2 L domains per chain.

domains. Igs perform many functions that are consequences of antigen binding, and these functions are associated with this unique structural motif. The manner in which structure is used in function in the antibody molecule will be discussed in Chapters 4 and 7.

Three-Dimensional Structure

From the voluminous work that followed the pioneering chemical studies on Ig structure, we now have a reasonably complete picture of the overall shape and structure of the Ig molecule. X-ray crystallographic analysis is now beginning to reveal the three-dimensional picture of the molecule. Figure 7 shows the orientation in space of an entire human Ig. The resolution of this crystal

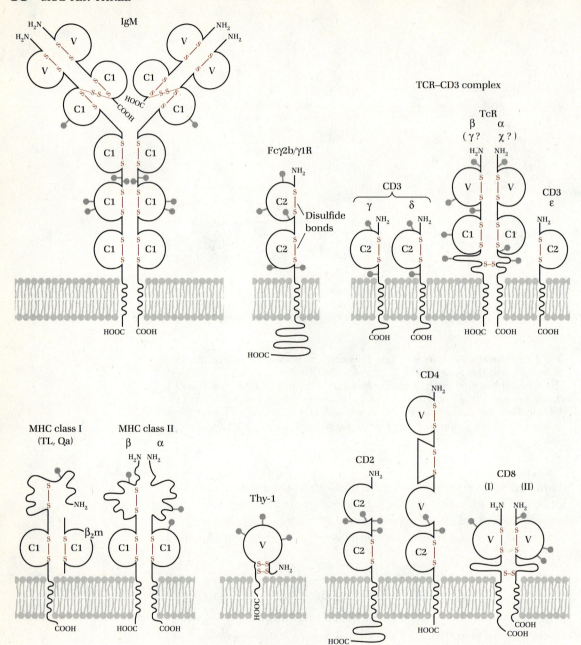

6   **The Ig Superfamily.** Some representative molecules of the Ig superfamily. Note that all members contain the distinct loop formed by the intrachain disulfide bond. [Redrawn from Williams and Barclay, 1988. *Annu. Rev. Immunol.* 6: 381]

structure by David Davies and his coworkers at NIH was a major step in both immunology and crystallography. In carrying out this study, the NIH group had to face a very difficult technical problem. The only complete Ig that would form crystals was the protein called Dob (after the multiple-myeloma patient from which the protein came). But Dob is a unique molecule because it lacks the hinge region. Molecules that have intact hinge regions have proved to be very difficult to crystallize, and so Davies and his colleagues chose to get the crystallographic solution to the *best* available molecule that could be crystallized. This representation of the molecule was shown by later work to be essentially correct.

Table 1 Some members of the immunoglobulin superfamily.

Location	Ig superfamily members
Immune system	Ig
	T-cell receptor
	CD3
	MHC
	β_2-microglobulin
	CD2
	LFA-3
	CD4
	CD8
	CTLA4
	Poly Ig receptor
	Fc receptor
Hemopoietic system receptors	PDGF receptor
	CSF-1 receptor
Nervous system	Thy-1
	MRC Ox-2
	N-CAM
	Myelin-associated glycoprotein
	P_0 myelin protein
	Opioid-binding protein
	Axonal glycoprotein
Miscellaneous	Carcinoembryonic antigen
	Basement membrane link protein
	α_1 B-glycoprotein

Source: Adapted from Williams and Barclay, 1988. *Annu. Rev. Immunol.* 6: 381.

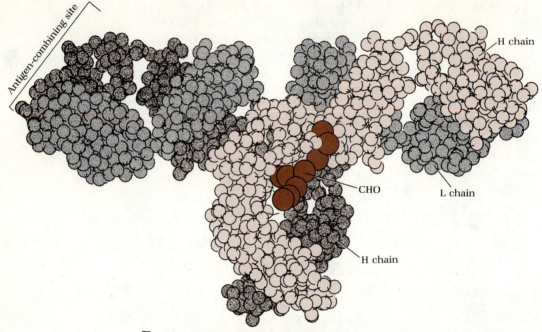

7 Three-Dimensional Structure of Human Ig. The schematic drawing is based on a pioneering X-ray crystallographic analysis of the myeloma protein called Dob. The H chains are represented by tan and dark brown. The L chains are gray. The large brown spheres are the carbohydrate moieties that lie between two of the H-chain domains. [From Silverton et al., 1977. *Proc. Natl. Acad. Sci. U.S.A.* 74: 5140; reprinted with permission]

Plate 3-1 is a computer-generated model by Arthur Olsen and his colleagues at Scripps of the α-carbon backbone of the Ig molecule. From this depiction of the molecule, it is easy to see the division of the molecule into (Fab)₂ and Fc. What leaps out from this picture is the fact that the vision of the molecule that we had arrived at from chemical studies has been fully confirmed by the X-ray studies. It takes very little imagination to see the structure that is depicted in the diagrams in the early part of the chapter embodied in the computer-generated model from the physical studies.

The reader should keep in mind that this represents two *functional* divisions as well. Antigen binding is the function of the (Fab)₂ portion, and various effector functions are carried out by Fc. These two functions will be discussed in detail in Chapters 4 (binding) and 7 (effector functions).

SYNTHESIS
The Structural and Functional Domains of the Antibody Molecule

The relatively simple four-chain structure of the antibody molecule is composed of structural domains. We first saw that the molecule can be divided into Fab and Fc portions and then that the intra-chain disulfide bonds cause loops that define domains. The question that the reader should now be asking is this: How can such a fairly simple molecule possibly have enough plasticity in structure to be able to bind specifically with all the antigens that clonal selection says it should? We will begin to take up this question in the next chapters.

Summary

1. Antibodies are found in the globulin fraction of serum proteins, the immunoglobulins (Igs).
2. Treatment of Ig with papain gives two fragments that bind antigen (Fab) and one fragment that does not (Fc). Treatment with pepsin gives one fragment that binds antigen [(Fab)$_2$] and many small pieces.
3. Reducing and alkylating the interchain disulfide bonds of Ig results in two heavy (H) chains and two light (L) chains.
4. The structural division into (Fab)$_2$ and Fc is a reflection of the functional divisions. The Fab portion binds antigen and the Fc carries out effector functions.
5. The intrachain disulfide bonds confer a unique motif to the Ig molecule. The loop caused by the disulfide bond defines a motif common to the Ig superfamily and is found in many molecules associated with the immune response.

Additional Readings

Davies, D. R. and H. Metzger. 1983. Structural basis of antibody function. *Annu. Rev. Immunol.* 1: 87.

Glynn, L. E. and M. W. Steward, eds. 1981. *Structure and Function of Antibodies*. Wiley, Chichester.

Kindt, T. J. and J. D. Capra. 1984. *The Antibody Enigma*. Plenum, New York.

Wall, R. and M. Kuehl. 1983. Biosynthesis and regulation of immunoglobulins. *Annu. Rev. Immunol.* 1: 393.

Williams, A. F. and A. N. Barclay. 1988. THe immunoglobulin superfamily—domains for cell surface recognition. *Annu. Rev. Immunol.* 6: 381.

THE STRUCTURAL BASIS OF ANTIBODY ACTIVITY

CHAPTER

4

Overview Up to now we have seen that the body can respond to a very large number of antigens by producing antibodies that react specifically with each of them. Since each antibody molecule is specific for only one antigen, the antigen-combining part of the antibody molecule must be a structure that can assume many shapes to interact with the many antigens. But we saw in the last chapter that the molecule is, if anything, remarkably unremarkable, consisting of two identical H chains and two identical L chains organized into repeating domains. In this chapter we will see that one of the domains in both H and L chains has great variability in its amino acid sequences. The remaining domains are relatively constant. We will see that the variation in the size and shape of the variable regions confers the ability to react specifically with antigen.

In the next chapter we will address the question of the genetic mechanism underlying this remarkable system.

Complementarity Determining Regions

Constant and Variable Regions

Up to now we have covered the evidence leading to the chain structure of the basic Ig molecule and the organization of the molecule into structural domains. But describing this structure explains neither the structural basis for the diversity of the antibody molecule nor how the molecule functions to combine with antigen. The discovery that was crucial to solving these problems was the finding that there are CONSTANT and VARIABLE regions of amino acid sequence in the Ig molecule. The announcement of the discovery was one of those rare moments in science when everyone is aware of an important advance. Russell Doolittle describes the moment[1]:

> Early in 1965 a meeting of the Antibody Workshop was held at Warner Springs, California, a small resort community about 60 miles east of San Diego. The meeting, with about 80 persons in attendance, was unique on several counts. Largely organized by Melvin Cohn (of the Salk Institute), a determined effort had been made to infiltrate the immunologic ranks with a galaxy of stellar molecular biologists, including James Watson, Francis Crick, Christian Anfinsen, Max Delbrück, Seymour Benzer, and a dozen other nonimmunologists of high repute. The program was simple enough—a few talks on immunologically competent cells, immunogenetics, antibody structure, and the like. For the first two days everything went according to schedule, predictable progress—but not much more—being reported, and the sessions were only slightly lengthened by the presence of the imported Brain Trust. On the third morning, however, the assemblage was electrified by the unexpected announcement from Norbert Hilschmann, reporting on work he had done in Lyman Craig's laboratory, that he had virtually completed the amino acid sequences of two very different Bence-Jones proteins (the equivalent of antibody light chains) and, with one quite explicable exception, had found that all the many amino acid replacements had occurred in the amino-terminal half of the molecules. Clearly, immunoglobulin light chains had a variable half and a constant half.
>
> The impact on the meeting was instantaneous, something very close to pandemonium ensuing. Francis Crick made his way to the chalkboard and drew a flurry of twisted loops, implying that simple DNA rearrangements could now explain antibody diversity; Seymour Benzer declared that at last immunology had become a science. It was one of those rare moments when an entire group senses that a solution to a major problem is directly at hand, but no one is quite sure of how to put the last piece in the puzzle, or even how to find it. Surely, if only a few more sequences were obtained the pattern would become absolutely clear. [R. Doolittle, 1974. *Science* 183: 190]

In other words, when the first amino acids from the amino-terminal end of Bence-Jones protein A and protein B are compared, they are found to be different. Similarly, when the second, third, and following amino acids are compared, the amino acids

[1] These moments when the confusion of a field is suddenly cleared away by a single experiment have been called *epiphanic moments* [see Golub, E. S., 1990. *Cell* 61: 1167]. It is unfortunate that we do not have published remembrances of other epiphanic moments comparable to Doolittle's.

at each of these positions in one protein are different from those in the other protein. This difference at each position continues until roughly the midpoint of the L chain. From that point on there is almost complete correspondence of amino acids, position for position (except for the genetically controlled allotypic variation that will be discussed in Chapter 6). Thus the first amino acid beyond the midpoint in proteins A and B is identical in both proteins, and this correspondence continues through to the carboxy-terminal end of the chain. The L chain can therefore be divided into a variable half and a constant half. The VARIABLE REGION, or V REGION, starts at the amino-terminal end of the L chain and comprises the first 110 or so amino acids. The CONSTANT REGION, or C REGION, begins at about residue 111 and continues to the carboxy-terminal end of the chain. Analysis of the H chains soon showed that they too are divided into C and V regions.

The chains of the Ig molecule can thus be divided into V_L and V_H (variable region of L chain and variable region of H chain) and C_L and C_H (constant region of L and H chains). The importance of this discovery cannot be overstated. For the first time the structural basis for the diversity of the antibody molecule could be visualized. If each antibody molecule can differ from other antibody molecules at a large number of amino acid positions, we can then see how the basic four-chain structure can give rise to an astronomical number of different functional molecules. Clearly, the variation of a few amino acids in the V region of an Ig must be responsible for antibody diversity and specificity (Figure 1).

Hypervariable Regions

With the realization that the Ig molecule contains variable regions, it became clear that these regions could be the structural basis for diversity. If there were total variability at all the 100 or so amino acids in the V region, the permutations of possible antigen-binding structures would be enormous. However, as more L chains were

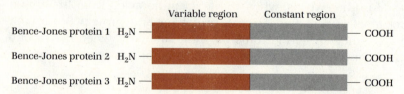

1   Diagram of Constant and Variable Regions. The diagram shows the comparison of amino acids between three Bence-Jones proteins (antibody L chains). The color areas had great variability in amino acid sequences, and the gray areas did not. These are the variable (V) and constant (C) regions.

sequenced, it became clear that there is not total variability in the V regions. Comparisons of sequences of L chains revealed that there are large stretches that are invariant even within the V region.

In 1970 Wu and Kabat compared all the then-known V_L sequences and came to the conclusion that there were "hot spots" of variability in the V regions. They defined the VARIABILITY RATIO V as

$$\text{Variability} = \frac{\text{number of different amino acids at a given position}}{\text{frequency of the most common amino acids at that position}}$$

Wu–Kabat plots for H and L chains are shown in Figure 2. The

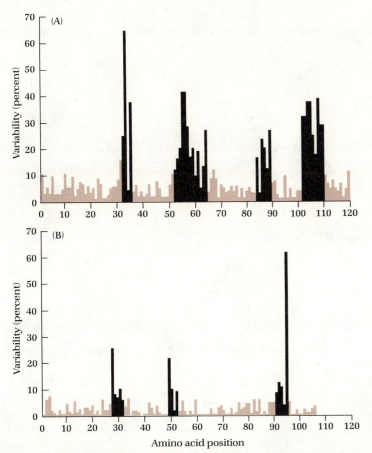

2   Hypervariable Regions of Igs. Wu–Kabat plots of amino acid positions of Ig (A) H chains and (B) L chains. The hypervariable regions, or CDRs, are clearly seen and are indicated in black. The method of calculating the variability is given in the text. [Redrawn from Kindt and Capra, 1984. *The Antibody Enigma*, p. 83, with permission]

areas of variability were called the HYPERVARIABLE REGIONS and the areas with little variability are called the FRAMEWORK REGIONS (FRs). Recent terminology calls the hypervariable regions COMPLEMENTARITY DETERMINING REGIONS (CDRs) because we now know that it is these regions that form the antigen-binding site (see below), that is, have a complementarity with the antigen that allows the binding. The location of FRs and CDRs is shown schematically in Figure 3.

Structural Domains Revisited

We mentioned earlier that the structural domains of the Ig molecule are formed by the disulfide loop motif characteristic of the Ig superfamily. We said then that the L chain has two of these motifs and the H has four. Now that we have introduced the variable and

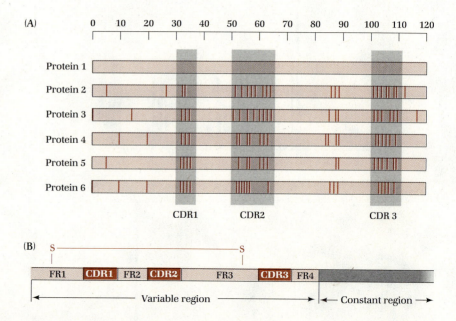

3 Complementarity Determining Regions. (A) Constant and variable regions. The diagram shows the essence of the Hilschmann and Craig experiment by comparing amino acid residues at each position of six different H chains. Each of the six is compared with protein 1, and a line indicates a difference at that residue from protein 1. [Redrawn from Capra and Kehoe, 1974. *Proc. Natl. Acad. Sci. U.S.A.* 71: 4032] (B) Schematic representation of CDR in the variable region. The diagram shows the location of framework regions (FRs) and CDRs in the region. The same pattern holds for both H and L chains.

constant regions, the reader is no doubt wondering how this information is to be incorporated into the domain structure. As can be seen in Figure 4, the first domain in each chain is the variable domain, and is followed by one or more constant domains. Thus an L chain is composed of V_L and C_L. An H chain is composed of V_H and C_H1, C_H2, and C_H3. (Some classes of Igs have an additional C_H.)

SYNTHESIS
The Strategy of Antibody Diversity

The basic strategy of antibody diversity is now apparent. Portions of the amino acid sequence of the Ig molecule remain constant but they do not determine the antigen-binding capacity of the antibody molecule. Rather, antigen-binding ability resides in the portions of the molecule that are variable. Compare this strategy with that of the enzyme cytochrome c. Figure 5A shows Wu–Kabat

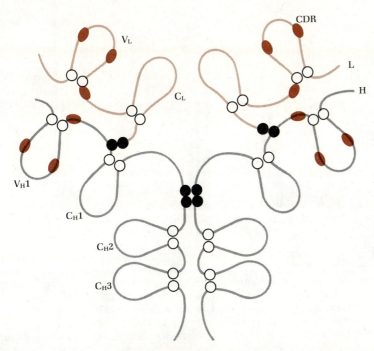

4   Domains and CDRs of an Ig Molecule. This diagram illustrates the location of the CDRs within the domain structure of an Ig molecule.

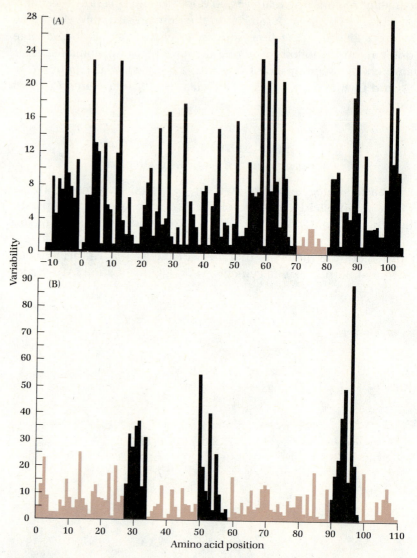

5 **Comparison of Variability Between Ig and Cytochrome _c_**. Wu–Kabat variability plots of (A) cytochrome _c_ of various species and (B) human L chains illustrate the different evolutionary strategies for conserving or generating variations. It can easily be seen that there is between-species variability in all the cytochrome _c_ molecules except in residues 70–80. This is the active site of the cytochromes and is the only part of the molecule that has been conserved in evolution. In contrast, there are only three variable areas in the Ig L chain; the rest of the molecule has been conserved. [After Kabat, Wu and Bilofsky, 1979. _Sequence of Immunoglobulin Chains_. U.S. Department of Health, Education, and Welfare, P.H.S., N.I.H., p. 121]

variability plots of cytochrome *c* from various species. Note that there is variability everywhere *except* in residues 70 to 80. These are the residues that constitute the active site of the enzyme. So, in contrast to Ig (Figure 5B), the active site is maintained as an invariant, or constant, region and the rest of the molecule is variable. This makes sense because all cytochrome *c* molecules in all species must carry out only one function, and the sequence required for that function is maintained. Antibodies, in contrast, must be able to bind with an enormous number of antigens, so the active site varies to allow this to happen.

Nature of the Antigen-Combining Site

The Lock and Key Metaphor

Up to now we have been developing the evidence that shows the structural basis of the combination of antibody with antigen and have stated that the CDRs are responsible for the reaction. Obviously, the specificity of the antigen–antibody reaction was known before we had much idea of the chemical nature of the reactants. In fact, as Arthur Silverstein points out in *A History of Immunology*, Paul Ehrlich was influenced by the similarity between the interaction of enzyme with substrate and antigen with antibody. The great biochemist Emil Fischer in 1892 made the analogy of a lock and key for the enzyme–substrate interaction. "To use a picture, I will say that enzyme and glucoside must join one another as *lock and key* [emphasis added] in order to be able to exert a chemical effect." Ehrlich introduced this metaphor into immunologic thought, where it has clung tenaciously. Metaphors are valuable because they allow us to form our thoughts more concretely or clearly, but there is always the danger that the metaphor will begin to color our view of what is real. The lock and key metaphor was useful to get us to where we are now, but X-ray crystallography and computer-generated graphics have allowed us to break free of this metaphoric view of the antigen–antibody combination. We will see as this chapter unfolds that a more apt visualization of the combination of antigen and antibody is one of two *surfaces* coming together rather than one structure fitting into a precise cavity in the other.

Electron Microscopic Studies

The structural studies discussed in Chapter 3 indicated that the antibody molecule has two combining sites. This was confirmed visually in 1967 when electron micrographs were made of antigen–antibody complexes. In these studies a bivalent hapten of 2,4-dinitrophenol (DNP) was constructed and reacted with anti-DNP antibody. Figure 6A is a micrograph in which clear Y-shaped structures can be seen. Figure 6B is the diagrammatic interpretation of this picture, showing the Fab portions of the molecule bound to the hapten.

Size of the Combining Site

Some of the earliest attempts to determine the *size* of the combining site were experiments involving inhibition of antigen–antibody reactions, experiments logically similar to those involving competitive inhibition of enzyme–substrate interactions. In the classic studies by Kabat and his coworkers, a dextran–anti-dextran system

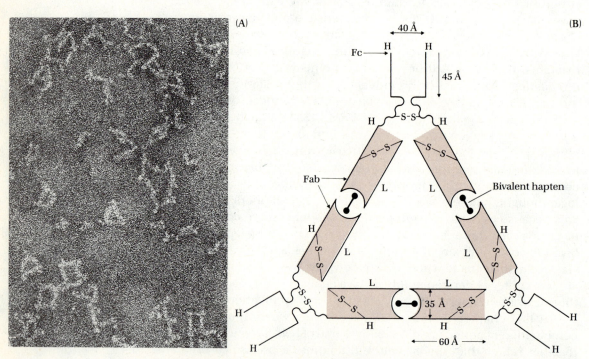

6   Antigen–(Fab)₂ Complexes. These two illustrations show the interaction of (Fab)₂ fragments made from rabbit anti-DNP with the hapten DNP conjugated in a manner that makes it divalent. (A) An electron micrograph. Note the Y shape, which is the two arms of the Fab bound to the bivalent hapten. (B) A schematic diagram of the interaction. [From Valentine and Green, 1967. *J. Mol. Biol.* 27: 615, with permission]

was used. Dextran is a large molecule of repeating sugar subunits. Smaller subunits of dextran (3, 4, 5, ... sugar subunits) were added to the anti-dextran antibody to determine whether they could *inhibit* the binding of the antibody to the dextran. If the small molecule could react with the combining sites on the antibody molecule, then when the large dextran molecule was added, the combining site would be occupied by the small molecules and the large molecules would be prevented from reacting. By using a graded series of sizes of dextran subunits, it was found that in general each site was fully occupied (inhibition approached maximum) by a molecule containing seven sugar moieties. Similar experiments with other antigen–antibody systems using small subunits of the various antigens showed that the combining sites have dimensions of about $30 \text{Å} \times 10 \text{Å} \times 6 \text{Å}$. This estimate was subsequently confirmed by X-ray diffraction studies that also revealed a number of other structural features.

X-Ray Diffraction Studies

The Barrel and Loop Structure of the Domains

Studies of the three-dimensional configuration of the antigen-combining sites of antibodies come primarily from X-ray diffraction studies of Fab fragments. From these X-ray crystallographic studies, we now know that the domain structure of Ig consists of a β-barrel with varying numbers of β-pleated sheets and a series of loops. This motif is known as the IMMUNOGLOBULIN FOLD and is seen diagrammatically in Figure 7A.

In Figure 7B it can be seen that the two β sheets of the Ig fold consist of anti-parallel β strands. Each of these contains between 10 and 15 amino acids. The overall structure is stabilized by the disulfide bond. The prevalance of the resulting loop structure was seen in Chapter 3 when the Ig superfamily was discussed.

The Antigen-Combining Surface

Before the advent of monoclonal antibodies, myeloma proteins were the only source of homogeneous antibody molecules. The binding of small molecules (phosphocholine, DNP, and vitamin K) showed that antigen bound to the CDRs of both H and L chains. With the advent of monoclonal antibody technology, it became possible for investigators to get large amounts of homogeneous antibody for almost any system that they wanted to study. The results of these studies have given us a new view of the nature of

(A)

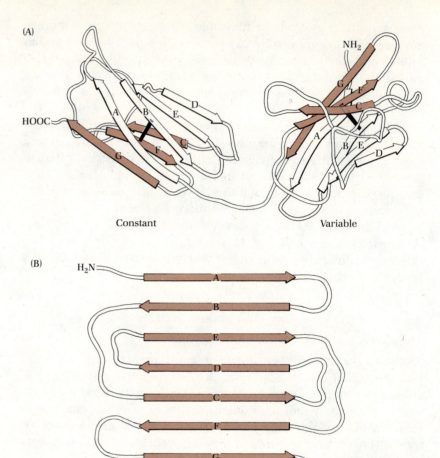

Constant   Variable

(B)

7   Folding Patterns of V and C Domains of Immunoglobulins. The immunoglobulin domains are composed of β-pleated sheets. (A) The path of the polypeptide chain is shown. The CDRs are formed by the loops at the end of the variable domain. (B) The anti-parallel β-strands of the sheets are shown in this diagrammatic representation. (A redrawn from Schiffer, Girling, Ely and Edmunson, 1973. *Biochemistry* 12:4620; B redrawn from Amzel and Poljak, 1979. *Annu. Rev. Biochem.* 48:961)

the interaction. To date the most complete studies have been carried out on lysozyme–anti-lysozyme and on hapten–anti-hapten complexes.

Plate 4-1 shows the epitope structure of lysozyme as determined by X-ray crystallography by Davies and his colleagues. It is immediately clear from this picture that the epitopes (antigenic determinants) cover large surfaces of the molecule. Plate 4-2 shows the "docking" of the Fab fragment of an antibody and one of the determinants. From this dramatic picture it is clear that the antigen-combining site of the antibody is really a large surface that is able to interface with the *surface* of the epitope.

This is also seen in the space-filling models of Roberto Poljak and his associates (Plate 4-3). This is especially clear in Plate 4-3C in which the antigen and antibody have been rotated 90° so that we are looking into the combining surfaces. It can easily be seen that residues on both H and L chain CDRs contact residues of the antigen and that the interaction is one of two surfaces coming together.

From these studies we now see that the antigen-combining site is really an irregular, rather flat surface with protuberances and depressions, formed by the CDRs of both H and L chains. The strength of the reaction between antigen and antibody is determined by how well the two surfaces can come together.

The Lock and Key Metaphor Revisited

It seems appropriate that we should now be thinking of antigen-combining *surfaces* rather than antigen-combining *sites*. Figure 8 shows the evolution of the metaphor of the antigen–antibody interaction from the lock and key to the current view. It may seem that the distinction between the models in Figure 8 are subtle. However, when one considers the thermodynamics of the antigen–antibody interaction, the implications of the differences are profound.

SYNTHESIS
The Antigen-Combining Surface of the Antibody

The ability of the simple four-chain structure of the Ig molecule to be able to react with enormous numbers of antigens is achieved by the variability of amino acid sequence in the variable regions. The parts of the variable region responsible for antigen interaction are the CDRs of both the H and L chains, and these are arranged in space in such a manner that they form a unique surface. The epitope on the antigen is also a surface, and the two are able to bind if there is sufficient complementarity between them. The fact that there are so many different specificities of antibody confirms the work of Landsteiner because it tells us that small changes in the surface of either the antigen or the antibody can lead to a change in the ability of the two surfaces to come together.

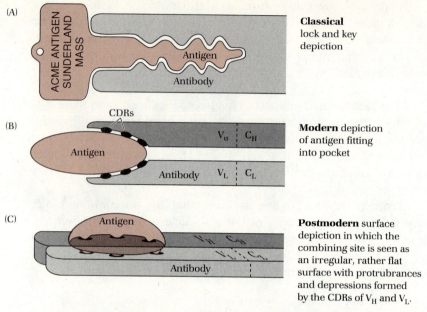

(A)

ACME ANTIGEN SUNDERLAND MASS

Antigen

Antibody

Classical lock and key depiction

(B)

CDRs

V_u | C_H

Antigen

Antibody V_L | C_L

Modern depiction of antigen fitting into pocket

(C)

Antigen

V_R C_R

V_L C_L

Antibody

Postmodern surface depiction in which the combining site is seen as an irregular, rather flat surface with protrubrances and depressions formed by the CDRs of V_H and V_L.

8   The Lock and Key Metaphor Revisited. The three drawings show the evolution of our thinking about the nature of the interaction of antigen and antibody. (A) Until the two-chain nature of the combining site was discovered, all immunologists used the metaphor as stated by Ehrlich and thought of the antigen as a key fitting into the correctly shaped keyhole. (B) This drawing is adapted from recent books on both immunology and cell biology and shows that even though we knew about the nature of the CDRs in the two chains, we still thought about the interaction in the lock and key mode with the antigen fitting into the keyhole and the CDRs acting as the tumblers. (C) A view that attempts to bring the earlier metaphor into line with the visual data from X-ray crystallography. Now the antigen is seen as fitting both onto and into the grooves and elevations of the *antigen-combining surface*.

Summary

1.   H and L chains contain constant (C) and variable (V) regions called V_H, V_L, C_H, and C_L.

2.   Wu–Kabat plots of variability show that there are three regions of hypervariability in the V regions. These areas are called complementarity determining regions (CDRs), and the areas between them are called framework regions (FR).

3.   X-ray crystallographic studies show that for protein antigens the CDRs form an antigen-reactive surface.

4.   The traditional lock and key metaphor of antigen–antibody interaction must now be modified to describe two surfaces coming into contact.

Additional Reading

Amit, A. G., R. A. Mariuzza, S. E. V. Phillips and R. J. Poljak. 1986. Three-dimensional structure of an antigen–antibody complex at 2.8 Å resolution. *Science* 233: 747.

Bentley, G. A., G. Boulot, M. M. Riottot and R. J. Poljak. 1990. Three-dimensional structure of an idiotope–anti-idiotope complex. *Nature* 348: 254.

Chothia, C., A. M. Lesk, A. Tramontano, M. Levitt, S. J. Smith-Gill, G. Air, S. Sheriff, E. A. Padlan, D. Davies, W. R. Tulip, P. M. Colman, S. Spinelli, P. M. Alzari and R. J. Poljak. 1989. Conformations of immunoglobulin hypervariable regions. *Nature* 342: 877.

Colman, P. M., W. G. Laver, J. N. Varghese, A. T. Baker, P. A. Tulloch, G. M. Air and R. G. Webster. 1987. Three-dimensional structure of a complex of antibody with influenza virus neuraminidase. *Science* 326: 558.

Davies, D. R. and H. Metzger. 1983. Structural basis of antibody function. *Annu. Rev. Immunol.* 1: 87.

Davies, D. R., S. Sheriff and E. A. Padlan. 1988. Antigen–antibody complexes. *J. Biol. Chem.* 263: 10541.

Glynn, L. E. and M. W. Steward, eds. 1981. *Structure and Function of Antibodies*. Wiley, Chichester.

Kindt, T. J. and J. D. Capra. 1984. *The Antibody Enigma*. Plenum, New York.

Silverton, E. W., M. A. Navia and D. R. Davies. 1977. Three-dimensional structure of an intact human immunoglobulin. *Proc. Nat. Acad. Sci. U.S.A.* 74: 5140.

Stanfield, R. L., T. M. Fieser, R. A. Lerner and I. A. Wilson. 1990. Crystal structures of an antibody to a peptide and its complex with peptide antigen at 2.8 Å. *Science* 248: 712.

Wall, R. and M. Kuehl. 1983. Biosynthesis and regulation of immunoglobulins. *Annu. Rev. Immunol.* 1: 393.

THE GENERATION OF DIVERSITY
The Variable Region

CHAPTER

5

Overview According to clonal selection, there are cells present in the body able to synthesize antibodies with specificity for a great array of antigens that the individual might come into contact with. We saw in the last chapter that the antibodies are composed of four chains, two H and two L, and that the CDRs in each chain form the antigen-reactive surface of the molecule. The question we address in this chapter is this: What is the nature of the genes that encode all these specific antibodies? If a given antibody-producing cell within an animal makes antibody molecules of only one specificity, and that animal can respond to perhaps 10^9 antigens, how is the information for all these antibodies encoded and distributed?

The answer to this question is both surprising and fascinating. We will see that fewer than 10^4 gene segments encoding antibodies are carried in germ cells (sperm and egg) and that these gene segments become rearranged in certain somatic cells (lymphocytes). A complete antibody gene is made as a result of this rearrangement of the gene segments.

Gene Rearrangement Causes Diversity

Germ Line versus Somatic Mechanisms

Before advances in molecular biology made it possible to directly answer the question of how V regions and C regions are generated, one of those seemingly interminable arguments in which immunologists specialize was raging over how much information for antibody specificity can be carried in the germ line (sperm and egg) and how much is generated in somatic cells (lymphocytes). The two sides were divided into camps; one championed the notion that all the genes are carried in the germ line, and the other championed the idea that there is some form of variation in the somatic cells.

The *germ-line* side argued that the genes for every antibody specificity are transmitted via the germ line, so that each cell has all the genes for the entire antibody repertoire. Each cell would thus have the genes for all the variable regions for H and L chains but by some unknown means would use only one of them.

The *somatic diversification* camp argued that, given the fact that there must be at least 10^6 and perhaps even 10^9 specificities and that most of the response repertoire is under no selective pressure for survival (the responses to such diverse antigens as DNP and camel erythrocytes are intact in all members of the human species but have no obvious survival value), there should have been genetic drift resulting in the loss of some specificities in some individuals. This does not normally occur. Furthermore, they argued, if the repertoire of responses exceeded 10^9 (which is certainly possible), the amount of DNA required to be conserved and transmitted would be too great to make biological sense. They argued that there must be a small number of germ-line genes that are highly conserved because of their survival value to the species that are transmitted from generation to generation via the germ cells. This number, they argued, must be far too small to account for the entire repertoire; so during differentiation into lymphocytes, these genes must undergo some sort of somatic variation. This variation in the somatic cells would result in the enormous diversity of the response.

With the discovery that there are variable and constant regions, each of the models had to explain how the V regions attain (or retain, depending on your persuasion) such a high level of diversity while the C-region genes retain such constancy.

Two Genes–One Polypeptide Chain

It was known from studies of human allotypes (constant region markers; see Chapter 6) that C-region genes are inherited in a simple Mendelian fashion. This finding presented a paradoxical situation: How could the same molecule have a C region inherited as a single gene and any one of 10^8 variable regions? In 1965 W. Dreyer and J. Bennett proposed that in light of these facts, V regions and C regions must be products of two genes. In other words, there are *two genes for one polypeptide chain* in antibody formation. To quote from their paper:

> These facts rule out the possibility that each of the complete
> polypeptide chains is synthesized under the genetic control of
> a separate and independent gene contained in the germ line. It
> appears that immunologically competent cells have evolved a

pattern of somatic genetic behavior which is radically different from anything normally found in modern molecular biology. [Dreyer, W. and J. Bennett, 1965. *Proc. Natl. Acad. Sci. U.S.A.* 54: 864]

The idea of two genes for one polypeptide chain ran counter to the dictum of one gene–one polypeptide chain and was met with a good deal of resistance. However, it was that creative leap that provided the framework for further thinking about the problem.

Shortly after the discovery of the V and C regions, experiments showed that there is only one "growing point" on the L chain as it is being synthesized, thus demonstrating that the mRNA for the chain is a continuous molecule. If this is so, then how do the two genes code for a single RNA molecule? The test of the two-gene model must somehow show that this mRNA can be coded for by two separate genes but be read as a single gene.

Genetic Reorganization

The discovery that the V and C regions are indeed coded for by two separate genes was made by Sosumu Tonegawa and his associates in Basel and is one of the most elegant and definitive series of experiments in the history of immunology. This seminal discovery came at a time when the idea and definition of a gene were changing and DNA sequencing techniques were in their infancy. Work on adenovirus-infected cells had shown that the genes of eukaryotic cells, unlike those of bacteria, are not uninterrupted sequences coding in a sequential manner for the amino acids of the peptide. Surprisingly, the coding sequences in a stretch of DNA were found to be interspersed among noncoding sequences, resulting in interruptions of informational material in the gene. The sequences that are used for coding are called EXONS (because they are **ex**pressed), and the noncoding **inter**vening sequences between them are called INTRONS.

The first step in the experimental process of testing the two gene–one polypeptide hypothesis was to isolate L-chain mRNA from a murine myeloma cell line (Box 1). The full-length mRNA contained the coding information for both the V and C regions. The 3' half of the mRNA contained the coding information for the C region only (Figure 1).

When radiolabeled, RNA can serve as a probe in hybridization experiments to detect and isolate DNA fragments containing sequences that are complementary to the RNA used. Hozumi and

BOX 1

Cloning an Antibody Gene

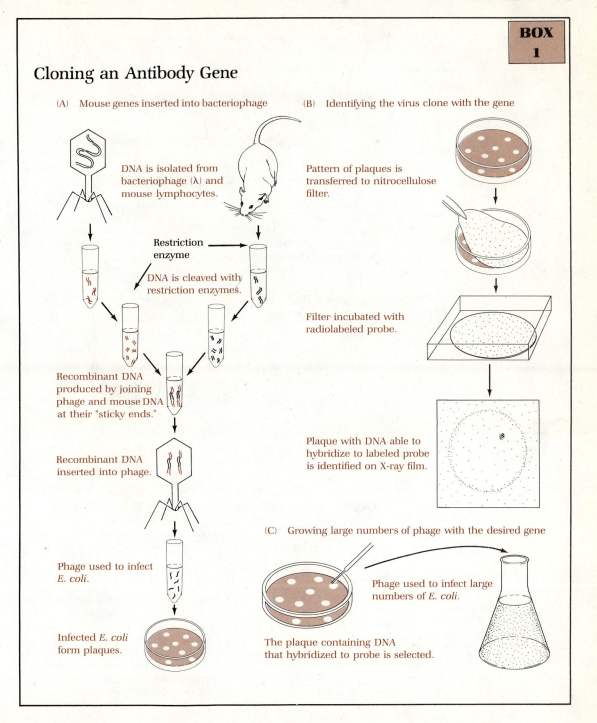

(A) Mouse genes inserted into bacteriophage

DNA is isolated from bacteriophage (λ) and mouse lymphocytes.

Restriction enzyme

DNA is cleaved with restriction enzymes.

Recombinant DNA produced by joining phage and mouse DNA at their "sticky ends."

Recombinant DNA inserted into phage.

Phage used to infect *E. coli*.

Infected *E. coli* form plaques.

(B) Identifying the virus clone with the gene

Pattern of plaques is transferred to nitrocellulose filter.

Filter incubated with radiolabeled probe.

Plaque with DNA able to hybridize to labeled probe is identified on X-ray film.

(C) Growing large numbers of phage with the desired gene

Phage used to infect large numbers of *E. coli*.

The plaque containing DNA that hybridized to probe is selected.

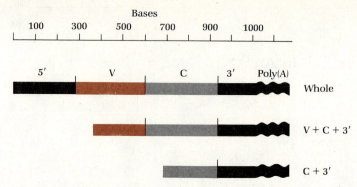

1   Light-Chain mRNA and Its Specific Fragments. Light-chain mRNA is about 1250 nucleotides long. It consists of five regions, including the poly(A) sequence at the 3′ end. These regions are designated by 5′, V (variable region, colored brown), C (constant region, colored gray), and 3′. [From Tonegawa et al., 1976. *Cold Spring Harbor Symp. Quant. Biol.* 41: 877]

Tonegawa treated DNA obtained from myeloma cells or from whole mouse embryos with restriction endonucleases and then reacted the resulting fragments with either the probe for V-C or that for C alone. They found (Figure 2) that both probes reacted with DNA fragments of the same size in the DNA obtained from the myeloma. However, the two probes reacted with different DNA segments in the DNA obtained from the embryo. This finding implies that in the myeloma cell there is one gene that codes for the V and C regions, and in the embryo there are two genes, one coding for V and one coding for C.

SYNTHESIS
Gene Rearrangement in Antibody Formation

The work of Hozumi and Tonegawa showed that the Dreyer–Bennett prediction is correct. We saw that there are two separate

2   Classic Experiment Showing Gene Rearrangement of Lymphocyte ▶ DNA. DNA from germ line (embryo) and lymphocytes (myeloma cells) is extracted and cleaved with restriction endonucleases, and the fragments are reacted with probes for V–C or C from Figure 1. Both probes bind to the same fragment in DNA from the lymphocyte source but to different fragments in the DNA from the embryo source. This shows that the gene segments for V and C regions are separate in the embryo but are rearranged in the lymphocyte. [Redrawn from Tonegawa et al., 1976. *Cold Spring Harbor Symp. Quant. Biol.* 41: 877]

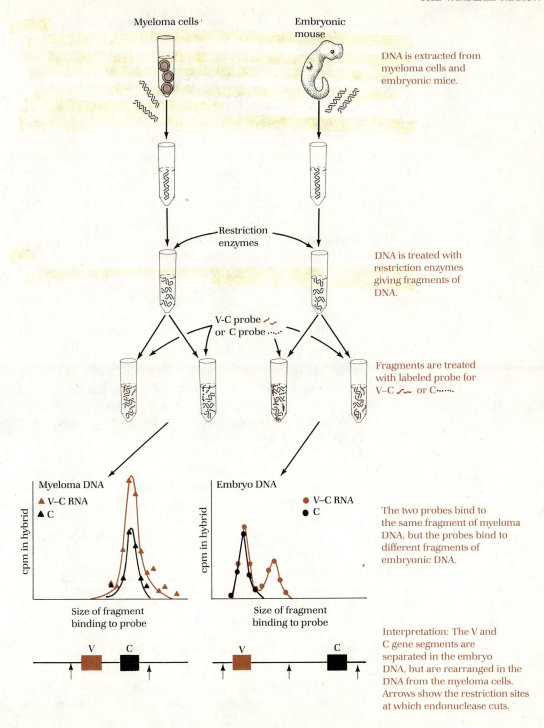

Myeloma cells

Embryonic mouse

DNA is extracted from myeloma cells and embryonic mice.

Restriction enzymes

DNA is treated with restriction enzymes giving fragments of DNA.

V-C probe 〜 or C probe ⋯⋯

Fragments are treated with labeled probe for V–C 〜 or C ⋯⋯

Myeloma DNA
▲ V–C RNA
▲ C

cpm in hybrid

Size of fragment binding to probe

Embryo DNA
● V–C RNA
● C

cpm in hybrid

Size of fragment binding to probe

The two probes bind to the same fragment of myeloma DNA, but the probes bind to different fragments of embryonic DNA.

V   C

V   C

Interpretation: The V and C gene segments are separated in the embryo DNA, but are rearranged in the DNA from the myeloma cells. Arrows show the restriction sites at which endonuclease cuts.

genes that code for a single chain of an antibody molecule. In the *germ line*, the DNA encoding the V region is separated from the DNA that codes for the C region. However, in *differentiated cells* able to produce antibodies (myeloma cells and B lymphocytes), the two segments are brought together to form a V-C segment. This is diagrammed in Figure 2; the V and C regions are seen to be separated in the germ line but are joined in the myeloma cell. When the germ-line DNA was cut with restriction endonucleases, the V and C segments were found on different fragments. But the site between the V and C segments that was cut to give these two fragments was no longer present in the myeloma cell. This indicates that the genes had been rearranged so that the V and C segments were now found on the same DNA fragment.

This Ig gene rearrangement has been extensively studied and is known to be the mechanism for the generation of diversity. All B cells contain rearranged Ig genes. The germ-line or unrearranged form is found in all other tissues.

Mechanisms of Ig Gene Reorganization

V–J Joining Forms the L-Chain Variable Region

Sequence analysis of the DNA in the V region of the L-chain (V_L) gene showed that the situation is more complex than it had at first appeared. A set of gene segments called J SEGMENTS (for *joining*), that are separated from the germ-line V gene segments by a large region of DNA, were discovered. The V segments and J segments are joined to form the functional V region of an L chain gene. Thus the V_L regions of the proteins that we have been discussing up to now are encoded by a V-region gene that is the result of the rearrangement and joining of two gene segments, a V_L segment and a J_L segment.

Figure 3 shows the organization of the L-chain genes. The L-chain gene sequences contain LEADER SEQUENCES that are transcribed and translated but excised from the protein before it is secreted from the cell. This leader sequence may be used for the transport of the molecule within the cell, because the L and H chains are encoded and synthesized on different chromosomes.

V–D–J Joining Forms the H-Chain Variable Region

The H-chain gene, like that of the L chain, has a tandem array of V segments, each separated by 5 to 15 kilobases (kb) of DNA. At an undetermined distance from the V segments of the H-chain gene,

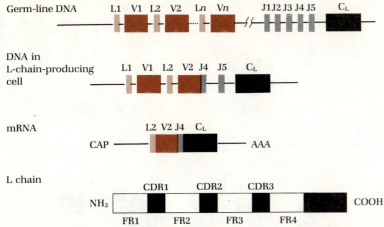

3 **Organization of L-Chain Genes.** A schematic representation of the organization of the germ-line L-chain gene segments is shown. This is the form present in all cells except B cells. As B cells develop, DNA rearrangement occurs (one *possible* rearrangement is shown by the dotted line). The intervening DNA is deleted during this event to bring one V_L and one J_L gene segment together in the genome of a L-chain producing cell. By RNA splicing the leader and C regions are joined to the VJ to produce the mRNA as shown. This encodes a complete L chain. [Alt et al., 1987. *Science* 238: 1079]

however, there are 5 to 15 segments of DNA that are not present on the L-chain gene; each of these segments codes for only about 10 amino acids. These additional elements of variation are the D SEGMENTS (for diversity), and there are more than 10 of them. Each of the D segments is separated from its neighbors by about 10 kb of DNA. In the formation of an H-chain V-region gene (V_H), first a D-J segment is formed, and then a V segment is transposed to the rearranged D-J segment. Thus, to form a functional V_H-region gene, there is rearrangement and joining of V-D-J segments. This is depicted in Figure 4.

Gene Reorganization Results in Diversity

So far we have seen that the variable regions of both H and L chains (V_H and V_L) are formed by the rearrangement of gene segments. We will see that there are a variety of different gene segments and that the rearrangement and joining of them results in a unique DNA sequence for each combination of segments. The actual number of specificities that can be generated in this way depends, of course, on the number of gene segments in the germ line.

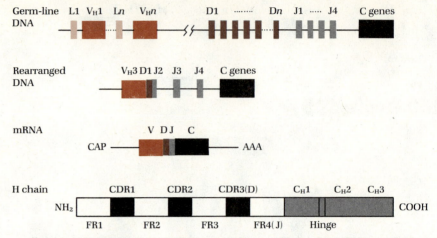

4 **Organization of H-Chain Genes.** The germ-line DNA is rearranged so that V–D–J joining results in a V region. In the mRNA this is joined to one of the C genes, which encodes a complete H chain. L1 and L*n* are leader sequences.

Recall that the germ-line proponents argued that all the V regions should be encoded in the DNA of the germ line, while the somatic-variation proponents argued that there are only a limited number of germ-line V-region genes and that there must be some somatic variation. Using hybridization techniques, the number of V, D, and J gene segments has been estimated. Table 1 gives a recent estimate of each of these. Note that there is a great uncertainty about the number of V segments in the mouse, and depending on the correct number, the number of antibody specificities that can be generated will be quite different.

In the mouse, the V_H segments have been divided into 15 *families* on the basis of the relatedness of their nucleotide sequences. In humans, at least 6 different distinct V_H families have been identified, and most of these are related to the murine families. One difference that is apparent is that the V_H genes in the mouse are found in discrete clusters, whereas in the human they are interspersed with one another.

SYNTHESIS
Potential for Diversity

One of the central questions in immunology has always been how the system can generate antibodies of any specificity. With the discovery that there are germ-line gene *segments* that become

Table 1 Estimates of the number of V, D, and J gene segments in human and mouse.

	Human		Mouse	
	H	L	H	L
V segments	100–200	90–100	250–1000	250
D segments	~30	—	10	—
J segments	6	5	4	4
V-region combinations	$(150 \times 30 \times 6)$ 2.7×10^4	(95×5) 4.7×10^2	$(625 \times 10 \times 4)$ 2.5×10^4	(250×4) 10^3
H and L V regions	1.27×10^7		2.5×10^7	

Source: Human from Strominger et al., 1989. *Cell* 57: 895. Mouse from Davis and Bjorkman, 1988. *Nature* 334: 395.

rearranged in the lymphocyte (but not in any other cells in the body), we have the solution to that problem. It now seems clear that by rearranging fewer than 1000 different gene segments, over 10 million different genes can be created. For example, if there were in the genome 200 V_L and 4 J_L segments, approximately 10^3 V_L regions $(200 \times 4 = 800)$ would be available through somatic generation. Similarly, if there were 250 V_H, 10 D, and 4 J_H segments, approximately 10^4 V_H regions $(250 \times 10 \times 4 = 10,000)$ would be available. If the 10^3 V_L regions were able to associate with the 10^4 V_H regions, there would be 10^7 possible antigen-combining sites. Of course all the possible combinations may not occur, but it is still clear that this *recombinatorial* mechanism allows a small number of gene segments to be combined into 10^7 genes.

This mechanism of gene rearrangement is very rare and would not have been discovered without the methods of molecular biology. But it is important to remember that the methods could not have been applied to this question without the decades of work that went into defining the immunologic problem.

The Generation of Diversity

We have seen that by rearranging a small number of germ-line gene segments it is possible to generate a very large number of antibody genes in somatic cells. In this section we will discuss the mechanisms by which this rearrangement and joining confers diversity.

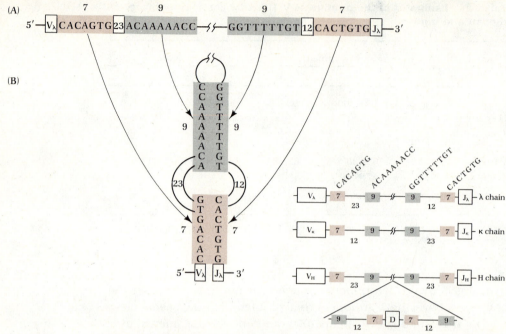

5 **V–J Joining in λ Chain.** V–J joining in λ chain by the heptamer–nonamer and 12/23 base pair rule. The shaded DNA segments in A separate the Vλ and Jλ segments that are to be rearranged by joining. Because they are palindromes, they can associate (as in B) to bring the V and J regions together. Inset: The heptamer–nonamer and 12/23 base pair rule in H and L chains. [After Tonegawa, 1983. *Nature* 302: 575]

Recombinatorial Diversification

Because the V_L and V_H regions are encoded by two (V and J) or three (V, D, and J) gene segments, with each segment existing in multiple forms, they can join in many combinations. The coming together of these gene segments to form the complete V-region gene introduces a level of diversity called RECOMBINATORIAL DIVERSITY.

The mechanism for the joining of one V and one J segment follows what is called the HEPTAMER–NONAMER AND 12/23 RULE. In the L chain, for example, each V region contains a palindromic seven-nucleotide sequence (the heptamer) 23 bases away from a nine-nucleotide adenine- and thymine-rich sequence (the nonamer) (Figure 5). Note that this is a palindrome in which T and G become A and C at the opposite end.[1]

[1] Palindromes are traditionally words or phrases that read the same forward and backward. The first words in courtly love were palindromic: "Madam, I'm Adam." In molecular biology, DNA sequences on the same strand that can complement each other are called palindromic (e.g., CACAGTG—CACTGTG, forming the base of the stem in Figure 5.

To the 5′ side of the J-region DNA is an inverted repeat of the heptamer and nonamer sequences, separated in this case by 12, not 23, bases. As shown in Figure 5, the V and J regions can be joined together, and the noncoding sequences are looped out and excised by appropriate enzymes. In this joining, the 12-base-pair spacer always matches with a 23-base-pair spacer. The predicted structure is called the LOOP–STEM STRUCTURE.

From the diagram it is easy to see why this is called the heptamer–nonamer and 12/23 base pair rule. A form of this rule applies to L-chain and H-chain gene segments, as shown in the inset in Figure 5 (in the figure, κ and λ are two L-chain types and will be discussed later.). The spacers differ between κ, λ, or H, but a 12-base-pair spacer rearranges only to a 23-base-pair spacer.

Junctional Site Diversity

Generally the first 100 to 110 amino acids comprise the variable regions. If there are 200 V_L gene segments that encode to amino acid 95 and 4 J_L gene segments encoding positions 96 through 108, then there could be 800 sequences for the L-chain variable region. In fact the number is even higher because of diversity at the site at which the two segments join. When the amino acid sequences of L chains were compared with the germ-line DNA sequences of J1, J2, J4, and J5, one amino acid in the protein—number 96— showed variability. This was found to be due to slight differences at the precise point of joining between V and J. The result of this imprecision is a new codon at the junction of the V-J region in the L chain and at V-D-J in the H chain. The result of this is JUNCTIONAL SITE DIVERSITY in CDR3 of the protein.

A possible mechanism for the generation of junctional site diversity is seen in Figure 6. At stage I, the two gene segments are lined up for joining. Presumably this is done with the help of DNA-binding proteins. The four strands are cut at the signal heptamer adjacent to the coding sequences. In stage II, the two heptamers are joined tail to tail, but the coding sequences do not join. Instead they are held by protein and retain their proximity. At stage III, exonucleases remove some nucleotides from the ends of the coding sequences. In stage IV, it is hypothesized that terminal transferase (which is found in bone marrow, where this rearrangement is going on) adds one or more nucleotides to these ends. Stage V is the final joining process. DNA polymerase replicates the added bases and a ligase seals the structure. The new codon(s) are represented by *N* in the figure.

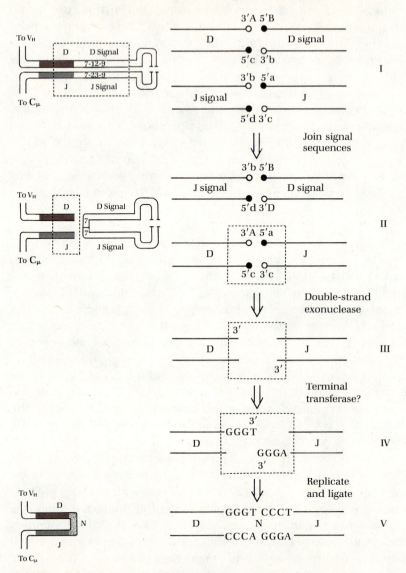

6 **Hypothetical Model for the D–J Recombination in H Chains.** Stage I: The D and J segments are lined up for joining and cut at the signal heptamer adjacent to the coding sequences (dark areas). Stage II: The heptamers that form the signal sequences are joined, but the coding sequences are held by a protein. Stage III: An exonuclease excises some of the coding sequences. Stages IV and V: A terminal transferase adds bases to the 3′ ends, which are joined by a ligase. [From Alt and Baltimore, 1982. *Proc. Natl. Acad. Sci. U.S.A.* 79: 4118]

Combinatorial Diversification

We have seen that H and L chains are generated by random gene rearrangement mechanisms. In an antibody-forming cell, the two come together to form a complete antibody molecule (H_2L_2). Since each of the chains is synthesized separately, when they come together the resultant antibody may have antigen-binding capacity for some antigen. If one calculates the possible random combinations of H and L that are possible, one finds that the number is enormous. This matching of one H and one L chain per cell is called COMBINATORIAL DIVERSIFICATION.

Somatic Mutation

Another level of diversity is added by SOMATIC MUTATION of the rearranged genes. There is good evidence that point mutations occur in the variable regions of rearranged V genes and contribute to some of the diversity. As we will see later, the major role of somatic mutation comes into play when clonal selection drives the development of increased affinity of antibodies for the antigen. This very important topic of affinity maturation will be discussed in detail in Chapter 21.

SYNTHESIS
Processes of Generating Diversity

We have seen that if a relatively small number of germ-line gene segments are rearranged, a very large number of different antibody genes can be generated (recombinatorial diversity). Even greater diversity can be introduced by slight changes in the way these segments are joined (junction site diversity) and to a lesser extent by somatic mutation. These events result in highly diverse H and L chains that are then combined to make an antibody (combinatorial diversity). Taken together, these mechanisms allow the immune system to make antibodies with an enormous range of specificities and show how the immune system can react to such a large number of antigens. Table 2 lists the various processes and the kind of diversity in which each results.

Allelic Exclusion

ALLELIC EXCLUSION is the phenomenon in which only the gene segments for one H chain and one L chain of an Ig molecule in a cell

Table 2   The generation of antibody diversity.

Process	Diversity
Large numbers of V genes	Genetic
Random choice of V(D)J	Recombinatorial
Imprecise joining of segments	Junctional
Independent diversification of H and L	Combinatorial
Somatic mutation	Mutational

are expressed. B lymphocytes—the cells that synthesize and secrete Igs—have the possibility of rearranging gene segments for two Ig genes, one on each of the two homologous chromosomes (one chromosome from each parent). If each of the chromosomes underwent independent rearrangement, the cell would synthesize products from both pairs. Allelic exclusion prevents this from happening.

The mechanism of allelic exclusion is not known. One of the theoretical explanations holds that because gene rearrangement is random, there is a probability that only one of the alleles will be functionally rearranged. This explanation is known as the STO-CHASTIC MODEL. Analysis of L-chain-producing cells, however, shows that the second allele is very often in its germ-line configuration, indicating that both alleles are not simultaneously undergoing rearrangement. Furthermore, there have been some cases in which both L-chain alleles are rearranged, transcribed, and even translated. But when this happens, only one of the transcripts combines with an H chain. To explain this, a REGULATED MODEL has been proposed. According to this model, H-chain rearrangement occurs first, and as soon as a productive rearrangement occurs, H-chain rearrangement stops and L-chain rearrangement is initiated. As soon as an L chain that is able to combine with an H chain is produced, the cell generates a signal that stops further rearrangement of the L-chain gene segments on the other allele. The result is one rearranged gene and one germ-line gene. If the first product made is unable to combine, then the second allele will be rearranged.

Generation of Diversity in Nonmammalian Species

In mammals, the antibody diversity we discussed above is generated in continuously produced B lymphocytes in the bone marrow (these will be discussed in detail in the chapters on cellular immunology). Each developing B cell undergoes random rearrangement of V, D, and J gene segments so that the antibody repertoire is constantly being created. Nonmammalian species that have immune systems have the same need to generate diversity of their immune repertoire, but they have evolved different, though related, strategies from the one we have described in humans and rodents. The study of these systems is beginning to give us great insight into the evolution of the immune system.

Shark

Multiple germ-line and mammalian-like recombination sequences are found in the V_H family of the horned shark (*Heterodontus francisci*), a primitive elasmobranch. This lower vertebrate is known to have a more restricted antibody response than mammals in that it does not discriminate between closely related haptenic structures in a Landsteiner-like experiment. When Gary Litman and his colleagues analyzed the genetic organization of the shark H-chain gene segments, they found that there is a very close linkage between the V_H, D_H, J_H, and C_H segments. Figure 7 compares the mammalian and elasmobranch (shark) gene components. In mammals the 200 or so V_H gene segments occupy approximately 2000 kb; D_H, J_H, and C_H segments occupy a total of about 260 kb. Thus the size of the region is enormous. In the shark, however, V_H, D_H, and J_H gene segments occur within approximately 1.3 kb, and

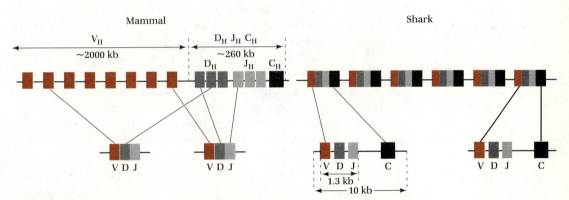

7   **Comparison of Genetic Organization of Shark and Mammalian Ig Genes.** A schematic depiction of the relative amounts of DNA occupied by mammalian and shark Ig gene segments. Because of the space occupied by the mammalian gene segments, many combinations can occur. The shark segments are in such close proximity that adjacent V–D–J segments preferentially combine. [After Hinds and Litman, 1986. *Nature* 320: 546]

even with the C_H segment occupy only 10 kb. It has been postulated that this organization favors the joining of *adjacent* V_H, D_H, and J_H segments and thus lowers the possibility that recombinatorial diversity will play a large role in the generation of diversity in these animals.

Thus, in this species the choice of germ-line segments to be combined and expressed would be the major contributor to antibody diversity, and this would account for the more restricted antibody response the species makes.

Bird

In the chicken, B cells are generated in the bursa (see page 216). The cells that give rise to B cells colonize the bursa about 8 days before hatching. In the bursa they induce the formation of bursal follicles, inside which they multiply and begin to express Ig on their surface. After hatching, the B cells, whose numbers have been expanded in the bursa, migrate out and constitute the peripheral B cells of the chicken (see Chapter 14 for a discussion of central and peripheral lymphoid tissue). At this stage the bursa involutes and no more B cells can be generated from the early precursor. This is in contrast to mammals, in which an early precursor cell is always present and continuously gives rise to new B cells. Thus at the time of bursal involution, the B-cell repertoire of the chicken is established.

There is another, even more striking, difference between avian and mammalian immune systems. It came as a great surprise to find that there is only one V_L- and J-region segment for chicken L chains. (The H-chain genes have been difficult to clone and sequence, but to date the same seems to be true for them as well, that is, one V_H, one D_H, and one J_H segment). How then can the chicken generate a full antibody response repertoire with this limited number of genetic elements to rearrange? The answer appears to be by GENE CONVERSION, the process by which an existing gene incorporates parts of nearby genes into itself.

Upstream from the single chicken L-chain V region lies a V-segment subgroup that contains 25 PSEUDOGENES in a 19-kb cluster. These pseudogenes, which interestingly have both transcriptional orientations, cannot encode a functional V region because they have either truncated 5′ or 3′ coding regions or an incorrect heptamer–nonamer recombination site. This organization is seen in Figure 8A.

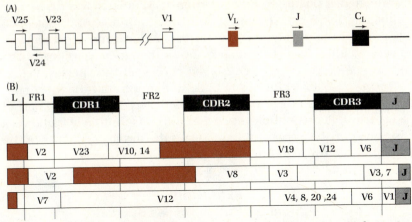

8 **Organization of Chicken L-Chain Genes.** (A) There is a single V_L, J_L, and C_L, but upstream of these is located a series of pseudogenes. The arrow indicates the coding orientation. (B) A schematic proposal for the generation of L-chain genes 3 weeks after hatching. Colored areas indicate unchanged V_L segments. Note that parts of the various pseudogenes are found in the V_L segment. [Modified from Weill and Reynaud, 1987. *Science* 238: 1094]

To generate diversity, several segments of the pseudogenes become incorporated into the one functional V_L region, resulting in a new specificity for the L chain. It is assumed that the same happens for the H chains. The kinds of diversity that result are seen in Figure 8B.

Thus the chicken uses the same basic mechanism of gene rearrangement as do the mammal and elasmobranch, but in this case the segments that are drawn upon are nonfunctional, so gene conversion is used. Nevertheless, like mammals and sharks, the chicken still requires a gene rearrangement that brings V and J together.

Amphibian

There are at least 80 V_H gene segments in the Ig gene complex of the primitive amphibian *Xenopus laevis*. There are also a number of J_H and putative D_H segments. All this suggests that recombinatorial and junctional site diversity are the mechanisms for diversity in this primitive species.

Conservation of V_H Sequences Across Species

Frederick Alt and his colleagues have recently compared the amino acid sequences of V_H chains of several species. These sequences were aligned (Figure 9), and a consensus sequence was derived by choosing the most frequently occurring amino acid at that position. Shark, caiman (crocodile), human, mouse, and *Xenopus* were used. Examination of the figure shows that some portions of the sequence are fairly well conserved across all the species. Figure 9B is a Wu–Kabat plot of the data and shows that the most *conserved* portions of the V regions are clustered in FR2, the end of FR3, and J. These authors argue that the conservation of framework regions may be important to maintain the tertiary structure of the Ig molecule through evolution.

SYNTHESIS
Clonal Selection Across Species

For clonal selection to work, it is necessary for lymphocytes to have receptors for antigen. Antibodies have both secreted and cell-surface forms, the latter acting as the antigen receptors. Thus, in the immune system, the generation of diversity allows the process of clonal selection to occur. Through the mechanisms we have discussed, each lymphocyte can bear a different antigen receptor to serve as a target for selection. Although the mechanisms of diversity differ among species, the result is the same: clonal selection can proceed.

It is interesting, however, that despite these differences, all the "solutions" to the problem of generating diversity have depended upon gene rearrangement. Not only are Ig genes generated by rearrangement in all the species studied, but in all cases these rearrangements have been found to obey the heptamer–nonamer and 12/23 rule. This finding suggests that the enzymatic complex responsible for DNA rearrangement is highly conserved in the vertebrates. It may be that the evolution of a mechanism for gene rearrangement of the sort we have discussed was necessary for the evolution of clonal selection and, in turn, the vertebrate immune response.

V(D)J Recombination-Activating Genes

We have seen in this chapter that the V(D)J recombination process generates the large numbers of V-region specificities required for clonal selection to operate. The rearrangements are mediated by the heptamer–nonamer and 12/23 recombination signal sequences (RSSs). The RSSs are conserved at each of the different loci that rearrange in the generation of diversity in antibody and across the

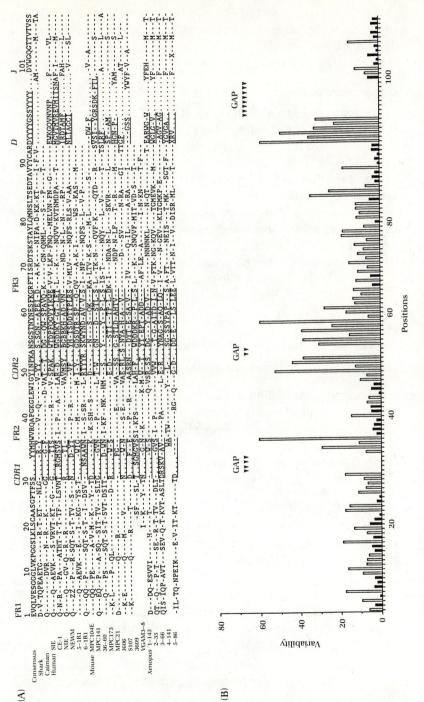

9   Comparison of V$_H$ Genes from Different Species. (A) The sequence of shark, caiman, human, mouse, and *Xenopus* are compared with a consensus sequence. (B) Variability of residues of V$_H$ region. Solid bars denote conserved positions. The picture that emerges is one of highly conserved regions between the variable regions across the species. [From Hsu, Schwager and Alt, 1989. *Proc. Natl. Acad. Sci. U.S.A.* **86:** 8010]

species. This suggests that the joining reaction is catalyzed by a single, evolutionarily conserved V(D)J RECOMBINASE. Two genes called *RAG-1* and *RAG-2* (*recombination activating gene*) that function as V(D)J recombinases have recently been identified.

The Discovery of *RAG-1*

David Schatz and David Baltimore at MIT used a retroviral construct containing germ-line Ig gene segments, a marker that signals rearrangement of the gene segments, and an independent marker for selection of cells that have integrated the retrovirus. A large number of murine cell lines were infected with the retrovirus, and those that were able to rearrange the gene segments were selected. As seen in Table 3, pre-B[2] cells were able to support the stable rearrangement of the gene segments. The fact that the nonlymphoid cell line was not able to support rearrangement was not surprising. But the fact that the cell lines derived from a lymphoid precursor or a differentiated B cell were unable to support rearrangement indicates that V(D)J recombinase activity is in the cells of the B-cell lineage only during a limited time of B-cell development.

Having found that the artificial substrate could undergo rearrangement in pre-B cells, Schatz and Baltimore then attempted to isolate the gene(s) responsible. They were able to transfer recombination activity into a line of fibroblast cells by transfecting these cells with genomic DNA from a cell line that exhibits recombinase activity. From these cells they were then able to isolate a gene that is responsible, that they called *RAG-1*. This group then went on to show that *RAG-1* is expressed in pre-T cells as well as pre-B cells and is conserved in chickens and frogs.

The Discovery of *RAG-2*

Marjorie Oettinger in Baltimore's lab then carried the work further. They had been puzzled by the fact that the *RAG-1* cDNA and an 18-kb genomic clone induced recombination no more efficiently than did total genomic DNA. Because this was an isolated and enriched gene, an increase in efficiency of at least 100-fold would have been expected. In an attempt to explain this situation, the researchers compared the sequences of the cDNA and genomic clones. They found that most, if not all, of the *RAG-1* was encoded

---

[2] As we will see in later chapters, the T cell is also a cell that contains rearranging gene segments.

Table 3   Patterns of expression in *RAG-1* and *RAG-2.*

POSITIVE CELL LINES	NEGATIVE CELL LINES
Pre-B	Mature B cell
Pre-T	Mature T cell
	Erythroid
	Macrophage
	Fibroblast
POSITIVE TISSUES	NEGATIVE TISSUES
Thymus	Spleen
Bone marrow	Brain

Source: From Schatz et al., 1989. *Cell* 59:1035; and Oettinger et al., 1990. *Science* 248:1517.

in a single exon confined to 6.6 kb of genomic DNA. The genomic clone therefore contained 12 kb of sequence whose function was not known but which may have been important in solving the paradox of the inefficient transfer of recombinase activity. One possibility was that located in this 12 kb of DNA was a second gene that was tightly linked with *RAG-1*. If this were true, then the reason for the lack of increase in efficiency would be explained by the fact that in all cases they were studying *RAG-1* plus another closely linked gene.

The first test of this two-gene hypothesis was to cotransfect fibroblasts with the *RAG-1* cDNA alone, the genomic DNA alone, or a mixture of the two. The reasoning was that if there was a second gene in the genomic DNA that complemented *RAG-1*, one would now see an increase in the number of transfectants with recombination. This is the very result that was obtained. The transfection with genomic DNA or cDNA alone gave about 30 recombination-plus transfectants, but transfection with the combination of genomic and cDNA gave 500. The second gene was called *RAG-2*.

Characteristics of *RAG-1* and *RAG-2*

From the above experiments it is clear that the first two candidates for rearrangement activation genes have been identified. *RAG-1* and *RAG-2* are closely linked but have no sequence homology. This indicates that unlike so many other closely linked and functionally related genes, they did not arise by gene duplication. Perhaps their most striking feature is that they contain no introns. It will be recalled that the intron–exon structure of genes is characteristic of eukaryotic cells, in contrast to prokaryotes, which lack introns. This has led Oettinger and her colleagues to suggest that these genes, which seem to be conserved in all species that can rearrange lymphoid gene segments, arose by viral or fungal infection into vertebrates or even protochordates. The recombination system could then have evolved to play the role that it currently does in V(D)J recombination.

Summary

1.   To explain the large number of V regions and the small number of C regions it was postulated that there must be two genes for one polypeptide chain of Ig.
2.   The genes for V and C regions were found to be separated from each other in nonlymphoid cells. However, in lymphoid cells there is a rearrangement of these genes so that they are adjacent. Thus the prediction that there are two genes for one polypeptide chain in antibody is correct.
3.   The V region of a heavy chain is formed by the rearrangements of variable (V) segments, diversity (D) segments, and joining (J) segments. Light-chain V regions result from the rearrangement of V and J segments.
4.   By gene rearrangement, under 1000 gene segments can give rise to 10^7 combinations of H- and L-chain V regions.
5.   V–J joining is mediated by recombination sequence signals (RSSs). These are a heptamer and nonamer and an intervening sequence of either 12 or 23 base pairs. Additional diversity is introduced by junction site diversification.
6.   Non-mammalian species such as the shark and chicken use variations of the mammalian theme of gene rearrangement to generate diversity in their Igs.

Additional Readings

Blackwell, T. K. and F. W. Alt. 1988. Immunoglobin genes. In B. D. Hanes and D. M. Glover, eds. *Molecular Immunology*. IRL, Oxford, pp. 1–60.

Blackwell, T. K. and F. W. Alt. 1989. Mechanism and developmental program of immunoglobulin gene rearrangement in mammals. *Annu. Rev. Genet.* 23: 605.

Golub, E. S. 1987. Somatic mutation: Diversity and regulation of the immune repertoire. *Cell* 48: 723.

Hinds, K. R. and G. W. Litman. 1986. Major reorganization of immunoglobulin V_H segmental elements during vertebrate evolution. *Nature* 320: 546.

Honjo, T. 1983. Immunoglobulin genes. *Annu. Rev. Immunol.* 1: 499.

Hsu, E., J. Schwager and F. W. Alt. 1989. Evolution of immunoglobulin genes: V_H families in the amphibian *Xenopus*. *Proc. Natl. Acad. Sci. U.S.A.* 86: 8018.

Kokubu, F., K. Hinds, R. Litman, M. J. Shamblott and G. W. Litman. 1987. Complete structure and organization of immunoglobulin heavy chain constant region genes in a phylogenetically primitive vertebrate. *EMBO J.* 7: 1979.

Oettinger, M. A., D. G. Schatz, C. Gorka and D. Baltimore. 1990. *RAG-1* and *RAG-2*, adjacent genes that synergistically activate V(D)J recombination. *Science* 248: 1517.

Schatz, D. G. and D. Baltimore. 1988. Stable expression of immunoglobulin gene V(D)J recombinase activity by gene transfer into 3T3 fibroblasts. *Cell* 53: 107.

Schatz, D., M. A. Oettinger and D. Baltimore. 1989. The V(D)J recombination activating gene, *RAG-1*. *Cell* 59: 1035.

Tonegawa, S. 1983. Somatic generation of antibody diversity. *Nature* 302: 575.

Wall, R. and M. Kuehl. 1983. Biosynthesis and regulation of immunoglobulins. *Annu. Rev. Immunol.* 1: 393.

Weill, J.-C. and C.-A. Reynaud. 1987. The chicken B cell compartment. *Science* 238: 1094

Wysocki, L. J. and M. L. Gefter. 1989. Gene conversion and the generation of antibody diversity. *Annu. Rev. Biochem.* 58: 509.

THE CONSTANT REGION

CHAPTER

6

Overview We began our discussion of antibody molecules by showing that they have a fairly simple four-chain structure but that the variable regions of each chain provide the structural basis of diversity. We then saw that this variable region diversity is achieved by the rearrangement of gene segments. It is this remarkable mechanism that allows lymphocytes that express the rearranged genes to be selected by antigen according to clonal selection. In the next two chapters we will focus on the constant region of antibodies. In this chapter we describe the structural basis of the heterogeneity and in the next the effector functions associated with the constant regions.

The constant region has not received as much attention as the variable region until recently because of the urgency felt by immunologists to solve the problem of the generation of diversity, even though it has been known for a long time that the constant region is not without interest. We will see that there are five classes of Igs, all defined by the constant region, and that virtually all the effector functions of antibody are mediated through the constant region. In fact, now that the mechanism of the generation of diversity seems to be essentially solved, more attention is being turned to the structure and function of the constant region.

Heterogeneity of Igs

Antibody activity is found in a broad spectrum of Igs. When analyzed by ultracentrifugation, antibody activity is found in molecules with sedimentation coefficients ranging from 7 to 19 S. This indicates great heterogeneity in *size* since these sedimentation coefficients correspond to molecular weights ranging from approximately 150,000 to a million. Heterogeneity is also seen when antibody molecules are analyzed by electrophoresis, indicating there is also great heterogeneity in *charge*.

When Igs of one species are injected into an animal of another species, they act as antigens. The antibodies raised against the Igs can be used as reagents to study the heterogeneity of the Ig. This heterogeneity has proved very important in the study of Igs because it defines *classes* or *isotypes* as well as *allotypes* and *idiotypes*.

Classes (or Isotypes) of Igs

Definition of Class

The Igs were originally classified according to their antigenic properties. Antibodies against the Igs of a species (human, for example) can be raised in another species (rabbit). Because there is great heterogeneity among Ig molecules, such an antiserum will contain antibodies against all the classes of Ig in the serum. Because the classes also differ in charge, the different reactivities can be visualized by immunoelectrophoresis (see Chapter 11). In a typical electrophoretic pattern there are several bands of precipitate, each representing a class of Ig. All normal individuals have molecules of each class in their serum.

Classes, or Isotypes

The CLASS, or ISOTYPE, of an Ig is determined by properties of the C_H. The five classes of Ig are designated by capital Roman letters: IgG, IgM, IgA, IgD, and IgE (a good mnemonic device is *Ig MADE*). Each of these differs in the H chain used, and the chains associated with each class are designated by a small Greek letter corresponding to the Roman letter of the class. Thus the H chain of IgG is a γ chain, and the H chain of IgM is a μ chain; IgA has an α chain, IgD has a δ chain, and IgE has an ϵ chain. As we will see, each of these is encoded by a different C_H gene segment. These gene segments are designated $C\mu$, $C\delta$, and so forth.

Some of the Ig classes are composed of polymers of the basic four-chain structure described up to now. Different classes have different molecular weights and diverse biological properties. None of these qualities, however, define class. The class of an Ig is always determined by the structure of the C_H.

There are two varieties of L chains called KAPPA (κ) and LAMBDA (λ). All of the Ig classes use these two types of L chains. Each monomeric Ig molecule has two H chains of the same class and two L chains of the same type. The monomeric form of any class of Ig can be therefore be described by its chain structure. An IgG molecule, for example, will always have two γ chains and either two κ chains or two λ chains. It would thus be $\gamma_2\kappa_2$ or $\gamma_2\lambda_2$.

We said earlier that the molecular weights of the Igs vary from 150,000 to a million. This variation in molecular weight is due to *polymerization* of the basic monomeric unit. An IgM molecule, for example, has a molecular weight of a million. IgM is a pentamer, but it is *not* a polymer of five IgG monomers. Rather it is formed by the polymerization of five $\mu_2\kappa_2$ or $\mu_2\lambda_2$ monomers. Thus an IgM is defined as $(\mu_2\kappa_2)_5$ or $(\mu_2\lambda_2)_5$. Similar notation can be used for all the classes, which will be discussed below.

Subclasses

Antisera that distinguish between molecules within a class can be made. For example, antisera that have been produced to detect differences *within* the IgG class will detect differences in the γ chains. These differences define SUBCLASSES of H chains and thus subclasses of Igs. Two IgG molecules will both contain two γ chains, but the H chains of one may differ in antigenic properties as well as in biological properties because of subclass differences. In all cases in which subclasses of Ig molecules have been found, the differences have been located in the C_H. As with class, each subclass is encoded by a different H chain gene segment. For example, in humans there are four known subclasses of IgG, cleverly called IgG1, IgG2, IgG3, and IgG4. These are encoded by $C\gamma_1$, $C\gamma_2$, $C\gamma_3$ and $C\gamma_4$. It is important to remember that all classes and subclasses of Ig are found in the serum of every normal individual.

There is enough sequence homology between the classes (~30%) that this has been used as an argument for the common evolutionary origins of C_H. There is great homology (~95%) between subclasses (e.g., IgG1 and IgG2). The areas of homology are found clustered in areas of β-pleated sheets, especially around the two cysteines that form the intrachain disulfide bond.

Properties of Ig Classes

Each class of Ig has the ability to carry out the primary function of antibody molecules—the combination with antigen—but they each have specialized functional ways of acting as *effector molecules*. These effector functions will be discussed in the next chapter. The properties of each of the classes and subclasses of human Igs are seen in Table 1. Although this list may be boring to some readers, the information is very important, and you may find yourself often returning to this section.

Table 1   Human immunoglobulins.

	IgG1	IgG2	IgG3	IgG4	IgM	IgA1	IgA2	IgA$_{sec}$	IgD	IgE
H chain	γ1	γ2	γ3	γ4	μ	α1	α2	α1, α2	δ	ε
Sedimentation constant(s)	7	7	7	7	19	7	7	11	7	8
Molecular weight (in thousands)	146	146	170	146	970	160	160	385	184	188
Mol. wt. of H chain (in thousands)	51	51	60	51	65	56	52	52–56	70	73
Number of H chain domain	4	4	4	4	5	4	4	4	5	5
Carbohydrate (%)	2–3	2–3	2–3	2–3	12	7–11	7–11	7–11	9–14	12
Serum conc. (mg/ml)	9	3	1	0.5	1.5	3	0.5	0.05	0.03	0.00005
Classical C fixation	++	+	+++	−	+++	−	−	−	−	−
Alt. pathway C activity	−	−	−	−	−	+	+	−	−	−
Placental transfer	+	+	+	+	−	−	−	−	−	−
Binding to mono-nuclear cells	+	−	+	−	−	−	−	−	−	−
Binding to mast cells and to basophils	−	−	−	−	−	−	−	−	−	+++
Reaction with Staph A	+	+	−	+	−	−	−	−	−	−
Half-life (days)	21	20	7	21	10	6	6	—	3	2
Distribution (% intravascular)	45	45	45	45	80	42	42	—	75	50
Fractional catabolic rate (% intravascular pool catabolized/day)	7	7	17	7	9	25	25	—	37	71
Synthetic rate (mg/kg/day)	33	33	33	33	3.3	24	24	—	0.4	0.002

Source: From many sources, but heavily from Turner, 1981. In Glynn and Steward, eds., *Structure and Function of Antibodies.*

IgG

IgG is a monomer and has the properties of the basic Ig monomer described in Chapter 3. It consists of two γ chains and two L chains (either κ or λ). Human IgG has a sedimentation coefficient of 7 S and a molecular weight of approximately 150,000. In the serum of normal human adults, it is the major class of Ig, constituting approximately 70% of the total Ig.

In humans there are four subclasses of IgG, each with a slight structural variation. These are shown in Figure 1. IgG1 constitutes 70% of the IgG, and IgG2 20%; IgG3 and IgG4 make up only 8 and

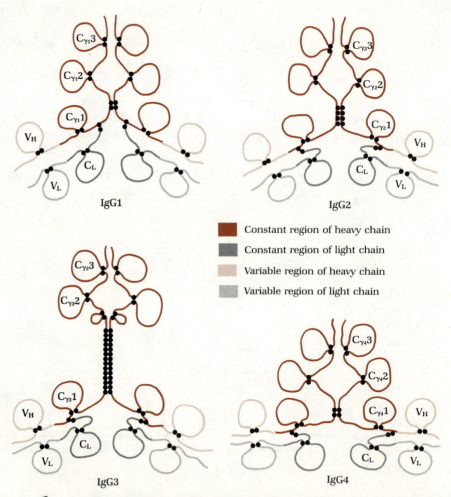

IgG1

IgG2

■ Constant region of heavy chain

■ Constant region of light chain

■ Variable region of heavy chain

■ Variable region of light chain

IgG3

IgG4

1   Structures of the Four Subclasses of Human IgG. The four subclasses of human IgG are diagrammed. The subclasses each have the same domain structure but differ in the number of interchain disulfide bonds as well as antigenic determinants. [From Turner, 1981. In Glynn and Steward, eds. *Structure and Function of Antibodies*]

2%, respectively. IgG3 has a rapid *catabolic rate* (the rate at which it is catabolized in the serum), with a half-life of 1 week; the other classes have half-lives of 3 weeks.

IgG is the only class of Ig that is able to cross the placenta; it is therefore the class of maternal antibodies that protects the newborn. IgG2, however, crosses more slowly than do the other subclasses. Recall from Chapter 2 that after the first Rh^+ pregnancy in an Rh^- mother, subsequent pregnancies are at risk because anti-Rh IgG antibodies are able to cross the placenta and react with the fetus.

IgM

IgM makes up approximately 10% of normal human serum Ig. It has a sedimentation coefficient of 19 S, which corresponds to a molecular weight of approximately 850,000 to a million. The molecule is rich in carbohydrate, which constitutes approximately 12% of its weight.

IgM is a pentamer of monomeric units composed of μ and L chains (see Figure 2). Each monomer has a molecular weight of approximately 180,000. IgM, unlike all other Ig classes except IgE, has a fourth C_H domain. The monomers are joined together through disulfide bridges. The entire pentamer assumes the circular shape seen in Figure 2. It was not known for some time what is responsible for this configuration. One alternative was that the entire circle is composed of the monomers joined together by disulfide bonds to form a "bracelet." Another alternative, called the CLASP MODEL, was that four of the monomers are attached to each other by disulfide bonds but the start and the end of the ring are attached to a structure called the J PROTEIN, which acts as a "clasp." Data favor the clasp model, and the J-chain clasp can be seen holding the circle of monomers together in Figure 2. It is important to keep in mind that the J chain is not an Ig and must not be confused with the *J segment* of Ig genes.

IgA

Serum IgA. IgA constitutes approximately 20% of the serum Ig. Of this, 80% is in the form of a monomer of molecular weight 160,000. The remaining 20% are dimers with a molecular weight of 415,000. The dimers are held together by the same J protein as in IgM.

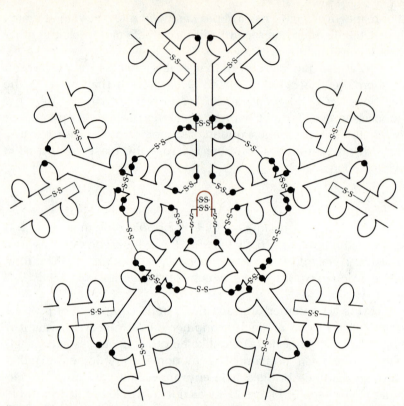

2   Structure of Human IgM with Location of the J Chain. The penta-meric structure of IgM is shown. Note that the monomers are held together with inter-H-chain disulfide bonds, and note the tentative location of the J chain. The black circles represent carbohydrate side chains. [From Turner, 1981. In Glynn and Steward, eds. *Structure and Function of Antibodies*]

Secretory IgA.   Secretory IgA is the predominant Ig in *seromucous secretions* and is found in external secretions such as saliva, tracheobronchial secretions, colostrum, milk, and genitourinary secretions. (The IgA in internal secretions such as synovial, amniotic, pleural, and cerebrospinal fluids is the serum type rather than the secretory type.)

Secretory IgA has four components: a dimer of two monomeric molecules, a 70,000-dalton SECRETORY COMPONENT, and the 15,000-dalton J chain. The J chain is produced by the same cells that produce the IgA and is probably linked in the same manner as in IgM (see Figure 2). The secretory piece, in contrast, is synthesized by epithelial cells and is covalently linked to the Fc of the IgA–J chain dimer as it passes through the epithelial cells of the mucosa. A schematic diagram of the association of secretory components and J chain with the IgA molecule is shown in Figure 3.

It is of interest that the combined quantities of serum and secretory IgA make this class the most abundant in the human body (even though IgG is the most abundant in the serum).

IgD

The concentration of IgD in the serum is very low, approximately 0.03 mg/ml. Because the concentration of IgD is so low, study of this molecule is very difficult and is complicated even further by the fact that the molecule is extremely labile. It is much more sensitive to proteolysis and heat than are other Ig classes, and proteolytic enzymes in serum may be sufficient to fragment the molecule during isolation procedures.

The molecular weight of IgD is approximately 180,000. The δ chain has a molecular weight of 60,000 to 70,000, with approximately 12% carbohydrate associated with this chain.

IgD is found to be present in association with IgM on the surface membranes of B lymphocytes. A cell that expresses both IgM and IgD is a mature but "virgin" B cell. The IgM and IgD

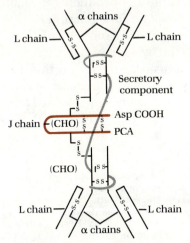

3   **Human Secretory IgA.** Diagram showing the possible arrangement of the two IgA monomers in relation to the secretory component and the J chain. The secretory component is synthesized by epithelial cells and is linked convalently to the Fc of the α chains (which are joined by the J chain) as it passes through the epithelial cells of the muscosa. [From Turner, 1981. In Glynn and Steward, eds. *Structure and Function of Antibodies*]

molecules on the same cell have the same antigen-binding specificity.

IgE

IgE is the HOMOCYTOTROPIC, or REAGINIC ANTIBODY, involved in immediate hypersensitivity and allergy (see Chapter 34). It has the lowest concentration in serum, approximately 0.00005 mg/ml; yet it has profound effector function.

IgE was discovered in 1966 in an ingenious experiment done by the Ishizakas while in Denver. They produced a reaginic-rich fraction of serum from an allergic patient and injected the fraction into a rabbit to produce anti-reaginic antibody. At the time, the known classes of Ig were IgG, IgM, IgA, and IgD. The antiserum was reacted with myeloma proteins of each of the known classes in an attempt to determine the class of the reaginic antibody by removing its activity. The antiserum against the human reaginic serum, now depleted of antibody to all *known* Ig classes, should have been devoid of any reactivity. However, this "empty antiserum" was able to form a precipitate with the reaginic-rich fraction of the patient's serum. In this way, they showed that an as-yet-unknown class of Ig was responsible for allergic reactions; but it was in such low concentration in the serum that it had been previously unidentified. It was not until IgE-producing myelomas became available that structural work became possible.[1]

The IgE molecule exists as a monomer ($\epsilon_2\kappa_2$, $\epsilon_2\lambda_2$) with a molecular weight of 180,000. The ϵ chain has a weight of 72,000 and, like IgM, has four C_H domains. The Fc portion binds strongly to a receptor on mast cells and in this manner carries out the molecule's effector function. The consequences of this binding are allergies due to mast cell degranulation and release of pharmacologically active substances. This whole fascinating story is covered in detail in Chapter 34.

[1] The scientific community was not quick to embrace this important discovery. The Ishizakas fought tremendous skepticism over the idea that an Ig isotype that was present at such low concentrations in serum could be responsible for allergy. This skepticism persisted for four years, despite the replication of the experiment in other laboratories. In an interview with one of us (DRG), Teruko and Kimishige Ishizaka explained that had it not been for the moral support of a few influential immunologists, especially Dan Campbell, Frank Dixon, and Merrill Chase, they might not have been able to proceed with their studies. The demonstration by the Ishizakas that IgE specifically interacts with mast cells and basophils to induce allergic responses (see Chapter 34) converted many of their detractors. With the identification of IgE-secreting myelomas (providing overwhelming experimental evidence that IgE is an antibody), the great insight and demanding technical expertise that led to the Ishizakas' discovery of IgE and its function were finally appreciated.

Genetic Variation in Igs (Allotypes and Idiotypes)

Allotypic Variation

ALLOTYPIC VARIATION is the variation between Ig molecules due to genetically controlled antigenic determinants (allotypic determinants) in the constant region.[2]

Ig molecules that exhibit allotypic variation are called ALLOTYPES. The name derives from the fact that these markers are due to *allelic* differences in C_H genes, genes that are inherited in a Mendelian fashion. Although every normal individual of a species has all Ig classes, each individual has only one or two allotypes. Allotypes are codominantly expressed, but an individual B lymphocyte secretes Ig molecules bearing only one of the parental allotypes because of allelic exclusion (see Chapter 5).

Both human and rabbit allotypes were discovered in 1956 and have been extremely useful in studying the genetics of Igs and as markers in linkage studies in cellular immunology. They have also been useful tools to anthropologists and population geneticists because they have unique distributions among ethnic groups.

Idiotypic Variation

Each normal member of a species has all of the Ig classes (isotypes) in its serum. Individual members of a species may differ in the allotypic markers present on their Igs. There is yet another kind of variation between Ig molecules that is unique to individual Igs. These are called IDIOTYPIC DETERMINANTS. (The word *idiotypic* derives from the Greek *idio*, which means "individual.") Unlike isotypic and allotypic differences that are coded in the C region, idiotypic differences are encoded in the V region.

It may not be surprising that anti-idiotype antibody is often directed against the antigen-combining site of the antibody molecule since this is the part of the molecule that is most individual. That this is the case was shown by reacting antibody with specific antigen and showing that when the combining site is occupied there is no reaction with its anti-idiotype antibody.

In most cases, response to an antigen results in a mixture of antibody molecules with several idiotypes. This is another way of saying that there are many idiotypes (id) for a given antigen specificity. This in turn indicates that there is heterogeneity in the composition of the combining site. However, the response to certain antigens results in a predominant idiotype on the antibody

---

[2] In the rabbit there are also V-region allotypes.

molecule. Production of a particular dominant idiotype to an antigen is an inherited quality. These inherited idiotypes are called DOMINANT, CROSS-REACTIVE, or PUBLIC IDIOTYPES. The very important role of id and anti-id in the regulation of the immune response will be seen in Chapter 29.

It was through the use of anti-isotype and anti-idiotype antibodies that it was shown that a single variable region can be associated with different constant regions. This is called the *Todd phenomenon* and led to the concept of class switching addressed later in this chapter.

C-Region Genes

Organization of C-Region Genes

The C-region genes are located on the 3′ side of the V, D, and J regions. L chains of both human and mouse are encoded by one Cκ and four Cλ genes (corresponding to the number of κ and λ families). Obviously, there are as many C_H genes as there are classes and subclasses of Igs, because isotype is determined in the constant region. All the C regions are coded in a single stretch of DNA. This is shown in Figure 4.

Formation of a Complete Ig H chain

A complete H-chain gene is of course composed of a V region and a C region. After the V-region gene segments are rearranged, transcription is initiated and continues through the V region to the μ and δ-region genes. mRNA encoding Cμ and Cδ is then produced by splicing the RNA as shown in Figure 5A. Thus the first complete H chains produced are μ and δ. Note that both have the same V region (and thus the same idiotype and specificity). We will see in Chapter 21 that both IgM and IgD act as surface receptors on B cells; the mechanism of processing to the membrane and secreted forms will be described at that time.

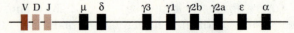

4 **Organization of C-Region Genes of H Chains.** The C-region genes of the H chain are encoded in a single stretch of DNA located 3′ of the V, D, and J genes. The C genes are multi-intron genes, but the separations are not shown in order to simplify the diagram.

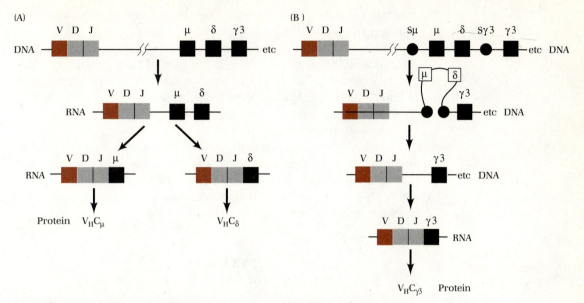

5   Generation of a Complete H-Chain Gene. (A) Generation of a μ H chain. After the V–D–J rearrangements occur, transcription begins. The first RNA transcript contains both the μ and the δ genes and is then processed so that there are separate μ and δ mRNAs. This results in μ and δ H chains. (B) Class switch. During the antigen-driven part of the immune response, another rearrangement occurs. A C-region gene (Cγ3 in the figure) moves into the position formerly occupied by Cμ and Cδ, which are excised and degraded. This results in a γ3 H chain. In the figure the black dot represents the switch regions of μ and γ3.

Class Switching

We will see in the chapters on cellular immunology that the intro-duction of antigen into an animal results in the appearance of newly synthesized antibody in the serum. As we saw above, the genes for the μ chain are the first ones in the line of C-region genes, and it is for this reason that the first antibodies that appear in the serum are of the IgM class. (Recall that IgD is in extremely low concentration in the serum.) However, as the response contin-ues there is usually a class switch. CLASS SWITCHING refers to the phenomenon by which the class, or isotype, of an antibody changes from IgM to one of the other classes. This class switch is mediated by yet another DNA rearrangement.

In the DNA rearrangement involved in class switching, the V region that was associated with the Cμ becomes associated with another C$_H$ gene segment—for example Cγ$_1$ or C$_α$. The V region remains the same during this switch.

The recombination required for class switching takes place in an intervening sequence between the V$_H$ and C$_H$ genes (Figure 5B). These stretches of DNA, called the S REGION (for **s**witch), are found in the 5′ flanking regions of each C$_H$ gene (except Cδ). Unlike the gene rearrangement in the last chapter, these do not obey the heptamer–nonamer and 12/23 rule.

A most interesting fact is that a DNA fragment with a nucleotide sequence almost identical to that of the S region of the mouse Cμ but with unknown function has been isolated from *Drosophila* DNA. This could mean that Ig genes have used a system already in place in other biological systems.

SYNTHESIS
Two Kinds of Gene Rearrangement

We saw earlier that the diversity of the antigen-binding sites in antibody molecules is generated by the rearrangement of V, D, and J gene segments. Class switching is another form of rearrangement that leads to another more limited kind of diversity. These two types of rearrangments occur by different mechanisms involving the heptamer–nonamer in the case of V–D–J and the switch region in the case of class switch. We will see in the next chapter that the effector function of an antibody molecule is determined by its constant region. Class switching allows the same antigen-binding specificity to be expressed with several different constant regions. This gives a wider range of effector functions to the specificities. Gene segment rearrangement leading to V regions occurs during development of the cells (before antigenic stimulation) but class switching occurs after the B cell has reacted with antigen.

Tissue-Specific Regulation of Ig Gene Expression

Promoters and Enhancers

Two DNA-binding elements, called PROMOTERS and ENHANCERS, are required for the regulation of gene expression in higher eukaryotic organisms. The promoter is required for accurate and efficient initiation of transcription, and the enhancers increase the rate of transcription from promoters. Promoters are located immediately upstream from the start site of transcription and are typically about

100 base pairs in length. The enhancers can act on the promoters from a distance and can be far downstream from the transcription unit.

   In Igs, the promoters are 5′ of each of the V-gene segments, and the enhancers are located in the introns between J and C (i.e., 5′ of C and 3′ of J). Figure 6 depicts the locations of the murine H- and L-chain promoter and enhancer. Note in the figure that the promoter region (*Prom*) and the enhancer region (*Enh*) are distant from each other. The function of the newly discovered additional Enh region 3′ of the Cκ coding region is not known. Since both promoter and enhancer elements are necessary for optimal transcription, the rearrangement of the V region (and its promoter) to the DJ region with its enhancer brings the promoter and enhancer into relative proximity and activates transcription (see Figure 6).

B Cell-Specific Transcription of Ig Genes

In Ig genes, both the Ig promoter and the IgH enhancer contain a highly conserved 8-base-pair sequence (octamer). At first it was thought that these sequences were responsible for B cell–specific transcription of Ig genes or perhaps coordinated H- and L-chain

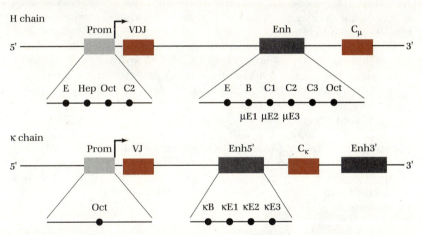

6   Components of the IgH, V$_H$, κ, and V$_κ$ Enhancer and Promoter. The figure depicts the arrangements of the promoter (Prom) and enhancer (Enh) sequences for the H chain and the κ chain. The coding sequences for VDJ, C$_μ$, VJ, and C$_κ$ are shown in color. The expanded portion of the promoter and enhancer areas show the binding sites for some of the DNA-binding proteins. The letters below the line in the H-chain enhancer section are alternative names of the binding proteins named above. [Redrawn after Calame, 1989. *Trends Genet.* 5: 395]

transcription. But the discovery that the deletion of the sequence in the IgH enhancer reduces but does not abolish activity, and the fact that the same octamer sequence appears in non-Ig gene promoters, indicates that the problem is very complex.

Proteins that bind to the promoters and enhancers cause tissue-specific regulation of transcription, and there have been several well characterized DNA-binding proteins identified in B cells. These are seen in Figure 6.

The ongoing discoveries of factors that bind both specifically and nonspecifically to the Ig enhancer and promoter sequences have made it impossible to give any model in a text of this level. It is clear that this important question will become more complex before the answer is obvious. However, we will return to the question of enhancers, promoters, and DNA-binding proteins when we discuss lymphocyte activation in Chapter 26.

Summary

1. Igs are heterogenous, varying in molecular weight and electrophoretic mobility.
2. Igs are divided into five classes, or isotypes, called IgG, IgM, IgA, IgD, and IgE. These classes and their subclasses are encoded by different C_H gene segments. All normal individuals produce all the classes and subclasses.
3. Allotypes are markers found on Ig molecules. These markers are controlled by allelic differences in C_H chains so that any individual expresses only a limited array of the total allotypes in the species.
4. Idiotypes are markers found on Ig molecules and are associated with the antigen-binding region.
5. Constant region genes are located 3' of the V region genes. After the gene rearrangements leading to a V region, there is an additional rearrangement leading to a complete H or L chain.
6. During the antigen-driven portion of the immune response, there is another gene rearrangement. In this one the V region that was associated with $C\mu$ becomes associated with another C_H region (γ3, for example).

Additional Readings

Calame, K. L. 1989. Immunoglobulin gene transcription: Molecular mechanisms. *Trends Genet.* 5: 395.

Ephrussi, A., G. M. Church, S. Tonegawa, and W. Gilbert. 1985. B lineage-specific interactions of an immunoglobulin enhancer with cellular factors in vivo. *Science* 227: 134.

Glynn, L. E. and M. W. Steward (eds.). 1981. *Structure and Function of Antibodies*. Wiley, Chichester.

Hanes, B. D. and D. M. Glover, eds. 1988. *Molecular Immunology*. IRL, Oxford, pp. 1–60.

Ishizaka, K. 1983. Structure and biological activity of immunoglobulin E. In F. J. Dixon and D. W. Fisher, eds., *The Biology of Immunologic Disease*. Sinauer, Sunderland, Mass. p. 13.

Janeway, C., E. E. Sercarz and H. Wigzell, eds. 1981. *Immunoglobulin Idiotypes*. Academic Press, New York.

Koshland, M. E. 1985. The coming of age of the immunoglobulin J chain. *Annu. Rev. Immunol.* 3:425.

Maniatis, T., S. Goodbourn and J. A. Fischer. 1987. Regulation of inducible and tissue-specific gene expression. *Science* 236:1237.

Metzger, H. 1970. Structure and functions of IgM immunoglobulins. *Adv. Immunol.* 12:57.

Muller, M. M., S. Ruppert, W. Schaffner and P. Matthias. 1988. A cloned octamer transcription factor stimulates transcription from lymphoid-specific promoters in non-B cells. *Nature* 336:544.

Nisonoff, A. 1984. *Introduction to Molecular Immunology*, 2nd ed. Sinauer, Sunderland, Mass.

Ptashne, M. 1988. How eukaryotic transcriptional activators work. *Nature* 335:683.

Scheidereit, C., J. A. Cromlish, T. Gester, K. Kawakami, C.-G. Balmaceda, R. A. Currie and R. G. Roeder. 1988. A human lymphoid-specific transcription factor that activates immunoglobulin genes is a homeobox protein. *Nature* 336:551.

Tomasi, T. B., Jr. 1976. *The Immune System in Secretions*. Prentice-Hall, Englewood Cliffs, N.J.

EFFECTOR FUNCTIONS OF IMMUNOGLOBULINS

CHAPTER

7

Overview Up to now we have focused on the antigen-binding properties of antibodies. We saw that the specificity of any antigen-reactive surface formed by the CDRs allows the specific antibody and antigen to come together. There are many consequences of this specific binding, and many of these are controlled by the constant region of the molecule. These include the activation of complement, which results in the lysis of target cells, opsonization, and mast cell degranulation. These last two reactions occur through the interaction of the Fc portion of the antibody molecule with an Fc receptor on the surface of a cell. The varied effector functions of antibody molecules are due to differences in their Fc portions, and this underscores the importance of class switching.

Flexibility of the Ig Molecule

It is clear from the last chapter that antibodies, although they have the same basic plan of two H and two L chains, come in a variety of shapes and sizes. What is not clear from the usual descriptions and diagrams of the antibody molecule is the great flexibility of the molecule. This is illustrated in Figure 1.

There is flexibility of the Fab around the hinge region (FAB ARM ROTATION and WAGGING) as well as within the Fab (FAB ELBOW BENDING) that allows the antigen-binding portion of the molecule to move. The reader will recall that electron micrographs of the antibody molecule (Figure 6 in Chapter 4) show a Y, but the X-ray diffraction picture (Figure 7 in Chapter 3) of the only complete Ig molecule that has been resolved in this manner shows a T. The myeloma protein used for the X-ray studies (a protein called Dob) lacks a hinge region, and it is thought that this deletion results in the molecule's permanent T shape. Intact molecules probably are in constant transit between the Y and the T shape, and the Fab arm

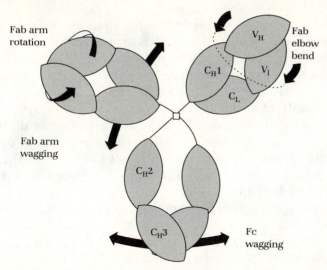

1   Flexibility of the Ig Molecule. Diagram of the Ig molecule showing the potential for *rotating*, *bending*, and *wagging*. [Courtesy of Dennis Burton]

rotation allows the molecule to move between a Y and a T shape. The Fab elbow bending gives the molecule great freedom to react with antigens that are fixed on surfaces, and the flexibility around the Fc (FC WAGGING) is very important for complement activation (see below and Chapter 8) as well as Fc-receptor binding.

Effector Functions of Antibody Molecules

Neutralization

There is at least one group of reactions in which the act of the antibody binding to antigen has a biological function. These are cases in which the antigen has its biological function neutralized by the antibody. The two most common cases are the neutralization of toxins and of virus (discussed further in Chapter 32). We will see in the chapter on autoimmunity (Chapter 35) that the binding of an antibody to a hormone or to a receptor can block biological function with deleterious effect to the host. But when the antibody is directed to a toxin or an invading virus it acts in a protective manner.

When dilutions of serum containing antibody to a virus are added to a constant number of virus particles, the antibody causes a reduction in the number of infective particles. This is seen in

Figure 2, which is Renato Dulbecco's classic experiment with polio-virus. In this experiment various concentrations of an anti-polio antiserum were incubated with virus for periods of time, and the remaining infective virus was then determined. A clear concentration-dependent neutralization can be seen. This neutralization of infectivity can be shown to be due to the combination of the antibody with the structure on the virus that reacts with the receptor on the surface of the cell. The virus particle is not destroyed, but its ability to infect is. Alternatively, if the antibody is directed at a determinant on the virus that is not used in infectivity, the resulting antigen–antibody complex may be cleared from the circulation. The formation of a complex can be seen to scale in Plate 7-1, which is a computer-generated graphic of antibody reacting with poliovirus.

The same phenomenon is true for toxins. Tetanus and diphtheria, for example, are caused by bacteria that elaborate exotoxins. When an animal is immunized with detoxified molecules, it devel-

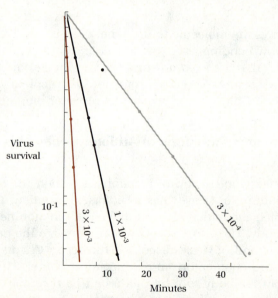

2   **Neutralization of Viruses by Antibody.** The results of a classic experiment by Renato Dulbecco showing that poliovirus is inactivated by anti-poliovirus antiserum. The virus was treated with antibody at various dilutions. At the indicated time intervals the number of surviving virus particles was determined by plating on appropriate target cells. The result is an exponential inactivation. Dilutions used were 3×10^{-3} (color trace); 1×10^{-3} (black trace); 3×10^{-4} (gray trace). [Redrawn from Dulbecco et al., 1956. *Virology* 2: 162]

ops antibody that reacts with the toxin in vivo. This results in the neutralization of the toxin and prevents it from combining with the appropriate cellular component so that it cannot cause disease.

Complement Fixation

In Chapter 8 we will discuss the complement system in detail. In that chapter it will be seen that one of the consequences of the combination of antigen and antibody is to allow the activation of the COMPLEMENT CASCADE. This cascade begins with the binding of one of the components of complement to the Fc portion of the Ig. When antibody (via its Fab) reacts with an antigen on the surface of a cell, the consequence of the activation of the complement cascade is the lysis of the cell. Obviously, if the cell is a bacterium, its destruction by lysis is a means of host defense. In this case, we can think of the specificity of the antibody molecule being used to guide the whole Ig molecule to the appropriate surface and the protective function being carried out by the Fc portion, the part with no specificity. IgM and all the IgG subclasses except IgG4 are able to bind complement and initiate the cascade. The other classes generally do not. Because it is a pentamer, IgM has much greater activity in complement fixation.

For many years it was thought that the binding of the Fab portion of the molecule to antigen caused a steric change in the Fc portion allowing the complement cascade to be initiated. We now know that this is not the case, and complement can bind to Ig molecules that are not reacted with antigen. But to initiate the activation of complement, it is necessary for *two* molecules of monomeric antibody to bind antigen, and then the complement component C1q reacts with *both* of them, as will be seen in Chapter 8. The fact that there is flexibility of the Fc portion of the antibodies allows easier reaction of the complement component with them. IgM is a much more efficient activator of complement because it is a pentamer and has a higher probability of having the Fc portions near each other. The C1q molecule binds to the C_H2 domain of IgG molecules (see Figure 1).

Opsonization

Phagocytosis, the ingestion of particles by a cell (*phagos*, from the Greek for "to eat") is one of the oldest and most efficient primary defenses of the body. It has been conserved in evolution and is probably the main defense of most of the animal world. It is nonspecific, and vertebrates have added to it the specificity of the immune response. Antibody is known to facilitate the phagocytic process. If an individual has specific antibody to an invading organism, the invaders are cleared from the bloodstream at a faster rate than in an unimmunized host.

The mechanism by which antibody enhances the phagocytic process is well understood. The initial event is known to depend on the specific binding of the antibody, through its Fab portion, to the particulate antigen. The Fc portion of the antibody molecule then binds to a receptor on the surface of the phagocytic cell. By binding to these cellular Fc RECEPTORS (FcRs), the antibody brings the antigen to the membrane of the phagocytic cell and the process of phagocytosis is initiated. This process is carried out by MEM-BRANE-ZIPPERING, as seen in Figure 3. The particle to be ingested has antibody over its surface with the Fc portions available to react with the cellular Fc receptors. As the phagocyte (a macrophage in the diagram) reacts with the Fc receptors, the membrane moves over the surface and engulfs the particle, essentially "zippering" the membrane closed around it. The ingested particle is now inside the phagocytic cell, but enclosed in a membrane, originally the surface membrane, and degradation of the particle begins.

Until very recently it was thought that the binding of the FcR to the Fc was in the C_H3 domain of the Ig. There is now growing evidence that the binding occurs in the C_H2 domain.

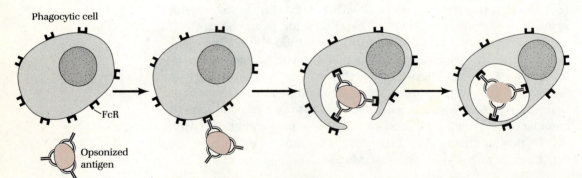

Phagocytic cell

FcR

Opsonized antigen

3   **Opsonization and Phagocytosis.** The antibody reacts with the antigen via the Fab portion, leaving the Fc portion exposed. The Fc of the antibody reacts with the FcR on the phagocytic cell. As more FcR reacts with bound Ig, the membrane "zippers" closed around the antigen particle, resulting in the internalization and ultimate destruction of the particle.

Antibody-Dependent Cell-Mediated Cytotoxicity

There is a defense mechanism called ANTIBODY-DEPENDENT CELL-MEDIATED CYTOTOXICITY, or ADCC, that may be of importance in the destruction of virus-infected cells and tumors. We will see in Chapter 28 that specific cell killing, or cytotoxicity, is a function of one class of lymphocytes called cytotoxic T cells. Other cells such as neutrophils, macrophages, and some other lymphocytes bearing Fc receptors on their surfaces also display cytotoxic function. In the case of ADCC, specificity for target cells is imparted by the Fab portion of the antibody molecule bound to the Fc receptor. If an animal makes an antibody response to an aberrant cell (either virus-infected or a tumor), the antibodies will bind via their Fab portion leaving their Fc facing outward. If the binding has been such that the Fc portions are clustered or aggregated, they can react with an FcR-positive cell via the Fc receptors. As a result of this binding, some FcR-positive cells are able to release the contents of their granules and cause the lysis of the target cells. This is diagrammed in Figure 4.

Mast Cell Degranulation

One very important consequence of the binding of antibody to antigen that is very unpleasant and can be life-threatening is the degranulation of mast cells and basophils. We mentioned earlier that allergy is mediated by the IgE class of Igs. We will discuss this in detail in Chapter 34. Mast cells contain large granules filled with biologically active molecules (histamine, serotonin, prostaglandins, leuokotrienes, etc.). They also have a high concentration of surface

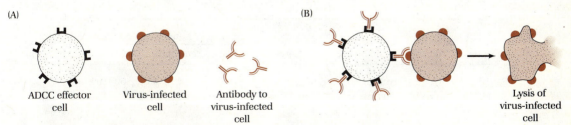

(A)

ADCC effector cell   Virus-infected cell   Antibody to virus-infected cell

(B)

Lysis of virus-infected cell

4 Antibody-Dependent Cell-Mediated Cytotoxicity (ADCC). (A) *The players*. (Left) ADCC effector cell with FcRs. (Center) Virus-infected cell with virus antigen on surface. (Right) Antibody to virus-infected cell. (B) *The drama*. (Left) The Fc of the antibody has reacted with the FcRs on the ADCC effector cell, leaving the antigen-binding sites available at the cell surface. (Center) The virus-infected cell reacts with the available antibody on the surface of the effector cell. (Right) The reaction results in the death of the infected cell.

receptors specific for the Fc of IgE. An "allergic individual" is one who has responded to an allergen with an IgE response. The IgE (against ragweed, for example) circulates through the bloodstream and reacts with the mast cells *via the FcRs*. The mast cells are thus coated with IgE molecules anchored by their Fc and with their antigen-reactive surfaces exposed. When ragweed binds with the Fab, the result is the degranulation of the mast cell with release of the granular contents, leading to the symptoms of allergy.

This, then, is a case of the antibody molecule being trapped at a site by nonspecific methods (binding of IgE and FcR) and the specific binding of the allergen causing the mast cells to degranulate. The mechanisms of degranulation are discussed in Chapter 34.

The Nature of the FcR

In the sections above we focused on the key role of cell-surface FcR in the effector function of antibodies. In the last few years a great deal has been learned about FcRs, so our understanding of how the antibody molecule can initiate the effector functions is growing. There are FcRs on many cell types, and there are several kinds of FcRs. Thus the term is really an operational one, and it should not be assumed that the same molecule is being discussed every time it is used.

The FcRs can be divided into at least two groups by the affinity with which they bind the Fc domain of Ig. See Table 1 for some properties of FcRs binding to IgGs (Fc$_\gamma$R). High-affinity receptors,

Table 1   Properties of Fc receptors.

Receptor	Mol. wt. (kd)	Subclass binding	Affinity	Receptors per cell			
				Monocyte	Neutrophil	Macrophage	Eosinophil
Fc$_\gamma$RI	70	Human IgG1 Human IgG3 Mouse IgG2a Mouse IgG3	High (10^{-9})	15–40	2	50–100	3
Fc$_\gamma$RII	40	Complexes	Low (10^{-6})	30–60	30–60	30–80	25–35
Fc$_\gamma$RIII	55–70	Complexes	Low	1–5	100–200	40–100	5–15

Data from Fanger, Shen, Graziano and Guyre. 1989. *Immunol. Today* 10:92.

called FcRI, bind with an affinity of 10^8 to 10^{10} M^{-1} Fc receptors designated FcRII bind with lower affinity, $<10^6$ M^{-1}. IgE binds with very high affinity to mast cells and basophils via their Fc_ϵ receptors. This $Fc_\epsilon RI$ has been cloned and shown to consist of three chains, called α, β, and γ. With the receptor now cloned, it can be expressed in a variety of cells, and these can be used to screen molecules that block or diminish the binding of IgE, an important advance for the development of drugs in the classical manner. IgE is also bound by eosinophils; however, this binding is of much lower affinity than that to mast cells and basophils. The binding to eosinophils is via an $Fc_\epsilon RII$.

SYNTHESIS
Division of Labor between Antibody Domains

We have seen so far that the V regions of Igs contain the antigen-combining surface and the idiotype. This is the portion of the molecule that confers specificity. We have also seen that the Fc domains of the molecule have effector functions such as binding of complement and FcRs leading to opsonization and degranulation. Thus we see the strategy that has evolved: Ig molecules react with a specific structure through the Fab domain and carry out nonspecific effector functions through the Fc domains.

To understand the physiological roles that antibodies can play, one must take into account the location of the antibody in the body, its physiochemical properties and the biological function of the receptors (C or Fc) that specifically interact with it. IgM, for example, is an efficient effector molecule by virtue of its interaction with complement and FcR receptors, but it is too large to penetrate deep into tissues. IgA is present in mucosal secretions and performs most of its effector function through neutralization or interaction with FcRs.

Summary

1. Most of the effector functions of Igs are mediated through the Fc domains of the molecule. There is thus a division of labor within the molecule: antigen binding in the Fab portion and effector functions in the Fc.
2. To accommodate the two functions, the Ig is flexible. There is Fab arm rotation, arm wagging, and elbow bending as well as Fc wagging. The hinge region contributes the structure for flexibility.

3. The complement cascade is activated when two antibody molecules are bound to antigen and are spatially close enough so that complement can bind. The C1q binding site is in the C_H2 domain.

4. Opsonization, antibody-dependent cell-mediated cytotoxicity (ADCC), and mast cell degranulation are associated with binding of the Fc portion of the Ig molecule to FcRs on effector cells.

Additional Readings

Burton, D. R. 1987. Structure and function of antibodies. In F. Calabi and M. S. Neuberger, eds. *Molecular Genetics of Immunoglobulin*. Elsevier Science, p. 1.

Metzger, H. and J.-P. Kinet. 1988. How antibodies work: Focus on Fc receptors. *FASEB J.* 2:3.

COMPLEMENT

Overview The complement system consists of two pathways, the classical and alternative pathways, that lead to cell lysis and the liberation of biologically active molecules. Both these systems are characterized by a cascade of enzymatic events in which one molecule becomes activated and in turn activates another. The classical pathway is initiated by the binding of the first component in the pathway to the Fc portion of an antibody–antigen complex. The alternative pathway is activated in the absence of antigen–antibody complexes by molecules on invading organisms. The two converge at the point where they generate two molecules called C3 convertase and C5 convertase. These molecules initiate the membrane attack complex on the surface of a cell that leads to the lysis of the cell.

CHAPTER

8

The complement system is a beautifully balanced and complex series of interactions that is of great importance in immunity and is a good example of the interaction of specific and nonspecific factors in immunity. Products of the cascade also act as opsonins and chemotactic factors in immunity.

Discovery of the Complement System

The realization that in addition to antibodies there is some component in antiserum that is important in immune reactions came about at the end of the nineteenth century (which is known as the Golden Era of microbiology). The initial observation was made in 1893 by Buchner, who noted that antisera that could kill bacteria lost their lytic activity when heated to 56°C. Jules Bordet followed this observation with the discovery in 1895 that the heat-labile substance was not antibody. He did this by showing that the lytic activity of a heat-inactivated anti-cholera antiserum could be restored by the addition of unheated *normal* serum. Bordet correctly concluded that antibodies are heat-stabile but that this other serum substance, which he called alexin, is heat-labile. (Ehrlich later renamed alexin COMPLEMENT.) Bordet also introduced the erythrocyte–anti-erythrocyte system as the experimental lytic system, a technical advance that significantly enhanced the study of complement. In 1919 Bordet received the Nobel prize for his work on complement.

The realization that complement is more than one substance came about over the next few decades. First it was found in 1907 that when fresh serum, which is used as a source of lytic complement, was dialyzed against water, a precipitate formed. Neither the precipitate (after being redissolved in saline) nor the dialysis fluid had complement activity (that is, neither solution could restore lytic activity to a heat-inactivated serum). But when the two fractions were mixed together, activity was restored. This finding showed that complement has at least two components.

The two components then were shown to act sequentially. When erythrocytes were first reacted with heat-inactivated anti-erythrocyte antiserum (so that the antibody would coat the red cells), the factor in the supernatant fluid was able to react only when the factor in the precipitate had reacted first. This finding showed that the reaction was sequential: antibody reacted with the antigen (forming what we now know to be an antigen–antibody complex), followed by the component in the precipitate, followed by the component in the supernatant fluid. Logically, the particulate factor (in the precipitate) was called "midpiece," and the soluble factor (in the supernatant fluid) was called "endpiece." Both midpiece and endpiece were heat-labile, so it seemed safe to conclude that—to use language that was appropriate at the time—"the heat-labile lytic factor in serum had two components, midpiece and endpiece." Midpiece was later renamed C1, and endpiece was renamed C2 (and we will now start using the modern terminology.)

The realization that things were more complicated than this came a few years later with the discovery that cobra venom destroyed the lytic activity of complement. The activity could be restored by addition of fresh normal serum (which was not surprising), but it could also be restored by addition of *heat-inactivated* normal serum. Because it was already known that C1 and C2 are heat-labile, this result meant that the cobra venom-labile but heat-stabile substance was another complement component; it was named C3. But now the easily visualized picture of midpiece–endpiece–lysis was replaced by a more complicated picture. Where did C3 fit into the reaction scheme? And, to paraphrase a song of the time, "Are there any more [components] at home like you?"

The answer to the question in the song was yes. It was noted that, believe it or not, when serum was mixed with yeast cells, the C3 was removed but *another* heat-stabile component remained. This component was named C4, and it was found to be inactivated by treatment with ammonia. It could be shown that the components react with the antigen–antibody (Ag–Ab) complex in the sequence C1, C4, C2, C3.

The situation remained like this until the late 1950s. At that time the modern era of complementology begins, as techniques of protein chemistry had advanced to the point where they could be applied to this obviously complex and important problem. The reader should once again be aware that although the advances in the modern era were possible because of advances in other areas, if the question had not been asked in terms of immunology up to that point, there would have been no problem on which to apply the new methodology.

As we progress through this chapter we will see that there are two pathways leading to lysis. One is called the classical pathway, and the second is called the alternative pathway. The pathways converge at the C3 step (Figure 1), and it would be wise for the

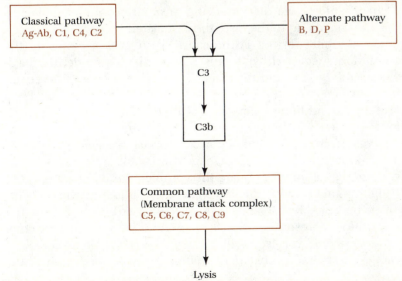

1   Overview of the Complement Events Leading to Lysis. The classical and alternative pathways converge at the C3 → C3b step and lead into the common pathway, which ends with lysis.

reader to keep this point in mind while reading about the events in the complement cascade.

The Classical Pathway

The Need For Multivalency to Activate Complement

The classical complement pathway begins when the first component of complement (C1) binds to the Ag–Ab complex. The pathway is obviously not triggered by the association of C1 with unreacted IgG, which is in high concentration in the serum. We will see below that the first complement component to react with IgG is a subcomponent of C1 called C1q. C1q has the form of a "bouquet of tulips" (see Figure 2) with six "stems." Each of these stems can react with the C_H2 domain of IgG and the C_H3 (and possibly C_H4) of IgM. It is this multivalency of C1q that is the key to why only Ig in an Ag–Ab complex or in aggregated form can initiate the cascade. Binding of C1q to monomeric Ig is very weak (a binding constant of $\sim 10^4\ M^{-1}$). In contrast, the binding to "associated" Ig (in the complex) is strong ($K_a \sim 10^8 M^{-1}$) and allows the activation process to proceed.[1] This mechanism is in sharp contrast to the older idea that the binding of antigen to antibody in the Fab portion caused a steric change in the Fc portion of the antibody that allowed C1q to bind.

In Chapter 7 we discussed the flexibility of the Ig molecule. The binding of C1q to the Fc of the associated Ig may be enhanced by the flexibility of the Fc domain. Figure 3 is a model of the interaction suggested by Dennis Burton. In this model the flexibility of the IgG around the hinge region allows Fc–Fc interaction that can occur by the change of the plane in which the Fc is located. The additional flexibility of the C1q molecule gives additional efficiency to the interaction. Thus, the binding of Ig to a multivalent antigen (optimally a cell-surface antigen) places two monomeric Igs in close enough proximity that C1q can interact with enough affinity to initiate the complement cascade.

IgM is much more efficient than IgG in initiating the cascade. This is because the molecule is a pentamer and provides a higher probability of presenting two sites for C1q binding. To achieve that higher probability, it is postulated that the molecule undergoes a change in spatial arrangement that allows easier reaction of the

---

[1]This is the first time that we are discussing equilibrium constants. For more details, the interested reader should refer to Chapter 10.

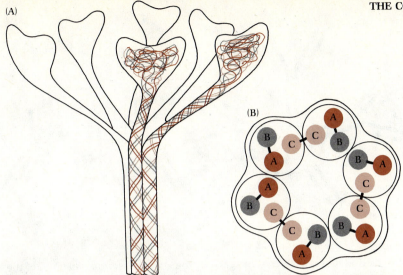

2   Structure of the C1q Component of Human Complement. (A) The molecule consists of 18 chains and has a "bouquet of tulips" appearance. (B) Cross section through the "stalk" showing the six "stems" composed of A, B, and C peptides. The A and B chains in each stem are connected to each other by disulfide bonds. The C chain of one stem is connected to the C chain of another stem by disulfide bonds.

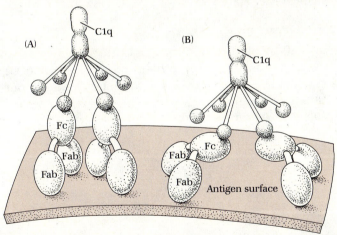

3   Possible Association of C1q with IgG. The figure shows two possible modes of interaction of C1q with two molecules of IgG on a cell surface. (A) Standard diagram. (B) View showing the flexibility of the Fc domains allowing easier contact of the C1q to the associated IgG, thus raising the binding constant of the C1q–IgG complex to allow the activation of the complement cascade. [After Burton, 1987. In Calabi and Neuberger, eds., *Molecular Genetics of Immunoglobulin*]

(A) Star

(B) Staple

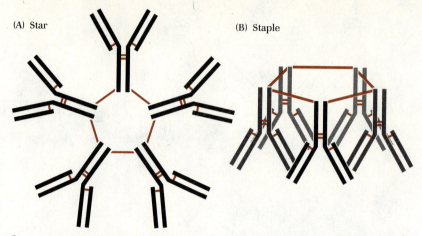

4 Two Structural Forms of IgM. (A) The standard *starlike* diagram of the pentameric IgM molecule. (B) The molecule with the (Fab)₂ arms rotated 90° about the twofold axis of symmetry, giving the associated IgM a *staplelike* quality. [Redrawn from Burton, 1987. In Calabi and Neuberger, eds., *Molecular Genetics of Immunoglobulin*]

Cμ3 or Cμ4 domain with C1q. The postulated change from the "star" form to the "staple" form of IgM is seen in Figure 4.

The Recognition Unit

The result of the binding of C1q to Ig is the formation of activated C1. C1 is a complex of three protein molecules called C1q, C1r, and C1s. Of these three proteins, C1q binds to the Fc portion of the antibody molecule.

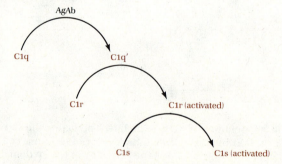

C1q is composed of six sets of peptide chains, each set having three members, so that the whole molecule is composed of 18 chains. The three types of chains, called A, B, and C, associate to form the tulip structure seen in Figure 2. The other two molecules of C1 (C1r and C1s) become altered after C1q combines with Fc. It has been postulated that the reaction of C1q with Fc causes a conformational change that distorts one of the C1r chains. This distortion exposes an enzymatic site on C1r, which in turn causes the cleavage of the second chain. The now-activated C1r then cleaves the C1s chain, thereby generating two active fragments. This sequence is diagrammed in Figure 5. As a result of this reaction, the next components in the cascade, C4 and C2, can become activated.

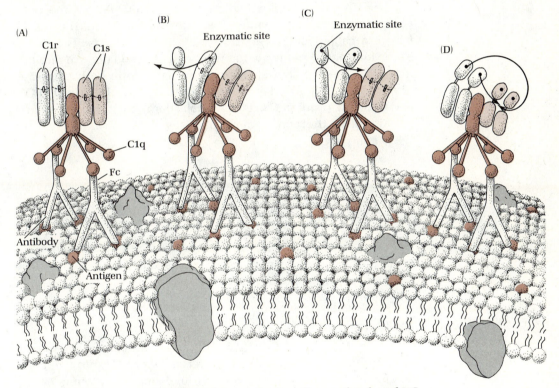

5   Recognition Unit of the Complement System. Two molecules of IgG are shown bound to the surface of a cell. (A) The C1q component of complement binds to the Fc portion of the Igs. This is the first step in the activation of the other C1 components. (B) Fc binding causes a change in the configuration of C1q, which then distorts one of the two polypeptide chains of C1r. This distortion exposes an enzymatic site on one of the C1r chains and leads to cleavage of the other chain. (C) The cleavage of the C1r chain opens an enzymatic site on the other C1r chain and cleavage of the second C1r chain occurs. (D) The activated C1r cleaves the C1s chains, thereby generating two activated fragments.

The Activation Unit: C4 and C2

The first set of reactions generates activated C1s, which acts as the enzyme to catalyze the next reaction in the cascade:

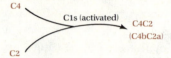

C1s cleaves low-molecular-weight peptides from C4 and C2 and exposes their active forms, C4b and C2a, which then fuse. These reactions are depicted in Figure 6.

The C4bC2a complex (which we will abbreviate as the C4C2 complex) acts as an enzyme whose substrate is C3. For this reason it is also called C3 CONVERTASE. Another C3 convertase is involved in the alternative pathway that will be discussed later. We mention it now to emphasize that this is a crucial step in both pathways. The enzyme C3 convertase splits C3 into two products, called C3a and C3b. The product C3b is the crucial component in the cascade, remaining in the complement pathway by associating with the C4C2 complex.

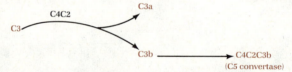

This is diagrammed in Figure 6C and 6D. The C4C2C3b complex is an enzyme that reacts with the next component, C5, in the common pathway (Figure 7). For this reason, the complex is called a C5 CONVERTASE.

The Crucial Role of C3

C3 is the major constituent of the complement system (serum concentration of 1 mg/ml). C3 convertase splits C3 into two components, C3a and C3b. This is the pivotal step in the complement activation cascade. The uncleaved C3 molecule consists of two chains. The α chain contains a thioester bond that becomes unstable after cleavage of C3 into C3a and C3b. The unstable C3b is called C3b* and is highly reactive. Most of the C3b* molecules react with water, but a few react with hydroxyl and amine groups of proteins and carbohydrates, forming covalent bonds at the cell surface (Figure 6C). Some of these are adjacent to the C4C2 complex, and the result is a C4C2C3b complex.

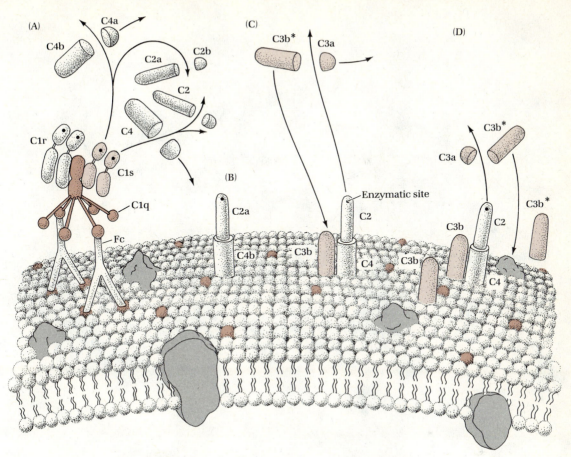

6 Assembly of the Activation Unit. (A) Activated C1s attacks C4 and then C2, cleaving a small activation peptide from each. (B) Formation of a bimolecular C4C2 complex occurs, and the complex attaches itself to the cell surface. This complex is known as C3 convertase (see next panel). (C) The C4C2 complex acts on C3 in the serum, splitting off C3b, which forms a trimolecular complex C4C2C3b on the cell surface. (D) The C4C2 complex continues to act on serum C3, and many C3b molecules accumulate on the cell surface.

At this point the classical and alternative pathways converge to form the MEMBRANE ATTACK COMPLEX, which leads to the actual lysis of the cell. We will pick up the narrative at the membrane attack unit after we examine the events in the alternative pathway that lead to the generation of C3b in a form that is also a C5 convertase.

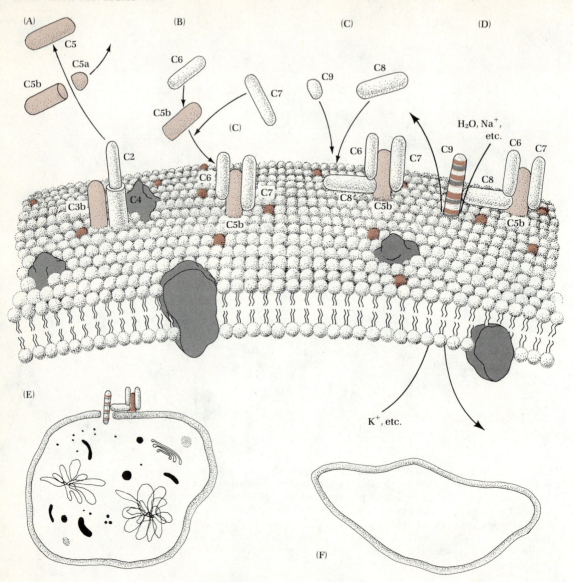

7 **C4C3C3b Complex as C5 Convertase.** (A) The C4C2C3b complex cleaves C5 in serum to C5a and C5b. (B) C5b, C6, and C7 combine and form a complex on the cell surface. (C) C8 combines with C5bC6C7, and C9 binds to the membrane. (D) C9 is polymerized by the C5b–C8 complex, and the larger complex attaches to the membrane. (E) The polyC9 opens a transmembrane channel that allows potassium ions to leave the cell and allows water and sodium to enter. The cell swells, thereby allowing the intracellular contents to leave. (F) Only an empty sac remains.

The Alternative Pathway

We saw above that the cleavage of C3 to C3b can be initiated by the interaction of Ag–Ab complexes with components of the classical complement pathway. As we will see, this process ultimately results in cell lysis. When the cells are infectious microorganisms, this is obviously an effector mechanism by which antibody destroys invaders. However, another complement pathway can be activated by some microbes, such that this effector mechanism functions in the absence of antibody. The steps in the process following the action of C3 convertase are identical in this ALTERNATIVE COMPLEMENT PATHWAY and in the classical pathway, as we will discuss. It is the formation of the C3 convertase that distinguishes the two pathways. Thus, the complement system can be utilized in antibody-dependent and independent ways to rid the body of pathogens.

The alternative pathway is associated with one of the tragic aspects of the scientific life. In the early 1950s Louis Pillemer, working at Western Reserve University in Cleveland, published papers in which he claimed to have discovered another complement pathway. This pathway did not need Ag–Ab complexes to be activated; instead it was activated by sugar moieties in yeast and bacterial cell walls. Pillemer argued that a substance in serum, which he called PROPERDIN, or P, is able to activate C3. This idea met with criticism and acrimonious debate. Pillemer was an unusual man with a history of academic brilliance and emotional problems and was apparently unable to withstand the pressures of this heated controversy. He took his own life a few years before his basic ideas were shown to be correct.[2]

The crucial points to be remembered about the alternative pathway are that the initiation can occur in the fluid phase rather than on a cell surface, that it does not require the presence of the Ag–Ab complex, and that it is an effective alternative method for producing C3b from C3.

Activation of the Alternative Pathway

The function of the activation unit in the classical pathway is to generate C3b. The C3b combines with the C4C2 complex to form the C4C2C3b complex, which connects to the membrane attack unit, a component common to both the classical and alternative

---

[2]The history of properdin and the controversy are covered in a brilliant essay by W. D. Ratnoff in *Perspectives in Biology and Medicine*, Summer 1980, p. 638. The essay was taken from Dr. Ratnoff's B.A. thesis at Harvard.

pathways. The alternative pathway generates C3b without the benefit of the Ag–Ab complex or the C1 recognition unit.

C3b is generated in the alternative pathway when C3 reacts with a serum component called FACTOR B, a reaction that produces a C3.B complex. The C3.B complex then reacts with FACTOR D, resulting in the cleavage of B to form C3Bb (and inactive Ba). Fluid-phase C3Bb acts as a C3 convertase to catalyze C3 to C3b*. The C3b* becomes bound to a cell surface where it can bind more Factor B. This cell surface C3bB now initiates a reaction called the AMPLIFICATION LOOP. Factor D acts on C3bB to form C3bBb, which then catalyzes the further conversion of C3 to C3b*.[3]

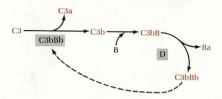

The formation of C3b apparently also occurs spontaneously in serum, but the C3b is inactivated as soon as it is formed by a C3b inactivator now called Factor I. In the presence of Factor I and another molecule called Factor H, the normal, very low serum level of C3b is maintained. This mode of C3b generation is called C3 TICKOVER.

Stabilization of the C3bBb Complex

The C3bBb complex is unstable unless it reacts with properdin to form a C3bPBb complex. Pillemer assumed that properdin was the *initiating* factor, but we now know that it is a *stabilizing* factor. (Most scientists would give a year's wages to be this close to being correct on a major discovery.)

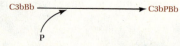

When a second C3b molecule is added to the C3bPBb complex, a conformational change occurs that makes the complex into a C5 convertase. At this step the alternative and classical pathways converge. (The reader can skip ahead to Figure 8 to see this convergence diagrammatically.)

[3]Molecules shown in boxes act as catalysts for this reaction.

SYNTHESIS
Why Two Complement Pathways?

The fact that the alternative pathway of complement can be directly activated by molecules on many types of invading organisms, including bacteria, fungi, and protozoans, leads one to speculate that rather than being the "alternative" pathway, this was the first complement-mediated defense mechanism to appear in evolution. So the reader might ask: "Why the *classical* pathway? One line of speculation has it that the binding of antibody to a foreign antigen is useful to host defense, but the system is faced with the problem of removing these complexes. The initial components of the classical pathway may have originally evolved to facilitate the clearance of Ag–Ab complexes from the system. When the results of an antigen–antibody interaction (i.e., the antigen–antibody complex) are coupled to the generation of C3 and C5 convertases, the specificity of the antigen–antibody interaction is now merged with the destructive power of the complement pathway. The immune system now has the capability of destroying parasites that might not ordinarily activate the complement pathway and can adapt to changes in those parasites by producing antibody of new specificity. This theme of joining specific immune mechanisms to nonspecific host defenses is one we will return to in Chapter 32.

The Common Complement Pathway

The Membrane Attack Complex: C5b, C6, C7, C8, C9

We saw earlier how a C5 convertase is generated in both the classical and alternative pathways. Both these C5 convertases can react with C5 to generate C5a and C5b. *C5b* forms a tetramolecular complex with C6, C7, and C8; this complex (C5b678) is attached to the target cell membrane (Figure 7).

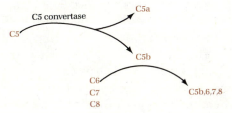

The C5b678 complex catalyzes the polymerization of approximately 16 molecules of C9 to form a 160 Å × 100 Å tube with a hydrophobic end that binds to lipids in the membrane. The polymerized C9 with the C5b678 complex is called the MEMBRANE ATTACK COMPLEX (MAC).[4] Manfred Mayer postulated a transmembrane channel that is active in lysis, and the MAC is probably the major component of this channel.

Figure 8 summarizes the classical, alternative, and common pathways.

The Role of Complement Components in Inflammation

One of the evolutionary "purposes" of the immune response is to defend the body from invading organisms, and specific antibody is the mechanism we have focused on so far. We will see later (Chapter 32) that INFLAMMATION, like phagocytosis, is a phylogenetically much older defense mechanism in which there is increased vascular permeability and release of mediators. Complement components play a role in both inflammation and phagocytosis.

In all the above discussion we have been dealing with the role of complement in lysis. Recall that in both the classical and alternative pathways both C3a and C3b are generated but that only C3b is used (C5 convertase). Similarly, in the common pathway, both C5a and C5b are generated but only C5b is used. For those readers who were wondering what happened to the C3a and C5a, the answer is that they play important roles in inflammation. Mast cells and basophils have receptors for both C3a and C5a. The reaction of these fragments with their receptors can cause degranulation of the cells with the release of histamine and other mediators of anaphylaxis (see Chapter 34). There are probably separate receptors for C3a and C5a, and C5a can cause a histamine-independent increase in vascular permeability of endothelial cells. These two biologically active split products of complement are called ANAPHYLOTOXINS.

Neutrophils have receptors for C5a. The reaction of C5a with these receptors induces CHEMOTAXIS (the directed migration of cells toward the region in which the complement cascade is occurring). In addition, bound C3 and C4 components act as OPSONINS, that is, agents that enhance phagocytosis (see Chapter 7). This is because phagocytes have receptors for complement products (e.g., C3b receptors) and can use these in much the same way as FcR (see Chapter 7).

[4]Many of our students call this the Big Mac Attack, for reasons that remain obscure to us.

Classical pathway

Ag + Ab ⟶ Ag-Ab

C1q → C1q′

C1r → C1r (activated)

C1s → C1s (activated)

C4 + C2 → C4C2

C3 → C3b + C3a

C4C2C3b

Alternate pathway

C3b + B → C3bB

C3b + C3a

$\overline{\text{C3bB}}$ ← D

C5 convertase

C5 → $\overline{\text{C5}}$

Common pathway

C6 → $\overline{\text{C56}}$

C7 → $\overline{\text{C567}}$

C8 → $\overline{\text{C5678}}$

C9 → $\overline{\text{C56789}}$

Lysis

8 **The Complement Cascade.** [Based on Mayer et al., 1981. *Crit. Rev. Immunol.* 2:33]

Summary

1. There are two complement pathways, classical and alternative. Both involve a cascade of enzymatic reactions leading to the production of a lytic complex and several biologically active molecules.

2. The classical complement pathway is initiated by antigen–antibody complexes (involving IgM or IgG) interacting with complement component C1. This leads (via C4 and C2) to the generation of a C3 convertase that acts upon C3 to generate C3a and C3b.

3. The alternative pathway is induced by carbohydrate structures on many bacteria, fungi, and protozoans. Through interaction with C3 and components B, D, and P, a C3 convertase is generated (which differs from that of the classical pathway).

4. The C3 convertase of either pathway acts on C3 to generate a C5 convertase. The action of this enzyme is to cleave C5 into C5a and C5b. At this point the two pathways converge.

5. The cleavage of C5 into C5a and C5b triggers a cascade (via C6–C9) to form the membrane attack complex (MAC). This complex produces a pore in the membrane of the invading organism, leading to lysis.

6. Many of the fragments produced during the cascade have other important functions. C3a and C5a act on mast cells, causing release of active mediators (e.g., which increase vascular permeability). C5a also induces chemotaxis in neutrophils. C3b and C4, bound to cell surfaces, act as opsonins by interacting with specific receptors on phagocytes.

Additional Readings

Burton, D. R. 1987. Structure and function of antibodies. In F. Calabi and M. S. Neuberger, eds. *Molecular Genetics of Immunoglobulin.* Elsevier, New York.

Goldstein, I. M. 1988. Complement: Biologically active products. In I. M. Goldstein and R. Snyderman, eds. *Inflammation: Basic Principles and Clinical Correlates*. Raven, New York, p. 55.

Hugli, T. E. 1986. Biochemistry and biology of anaphylatoxins. *Complement* 3: 111.

Müller-Eberhard, H. J. 1983. Chemistry and function of the complement system. In F. J. Dixon and D. W. Fisher, eds. *The Biology of Immunologic Disease*. Sinauer, Sunderland, Mass., p. 128.

Müller-Eberhard, H. J. and R. D. Schreiber. 1980. Molecular biology and chemistry of the alternate pathway of complement. *Adv. Immunol.* 29: 1.

Reid, K. B. M. 1988. The complement system. In B. D. Hames and D. M. Glover. *Molecular Immunology*. IRL, Oxford, p. 189.

ANTIGEN—ANTIBODY REACTIONS

Acta exteriora indicant interiora sereta.
Outward actions show inward intent.

Legal maxim

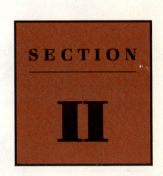

SECTION

II

In the three chapters in this section we will look at some of the uses of antibodies and how one measures the interaction of antigen and antibody. These chapters will differ slightly from the rest of the book because, for the most part, they do not follow the logical flow of ideas through experiments, but will be examining facts in a rather traditional way. The chapters on using antibodies as tools and the one on methods are of great practical importance and will probably be returned to often at later times.

ANTIBODIES AS TOOLS

Overview So far we have seen in some detail the structure and genetic organization of antibodies as well as some of their effector functions. This chapter is a brief look at some of the uses of antibodies. We will discuss the very important topic of the production of monoclonal antibodies and then show their potential use in immunosuppression, in imaging of tumors and infections, and as catalytic agents. Monoclonal antibodies are made in mice or rats, so it is obvious that for the principle of monoclonal antibodies to be used in human therapy, human molecules must be used. We will discuss the recent progress that has been made in generating both "humanized" and human antibody molecules.

Monoclonal Antibodies

Monoclonal and Polyclonal Antibodies

We learned from clonal selection (Chapter 1) that the repertoire of immune responses is distributed clonally among the lymphocytes. In other words, a given B cell is preprogrammed to respond to a single antigenic determinant. We will see in Part Two that the reaction of antigen with a cell-surface receptor on a lymphocyte leads to proliferation and clonal expansion that results in a large number of cells producing antibodies of the same specificity. But, as we saw in Chapter 2, most immunogens have multiple antigenic determinants (epitopes) and therefore induce the expansion of several clones of antigen-reactive cells (one clone for each determinant). The response of the individual to the whole antigen is therefore POLYCLONAL, but the response of each B cell is MONOCLONAL. A "conventional" antiserum (one raised by injecting antigen into an individual or immunizing cells in vitro) therefore almost always has antibodies directed against many determinants on the antigen molecule. In other words, conventional antisera are both multi-specific and polyclonal.

Immunologists have spent countless hours attempting to make multispecific antisera monospecific by *adsorbing* out as many of the unwanted specificities as possible. This is done by adding to the antiserum all the antigens except the one to which antibody is desired; the idea being that each antigenic determinant reacts with the specific antibody and forms an antigen–antibody complex. These complexes can then be removed, in theory leaving a monospecific antiserum (i.e., with antibody to only one determinant). The reader can imagine that this ideal situation was almost never achieved, even after exhaustive attempts to adsorb out all the unwanted specificities.

But if we could isolate antibodies from a single cell, we would have antibodies of only one specificity. We would have, in other words, MONOCLONAL ANTIBODIES. Unfortunately, even if there were a means available for selecting out those few cells producing the antibody to the desired determinant, no tissue culture methods exist for the long-term cultivation of normal antibody-producing cells.

This technical problem seemed insurmountable until Georges Köhler and Cesar Milstein in 1975 introduced a method for generating antibodies that are known to be monospecific because they are monoclonal. This monoclonal methodology has revolutionized the uses of antibody in all biology and medicine, and in 1984 Köhler and Milstein were awarded the Nobel prize for their work. The prize was shared with Niels Jerne, who introduced the concept of clonality of the immune response—the theoretical foundation upon which the method is based. Again we see a case in which the question was formulated in terms of immunology but the solution required methodological advances.

The Principle of Monoclonal Antibody Production

The principle of monoclonal antibody production is elegant. By applying it we can capture the specific synthesis of a single antibody-forming cell and "immortalize" it in tissue culture. Whereas normal antibody-forming cells cannot be grown and perpetuated in culture, tumors of the antibody-forming system, called MYELOMAS (Chapter 3), can be grown indefinitely in culture. In the jargon, they are "immortal." What is needed, then, is a method for bringing together in one cell the separate abilities to synthesize a specific antibody and to grow forever in culture. Köhler and Milstein achieved this by fusing an antibody-forming cell with a myeloma cell. The resulting hybrid cell is called a HYBRIDOMA. The problem of *selecting* the antibody-forming cell of the desired specificity is solved by fusing large numbers of antibody-forming cells and myeloma cells and then examining (or selecting) the resulting hybridomas for those that are synthesizing the antibody of the desired specificity.

Cell Fusion

The principle of generating monoclonal antibodies is seen in Figure 1. Monoclonal antibodies are achieved by fusing an antibody-forming cell (usually a spleen cell) with a myeloma cell (myelomas

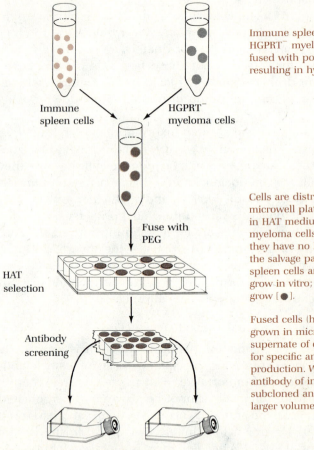

Immune spleen cells and HGPRT⁻ myeloma cells are fused with polyethylene glycol resulting in hybrid cells.

Immune spleen cells

HGPRT⁻ myeloma cells

Fuse with PEG

HAT selection

Cells are distributed in microwell plates and grown in HAT medium. Unfused myeloma cells die because they have no HGPRT to use the salvage pathway. Unfused spleen cells are unable to grow in vitro; only fused cells grow [●].

Antibody screening

Fused cells (hybridomas) grown in microwells and supernate of each well tested for specific antibody production. Wells making antibody of interest are subcloned and grown in larger volumes.

Subcloning

1   Production of Monoclonal Antibodies. Cells from an immunized mouse are fused with myeloma cells and undergo HAT selection. The fused cells, called hybridomas, are then screened for their ability to react to the antigen of interest. The clones of interest are then subcloned and expanded.

are tumors of B cells) in the presence of one of a variety of fusing agents; polyethylene glycol (PEG) is the most commonly used agent. This results in the hybridoma mentioned above. The problem of separating the fused hybridoma cells from the normal spleen cell population is easily solved because the spleen cells die off in culture after a short period of time. But both the unfused myeloma cells and the hybridoma cells are immortal, so a method is needed to get rid of the unfused myeloma cells. This is achieved by using myeloma cells that are killed in the presence of the drug aminopterin.

Myeloma cells, like most cells, use two pathways of nucleotide synthesis: the major synthetic pathway and a salvage pathway (Figure 2). Normal cells synthesize nucleotides using both pathways. When the drug 8-AZAGUANINE is added to normal cells, it is incorporated into DNA through a reaction catalyzed by the enzyme HYPOXANTHINE GUANINE PHOSPHORIBOSYL TRANSFERASE (HGPRT) via the salvage pathway. Such cells die because they cannot function with the altered base. A variant cell that cannot carry out the salvage pathway because it lacks HGPRT would be 8AzG RESISTANT and would therefore not be killed by the drug. Such HGPRT⁻ mutants can therefore be selected with this drug and are the myeloma cells used for fusion.[1]

---

[1] The best fusion partners are HGPRT⁻ cells that have also lost the ability to produce either the H or the L chain of Ig. These are called *nonsecretors*.

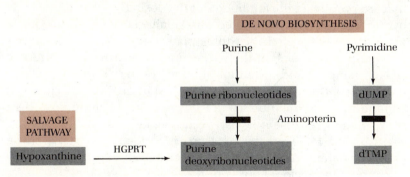

$$\text{DE NOVO BIOSYNTHESIS}$$

Purine   Pyrimidine

Purine ribonucleotides   dUMP

Aminopterin

SALVAGE PATHWAY

Hypoxanthine →HGPRT→ Purine deoxyribonucleotides   dTMP

2   Aminopterin Works by Blocking the Reduction of Dihydrofolate to Tetrahydrofolate. In pyrimidine biosynthesis $CoFH_4$ is oxidized to FH_2, thus using up FH_4. In purine biosynthesis $CoFH_4$ is converted to FH_4 nonenzymatically so that FH_4 can be reconstituted to $CoFH_4$. Aminopterin blocks the conversion of FH_2 to FH_4 so that no more FH_4 can be generated. As soon as it has depleted the existing FH_4, the cell can no longer function. As a consequence of the pyrimidine pathway now using up all of the FH_4, the purine pathway also stops; however, the cell still carries out DNA synthesis via the salvage pathway.

The drug AMINOPTERIN acts on the major synthetic pathway by interfering with the conversion of dihydrofolate to tetrahydrofolate and preventing a series of one-carbon transfers. Thus in the presence of aminopterin the cell cannot synthesize nucleotides via the main synthetic pathway and so must use the salvage pathway. A normal cell can still grow in the presence of aminopterin, but a HGPRT⁻ cell cannot, because HGPRT⁻ mutants cannot carry out the salvage pathway; HGPRT⁻ cells are therefore killed in the presence of aminopterin.

When HGPRT⁻ myeloma cells are fused with normal B cells, the resulting hybridomas are able to grow in the presence of aminopterin because the normal cell contributes functional HGPRT. When hypoxanthine and thymidine, which are the precursor molecules used by the enzyme HGPRT in the salvage pathway, are added to the medium, the hybridoma is able to use the alternate pathway to synthesize DNA. The unfused normal spleen cells die because they are unable to grow for long periods of time in tissue culture, and the unfused myeloma cells are killed by the aminopterin. Thus only the fused hybridomas are able to grow. This process is called HAT SELECTION (*h*ypoxanthine, *a*minopterin, *t*hymidine selection; Box 1).

Screening the Hybridomas

We still need a means of identifying and isolating those hybridomas that are producing the antibodies of the desired specificities. Single hybridoma cells are distributed into small wells in a tissue culture plate (these are called microtiter plates) and grown. The supernatant fluid over each of the wells containing growing hybridoma cells is sampled and tested for antibody of the desired specificity using any of the methods to be described in Chapter 11. The most commonly used method is the enzyme-linked immunosorbent assay (ELISA) because it is fast, accurate, and reasonably sensitive (see Chapter 11). The screening process requires a source of the antigenic determinant because one must be sure that the antibody is not only monoclonal but is of the desired specificity.[2]

Wells that contain cells producing antibody of the desired specificity are cloned, that is, grown out as single cells so that one is sure that all the cells to be used have the same origin. In this

---

[2] These facts are often overlooked by investigators who want to use monoclonal antibodies. In fact, the reason for failure to be able to use the technology is almost always because no reasonable screening procedure is available. Most investigators find that with some effort this problem can be overcome.

Principle of HAT Selection

BOX 1

1. When the main synthetic pathways are blocked by the folic acid analog AMINOPTERIN, the cell must use the salvage pathway. This pathway contains the enzyme HGPRT.

2. HGPRT$^-$ myeloma cells can be selected because they can grow in the presence of 8-azaguanine. HGPRT$^+$ cells incorporate 8-azaguanine into DNA. HGPRT$^-$ cells do not incorporate the toxic molecule. Thus, HGPRT$^-$ cells can grow in its presence.

3. HGPRT$^-$ cells die in the present of HAT (HYPOXANTHINE, AMINOPTERIN, THYMIDINE) because both the main pathway and the salvage pathway are blocked.

4. Fusion of the HGPRT$^-$ myeloma cells with HGPRT$^+$ spleen cells allows growth in HAT by providing the missing enzyme for the salvage pathway.

way the investigator is sure that there are cells of only one specificity present. The monoclonal antibody production method enables researchers to produce large amounts of antibody that is monospecific because it is monoclonal. It also opens up a whole new world of biological manipulation of the genes for antibody production.

SYNTHESIS
The Specificity of Monoclonal Antibodies

A common misconception is that because monoclonal antibodies by definition react with a single antigenic determinant, they are necessarily specific. As we pointed out in Chapter 2, the same or a similar epitope can appear in many places, leading to cross reactivity of antibodies directed against the epitope. Monoclonal antibodies are not an exception to this rule, and in fact a single monoclonal antibody may display unexpected cross reactivity. The problem is not with the monoclonal antibody, but rather that the antigenic determinant appears in more than one place. The advantage of monoclonals is that once a specificity is established, we can trust that it will not change.

The Uses of Monoclonal Antibodies

Monoclonal antibodies have been a great technological advance in experimental immunology. We will see in the chapters on cellular immunology that much of our understanding about cell interactions comes from studying the molecules at the cell surface, and the best tools for this have been antibodies. The exquisite specificity of monoclonal antibodies has allowed us to make great strides in this area of research. But monoclonal antibodies have also begun to have other uses as well. We will discuss only a few of the emerging areas of their utility.

Monoclonal Antibodies as Immunosuppressive Agents

The first (and so far only) monoclonal antibody to be approved for use in humans was developed by Patrick Kung and Gideon Goldstein in 1981. This antibody, called OKT3, is directed against an epitope on one of the chains of the CD3 molecule associated with the T-cell receptor and is found on virtually all T cells (discussed in Part Two). It has been possible to prevent rejection of kidney grafts by the injection of OKT3 because T cells are responsible for graft rejection. OKT3 reacts with the cells in vivo and prevents them from functioning. It is not clear if the antibody kills the cells, alters their homing pattern, or causes some kind of cellular anergy (loss of function) by some unknown mechanism. Monoclonal antibodies to other T-cell markers, particulary CD4 and CD8, are potentially very useful because they react with subsets of T cells (helper and effector, see Chapter 16). Because CD3 is present on all T cells, the use of OKT3 causes a general immunosuppression by eliminating the function of all T cells. Since CD4 and CD8 are on the helper and effector functional subsets, their elimination may have a more limited effect on the immune system.

One problem with monoclonal antibodies as they are now produced for use in humans is that they are made in mouse systems. The monoclonal antibodies described above therefore are mouse Igs that react with antigens on human T cells. Not surprisingly, mouse Igs are immunogenic for the humans into whom they are injected. Anti-isotype and anti-idiotype antibodies can be made by the treated patients, and this can reduce the usefulness of the antibodies if they have to be injected repeatedly because the anti-monoclonal antibody in the patient's serum is neutralizing the injected monoclonal antibody before it can react with the T cells. There is also the problem of developing allergies to the mouse Igs.

The production of human monoclonal antibodies may get around some of these problems.

Imaging

Another emerging use of monoclonal antibodies is in imaging. If a radioactive or radio-opaque label can be put on a monoclonal antibody, it should be possible to follow its location and distribution in the body after injection. If the specificity of the antibody is for a tumor or some other structure that the clinician is interested in, the great specificity of the monoclonal antibody can be used to find small pockets of the structure. The problem here is to find monoclonal antibodies specific for the tissue or structure that do not cross-react with other tissues. This is not a problem that monoclonal antibody technology can readily solve since the presence of similar antigens on different tissues is a reality that confronts the investigator.

Immunotoxins

At the turn of the century Paul Ehrlich had the dream of devising drugs with such great specificity that they would be "magic bullets." His dream of chemical drugs as magic bullets has not come to pass, but antibodies offer the means of delivering a drug to a specific site in the body. One of the first uses of the monoclonal antibody as a specific delivery system has been with IMMUNOTOXINS.

There are toxins produced by plants that inhibit protein synthesis in any cell that they can get into. These toxins have evolved as disulfide-bonded heterodimers. One chain, called the B chain, is usually a galactose-specific lectin, and the other chain, called the A chain, is the toxin but is inactive in the complexed form. If a cell has a receptor for the B chain, the A–B dimer binds to the cell and is internalized. Once the dimer is inside the cell, the disulfide bond is cleaved and the inactive A chain becomes active. The A chain of RICIN, one of the more commonly used toxins in immunotoxin technology, is an enzyme that inactivates the 60 S ribosomal subunit of eukaryotic cells by modifying one or two nucleoside residues of the 28 S ribosomal RNA. When the toxin A chain is covalently complexed to an antibody directed against a cell-surface antigen, the A chain can be delivered to a specific cell. The antibody acts in place of the sugar-specific B chain. The antibody–toxin dimer is internalized and the disulfide bond cleaved, freeing the toxin to kill the cell. The principle is diagrammed in Figure 3.

(A) Toxin

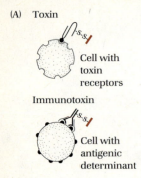

Cell with toxin receptors

Immunotoxin

Cell with antigenic determinant

(B)

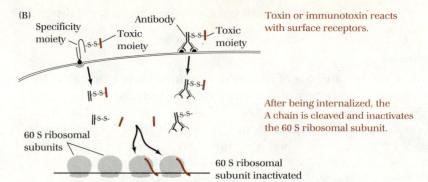

Specificity moiety

Toxic moiety

Antibody

Toxic moiety

60 S ribosomal subunits

60 S ribosomal subunit inactivated

Toxin or immunotoxin reacts with surface receptors.

After being internalized, the A chain is cleaved and inactivates the 60 S ribosomal subunit.

3   The Principle of Immunotoxins. (A) Some toxins consist of a toxic moiety, the A chain, and a specificity moiety, the B chain. The A chain is inactive while it is disulfide-bonded to the B chain. Interaction with a cell occurs through the B chain's reaction with cell-surface receptors (usually a galactose-containing molecule). In an immunotoxin, the A chain is linked to an Ig via a disulfide bond. The specific reaction at the cell surface is through the antigen-binding site of the antibody. (B) When the molecule is internalized, the disulfide bond is broken and the A chain exerts its toxic action by inactivating the 60 S ribosomal unit.

If the antibody is specific for an antigen on a tumor cell, this becomes a powerful tool for delivering toxins to specifically eliminate tumor cells. One drawback for this application is the difficulty of getting antibodies that do not cross react with antigens on normal tissue, that is, to find monoclonal antibodies that are truly specific for tumor cells. One application that has been very successful, however, is the treatment of acute graft-versus-host disease. In this case it is known that the effector cell is a T cell, and a ricin-conjugated murine monoclonal anti-T cell antibody eliminates the symptoms.

Catalytic Antibodies

We have already seen that antibodies bind to antigen, and we have examined some of the effector functions of the antibody that are carried out by the Fc portion of the molecule after the binding of antigen by the Fab portion. Recently two groups have shown that an effector function can be carried out *because* of the specific binding of an antibody to an antigen. Richard Lerner in La Jolla and Peter Schulz in Berkeley have been able to make antibodies function as enzymes, that is, carry out catalysis. These are called CATALYTIC ANTIBODIES or ABZYMES.

The principle is one that was predicted many years ago by Jencks, who proposed that if one could develop an antibody to a *transition state* of a molecule, the antibody might in fact act as an enzyme. To understand this we must first understand the nature of the transition state in the energetics of catalysis.

> Chemical processes can be described by energy surfaces in which stable molecules are defined by deep wells. For one molecule to be transformed into another, its atoms must travel across the energy surface from one well to another. The atoms must first gain energy until they reach a crest and then lose energy to fall into the stable product well. The highest point on the reaction path corresponds to a dynamic, unstable transition state in which bonds are only partially formed or broken. The transition state exists for just a fleeting instant during the journey from reactants to products. [R. Lerner, 1988. *Sci. Am.* March: 60]

This is illustrated in Figure 4.

The principle of the catalytic antibody is that the antigen is a transition-state analog, a molecule that mimics the transition-state molecule. If an antibody capable of binding to the transition state can be generated, then the combination of the antibody with the actual transition-state molecule might result in the stabilization of the molecule, and then the catalysis could occur. At almost the same time, the La Jolla and Berkeley groups produced antibodies that catalyzed the hydrolysis of an ester bond. More recently, the La Jolla group has been able to catalyze the hydrolysis of an amide bond, and there is great hope that by devising the proper antigens, that is, the proper mimics of transition states, we will be able to tailor enzymes to any specificity. It is not difficult, for example, to visualize the construction of a catalytic antibody that is specific for the amide bond in a given structure on a virus. Its binding to the virus would then cleave the bond and disrupt the protein, resulting in a whole new mode of antiviral therapy.

Human and "Humanized" Monoclonal Antibodies

Because of the potential immunogenicity of mouse monoclonal antibodies, the use of human monoclonal antibodies for injection

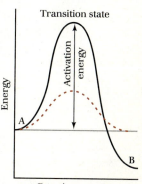

4 **The Energy Demands of a Hypothetical Chemical Reaction.** To go from substrate (A) to product (B) requires energy (activation energy) to get through the transition state. An enzyme or a catalytic antibody can lower the amount of energy required (*dotted lines*) and therefore catalyze the reaction.

into humans is obviously a desired goal. Most immunologists thought that the modification of the technology from mouse to human monoclonal antibodies would be a simple task. This has proved not to be the case, and the potential of human monoclonal antibodies has not been realized.

One of the problems has been the relative instability of immortalized human B-cell lines. Even in those cases in which the line has been reasonably stable, antibody production has been poor. But an even greater problem is the source of immune lymphocytes to fuse with the cell line. In the mouse system, one can inject the animal with any antigen one desires and then fuse the spleen cells of that mouse with the immortalized cell line. But what should one use as the source of immune cells in humans? Even if in vitro immunization techniques were efficient, which they are not, there would still be the problem of immune tolerance, the inability of an individual to make an immune response to its own antigens. (This will be discussed in great detail in Chapter 31.) Since all humans have structurally (and antigenically) identical CD3, CD4, and so forth, the human immune system cannot be immunized to such human antigens. To overcome these problems, the techniques of molecular biology have been applied to make chimeric human–mouse molecules and to graft mouse CDRs onto human framework regions.

Chimeric Mouse–Human Monoclonal Antibodies

Because it is desirable but difficult to produce human monoclonal antibody, one can compromise by producing a hybrid antibody that contains mouse V regions and human C regions. This mouse–human hybrid, or CHIMERIC ANTIBODY, has the advantage of retaining the specificity of the mouse monoclonal but is a human isotype. This eliminates the chance of an anti-isotype response, although the anti-idiotype response is still a problem.

5 Chimeric and CDR-Grafted Antibodies. Mouse–human chimeric: The ▶ genes encoding the Fab domains of the human antibody are replaced with the genes encoding the Fab from a mouse monoclonal antibody. This results in an antibody that has the mouse Fab (*black*) and the specificity of the monoclonal antibody and an Fc domain that is human. CDR-grafted molecules: The areas thought to represent the six CDRs of a murine monoclonal antibody are engineered into the genes of a human Ig. The resulting molecule has the specificity of the mouse monoclonal antibody, but the rest of the molecule is human.

Figure 5 shows a schematic representation of the creation of chimeric mouse–human monoclonal antibodies. This is done by cloning the H- and L-chain genes from a mouse hybridoma producing the monoclonal antibody of the desired specificity. These are then treated with restriction endonucleases so that the portions containing the V and C regions are separated. The same is done with a human Ig gene of any specificity (because it will be the source of the C region, the specificity of the human Ig does

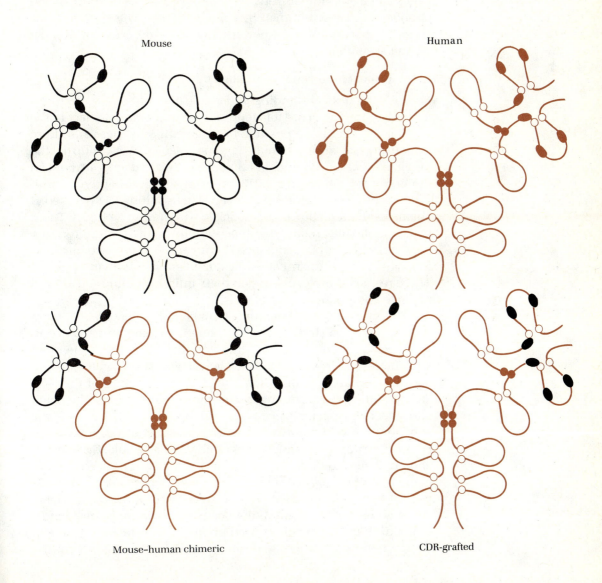

Mouse   Human

Mouse–human chimeric   CDR-grafted not matter). For both the H and L chains, the V-region gene of the mouse is then joined to a human C-region gene. The hybrid gene is then transfected into a suitable myeloma cell line and expressed. There have been some problems with differential expression of H and L chains and with levels of production of Ig by the cells, but these are technical problems that are being solved.

The first chimerics were made against haptens, but now any antibody that is being considered for use in humans is a good candidate to be "humanized." It is possible to make the humanized antibody even more human by using only the CDRs of the mouse engrafted onto human framework regions as described in the following section.

CDR-Grafted Monoclonal Antibodies

Because the antigen-binding surface of the antibody molecule is formed by the hypervariable loops at one end of the β-sheet of the Ig chains, it should be possible to transplant only these sites from a mouse gene into a human Ig gene (Figure 5). A group at the Medical Research Council in Cambridge, England, first introduced the genes for the H-chain CDRs from mouse anti-hapten or anti-protein into a human H-chain gene. The resulting CDR-grafted H chains were then allowed to associate with mouse L chains. These hybrid molecules retained antigen-binding activity. More recently the Cambridge group engineered both the H- and L-chain CDRs from a rat anti-human cell-surface antigen into human Ig genes. These reshaped molecules retain their antigen-binding activity and mediate complement lysis of cells.

The strategy for generating CDR-grafted molecules is more difficult than the strategy for the chimeric molecules discussed in the previous section. The first problem is to determine the exact nucleotides that make up the CDR genes. This is a delicate problem because a change in one amino acid at the juncture of the CDR and the framework area could alter the conformation of the chain and affect the packing of the H and L CDRs and therefore the configuration of the antigen-reactive surface. The computer models for this process are improving rapidly. For example, Cary Queen and his colleagues in Palo Alto have recently produced a CDR-grafted antibody against a molecule called Tac or CD25 (see Chapter 27) that has potential use as an immunosuppressive agent. Using a computer program, they constructed a molecular model of the anti–Tac V domains based on known crystal structure and energy minimization. They decided which amino acids from the mouse Ig were in the CDRs and which amino acids potentially interacted with the CDRs. The resultant molecule is seen in Plate 9-1. It had specificity for Tac and is now being used in clinical trials as an immunosuppressant.

Human Monoclonal Antibodies Expressed in Mouse Cells (Heterohybridomas)

The approaches described above, making chimeric and CDR-grafted antibody, attempt to get around the problem of injecting mouse Ig into humans by "humanizing" the mouse molecule. Another approach that has been taken is to make a human monoclonal antibody by expression of the entire gene for a human antibody in a mouse cell. This gets around the difficulty of the instability and low expression of human hybridoma cell lines by using stable mouse lines that are known to give high levels of expression of the molecules. The problem is still the source of immune lymphocytes to use as the source of the antibody. An anti-tetanus and an anti-microbial exotoxin have been successfully produced in this manner by using cells from immunized individuals.

The strategy is to transform antibody-forming cells from an individual immunized to the antigen with Epstein-Barr virus (EBV), a virus that specifically infects B cells. These transformed cells grow in culture and serve as the source of the human antibody genes but are poor producers of antibody. cDNA libraries are made from these cells, and clones encoding H and L chains are isolated. These genes can then be transfected into mouse cells that then secrete human antibodies.

With the heterohybridoma method, the antibody is fully human, but the method still has the problem of immunization. One is limited to only those antigens that a human can be immunized to or happens to make for pathologic reasons.

Human Ig in Transgenic Mice

Another approach that has recently been reported is to introduce human gene segments into the mouse germ line, that is, produce transgenic mice that express human Ig genes. A plasmid containing human V_H, D, and J segments as well as $C\mu$ was injected into the pronucleus of fertilized mouse eggs. It was found, when the transgenic mice were born, that this "minilocus" was rearranged in B cells and these B cells produced human Ig.

It will be very interesting to see if these animals can indeed make specific antibody after challenge with antigen. If they can, transgenic mice of this kind will be a convenient and important source of human monoclonal antibodies in the future.

Two groups have recently reported that the immunodeficient *scid* mouse (*s*evere *c*ombined *i*mmuno*d*eficiency) can be repopulated with either peripheral human lymphocytes or fetal human hemopoietic tissue. The animals become repopulated with human tissue, but to date they have only been shown to make secondary immune responses (i.e., responses to antigens to which the donor of the cells had already been exposed). If this system can be manipulated to support primary immune responses in human cells, it will be a valuable addition to the strategies we have discussed above.

Expression of the Human Immune Repertoire in *E. coli*

Two groups of immunologists independently began applying recent advances in biotechnology to the problem of human monoclonal antibodies. Gregory Winter and his colleagues in Cambridge, England and Richard Lerner and his colleagues in La Jolla began amplifying the genes for V_H and V_L in order to obtain large enough numbers of individual genes to work with. Both groups took advantage of the fact that there are conserved nucleotide sequences at each end of the V_H and V_L domains of both human and mouse Igs. By using these sequences to construct primers for the polymerase chain reaction (PCR), they were able to amplify almost all of the V_H and V_L genes.

The reasoning is that the frequency of a gene encoding any particular V_H or V_L in the lymphocytes of an individual is very low (one of the basic assumptions of clonal selection). The PCR procedure will amplify all genes that contain the conserved nucleotide sequences—even though these sequences are nowhere near those for the CDRs. Because the sequences are conserved, all genes in which they appear will be amplified. By expressing the genes in a bacteriophage, one can then infect the bacteria *E. coli* and take advantage of the ease with which large numbers of bacteria can be handled. The phage-infected bacteria are grown on plates, and the plates are screened with labeled antigen to identify those colony lysates that have the desired antibody. The V_H and V_L genes can then be recovered from the phage and joined to the gene for a desired Fc portion. By transfecting into an appropriate cell line, one gets production of the full monoclonal antibody.

The goal of this work is to generate fully human monoclonal

antibodies of therapeutic importance. Once the remaining technical barriers (mostly involving screening) are overcome, this method should provide a routine way of generating human monoclonal antibodies.

Summary

1.   Monoclonal antibodies are generated by fusing an antibody-forming cell with a myeloma. The resulting hybridoma produces identical antibody molecules. Because all the antibody-forming cells (hybridomas) are progeny of the same cell, they are a single clone (hence the term "monoclonal antibody").
2.   Monoclonal antibodies are used as immunosuppressive agents and vehicles for imaging and delivering toxins.
3.   Catalytic antibodies are monoclonal antibodies that bind to antigen and can affect the rate of a chemical reaction, i.e., catalysis.
4.   Progress toward making human monoclonal antibodies has been steady, but the problem has been immunization of the human cells.
5.   Mouse monoclonals can be "humanized" by making mouse $(Fab)_2$–human Fc chimeras or by engineering the genes for mouse CDRs into human Ig molecules. Other approaches include transgenic mice with a human transgene and mouse cells with transfected human antibody genes.
6.   Recently it appears that it may be possible to express the human H- and L-chain repertoires in *E. coli* and select H and L combinations that have a desired specificity. These will be purely human monoclonal antibodies and will eliminate the need for immunization.

Additional Reading

Bruggemann, M., H. M. Caskey, C. Teale, H. Waldmann, G. T. Williams, M. A. Surani and M. S. Neuberger. 1989. A repertoire of monoclonal antibodies with human heavy chains from transgenic mice. *Proc. Natl. Acad. Sci. U.S.A.* 86: 6709.

Gillies, S. D., H. Dorai, J. Wesolowski, G. Majkeau, D. Young, J. Boyd, J. Gardner and K. James. 1989. Expression of human anti-tetanus toxoid antibody in transfected murine myeloma cells. *Bio/Technology* 7: 799.

Goding, J. W. 1983. *Monoclonal Antibodies, Principles and Practice: Production and Application of Monoclonal Antibodies in Cell Biology, Biochemistry and Immunology*. Academic, New York.

Huse, W. D., L. Sastry, S. A. Iverson, A. Kang, M. Alting-Mees, D. R. Burton, S. J. Benkovic and R. A. Lerner. 1989. Generation of a large combinatorial library of the immunoglobulin repertoire in phage. *Science* 246: 1275.

Köhler, G. and C. Milstein. 1975. Continuous cultures of fused cells secreting antibody of predefined specificity. *Nature* 256: 495.

Morrison, S. L. and V. T. Oi. 1989. Genetically engineered antibody molecules. *Adv. Immunol*. 44: 65.

Mullinax, R. L., E. A. Gross, J. R. Amberg, B. N. Hay, H. H. Hogrefe, M. M. Kubitz, A. Greener, M. Alting-Mees, D. Ardourel, J. M. Short, J. A. Sorge and B. Shopes. 1990. Identification of human antibody fragment clones specific for tetanus toxoid in a bacteriophage λ immunoexpression library. *Proc. Natl. Acad. Sci.* U.S.A. 87: 8095.

Neuberger, M. S., G. T. Williams and R. O. Fox. 1984. Recombinant antibodies possessing novel effector functions. *Nature* 312: 604.

Orlandi, R., D. H. Gussow, P. T. Jones and G. Winter. 1989. Cloning immunoglobulin variable domains for expression by the polymerase chain reaction. *Proc. Natl. Acad. Sci. U.S.A.* 86: 3833.

Plückthun, A. 1990. Antibodies from *Escherichia coli. Nature* 347: 497.

Queen, D., W. P. Schneider, H. E. Selick, P. W. Payne, N. F. Landolfi, J. F. Duncan, N. M. Avdalovic, M. Levitt, R. P. Junghans and T. A. Waldmann. 1989. A humanized antibody that binds to the interleukin 2 receptor. *Proc. Natl. Acad. Sci. U.S.A.* 86: 10029.

Riechmann, L., M. Clark, H. Waldmann and G. Winter. 1988. Reshaping human antibodies for therapy. *Nature* 332: 323.

Yelton, D. E. and M. D. Scharff. 1981. Monoclonal antibodies: A powerful new tool in biology and medicine. *Annu. Rev. Biochem*. 50: 657.

THE ANTIGEN–ANTIBODY COMPLEX

Overview   Up to now we have discussed the nature of antigens and the structure of antibodies. In this chapter we will discuss the interaction between the two that leads to the formation of an antigen–antibody complex. It will become obvious that this reaction between antigen and antibody can be looked upon as a problem in physical chemistry in which reaction rates and affinities can be calculated and used to analyze the reaction. Our purpose is not to rigorously derive the equations that describe the reaction but only to provide the average reader with enough detail about the reaction to be useful in understanding some of the methods that will be described.

All methods of quantifying the antibody response depend upon analyzing the formation of the antigen–antibody complex. The reaction leading to the formation of the complex can be treated as an interaction between any two ligands. We will apply the laws of mass action to show that both an equilibrium constant and an affinity constant can be derived. The strength of the reaction can thus be described in exact physical terms. We saw in an earlier chapter that antibodies are heterogeneous, and this heterogeneity is seen in the binding to antigen. For this reason we will derive the equation to determine a heterogeneity index.

The interaction of an antibody with an antigen is no different in principle from any other bimolecular reaction between a ligand and a molecule that specifically binds that ligand. The reaction between enzyme and substrate is a bimolecular reaction and follows the same rules of physical chemistry as do antigen–antibody reactions. The difference between the two is that the substrate is changed in an enzyme–substrate reaction, but not in an antigen–antibody reaction. A reaction in which one of the reactants is altered will be a one-way, or nonreversible, reaction. Antigen–antibody reactions are reversible because the interaction does not result in permanent change to either of the reactants.

151

The Antigen–Antibody Complex

The reaction of antigen with antibody results in the formation of an antigen–antibody complex (AgAb):

$$Ag + Ab \rightleftharpoons AgAb \tag{1}$$

AgAb is formed by *noncovalent* interactions such as hydrogen bonding, polar or hydrophobic bonding, ionic or coulombic interaction, and van der Waals forces. Because the reaction is noncovalent and neither reactant is altered, the reaction is in theory a reversible one. All the methods used to quantify the antigen–antibody reaction depend upon the ability to measure AgAb.

We will see in the next chapter that the form taken by AgAb depends on the nature of the antigen. Soluble antigens such as proteins form complexes with antibody and become insoluble precipitates. Particulate antigens, such as cells, after reacting with antibody may form an AgAb that agglutinates. The reaction is analyzed by determining either the rate of formation or the quantity of precipitate or agglutinate.

Affinity of the Antigen–Antibody Reaction

Because the formation of AgAb can be treated as a chemical reaction between two ligands and because the reaction is reversible, the *affinity*, or strength, of the reaction can be determined. The law of mass action states that the rate of a reaction is proportional to the concentration of the reactants. By applying the law of mass action to Equation (1) we obtain

$$Ag + Ab \underset{k_d}{\overset{k_a}{\rightleftharpoons}} AgAb \tag{2}$$

$$k_a[Ab][Ag] = k_d[AgAb]$$

where [Ag] and [Ab] are the concentrations of free antigen and antibody; [AgAb] is the concentration of bound Ag and Ab, that is, the Ag–Ab complex; and k_a and k_d are the association and dissociation constants, respectively.

From Equation (2) we can arrive at the EQUILIBRIUM CONSTANT for the reaction:

$$K = \frac{k_a}{k_d} = \frac{[AgAb]}{[Ag][Ab]} \tag{3}$$

AFFINITY is the sum of the noncovalent attractive and repulsive forces stabilizing the complex and is therefore the same as the

EQUILIBRIUM CONSTANT K (which is expressed in liters per mole).

These reactions hold only for homogeneous binding sites (antibodies) and ligands (haptens). We know from the preceding chapters that antibodies are extremely heterogeneous; therefore these equations are only an approximation of the actual conditions. For monoclonal antibodies, however, these equations come very close to representing the actual interactions.

Determining Affinity

To determine the affinity of the reaction, we obviously need a means of determining the concentration of free and bound hapten. This is most conveniently accomplished by EQUILIBRIUM DIALYSIS. This method is diagrammed in Figure 1. Antibody and hapten are separated by a semipermeable membrane. The hapten, with a suitable label (such as a radioisotope), is placed on one side of the membrane and the antibody is placed on the other. The pore size of the membrane is such that the hapten freely passes through; but the antibody, being of higher molecular weight, does not. Samples are then taken from each side at various times to determine the amount of hapten on each side.

In Figure 1A the antibody is not directed to the hapten, so no AgAb forms and all the hapten is unbound. This condition serves as a control because it tells the rate at which the concentration of the hapten reaches equilibrium on both sides of the membrane. In Figure 1B the antibody reacts with the hapten, so that some of the hapten moving into the antibody compartment becomes bound and forms an Ag–Ab complex. The system will still come to equilibrium, of course, but at equilibrium the concentration of free or *unbound* hapten will be lower than in A. This happens because the equilibrium is established by the unbound molecules, even though the *total* amount of hapten on the antibody side is greater than the amount of hapten on the other side.

Other methods, such as FLUORESCENCE QUENCHING, can also be used. This method takes advantage of the fact that tryptophan absorbs light at 280 nm and emits the absorbed light at 350 nm. (*Fluorescence* is defined as absorption of light at one wavelength and emission of it at another; see Figure 12 in Chapter 11.) When a hapten is bound to an antibody, some of the tryptophan residues in the combining site are not accessible to absorb the ultraviolet light at 280 nm; hence emission at 350 nm will be reduced, or "quenched."

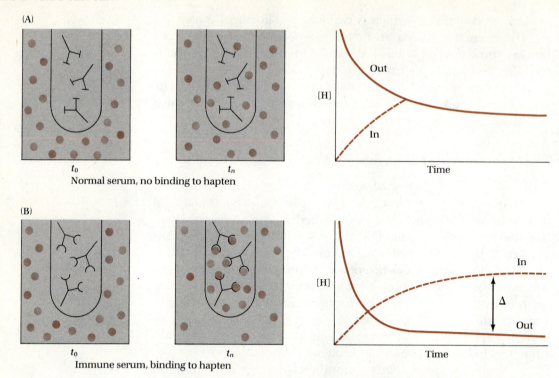

(A)

t_0

t_n

Normal serum, no binding to hapten

[H]

Out

In

Time

(B)

t_0

t_n

Immune serum, binding to hapten

[H]

In

Δ

Out

Time

1 **Equilibrium Dialysis.** Anti-hapten antibody and labeled hapten are separated by a dialysis membrane. With time the hapten molecules diffuse across the membrane and reach equilibrium. (A) In normal serum no binding of the hapten occurs when it crosses the membrane; and at equilibrium equal amounts of hapten are present on both sides of the membrane. (B) In immune serum the hapten is bound by the anti-hapten antibody, reducing the concentration of free hapten [H] inside. When the unbound hapten reaches equilibrium, there is a difference Δ between [H] in and [H] out. (C) The difference Δ is the amount of hapten bound.

Antibody Affinity and Valence

The reader with knowledge of thermodynamics will see that from Equation (3) a form of the Langmuir absorption isotherm may be derived.[1]

$$\frac{[AgAb]}{[Ab]} = r = \frac{nK[Ag]}{1 + K[Ag]} \tag{4}$$

[1] For the reader without knowledge of thermodynamics, trust us. We have relied very heavily for this section on the clearest discussion we know of the subject, which is in M. W. Steward's chapter in Glynn and Steward, *Immunochemistry: An Advanced Textbook* (1977).

2   Scatchard Plot of Ideal Hapten–Anti-Hapten Binding. The values of r are obtained from Equation (4) and $r/[Ag]$ from Equation (5). In this plot the slope K is equal to the affinity, and the intercept n is equal to the valence.

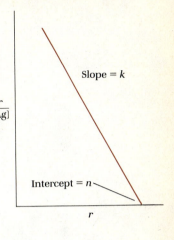

where r is moles of antigen bound per mole of antibody; [AgAb] is the concentration of bound antibody; [Ab] is the concentration of free antibody; [Ag] is the concentration of free antigen; and n is the valence of the antibody.

By algebraic manipulation one can convert Equation (4) into Equation (5).

$$\frac{r}{[Ag]} = nK - rK \tag{5}$$

By plotting $r/[Ag]$ versus r, we can derive the values of both K (which is the affinity) and n (which is the valence). Such a plot (Figure 2) is called a SCATCHARD PLOT. Figure 3 shows some actual data plotted according to Equation (5).

For bivalent antibody (i.e., where $n = 2$), the average intrinsic association constant (k_0) can be calculated from Equation (5). Diva-

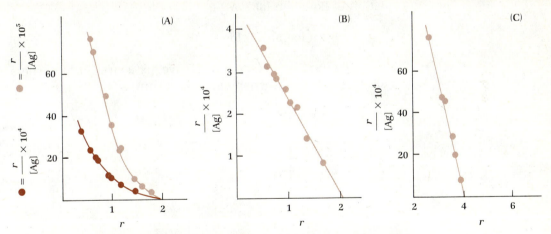

3   Scatchard Plots of Experimental Data. (A) Hapten–anti-hapten binding. Two antibody preparations (anti-DNP) that differ about 30-fold in affinity react with dinitroalanine. (B) Hapten–anti-hapten binding. A myeloma protein with anti-DNP activity reacts with dinitroalanine. Because the population of molecules is homogeneous, it gives a straight-line plot. (C) Enzyme–substrate binding. Muscle phosphorylase a binds AMP. [Redrawn from Eisen, 1974. *Immunology*]

lent antibody has two binding sites ($n = 2$), so when half of them are bound to antigen, $r = 1$. In that case Equation (5) becomes

$$\frac{1}{[Ag]} = 2K - K = K_0 \tag{6}$$

Affinity may also be calculated by the Langmuir plot by converting Equations (4) and (5) into Equation (7):

$$\frac{1}{r} = \frac{1}{n} \cdot \frac{1}{[Ag]} \cdot \frac{1}{k} + \frac{1}{n} \tag{7}$$

Plotting the data in this form results in a curve like that shown in Figure 4.

Heterogeneity of Binding

Because (as we already know) antigens and antibodies are not homogeneous, the actual curves obtained are not linear. It has been shown, however, that the distribution of affinities can be described by the Sips distribution function:

$$\frac{r}{n} = \frac{[K_0 Ag]^a}{1 + [K_0 Ag]^a} \tag{8}$$

where a is the heterogeneity index. By using the logarithmic transformation of Equation (8), we get

$$\log \frac{r}{n - r} = a \log K_0 + a \log [Ag] \tag{9}$$

Plotting $\log[r/(n - r)]$ versus $\log [Ag]$, we get a straight line where the slope is the heterogeneity index a (Figure 5).

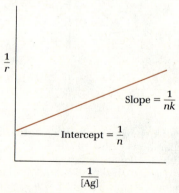

4 Langmuir Plot of Ideal Hapten–Anti-Hapten Binding. This plot was obtained by using Equation (7).

5   Sips Plot of Ideal Antigen–Antibody Binding. This plot was obtained by using Equation (9), in which a is the heterogeneity index.

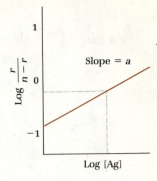

Kinetics of Antigen–Antibody Reactions

The combination of antigen and antibody is so rapid that it can only be studied with extremely sophisticated methods such as temperature-jump relaxation and stopped-flow techniques.[2] These methods show that the association rates for most hapten–antihapten systems studied are similar ($\sim 10^8\,M^{-1}\,sec^{-1}$). In contrast, the dissociation rate constants show great variation, which means that the stability of the complex is determined to a great extent by the dissociation rate.

Summary

1.   Antigen and antibody combine to form an antigen–antibody complex, AgAb, which is held together by noncovalent forces. This reaction obeys the laws of bimolecular reactions.

2.   The concentration of free and bound hapten can be experimentally determined by equilibrium dialysis. Using these values and applying the law of mass action to the basic equation, we can determine the affinity of the Ag-Ab reaction.

3.   The valence of antibody molecules can be determined from Scatchard plots. By using the Sips distribution function, we can calculate the heterogeneity index.

Additional Readings

Day, E. D. 1966. *Foundations of Immunochemistry*. Williams & Wilkins, Baltimore.

Eisen, H. N. 1974. *Immunology*. Harper & Row, Hagerstown, Md.

Steward, M. W. 1977. Affinity of the antigen–antibody reaction and its biological significance. In Glynn, L. E. and M. W. Steward, eds. *Immunochemistry: An Advanced Textbook*. Wiley, Chichester.

---

[2] For the reader without knowledge of thermodynamics and advanced physical chemistry who trusted us on page 154, you are now on your own.

MEASURING IMMUNE REACTIONS

<table>
<tr><td>

CHAPTER

11

</td></tr>
</table>

Overview In the preceding chapters we have examined some of the properties of antigens and antibodies and the nature of their interaction to form the antigen–antibody complex. We have mentioned at a few places that in addition to the humoral immune response that results in the production of antibodies, there are also cell-mediated reactions that are carried out by the cells themselves. In this chapter we will discuss some of the methods that are used to measure reactions of both types.

The most important point we will make in this chapter concerning the methods of identifying, localizing, or quantifying the antigen–antibody reaction is that all these methods rely on the study of the antigen–antibody complex. But very much like the Biblical instruction "By their fruits you shall know them," the only way to know about the interaction of the antigen and antibody is to know about their product. For this reason we will see that all the methods that examine antibody reactions are devised to look at the complex. In contrast, reactions that measure cell-mediated responses look at the response of an immunologically active cell to interaction with antigen. We will see that this can take the form of proliferation or killing.

The reader may prefer to browse through this chapter to get the general idea of how immunologic reactions are carried out. Later you will no doubt come back to look at specific reactions in more detail as they become important in order to understand an experiment.

ANTIBODY REACTIONS

The union of antigen and antibody results in the formation of an antigen–antibody (Ag–Ab) complex. All methods of measuring and quantitating antigen–antibody reactions take advantage of this fact and measure either the amount or the rate of formation of the complex. The complex takes one of several forms, depending upon the nature of the antigen. For example, soluble proteins react with antibody to produce an Ag–Ab complex that forms a precipitate, whereas with particulate antigens such as cells, the Ag–Ab complex agglutinates. But whether one is localizing an antigen on a cell surface, or within a cytoplasmic structure of a cell, or determining the concentration of a hormone in a body fluid, the assay systems all rely on the same principle: assay of the amount or rate of formation of the Ag–Ab complex.

The Precipitin Reaction

When the antigen is soluble (a protein, for example), the reaction of antigen and antibody results in the formation of an insoluble precipitate.

$$Ag + Ab \rightleftharpoons AgAb \text{ (precipitate)}$$

For a precipitate to form, both the antigen and the antibody molecules must be at least *bivalent* (i.e., have a minimum of two combining sites). One combining site on an antibody molecule can react with an antigenic determinant on one antigen molecule, and the other combining site can react with a determinant on another antigen molecule. If this happens often enough, a *lattice* will form and will grow until it becomes insoluble and forms a precipitate (Figure 1). For historical reasons this is called the PRECIPITIN REACTION and is probably the assay with the most variations that is used in immunology.

Precipitin reactions can be quantitative or qualitative; they can be carried out in solution or in semisolid support medium such as a gel. Traditional texts and methods books cover the *quantitative precipitin reaction* and its many variations in detail. Even though the quantitative precipitin reaction was very important in the development of immunology into a quantitative science, it has been supplanted by other methods. However, one very important theoretical point came out of this pioneering early work. The optimum amount of precipitate forms at the EQUIVALENCE ZONE. When either antigen or antibody is present in excess, less precipitate forms. This means that we cannot merely mix some antigen and some antibody together and get the maximum amount of precipitiate. Nor can we add extra antigen to ensure that all the antibody will be bound into an Ag–Ab complex and be part of the precipitate.

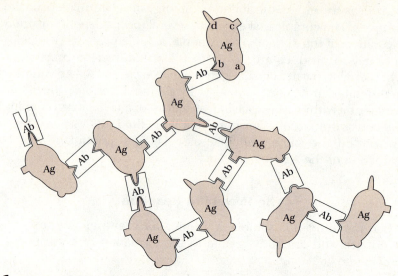

1   Cross-Linking of Antigenic Determinants and Antibodies. The soluble antigen has determinants a through d. Each determinant reacts with the specific antibody, which is bivalent. In this way the antigen molecules are cross-linked, forming a large complex that precipitates. [Redrawn from Nisonoff, 1984. *Molecular Immunology*, 2nd ed.]

While all the antibody may indeed be bound into the complex, the complexes at any given ratio of antigen and antibody may not be the one that gives the maximum amount of precipitate.

Reactions in Gels

In most precipitin reactions, there are many antigen and antibody reactions going on because most antigens have several antigenic determinants. For example, when we use human serum as the antigen in another species, antibodies are generated against all the components of the serum. Even when we use only one of the serum components (e.g., albumin) as antigen, it elicits the production of many different antibodies because it has many antigenic determinants. Fortunately, these complex reactions can be analyzed by carrying out the precipitin reaction in gels.

The Ouchterlony Assay

In this assay—named after its inventor—the antigen and the antiserum are placed in wells that have been cut in agar. The reaction is conveniently done in a petri dish but is often miniaturized and carried out on microscope slides. The antigen and antibody diffuse toward each other through the agar and at some point meet and react to form an Ag–Ab complex. A precipitate forms where the reactants are close to the equivalence zone. Because the complex is too large to diffuse through the gel, it is immobilized. Each antigen diffuses at its own rate, depending on characteristics such as size and shape; and when it meets its specific antibody, a precipitate forms. The pattern of lines that form can be interpreted to determine whether the reactants are the same or different, as illustrated in Figure 2.

The Mancini Assay

The Ouchterlony assay is qualitative. It tells us the minimum number of reactants involved but does not give information about the amount of the reactants present. A variant of the Ouchterlony assay that allows some quantitation of the antigen is called the MANCINI ASSAY. In this reaction the agar contains antibody, and antigen is placed in the well. As the antigen diffuses into the antibody-containing agar, the zone of equivalence is approached and a ring of precipitate is formed. The diameter of the ring is an indication of the concentration of antigen in the well, which is determined by comparing the diameter of the ring with the diameters of rings

(A) Line of identity

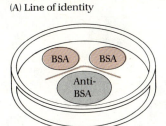

(B) Line of partial identity

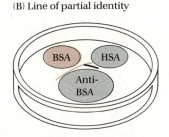

(C) No cross reaction

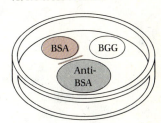

(D) No cross reaction

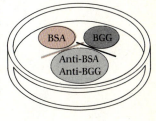

2 Ouchterlony Gel Diffusion Patterns. (A) Line of identity. The reactants (bovine serum albumin, BSA) are the same in both wells; hence a smooth line of precipitate forms. (B) Line of partial identity. The reactants are cross reactive, and the "spur" shows that there is some cross reaction between human serum albumin (HSA) and anti-BSA. (C,D) Lines showing no cross reactions. Because there is no cross reaction between BSA and bovine γ-globulin (BGG), the anti-BSA forms no precipitate with BGG, and anti-BGG and anti-BSA form separate lines of precipitate.

formed by a set of standards. The Mancini test is illustrated in Figure 3. This assay is useful when we know the qualitative nature of the antigen but need an easy means of quantitation.

Immunoelectrophoresis

A widely used variation of the precipitin reaction in a gel is IMMU-NOELECTROPHORESIS (IEP). In this case one of the reactants, usually the antigen, is placed in a well cut in the agar. However, the antigen is not allowed to diffuse passively. Instead, the agar slab is subjected to electrophoresis, and each molecule in the antigen preparation moves in the electric field according to its charge. In other words, the antigen is subjected to electrophoretic separation in the gel. To visualize the electrophoretically separated components, the investigator cuts a trough in the gel parallel to the direction in which the components have moved. Antiserum is placed in this trough and allowed to diffuse passively (*not* in an electric field) into the gel. When the antibody reaches the electrophoretically separated antigen, Ag–Ab complexes are formed. This test is illustrated in Figure 4.

This method allows the analysis of complex antigen–antibody systems such as serum (Figure 5). It can also be used as a means of identifying an unknown antigen, by determining whether the unknown has the same immunoelectrophoretic properties as a

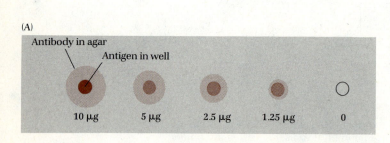

(A)

Antibody in agar

Antigen in well

10 μg   5 μg   2.5 μg   1.25 μg   0

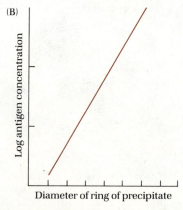

(B)

Log antigen concentration

Diameter of ring of precipitate

3 Mancini Assay. (A) Antigen diffuses into antibody-containing agar. The diameter of the ring of precipitate that forms is proportional to the log of the concentration of the antigen. (B) Standard curve. The concentration of antigen in an unknown sample is determined from a standard curve, which is prepared by using samples with known antigen concentrations.

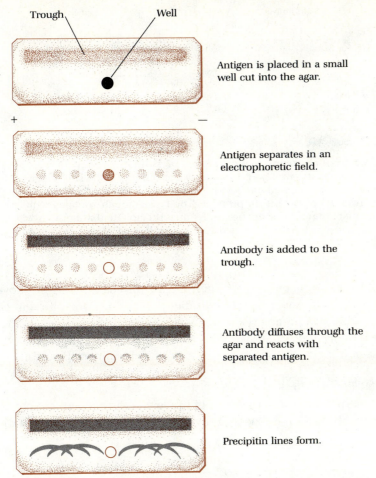

Trough   Well

Antigen is placed in a small
well cut into the agar.

+   —

Antigen separates in an
electrophoretic field.

Antibody is added to the
trough.

Antibody diffuses through the
agar and reacts with
separated antigen.

Precipitin lines form.

4   Principle of Immunoelectrophoresis. The distance that the antigen
in the well migrates in the electric field is proportional to the antigen's charge.
Antibody is added to the trough and diffuses through the agar. It reacts with
the electrophoretically separated antigen, and a precipitate is formed.

known antigen. One can also do gels in two dimensions (2-D gels).
The first dimension is usually IEP and the second SDS-PAGE (polyacrylamide gel electrophoresis). The second dimension separates
the components on the basis of size.

A variant of IEP, called ROCKET IMMUNOELECTROPHORESIS, is similar
to the Mancini test and allows some quantitation of the reaction.
Various concentrations of antigen are placed in wells that have
been cut in the agar. In this test, the agar already contains antibody.

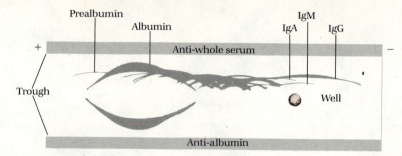

5 **Immunoelectrophoretic Pattern of Human Serum.** Human serum was placed in the well and separated electrophoretically. The upper trough contains rabbit antiserum to whole human serum; hence the lines of precipitate form for all the serum proteins. The lower trough contains rabbit anti-human albumin antiserum; hence the only precipitate that forms is with the human serum albumin. [Modified from Nisonoff, 1984. *Molecular Immunology,* 2nd ed.]

The slab is subjected to an electric field, and as the antigen moves in the field it reacts with the antibody in the agar, resulting in the formation of characteristic "rockets." By comparing the height of the rocket of an unknown with that of a standard, the concentration of antigen in the unknown can be determined (Figure 6).

Western Blotting

In recent years the separation of nucleic acids and proteins by gel electrophoresis has become a common analytic and preparative

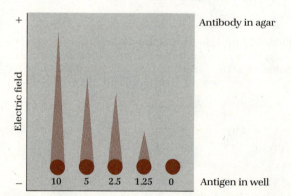

6 **Rocket Electrophoresis.** Varying concentrations of antigen are separated by electrophoresis in agar that contains antibody. By comparing the distance migrated by an unknown with data plotted on a standard curve, one can determine the concentration of antigen in the unknown sample.

tool in cell and molecular biology. But characterization of the bands or spots that are resolved by the technique has been difficult in both one- and two-dimensional gels. One very potent method for achieving characterization is called WESTERN BLOTTING.

In Western blots the protein that has been separated in the gel is transferred to a nitrocellulose membrane, usually by electro-elution, and the nitrocellulose filter is reacted with antibody. If the antibody is directed against one of the components on the filter, an Ag–Ab complex will form and be immobilized on the nitrocel-lulose filter. The Ag–Ab complex can then be identified with a labeled reagent that reacts with the complex, usually radiolabeled anti-Ig (Figure 7). (Labeled antibody methods will be described later.)

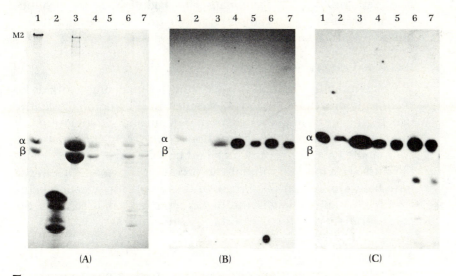

7   Western Immunoblot. Microtubule proteins were prepared from various tissues and animals and separated by discontinuous sodium dodecyl sulfate polyacrylamide gel electrophoresis, and probed with two different monoclonal anti-α-tubulin antibodies. (A) Gel stained with Coomassie blue. (B,C) Autoradiograms of Western blots. Gels were probed with two different monoclonal anti-α-tubulin antibodies; antibody binding was detected by ^{125}I-labeled protein A. Samples: 1, cow brain microtubule protein; 2, bull spermatozoa; 3, chick brain microtubule protein; 4, *Strongylocentrotus purpuratus* (a sea urchin) egg microtubule protein; 5, *S. purpuratus* sperm flagella; 6, *Lytechinus pictus* (another sea urchin) sperm flagella; 7, *Ciona intestinalis* (a tunicate) sperm flagella. The tubulins split into their α and β subunits. Brain microtubule protein also contains high-molecular-weight associated proteins, marked M2 in (A). [Courtesy of David Asai]

E. M. Southern introduced a method called Southern blotting in which electrophoretically fractionated DNA can be immobilized on nitrocellulose filters and used to analyze complementary sequences by hybridization in situ. An adaptation of this is to use complementary DNA to probe immobilized RNA. This method was amusingly called "Northern blotting" by its inventors. The method of analyzing antigen–antibody complexes on nitrocellulose was invented in Seattle by Burnette, who called it "Western blotting."

Agglutination Reactions

When the antigen is particulate (for example, a cell), it settles to the bottom of the container and forms a visible pellet. If the cells have been reacted with antibody, however, the pattern of settling is altered and the cells *agglutinate*. This agglutination can produce various forms of Ag–Ab complex, ranging from large clumps to fine material with the appearance of ground glass.

Red Blood Cell Typing

The agglutination reaction is useful only for qualitative work or for *relative* quantitation. Blood tests are the most common qualitative use of the agglutination reaction. The major blood groups of humans form the ABO system; donor and recipient must have compatible types for successful blood transfusion (Chapter 2). Simple and accurate methods of RED BLOOD CELL TYPING (RBC TYPING) have been worked out (Figure 8). In these tests the question being asked is usually, What is the blood type? and not, What is the concentration of anti-red blood cell antibody?

Antibody Titer

The relative concentration of antibody in an antiserum can be determined by *titrating* the serum. For this titration, serial dilutions of the antiserum are prepared and reacted with a constant concentration of antigen. The last dilution to give a positive agglutination reaction is considered the end point, and the serum is said to have a TITER equivalent to the final dilution (for example, 1/20 or 1/100). In this way the amount of antibody in the serum can be compared with the amount in another antiserum measured in the same way. This can be used in the opposite direction, to determine the relative concentration of antigen, as well. In this case, a constant amount of a given antiserum is reacted with various concen-

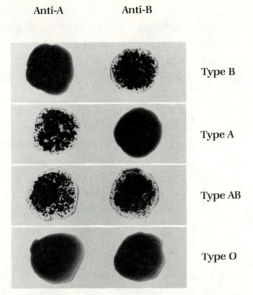

Anti-A   Anti-B

Type B

Type A

Type AB

Type O

8   RBC Typing. To test for the presence of A or B antigens on the surface of red blood cells, the investigator takes two small drops of blood by finger-prick, places them on a slide, and adds a drop of anti-A to one and a drop of anti-B to the other. A positive reaction is seen by a rapid agglutination of the cells. Agglutination in both drops indicates that the blood is type AB; no agglutination indicates that the individual is type O.

trations of antigen. The concept of antibody titer is a general one, and can be applied to any quantitation of endpoint dilution of antibody reactivity.

Labeled Antibody Techniques

Because the essential problem of immunochemistry is to identify the Ag–Ab complex, it is not surprising that there have been remarkable advances in the technology of labeling antibodies in order to identify them in the complex or to quantitate the complex. Radioactive, fluorescent, enzymatic, and electron-dense markers can be readily introduced onto an antibody molecule and are routinely used in both immunoassays and immunohistochemistry.

Primary and Secondary Antibody Methods

Two general methods are used to identify the Ag–Ab complex using labeled antibody (Figure 9). In the PRIMARY METHOD we label all the

Ig molecules in an antiserum, react the antiserum with antigen to form Ag–Ab complexes (in this case, with labeled antibody, AgAb*), and then remove the unreacted molecules. This procedure leaves only those Ig molecules that are part of the Ag–Ab complex; and because these are labeled, the complex can be identified and studied.

A more sensitive, and thus more widely used, method is the SECONDARY METHOD. The first reaction is carried out with unlabeled reactants, and unlabeled Ag–Ab complexes are formed. A second antibody, labeled anti-Ig, is mixed with the Ag–Ab complex formed in the first reaction. The labeled anti-Ig combines with all the Ig molecules (i.e., antibody) in the Ag–Ab complex and thereby labels them. This acts as an amplification step because several labeled anti-Ig can bind to one Ag–Ab complex.

Radioactive Labels

Radioactive labels have been used in immunology and immunochemistry for a very long time. ^{125}I or ^{131}I can be attached to the tyrosine residues in a protein in such a manner that the immunologic reactivity of the molecules is not altered. Because only a very small fraction of the Ig molecules in an antiserum are antibodies of the specificity being studied, it is not usually practical to label the primary antibody. Instead, a labeled second antibody is used (see preceding section). Radioactive labels are used for very sensitive assays called RADIOIMMUNOASSAYS (RIAs), which have become the most commonly used and most powerful tools of immunochemistry. They are also a very powerful tool for localizing antigens in tissue sections or on cell surfaces.

Radioimmunoassays are outgrowths of the assay developed in the 1960s by Solomon Berson (who died in 1973) and Rosalyn Yalow to immunologically quantify insulin. Rosalyn Yalow received the Nobel prize for their work in 1977.

The principle of the RIA is that a very small amount of antigen in an unknown sample will *compete* with the binding of a known amount of radiolabeled antigen for a known amount of antibody. In this manner the concentration of *antigen* in an unknown sample can be determined by its ability to compete with labeled antigen. The principle is illustrated in Figure 10.

To carry out an RIA, a known concentration of labeled antigen X (Ag*) is reacted with a known concentration of antibody (anti-X). The Ag*Ab that forms can be quantitated by determining the amount of radioactive label. When unlabeled antigen (Ag) is added,

(A)   Direct, or primary, method   (B)   Indirect, or secondary, method

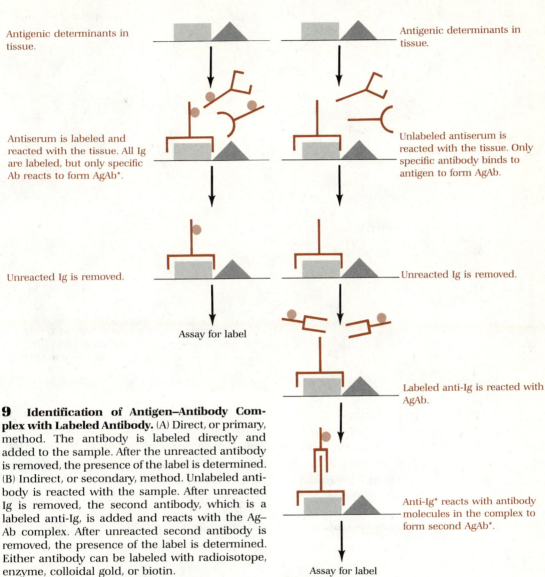

Antigenic determinants in tissue.

Antiserum is labeled and reacted with the tissue. All Ig are labeled, but only specific Ab reacts to form AgAb*.

Unreacted Ig is removed.

Assay for label

Antigenic determinants in tissue.

Unlabeled antiserum is reacted with the tissue. Only specific antibody binds to antigen to form AgAb.

Unreacted Ig is removed.

Labeled anti-Ig is reacted with AgAb.

Anti-Ig* reacts with antibody molecules in the complex to form second AgAb*.

Assay for label

9   Identification of Antigen–Antibody Complex with Labeled Antibody. (A) Direct, or primary, method. The antibody is labeled directly and added to the sample. After the unreacted antibody is removed, the presence of the label is determined. (B) Indirect, or secondary, method. Unlabeled antibody is reacted with the sample. After unreacted Ig is removed, the second antibody, which is a labeled anti-Ig, is added and reacts with the Ag–Ab complex. After unreacted second antibody is removed, the presence of the label is determined. Either antibody can be labeled with radioisotope, enzyme, colloidal gold, or biotin.

it competes with the labeled antigen (Ag*) for the constant number of combining sites on the antibody, thus *reducing* the amount of Ag* in the complex. By setting up standard curves, we can quantify the amount of antigen (Ag) in the sample.

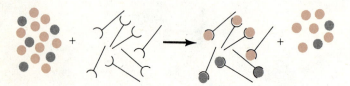

Control: A known amount of labeled antigen (●) is reacted with enough antibody (─◯) to bind 70% of the antigen.

Experimental: An unknown antigen (●) is added and competes for binding of labeled antigen.

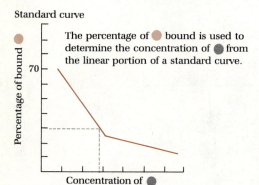

Standard curve

The percentage of ● bound is used to determine the concentration of ● from the linear portion of a standard curve.

Percentage of bound

70

Concentration of ●

10 The Principle of Radioimmunoassays. In radioimmunoassays, the concentration of antigen is assayed by determining its ability to compete with known amounts of a labeled antigen.

Radioimmunoassays are extremely sensitive (in the range of detection of nanograms per milliliter of antigen) and are widely used to quantify molecules present in very low concentration. They are especially useful for molecules in biological fluids, for example, insulin, steroid hormones, and neuropeptides. Commercial kits are available.

Enzyme-Linked Immunosorbent Assay (ELISA)

A variant of the enzyme-labeled localization technique used in histochemistry is the very popular ENZYME-LINKED IMMUNOSORBENT ASSAY, or ELISA. As the name suggests, the assay uses enzyme-linked methods. The test's uniqueness comes from the fact that one of the reactants, usually antigen, is immobilized (adsorbed) onto the surface of a test tube or microtiter well (Figure 11).

To determine the quantity of antibody in a sample, an aliquot of antiserum is reacted with the adsorbed antigen. The unreacted

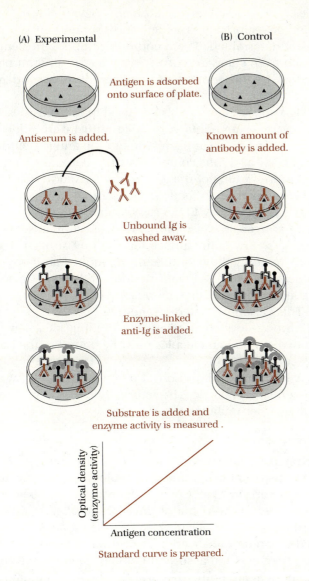

(A) Experimental

(B) Control

Antigen is adsorbed onto surface of plate.

Antiserum is added.

Known amount of antibody is added.

Unbound Ig is washed away.

Enzyme-linked anti-Ig is added.

Substrate is added and enzyme activity is measured .

Standard curve is prepared.

11 **The ELISA Assay.** *Experimental.* Antigen is adsorbed to the surface of a plate or microwell, and antibody is added. Some antibody binds to the adsorbed antigen, forming an antigen–antibody complex. The unreacted antibody is washed away, and an appropriate anti-Ig that has an enzyme linked to it is added. The labeled anti-Ig reacts with all the antibody that has reacted with the antigen, and when the substrate is added, the enzyme can be identified. *Control.* A known amount of antibody is added to the antigen on the plate and enzyme-linked anti-Ig is added. The standard curve is derived from this group.

molecules are washed away, and an enzyme-linked anti-Ig is added. Finally, substrate is added and the amount of color that develops is determined. The amount of antibody present can be determined from standard curves, because the amount of color is proportional to the amount of enzyme-linked second antibody reacted.

An INHIBITION METHOD can also be used in ELISA assays. In these reactions, varying amounts of soluble antigen are added to the antiserum. This soluble antigen binds to the antigen-binding sites on the antibody and thus competes with the immobilized antigen. A reduction in binding of the antiserum is used to determine the quantity of antigen or antibody in the sample.

There is another way ELISA assays can be used to quantify the amount of antigen in a sample. This is done by adsorbing unlabeled antibody to a solid surface followed by antigen. The Ag-Ab complex is quantified by adding enzyme-linked antibody directed against the antigen (i.e., labeled antibody of the same specificity as the unlabeled antibody already adsorbed to the surface, not an anti-Ig). This variation (called a *sandwich ELISA*) requires that the antigen have at least two accessible binding sites for antibody because two antibody molecules must be bound to the same antigen molecule.

ELISA kits for the detection of a very wide range of antigens are commercially available. The sensitivity of ELISA is in the range of nanograms per milliliter.

Fluorescent Labels

One of the great advances in the use of the immune system in diagnosis, histochemistry, and cell biology was made by Albert Coons at Harvard in 1944. Coons, who was a much-beloved figure in immunology, showed that a fluorescent label could be introduced into antibody molecules, so that when an Ag–Ab complex is formed it can be visualized by virtue of the fluorescence.

Fluorescence is the absorbtion of light of one wavelength and emission of light at another (Figure 12). The most commonly used fluorescent labels are fluorescein (which emits yellow-green light) and rhodamine (which emits red light). Figure 13 shows cells stained with fluorescein conjugated to anti-tubulin antibody.

The immunofluorescence technique takes advantage of the contrast between the emitted light and the nonemitting background. The method has a resolution limit of 200 nm. Higher resolution is achieved using electron-dense labels and electron microscopy.

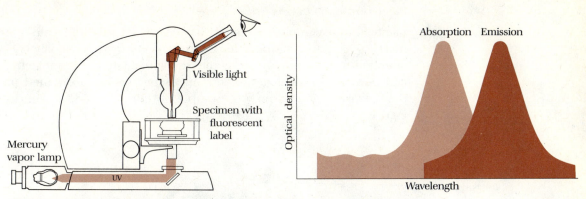

Visible light

Specimen with fluorescent label

Mercury vapor lamp

UV

Absorption   Emission

Optical density

Wavelength

12   Principle of Fluorescence Microscopy. Excitation light at one wavelength (ultraviolet) is absorbed by the label, and light of another wavelength (visible) is emitted and observed through the fluorescence microscope.

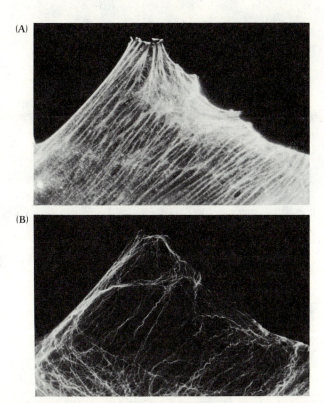

(A)

(B)

13   Fluorescence Microscopy. The same mouse fibroblast, stained with (A) an antibody that stains all microtubules and (B) another that stains a subset of chemically distinct mictrotubules. (A) Rabbit anti-tubulin rhodamine-labeled. (B) Mouse monoclonal fluorescein-labeled. [Courtesy of David Asai]

Electron-Dense Labels

Electron-dense molecules such as ferritin or colloidal gold are markers used in electron microscopy. When one of these labels is attached to an antibody molecule, the specificity of the molecule can be used to localize antigens in tissue sections examined in the electron microscope. An example of "immunogold" is seen in Figure 14.

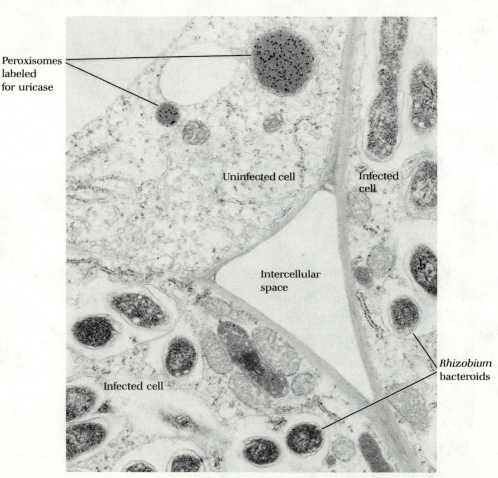

Peroxisomes labeled for uricase

Uninfected cell

Infected cell

Intercellular space

Infected cell

Rhizobium bacteroids

14 **Immunogold Label.** Electron micrograph (×17,280) of a 3-week-old soybean nodule. The thin sections were incubated with rabbit antibody against a subunit of nodule-specific uricase. This was followed by 20-nm gold particles conjugated to protein A. The gold particles are found over the large peroxisomes in uninfected cells adjacent to cells infected by *Rhizobium*. It is thought that the *Rhizobium* fixes the nitrogen, which is then assimilated into the plant's uninfected cells using the uricase. [Courtesy of K. A. Vanden Bosch]

Because electron-dense labels absorb electrons, a tissue structure that has reacted with labeled antibody can be visualized. A powerful new method called IMMUNOPHOTOELECTRON MICROSCOPY has a resolution of 5 nm.

Immunophotoelectron microscopy is essentially the electro-optical analog of immunofluorescence. In fluorescence microscopy the incident light stimulates the fluorescence emission from the dye, that is, light is emitted. In immunophotoelectron microscopy, the incident light has a shorter wavelength and stimulates the emission of electrons from the label, which is colloidal gold. The electrons are then accelerated to high velocity and imaged.

In Figure 15 the specimens were simultaneously prepared for both fluorescence and immunophotoelectron microscopy. The *primary* antibody is a monoclonal anti-tubulin, which is reacted with the tissue specimen. The *secondary* antibody is a fluorescence-labeled goat anti-mouse Ig. The *tertiary* antibody is colloidal gold-labeled rabbit anti-goat Ig. The final Ag–Ab complex can be visualized either in a fluorescence microscope or in a photoelectron microscope.

Nonspecific Binding to Ig

There are some molecules that can bind nonspecifically to Ig molecules. We take advantage of this fact by labeling these special molecules with one of the labels discussed above.

PROTEIN A is a cell wall protein from *Staphylococcus aureus*; it has the property of binding nonspecifically to the Fc portion of Ig molecules. Heat-killed staphylococci that express protein A can be used to precipitate Ig molecules from solution. Protein A can also be labeled and used as a probe for the Ag–Ab complex.

Feeding large quantities of egg white to animals produces a biotin deficiency. This reduction in biotin was found to be due to a molecule in egg white that binds to biotin with extraordinary affinity. The molecule, a basic glycoprotein of molecular weight 68,000, is called AVIDIN, and the biotin–avidin binding reaction has been exploited in immunological assays. Many biotin molecules can be put on an antibody molecule without altering the antigen-binding properties of the antibody.[1] Several molecules of avidin can bind to each biotin. When the avidin is labeled with an enzyme, this system can be used to examine the Ag–Ab complex.

---

[1] Thus there are two different interactions. The first is the binding of antibody to antigen and the second is the binding of the biotin (on the antibody) to avidin (carrying a label).

(A)

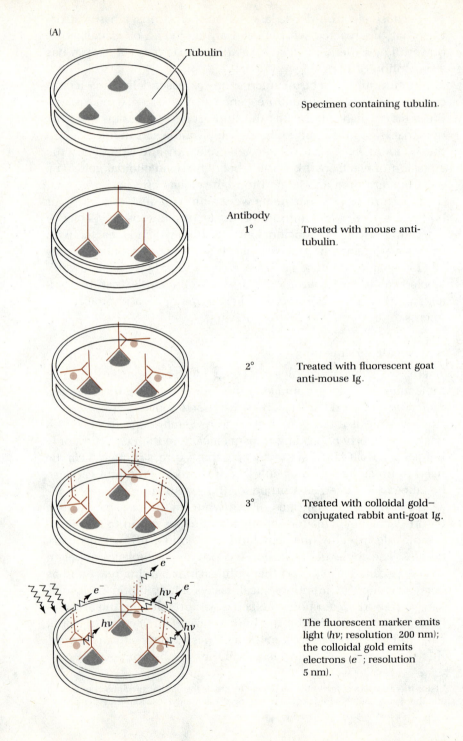

Tubulin

Specimen containing tubulin.

Antibody

1° Treated with mouse anti-tubulin.

2° Treated with fluorescent goat anti-mouse Ig.

3° Treated with colloidal gold–conjugated rabbit anti-goat Ig.

The fluorescent marker emits light ($h\nu$; resolution 200 nm); the colloidal gold emits electrons (e^-; resolution 5 nm).

(B)

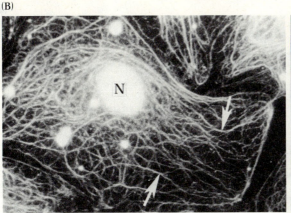
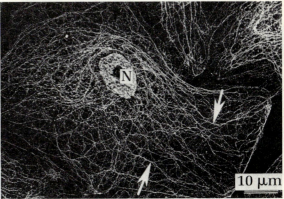

10 μm

15 **Comparison of Immunofluorescence and Immunophotoelectron Microscopy.** (A) Preparation of the samples (page 176). The sample is reacted with the primary antibody (monoclonal anti-tubulin), and antigen–antibody complexes form. A secondary antibody of fluorescence-conjugated goat anti-mouse Ig is reacted. The samples can now be used for fluorescence microscopy. A tertiary antibody of colloidal gold-conjugated rabbit anti-goat Ig is reacted. The samples can now be used for immunophotoelectron microscopy. (B) Immunofluorescence (*left*) and immunophotoelectron (*right*) microscope pictures of tubulin–anti-tubulin specimen prepared in (A). Arrows identify some of the many microtubules that can be seen in both the fluorescence and photoelectron micrographs. [Courtesy of O. H. Griffith]

Flow Cytometry

A significant advance in technology has been the ability to either sort or analyze cells on the basis of their surface antigens using the technology of FLOW CYTOMETRY (Figure 16A). Cells can be treated with an antibody conjugated to a fluorescent probe, so that when the cell passes through a laser beam fluorescent light is emitted. This light is collected, and the intensity of the light from the individual cell is analyzed, and/or the light is used to put a charge on the droplet that forms around the cell as it leaves the nozzle assembly. The cells pass through charge deflection plates, and charged drops are deflected and collected. This process is referred to as FLUORESCENCE-ACTIVATED CELL SORTING, or FACS.

Cells can also be sorted on the basis of the amount of light they scatter. Droplets that scatter predetermined amounts of light can have a charge placed on them and then be deflected.

One of the important applications of FACS is for analysis of the frequencies of cells in different populations (as defined by fluores-

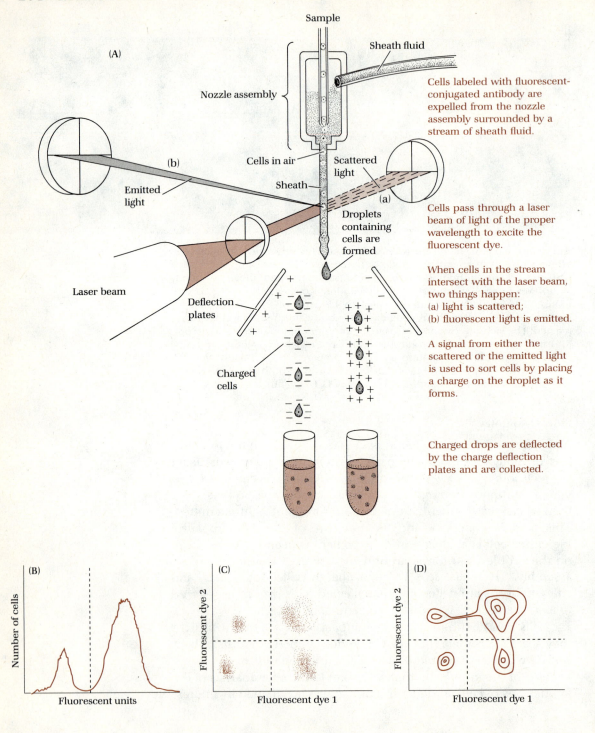

(A)

Sample

Sheath fluid

Nozzle assembly

Cells labeled with fluorescent-conjugated antibody are expelled from the nozzle assembly surrounded by a stream of sheath fluid.

(b)

Cells in air

Scattered light

Emitted light

Sheath

(a)

Droplets containing cells are formed

Cells pass through a laser beam of light of the proper wavelength to excite the fluorescent dye.

Laser beam

Deflection plates

When cells in the stream intersect with the laser beam, two things happen:
(a) light is scattered;
(b) fluorescent light is emitted.

Charged cells

A signal from either the scattered or the emitted light is used to sort cells by placing a charge on the droplet as it forms.

Charged drops are deflected by the charge deflection plates and are collected.

(B)

Number of cells

Fluorescent units

(C)

Fluorescent dye 2

Fluorescent dye 1

(D)

Fluorescent dye 2

Fluorescent dye 1

cent antibodies or other probes). Some common representations of such analyses are shown in Figures 16B–D.

The Jerne Plaque Assay

In 1963 Niels Jerne devised an assay to determine the number of antibody-forming cells *in a cell suspension*. This assay, called the HEMOLYTIC PLAQUE ASSAY or the JERNE PLAQUE ASSAY, made possible the quantitative study of the cellular events in antibody formation and was as important to the development of cellular immunology as the quantitative precipitin reaction was to immunochemistry.

When a cell that is producing antibody is immobilized in agar, the antibody molecules it produces will accumulate in the vicinity of the cell. If antigen is suspended uniformly in the agar, then an Ag–Ab complex will form in an area surrounding the antibody-producing cell. When the antigen is an erythrocyte or a molecule that has been conjugated to an erythrocyte, lysis of the erythrocytes surrounding the antibody-producing cell occurs when complement is added. This produces a clear space, or PLAQUE (Figure 17).

The number of antibody-forming cells in the starting suspension of cells can be determined because the experimenter knows the total number of cells per milliliter in the suspension and the volume plated into the antigen-containing agar. By counting the number of plaques in the agar, the number of PLAQUE-FORMING CELLS (pfc) can easily be calculated. This is usually expressed as either pfc/spleen or pfc/10^6 cells.

16 **FACS.** (A) Principle of flow cytometry. Cells can be analyzed or sorted. The cells enclosed in a sheath of fluid pass through a laser beam. The amount of light scattered and the fluorescent light emitted are recorded. Either of these signals can be used to place a charge on the droplet so the cell can be deflected. (B) FACS analysis: histogram. Arbitrary fluorescent units are plotted against the number of cells at each fluorescent intensity. The dashed line separates two populations that qualitatively differ in staining. (C) FACS analysis: two-dimensional dot plot. Cells are stained with two different fluorescent dyes (e.g., bound to antibodies) and the relative intensity of one dye is plotted against that of the other for each cell (represented by a dot). The dashed lines separate four populations differing in staining. Note that in this representation, the *density* of the dots is important. (D) FACS analysis: two-dimensional contour plot. Cells are stained as in (C), but the relative number of cells in each region is represented by contour lines. Each contour line connects points with equivalent cell numbers. You can imagine looking down at hilltops, the peaks of which represent the highest number of cells.

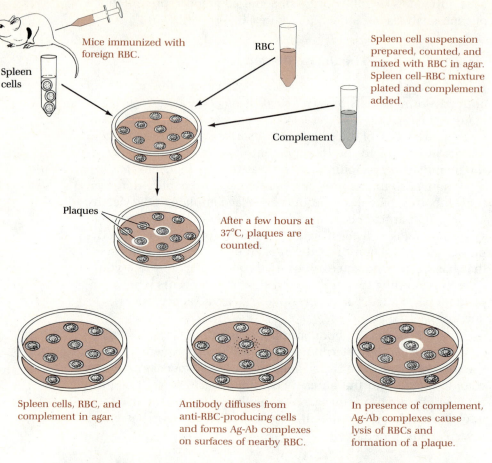

Mice immunized with foreign RBC.

Spleen cells

RBC

Spleen cell suspension prepared, counted, and mixed with RBC in agar. Spleen cell–RBC mixture plated and complement added.

Complement

Plaques

After a few hours at 37°C, plaques are counted.

Spleen cells, RBC, and complement in agar.

Antibody diffuses from anti-RBC-producing cells and forms Ag-Ab complexes on surfaces of nearby RBC.

In presence of complement, Ag-Ab complexes cause lysis of RBCs and formation of a plaque.

17   The Jerne Plaque Assay. An assay to determine the number of antibody-forming cells in a population. Mice are immunized with red blood cells, and the spleen cells are suspended in agar along with red blood cells. Complement is added, and after a few hours at 37°C the plaques are counted. Each plaque is caused by the specific antibody that is synthesized by antibody-forming cells.

The Complement Fixation Test

The binding of complement to the Ag–Ab complex is stoichiometric, so by determining the amount of complement bound (or *fixed*) to the complex we can determine the amount of complex. The principle of the complement fixation (CF) test is to determine how much lytic activity of complement has been removed from a sample of complement after an unknown amount of Ag–Ab complex is added. This is an absolute value that gives the relative amount of Ag–Ab complex present, although by using proper standard curves we can convert this number into the absolute amount of complex present.

Before the CF test is carried out, STANDARDS must be made: a sample of complement (usually normal guinea pig serum) is titrated by adding various amounts to a mixture of a known amount of red blood cells and a known amount of anti-RBC antibody. The red cell–anti-red cell mixture forms an Ag–Ab complex, which lyses when complement is bound. The titration is carried out to an end point (expressed as percentage of lysis; in practice 60% is often used). We now have a set of reagents (namely, a known amount of complement and a test system of red cells and anti-red cells) that always gives the same amount of lysis when mixed together.

To carry out the CF test (Figure 18), the sample to be tested (for example, a sample of serum that may contain antibodies against molecule X) is mixed with X. If the sample contains anti-X, a small amount of X–anti-X complex will be formed. To determine how much X–anti-X has been formed, the amount of standard complement solution that results in 60% lysis of the standard red cell–anti-red cell complex is added. If any X–anti-X complex is present, some of the added complement will be "fixed," and the complement activity of the standard complement solution will be reduced by this amount.

To determine how much of the standard complement solution has been fixed to X–anti-X, the test red cell–anti-red cell mixture is then added. Because the original amount of complement that was added was sufficient to lyse 60% of this test mixture, any *reduction* of lysis of the added red cells must be due to a reduction in the amount of complement available, that is, fixed to X–anti-X. The appropriate controls of standard complement plus X in the absence of the test serum must be done to rule out ANTICOMPLE-MENTARY EFFECTS in the serum (because the system is complex, the inactivation of one component in the cascade by some nonspecific factor could give a reduction in lysis that would be interpreted as a false positive).

CELL-MEDIATED REACTIONS

The reactions that we discussed above involve antibody, and all of them except the Jerne plaque assay measure the antibody in the absence of the cells that produce them. In cell-mediated responses

(A) Standard

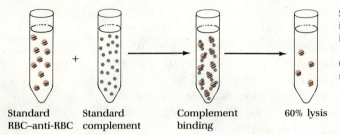

Standard | Standard | Complement | 60% lysis
RBC–anti-RBC | complement | binding |

Standardized complement is added to standardized RBC–anti-RBC (AgAb).

Complement binds to AgAb resulting in 60% lysis.

(B) Test for anti-X in unknown: reaction of unknown sample plus antigen to form AgAb

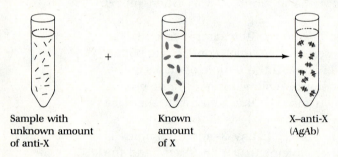

Sample with unknown amount of anti-X | Known amount of X | X–anti-X (AgAb)

Unknown amount of anti-X in the sample is reacted with X. If sample contains anti-X, a complex of X–anti-X will form.

(C) Test for anti-X in unknown: addition of standard system to determine whether complement is fixed

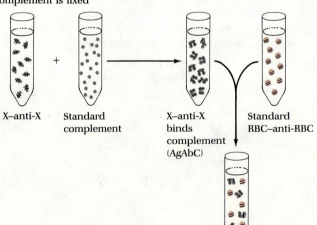

X–anti-X | Standard complement | X–anti-X binds complement (AgAbC) | Standard RBC–anti-RBC

Standard complement (as in A, above) is added to AgAb formed in B; AgAbC forms.

The standard RBC–anti-RBC is not lysed because all of the complement has been fixed by the unknown AgAb.

No lysis

the lymphocytes themselves are involved in the reactions. In the following we will describe some of the most commonly used methods of measuring cell-mediated responses.

In Vivo Reactions

Allograft Rejection

An ALLOGRAFT is a graft of tissue from one member of a species to a different member of the same species. For example, grafts from one human to another are allografts. A graft between members of two different strains of mice is also an allograft. If tissues from one strain of mouse are grafted onto animals of another strain, the tissues will begin to grow; but after several days the immune system will cause the graft to stop growing and die. This reaction is called GRAFT REJECTION. In humans, organ transplants (such as skin, kidney, and heart transplants) are allografts, and when rejection occurs, the immunologic mechanisms are the same as those seen in experimental animals. Graft rejection is a cell-mediated phenomenon because it can be transferred to normal animals only with lymphocytes and not with serum.

Delayed-Type Hypersensitivity

Delayed-type hypersensitivity (DTH) is the traditional form of cell-mediated response and is best exemplified by the TUBERCULIN TEST. If an individual has come in contact with *Mycobacterium tuberculosis* (the organism that causes tuberculosis), that individual becomes *sensitized* to antigens of the organism—that is, that individual has made an immune response to some of these antigens. Most individuals tend to make a stronger cell-mediated response than antibody response to this organism (which is why it was

◄**18**   **Complement Fixation.** (A) A mixture of known amounts of anti-RBC, RBC, and complement are added together so that a standard amount of lysis will occur. The concentrations of each of these must be experimentally determined. This serves as the control. (B) A known amount of antigen is added to a sample with an unknown amount of antibody to the antigen. The antibody that is present reacts with the antigen, forming antigen–antibody complexes. (C) The amount of complement that was used in A is added to the mixture from B. The complement reacts with the antigen–antibody complexes. When the same concentrations of RBC–anti-RBC that were used in the standard are added, there is a reduction in the lysis because some of the complement has been used in the reaction in B.

chosen as an example). To test for the presence of sensitized cells (i.e., to test for a cell-mediated response), a small amount of antigen (usually supernatant fluid from the medium in which the organisms were grown) is injected into the skin. If the individual has sensitized cells, these cells will accumulate and cause other cells to be attracted to the site of the injected antigen. The result is a lump, visible and palpable by 48 hours after injection. If the response were due to antibody (immediate hypersensitivity), the reaction would reach a maximum in 24 hours. In experimental animals, DTH reactions can be quantified by measuring the size of the lump that forms, or by injecting the antigen into the footpad of a mouse and measuring the amount of swelling after 48 hours. The footpad that received antigen is then compared with the other, which received a control injection of diluent without antigen.

Graft-versus-Host Reaction

In the allograft reaction the host is immunologically competent, and the graft, usually skin, does not contain immunologically competent cells. Therefore, the host recognizes the antigens of the graft as foreign and responds against them. In such a case, the host rejects the graft. In the graft-versus-host (GVH) reaction, the roles are reversed. As the name implies, it is the graft that recognizes the antigens of the host and responds against them. Therefore, the graft in a GVH reaction must contain immunocompetent cells.

The GVH reaction is widely used in the laboratory; but, like DTH and allograft rejection, it also has clinical implications, especially in bone marrow transplantation. If any immunocompetent lymphocytes have recirculated into the donor bone marrow, these cells will be transferred with the transplanted bone marrow cells (the graft); they can then react against the recipient (the host). In experimental situations the host is usually rendered immunologically incompetent either by treatment with X rays or by experimental design—that is, by the use of very young mice that have not yet acquired full immune competence. These immunologically incompetent hosts are injected with lymphocytes that can react against antigens of the host. As in all cell-mediated responses, the ability to carry out a GVH reaction is limited to cells; antibody does not play a role.

In the mouse, one of the consequences of a GVH reaction is the enlargement of the host's spleen. Interestingly, it is primarily the host's own cells that infiltrate and enlarge the spleen, although they do this because of the presence of the graft cells, which are carrying out a reaction against the host. The amount of spleen enlargement, or SPLENOMEGALY, is taken as a measure of the severity of the GVH reaction. Splenomegaly is expressed as the SPLEEN INDEX.

$$\text{Spleen index} = \frac{\dfrac{\text{weight of experimental spleen}}{\text{total body weight}}}{\dfrac{\text{weight of control spleen}}{\text{total body weight}}}$$

Control animals in a GVH reaction are recipients that are the same age and sex as the experimental recipients but are injected with cells of the same type of host, that is, syngeneic cells. Injecting syngeneic cells into a recipient should cause no effect, because the control cells will not recognize the host as foreign. If there is no splenomegaly in the experimental animal, it will have the same ratio of spleen to body weight as the control, and the spleen index will be 1.0. By convention, a spleen index of 1.3 or more is considered indicative of a positive GVH reaction.

In experimental situations, the recipients in the GVH reaction are usually F_1 mice and the donors one of the parental strains. In this manner the host does not recognize the transferred cells as foreign. This procedure is diagrammed in Figure 19A. Spleen cells of strain A are injected into $(A \times B)F_1$ hybrids. The A cells (the graft) induce a GVH reaction in $(A \times B)F_1$ hosts but not in the A host, because the immunocompetent cells of the A graft recognize the antigens of B on the $(A \times B)F_1$ host cells. The cells of the $(A \times B)F_1$, however, do not recognize anything as foreign on the A cells. To be sure, the A cells are different because they do not have the B antigens, but it is important to remember that the immune response is directed only to the presence of different antigen, not to differences resulting from the absence of antigen. This experiment is diagrammed in Figure 19B.

In Vitro Reactions

Mixed Lymphocyte Responses and Cytotoxic T Cells

The two most commonly used in vitro models for cell-mediated responses are diagrammed in Figure 20. Cells from the two strains of animals (or from two individual people) are mixed and placed into culture. Usually, cells from one source are irradiated or treated with agents to prevent their proliferation. This population is called the STIMULATOR, and the untreated population is called the RESPON-

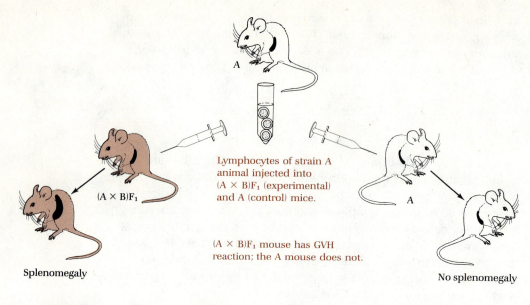

Lymphocytes of strain A
animal injected into
(A × B)F$_1$ (experimental)
and A (control) mice.

(A × B)F$_1$ mouse has GVH
reaction; the A mouse does not.

(A × B)F$_1$

Splenomegaly

A

No splenomegaly

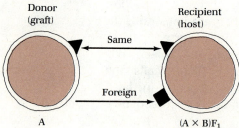

Donor
(graft)

Recipient
(host)

Same

Foreign

A

(A × B)F$_1$

19 **The Graft-versus-Host Reaction.** In the graft-versus-host reaction
(GVHR) the immunocompetent cells in the grafted tissue recognize and react
with the antigens of the host. The lymphocytes of a parental strain, A, react
with cell surface antigens, B, in the (A × B)F$_1$. The reaction (shown diagrammatically at the bottom of the figure) occurs because the cells of A recognize
and react with the B antigens on the F$_1$ cells. In contrast, because the F$_1$ has
both A and B antigens it does not recognize and react with the antigens on A.

DER. (This is a "one-way" response. If neither population is treated,
then it is a "two-way" response.) Two measurable consequences of
culturing the mixture of stimulator and responder cells are proliferation and the generation of CYTOTOXIC T CELLS or cytotoxic
lymphocytes (CTLs). Proliferation is measured by the addition of
radioactive thymidine ([^{3}H]TdR), which is incorporated into the
DNA of the responding cells. By extracting the DNA and measuring
the amount of radioactive label incorporated, a measure of the
degree of proliferation is obtained. This assay is called a MIXED

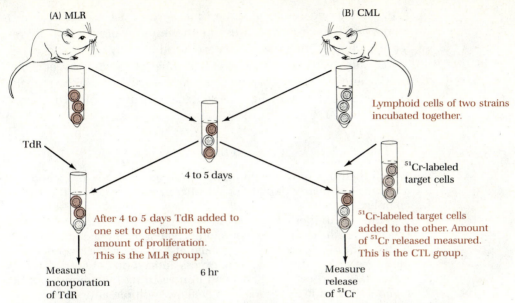

(A) MLR

(B) CML

Lymphoid cells of two strains incubated together.

TdR

4 to 5 days

^{51}Cr-labeled target cells

After 4 to 5 days TdR added to one set to determine the amount of proliferation. This is the MLR group.

^{51}Cr-labeled target cells added to the other. Amount of ^{51}Cr released measured. This is the CTL group.

Measure incorporation of TdR

6 hr

Measure release of ^{51}Cr

20 The MLR and CML Reactions. When lymphocytes of two strains are cultured together in vitro they react against each other. (A) The MLR (mixed lymphocyte reaction) is a proliferative response in which the incorporation of TdR is used to determine the amount of cell division. (B) The CML (cell-mediated lymphocyte reaction) results in the generation of cytotoxic lymphocytes (CTL) that are quantitated by a ^{51}Cr-release assay on appropriate target cells.

LYMPHOCYTE RESPONSE, or MLR. The generation of CTLs can also be assayed, in a reaction called CELL-MEDIATED LYMPHOLYSIS, or CML. After the cell mixture has been cultured for several days, the cells are recovered and mixed with different TARGET CELLS. These target cells are usually labeled with radioactive chromium (^{51}Cr), which has the fortunate property of entering cells rapidly but leaving them very slowly, as long as the cell membrane is intact. When the membrane is damaged, the chromium is rapidly released. Thus, by quantifying the amount of chromium released from the cells, we can determine how much membrane damage (killing) has been done by the sensitized responder cells. CTL data are expressed as a percentage, based on the following formula:

$$\frac{(\text{Experimental} - \text{Control})}{(\text{Maximum} - \text{Control})} \times 100\%$$

where "Experimental" represents the radioactivity recovered in the supernatant of the mixture of cells, "Control" represents the radioactivity released over the same time by the target cells cultured alone, and "Maximum" represents the amount of radioactivity released when all the target cells are lysed (e.g., by detergent).

Usually CTLs are assessed at a number of effector/target ratios (E/T's), and the results can be expressed as the slope of the straight line that is generated when percentage of killing is plotted against a range of E/T.

Summary

1.   All methods of determining the presence, amount, or location of antigen or antibody depend on identifying or quantifying the Ag–Ab complex.
2.   Antigen–antibody reactions in which the antigen is soluble form precipitates. In quantitative precipitin reactions the amount of antibody in the precipitate is determined at the equivalence zone. Complexes formed in the presence of excess antigen do not form as much precipitate, and caution is needed in measuring the amount of precipitate. Precipitin reactions in gels allow multiple antigen–antibody systems to be studied.
3.   When the antigen is particulate (for example, a cell), formation of the Ag–Ab complex results in an agglutination reaction. Agglutination reactions are usually qualitative only, the most common being the typing of red blood cells.
4.   Modern methods of quantifying and localizing the antigen–antibody reaction rely very heavily on labeling one of the reactants. Radioactive and enzyme-linked labels are the most commonly used, but electron-dense labels are very useful in immunoelectron microscopy.
5.   Radioimmunoassays (RIAs) and enzyme-linked immunosorbent assays (ELISAs) are very sensitive (nanograms per milliliter) and very commonly used assays.
6.   Flow cytometry allows the analysis of the concentration of molecules on the surface of cells after they have been reacted with specific antibody to the surface marker.
7.   Cell-mediated responses are measured by examining an effect on a cell. Graft-versus-host, delayed hypersensitivity, and graft rejection are commonly used in vivo methods for measuring cell-mediated responses. The mixed lymphocyte reaction and cytotoxic cells are in vitro reactions.

Additional Readings

Golub, E. S., R. I. Mishell, W. O. Weigle and R. W. Dutton. 1968. A modification of the hemolytic plaque assay for use with protein antigens. *J. Immunol.* 100: 133.

Jerne, N. K. and A. A. Nordin. 1963. Plaque formation in agar by single antibody-producing cells. *Science* 140: 405.

Kabat, E. 1961. *Kabat and Mayer's Experimental Immunochemistry*, rev. ed. Thomas, Springfield, Ill.

Lefkovits, I. and B. Pernis. 1979. *Immunological Methods*, Vols. 1, 2, and 3. Academic, New York.

Mishell, B. B. and S. M. Shiigi. 1980. *Selected Methods in Cellular Immunology*. Freeman, San Francisco.

Nowotny, A. 1979. *Basic Exercises in Immunochemistry*, 2nd ed. Springer-Verlag, New York.

Weir, D. M. 1985. *Handbook of Experimental Immunology*, 4th ed. Mosby, St. Louis.

Williams, C. A. and M. W. Chase. 1967. *Methods in Immunology and Immunochemistry*, Vols. 1, 2, and 3. Academic, New York.

CELLULAR IMMUNOLOGY

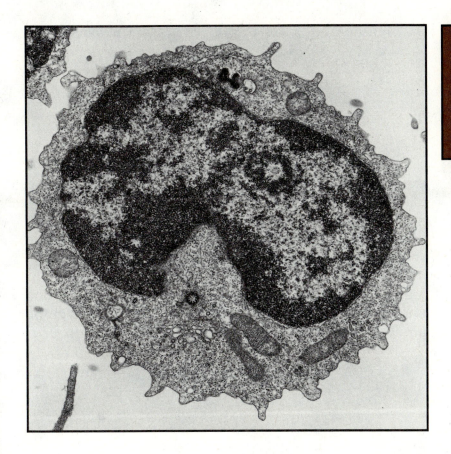

ORIGIN AND ORGANIZATION OF LYMPHOID TISSUE

SECTION

I

I must Create a System, or be enslaved by another Man's.

WILLIAM BLAKE

The cells carrying out specific immune functions are in the blood system. In the four chapters of Section I we will examine the origin of these cells in the bone marrow; follow their differentiation in the bone marrow and thymus; describe their organization in the secondary lymphoid organs, the spleen and lymph nodes; and examine some of their surface properties.

The basic understanding of the properties of the immune system cells covered in this section is crucial to the understanding of the nature of cellular interactions in the immune response, which will be covered in Section II.

HEMOPOIESIS

Overview The cells of the blood are constantly renewed during the life of an individual. The strategy that has evolved is one in which all the blood cells are derived from a very small number of multipotent cells called stem cells. Differentiation can be viewed as a series of binary "decisions" that a cell must make. Each decision closes off a large series of differentiative options, thus limiting the number of options left to the cell's progeny. The first decision of the stem cell is really one of life or death, because its options are either self-renewal or commencement of differentiation into a terminal end cell. This chapter will discuss the nature of the decision process, the concept of determination, and the nature of commitment. The reader should keep in mind that the rules of hemopoietic differentiation are only now beginning to be worked out. Even though we are ultimately concerned with lymphocytes, we will often use evidence from erythrocyte and neutrophil differentiation to make the general points.

CHAPTER

12

Hemopoiesis

The cells of the blood all have finite life spans and must be constantly renewed during the lifetime of the animal. When radiolabeled erythrocytes or neutrophils are injected into an animal, they disappear from the body. When the rate of disappearance is monitored, we see that the *proportion* of labeled cells gradually declines, but the *total* number of cells remains constant. This implies that there is a state of homeostasis in which the rate of production of new cells is equal to the decline of old cells. The different mature cell types each have characteristic life spans. The half-life of red cells, for example, is months, whereas granulocytes have half-lives of hours. The process of blood cell formation, called HEMOPOIESIS, is a differentiation process that must occur throughout the life of the animal.[1]

Hemopoiesis is of interest to us not only because the blood-forming system is physiologically important, but also because it provides a very good system for studying some of the fundamental problems of differentiation. One of these problems concerns the ability of a cell to give rise to progeny, each of which is committed to differentiate into a different kind of cell. The fertilized egg is the ultimate example of this; but the blood-forming system is a good one in which to study cellular differentiation because blood cell formation occurs constantly in the adult animal. The study of hemopoiesis has been facilitated by the fact that the blood-forming system is sensitive to X irradiation (e.g., a mouse exposed to approximately 800 rad will die in about 10 days because its blood-forming system has been destroyed).[2] But irradiated animals can be rescued with an injection of bone marrow cells (that is, by performing a bone marrow transplant), because the procedure leads to a repopulation of the entire blood-forming system. Repopulated animals have normal numbers of all the differentiated cells of the blood within a few days. Furthermore, the repopulated cells are of *donor* origin. This means that the cells of the injected bone marrow are able to reconstitute the entire hemopoietic system of the recipient.

How does this come about? We can imagine two possibilities. Either the bone marrow contains *separate* cell types able to differentiate into each of the various mature blood cell types, or there exists in bone marrow a *single* cell type that has the ability to give rise to all the different blood cells. This latter type of cell, one that can give rise to more than one type of cell and is self-renewing, is called a STEM CELL. We now know that the irradiated mice are repopulated with the progeny of multipotent hemopoietic stem cells, but the solution to the problem was only possible because of the development of clonal assays for stem cells and their progeny.

---

[1] *Hemo*, blood; *poiein*, to make. It is interesting that the word *poiesis* is also the root of the word *poetry*. To the Greeks, the poet was the maker of words. This common root may strike the reader's fancy in a later section when we discuss Niels Jerne's notion of the generative grammar of the immune system. We thank Professor Constance Jordan for pointing out the common origin to us.

[2] The rad is a unit of radiation; the unit of absorbed dose is equal to 0.01 joule/kg in any medium.

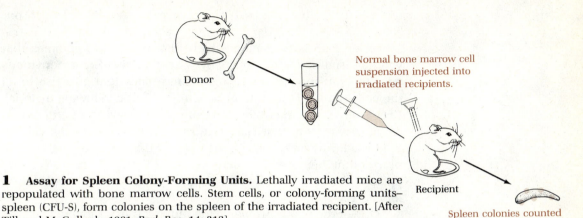

1 Assay for Spleen Colony-Forming Units. Lethally irradiated mice are repopulated with bone marrow cells. Stem cells, or colony-forming units–spleen (CFU-S), form colonies on the spleen of the irradiated recipient. [After Till and McCulloch, 1961. *Rad. Res.* 14: 213]

Normal bone marrow cell suspension injected into irradiated recipients.

Spleen colonies counted 7 to 10 days later.

Assay of Colony-Forming Units

An assay that allowed the problem of the origin of the cells of the blood to be studied experimentally was devised by Till and McCulloch in Toronto in 1961. In this assay (Figure 1) mice are lethally irradiated and repopulated by intravenous injection of a small number of bone marrow cells ($\sim 10^5$). When the spleens of these irradiated recipients are examined ten days later, discrete colonies can be seen on the spleen surface (Figure 2). The bone

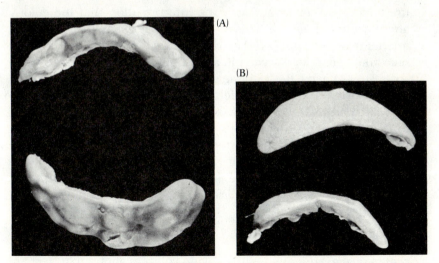

2 Spleen Colonies in the CFU-S Assay. (A) Two spleens from mice that received bone marrow show colonies. (B) Two spleens from uninjected controls. Note the single spontaneous colony on the upper control spleen.

marrow cells that give rise to these colonies are called COLONY FORMING UNITS, or CFUs. These are called COLONY-FORMING UNITS—SPLEEN or CFU-Ss to distinguish them from in vitro colonies that will be discussed later. For many years CFU-Ss were synonymous with the pluripotent hemopoietic stem cells that give rise to all the cells of the blood. But as we will see in the following material, CFU-Ss are multipotent, but do not meet the stringent criterion of being pluripotent, that is, they do not give rise to *all* the cells of the blood. However, even though the CFU-S is not the primordial pluripotent hemopoietic stem cell, the study of the CFU-S has opened the way for us to begin to study the earlier cell that is indeed the stem cell.

One of the major problems in studying the nature of the CFU-S is its extremely low frequency. In mouse bone marrow, for example, the frequency of the CFU-S is approximately 10^{-4}, or 1 CFU-S per 10,000 bone marrow cells. The rarity of this cell makes direct study extremely difficult, so experiments designed to determine whether the colony-forming cell is a stem cell (i.e., can give rise to multiple cell types and be self-renewing) were indirect.

Single-Cell Origin of Colonies

When bone marrow cells are injected into lethally irradiated mice as described above, the number of resultant spleen colonies is linearly related to the number of injected bone marrow cells (Figure 3). This is consistent with the interpretation that the colony arises from a single cell. This conclusion is strengthened by experiments using chromosome markers. The CBA/T6 mouse carries a naturally occurring karyotypic alteration (an altered chromosome structure). When CBA/T6 bone marrow cells are injected into irradiated normal CBA mice (which do not have the altered karyotype and are designated +/+), over 90% of the cells in each colony examined contain the marker. This result strongly suggests that the cells in a colony are derived from the T6 cells. In another experiment, various ratios of marked and unmarked cells were injected. When this was done, it was found that the proportion of colonies with marked cells varied with the proportion of injected marked cells.

Multipotency of the CFU-S

Cytological examination of the spleen colonies shows that they are composed of several types of blood cells. These include erythrocytes, granulocytes (also called neutrophils), monocytes, and

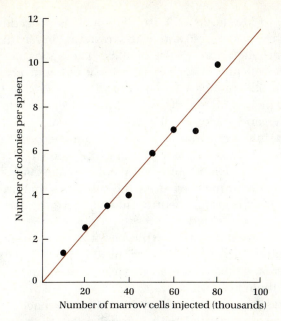

3 **Spleen Colonies from Injected Cells.** The relationship between the number of cells injected and the number of colonies. [After Till and McCulloch, 1961. *Rad. Res.* 14: 213]

megakaryocytes. The reader unfamiliar with blood cells may want to glance ahead at Figure 6 to get a feeling for the diversity of blood cell types. The fact that the colony is derived from a single cell and is composed of several cell types is the basis for the argument that a single cell type gives rise to different kinds of blood cells. In other words, the CFU-S appears to be a multipotent hemopoietic cell because it can give rise to multiple cell types. However, the direct test of this assertion is a difficult task. Also keep in mind that this kind of experiment does not address the question of self-renewal, the other requirement for a cell to be a multipotent stem cell.

The multipotency of the CFU-S has been tested in several ways, but the most convincing of the experiments uses *unique* and rare chromosome markers. The T6 marker discussed above is carried by every cell in the CBA/T6 mouse, so the colonies in the experiments showing 90% marker-bearing cells could conceivably have been formed by more than one marked cell. The use of unique markers would allow this problem to be overcome. Unique markers can be introduced at random in the cells of a mouse by subjecting the animal to low levels of X irradiation. This procedure causes breaks in chromosomes in some cells, resulting in rare and unique chromosome alterations. Most of these alterations are probably lethal to the cell, but an occasional cell has a unique chromosome pattern and still retains normal function. If such a rare marker were to occur in a stem cell, then all its progeny would have the same marker, and any cell in the colony that contained the marker almost certainly would be descended from the original marked cell. Therefore, the ideal test of the proposition that there is a multipotent hemopoietic stem cell would be to examine the cells in a colony to determine whether the cell types that are differentiating into erythroid and neutrophil cells have the same characteristic chromosome marker.

The experiment (Figure 4), while easy to conceive and describe, is very difficult to carry out for technical reasons. First of all, the number of marked cells is so low that they must first be enriched by growing them in a mutant mouse (called W/W^v) that is incapable of generating its own CFU-Ss.[3] Those W/W^v mice that can be shown to have been repopulated with marked cells are then used as a source of bone marrow cells for the experiment. The cells are injected into irradiated $+/+$ mice, and the spleen colonies of the recipients are examined 10 days later. If the CFU-S is in fact a multipotent stem cell that can give rise to both erythrocytes and neutrophils, then the cells differentiating into each of these types should have the marker. But now the second technical difficulty arises. It is not possible to do both a karyotype analysis to determine the presence of the marker and a histochemical analysis to determine cell type (erythrocyte, neutrophil) on the *same* cell. Therefore, many cells in the colony must be examined and the conclusion drawn from a statistical analysis of the data.

Typical data from this experiment are shown in Table 1. Because the same cell cannot be examined for both marker and function, the first information needed is the percentage of cells that do *not* have the marker. It is possible that two cells, one marked and one unmarked, could have lodged in the same place in the spleen and produced a colony that is actually composed of cells derived from both of them. The value in column 1 of Table 1 tells us the maximum percentage of cells in the colony that could not have come from the marked cell. Columns 2 and 3 of Table 1 give the percentage of cells in each colony that are differentiating

---

[3] Because of the very small numbers of cells involved, if these were injected into irradiated mice there would be insufficient numbers of stem cells to keep the mice alive. After expansion in the W/W^v the numbers are greatly increased.

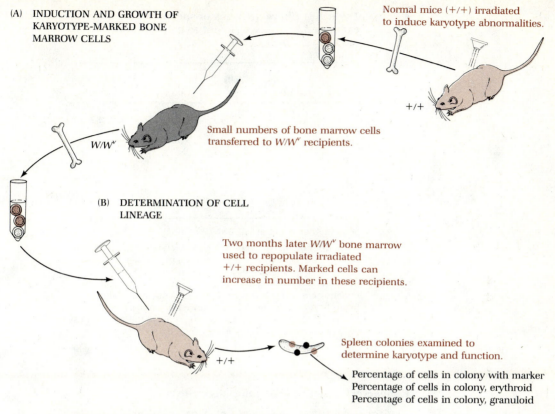

(A) INDUCTION AND GROWTH OF KARYOTYPE-MARKED BONE MARROW CELLS

Normal mice (+/+) irradiated to induce karyotype abnormalities.

+/+

Small numbers of bone marrow cells transferred to W/W^v recipients.

W/W^v

(B) DETERMINATION OF CELL LINEAGE

Two months later W/W^v bone marrow used to repopulate irradiated +/+ recipients. Marked cells can increase in number in these recipients.

+/+

Spleen colonies examined to determine karyotype and function.

Percentage of cells in colony with marker
Percentage of cells in colony, erythroid
Percentage of cells in colony, granuloid

4   Determination of Origin of Differentiating Cells. (A) Karyotypic markers are induced in normal bone marrow with X-rays. Bone marrow cells are expanded in W/W^v mice, and their bone marrow is used to repopulate +/+ mice. (B) Marked bone marrow is injected into +/+ mice; some cells from each colony are examined to determine whether the colony arose from a marked bone marrow cell (karyotype analysis). Cells from colonies with marked cells are tested for erythroid lineage (Fe incorporation) or granuloid lineage (presence of acid phosphatase). Because karyotype and function analyses cannot be carried out on the same cell, percentages of each are recorded from cells in the same colony. Typical results are shown in Table 1.

into erythrocytes and neutrophils. Now, if the percentage of cells differentiating along both lines is higher than the percentage of cells without the marker, it must mean that at least some of the marked cells had to give rise to *both* erythrocytes and granulocytes. Examination of the data in Table 1 shows that this is the result obtained. This experiment therefore shows that because some of the cells in the colony came from a common cell, the CFU-S is in fact a multipotent cell.

Table 1 Characteristics of spleen colonies examined in an experiment to determine the lineage of differentiating cells.[a]

Colony	Percentage of cells without markers	Percentage of granulocytes	Percentage of RBC
I	10	52	32
II	1	14	28
III	0	12	16
IV	2	12	12
V	0	20	16

Source: After Wu et al., 1976. *J. Cell Physiol.* 69: 177.

[a]Data from the experiment in Figure 4. The percentage of cells without the marker gives the maximum percentage of cells that could be in the colony from the host mouse (i.e., not the injected cells). Note that in each case the percentage of differentiating erythroid and granuloid cells is higher than the number of host cells in the colonies. Since the marker is so unique, this is a strong argument that at least some of these cells must have given rise to both kinds of differentiating cells.

Characterization of the Multipotent Stem Cell

In the early 1970s Dirk van Bekkum and Karl Dicke in the Netherlands began a series of experiments to isolate and characterize the stem cell. Using a combination of enrichment methods, they were able to achieve a significant enrichment of CFU-S. Their colleagues have since used antibodies and cell sorting to get even greater enrichment. Recently, the lab of Irving Weissman at Stanford has approached the problem using antibodies to differentiation markers and various clonogenic assays. We will discuss the Stanford group's data for didactic reasons.

The basis of these experiments is the ability to *negatively select* multipotent cells using monoclonal antibodies directed against differentiation markers. The concept of differentiation markers will be discussed in detail in the next chapter, but for now the reader should think of these as molecules expressed on the surface of some cells at certain times in differentiation. The reasoning behind these experiments is as follows: if differentiation markers appear on the surface of cells after they have become committed to differentiate along a cell lineage, by removing all cells that express differentiation markers for each of the lineages, one will be left with cells that do not express differentiation markers. This population should contain the cell that gave rise to all these committed cells, that is, the PRIMORDIAL PLURIPOTENT STEM CELL.

Using a panel of antibodies directed against markers on two kinds of lymphocytes (B cells and T cells; see Chapter 13), granulocytes, and monocytes, they treated bone marrow cells with monoclonal antibodies to each type of cell.[4] The cells that reacted with the antibodies were removed, leaving a population of cells that were B^-, T^-, G^-, M^- (corresponding to the lineages above), and were referred to as Lin^- (lineage marker-negative). When these cells were compared with unseparated bone marrow cells for their ability to form spleen colonies, it was found that it took only 10 of these cells to give a colony versus 7200 of the unseparated cells. This experiment is diagrammed in Figure 5.

In addition, the Stanford group was able to separate the Lin^- population into two groups according to expression of another marker. This marker was identified on several lineages of hemopoietic cells and was called Sca-1 (stem cell antigen-1) by Jan Klein and co-workers in Tübingen. When the Stanford group treated Lin^- cells with anti–Sca-1 antibody, they found that the portion of cells that were $Sca-1^+$ were enriched for multipotent cells. The fact that these cells were enriched in clonogenic assays that determine lymphoid and other progenitors showed that they met one of the criteria of the primordial pluripotent stem cell, that is, giving rise to all the blood cell lineages.

To determine if these cells met the second criterion, that is, that they also were self-renewing, they tested the ability of small numbers of the cells to grow and reproduce in animals (as determined by the ability of a small number of cells to keep an irradiated mouse alive for 30 days). As seen in Figure 5, it takes 30 Lin^- $Sca-1^+$ cells to keep 50% of the injected mice alive for 30 days. In contrast, it takes over 10^4 unenriched bone marrow cells to achieve the same result.

Taken together, these studies from Stanford and the Netherlands show that we are making progress toward isolating the primordial pluripotent hemopoietic stem cell. Methods for propagating the cells in vitro now await development. Some long-term bone marrow cultures allow the stem cell to grow in vitro, but other cells are needed in these cultures. So far the stem cell cannot

---

[4] The cells expressing the antigens that the antibodies react with will be referred to as B, T, G, and M.

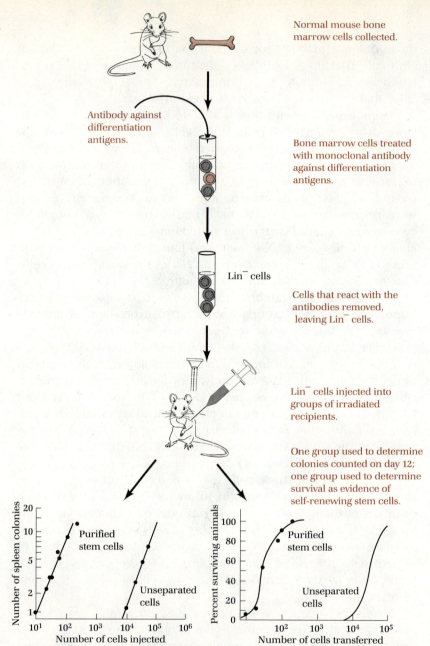

Normal mouse bone marrow cells collected.

Antibody against differentiation antigens.

Bone marrow cells treated with monoclonal antibody against differentiation antigens.

Lin⁻ cells

Cells that react with the antibodies removed, leaving Lin⁻ cells.

Lin⁻ cells injected into groups of irradiated recipients.

One group used to determine colonies counted on day 12; one group used to determine survival as evidence of self-renewing stem cells.

5   Purification of Stem Cells by Negative Selection. To enrich the hemopoietic stem cell, cells are treated with monoclonal antibodies against B cells, T cells, granulocytes and monocytes, and the reactive cells are removed. This leaves a (negatively selected) population of cells lacking any lineage-specific antigens; this population is called Lin⁻. When the Lin⁻ cells are injected into irradiated recipients (a Till-McCullogh assay), it can be seen that one colony is formed by 7200 unseparated bone marrow cells or by 10 enriched cells. [After Spangrude, Heimfeld and Weissman, 1988. *Science* 241: 58] be maintained free of these other cells in culture, and this offers an opportunity for a young investigator to make his or her reputation.

Proliferative Characteristics of the Hemopoietic Stem Cell

We will see that the cells derived from the stem cell are very sensitive to regulatory signals. The stem cells themselves, however, appear to be remarkably independent of these regulatory influences. The stem cell is a relatively quiescent cell with a very low rate of proliferation. This fact can be shown with "tritium suicide" experiments. In these experiments, tritiated thymidine of extremely high specific activity is added to cultures of cells. The proliferating cells incorporate the highly labeled precursors into their DNA, and the radioactive disintegrations damage the DNA and prevent further replication of the cell. This procedure only works if the cell is synthesizing DNA and therefore incorporating the labeled precursor. Suicide experiments have no effect on the stem cell, which shows that the cell is not actively dividing.[5] It replicates only often enough to maintain the normal physiological number.

SYNTHESIS
The Strategy of the Stem Cell

The stem cell as we have defined it faces two major problems. It must make cells like itself (self-renewal) and it must make different kinds of cells (differentiation). The experimental evidence shows that the differentiation process can happen quickly, but that the stem cell divides only infrequently. The problem appears to be solved by the very small number of primordial stem cells giving rise to cells that both rapidly proliferate and differentiate into all the cell types of the blood. In this manner the system is assured of large numbers of blood cells of all types under a wide range of physiological conditions.

This strategy is not unfamiliar to us; it is the same basic principle that we saw with antibody gene segments. In that case a small number of gene segments gives rise to a very large number of antibodies. In this case, a small number of stem cells gives rise to a large number of differentiating and therefore differentiated cells.

---

[5] The stem cells obtained from fetal liver, in contrast, are killed in the tritium suicide experiment and are thus actively proliferating cells.

Commitment and Differentiation

Normal homeostatic levels of mature blood cells are maintained by regulation of both the number of stem cells and the rate at which they give rise to progeny (which differentiate into the various cell types of the blood). Because the stem cell gives rise to all the mature cells, it and its progeny must have some mechanism for responding to changes in the body. This regulation involves obviously complex and delicate signal and feedback mechanisms of which, except for the red blood cell, we know very little.

At some point, the stem cells become ready to initiate the events of differentiation into more mature cells. This act is called DETERMINATION. How a cell is determined to follow certain lineages and not others is one of the central questions in biology. Once a determined cell actually starts the changes down the lineage pathway leading to a terminally differentiated cell, it is called a COMMITTED CELL. The pathways of differentiation in the blood are shown in Figure 6.

Cellular differentiation can be considered a process of choices by the cell.[6] It can be readily seen in Figure 6 that a cell can reach a certain point in its differentiation and still have several potential lineages to follow. By making a choice at such a branch point, the cell effectively closes off other potential lineages. Almost nothing is known about the decision-making process; it is widely (but not universally) agreed that it is *stochastic*, or random. But it is clear that in cellular differentiation, as in choosing a career or a lover, decisions made early in the process must be lived with for a long time. The cell's future is determined by its past.[7]

Differentiation of Stem Cells into Progenitor Cells

The earliest *committed* hemopoietic cells are called PROGENITOR cells. The frequency of these cells, which are now in an established

[6] The psychologist Steven Chorover has pointed out to us that by using the terms *choice* and *decision*, we seem to be attributing to the cell a level of consciousness. This is of course not the intent. The words are used by developmental biologists as a means of graphically describing the biochemical and molecular events that occur at a certain time. We feel that *why* the cell decides to do this might be its own business.

[7] We should point out here that there is another problem in differentiation, called morphogenesis. MORPHOGENESIS is the establishment of form and pattern, as in an embryo or a limb bud. In this process it seems quite certain that positional effects (i.e., the cell's location relative to other cells) is important. These two problems—cellular differentiation and morphogenesis—are usually treated as separate phenomena, but they may be variations on the same theme of lineage establishment.

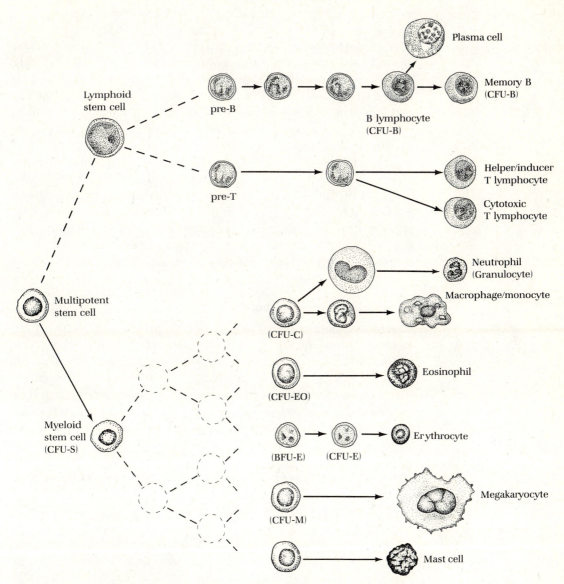

6   Hemopoietic Lineages. The path of lineage establishment of the hemopoietic system starts with the multipotent stem cell. The first lineages that are established are lymphoid and myeloid. In this version, differentiation is seen as a string of "branch point decisions." The dotted outlines indicate proliferation and decision events that are not able to be studied.

cell lineage, is about 10-fold higher than that of the stem cells (i.e., about 10^{-3}). Progenitor cells are assayed in vitro in soft agar. These assays take advantage of the dependence of the progenitor cells on certain growth factors (discussed below). Cytological examination of the colonies formed in agar in the presence of a given growth factor shows that they contain cells that are differentiating along one or a limited number of pathways. It is important to realize that these growth factors probably do not cause the cell to become determined; rather they induce a determined cell to undergo the changes of the differentiative pathway, that is, to become committed.

We assume that the process of becoming determined must result in the expression of receptors for the inducing molecule. Reaction of the inducing factor with the receptor then results in commitment and the initiation of the differentiation process. The strategy of producing many cells from the stem cell requires that a small number of cells carry the potential to become a large number of cells of many different types; so along with differentiation, there must also be proliferation.

Hemopoietic Inducing Factors

One of the most active areas of research involves the study of the factors that induce cells to differentiate and proliferate, since both normal function and cancerous growth are often controlled by these factors. Most of the known factors induce proliferation in many types of cells but induce differentiation in only a limited or specific subset of cells (Table 2). The picture will become more complicated as these studies progress because in some differentiating systems there is an inverse correlation between proliferation and differentiation, whereas in others the two are directly correlated. Identification of physiologically significant inducing and proliferation factors is very difficult because many molecules, some of which cannot possibly be used in normal physiological conditions, are able to induce both proliferation and differentiation. Some of the properties of the inducers are discussed in Box 1.

The mechanisms by which the various inducing molecules affect the cells are unknown, but an in vitro experiment has shown that the progenitor is sensitive to the *concentration* of one of the inducing molecules, granulocyte–macrophage colony-stimulating factor (GM-CSF). As seen in Figure 7, which summarizes an experiment done by Donald Metcalf in Australia, bone marrow cells

Table 2   Hemopoietic growth factors and their target cells.

Factor	Abbreviation	Target cells[a]
RELATIVELY MONOSPECIFIC FACTORS		
Granulocyte CSF	G-CSF	G (M)
Macrophage CSF	M-CSF (CSF-1)	M (G)
Erythropoietin	Epo	E (meg)
Interleukin-5	IL-5	Eo, B
RELATIVELY MULTISPECIFIC FACTORS		
Interleukin-3	IL-3	G, M, meg, mast, multi
Granulocyte-macrophage CSF	GM-CSF	G, M, Eo, meg, mast, multi

Source: From many sources, but see Metcalf, 1989. *Nature* 339: 27.

[a]G, granulocyte; M, macrophage; Eo, eosinophil; meg, megakaryocyte; mast, mast cell; multi, multipotent progenitor; B, B cell.

were cultured on soft agar in the presence of high (2500 units) or low (50 units) concentrations of GM-CSF. After 7 days, it was found that the low dose yielded almost exclusively monocyte colonies. In contrast, the high dose gave both granulocyte and monocyte colonies. To determine whether a single progenitor cell is sensitive to the concentration of GM-CSF or whether there are cells of two sensitivities in the progenitor cell population, the bone marrow cells were cultured in the presence of a high concentration of GM-CSF for 24 hours, after which the plates were examined and colonies containing two cells were identified and removed. The two daughter cells were placed in separate containers, one with a high and one with a low concentration of GM-CSF. Figure 7 shows that the daughter cells grown in low concentrations gave rise to monocytes and those grown in high concentrations gave rise either to mixed colonies of granulocytes and monocytes or to pure granulocyte colonies. This experiment indicates that the granulocyte–monocyte progenitor is indeed bipotential and that the choice of which differentiative pathway it will choose is a function of the concentration of the inducing agent.

Human Hemopoietic Growth/Inducing Factors

BOX
1

Granulocyte Colony-Stimulating Factor (G-CSF)

Originally purified from a human bladder carcinoma cell line, G-CSF has a molecular weight of 19,600. The G-CSF gene is located on chromosome 17, adjacent to a break point in the translocation of acute promyelocytic leukemia. It is produced by a variety of cells including monocytes, fibroblasts, and endothelial cells. These cells produce the factor after stimulation with a bacterial product (lipopolysaccharide) or cellular products (IL-1 or TNF; see Chapter 27), which suggests that it is produced in response to infection. The gene for the receptor has not yet been cloned, but it is estimated that, as is true of many growth factor receptors, the number of receptors per cell will be low. Cells in early granulocyte differentiation probably respond to G-CSF by proliferating, but mature granulocytes have increased superoxide formation in response to stimulation. Recombinant G-CSF is in clinical trials in several conditions of neutropenia and seems a very promising candidate for a therapeutic agent.

Erythropoietin (Epo)

Epo was first purified from the urine of patients with aplastic anemia. It is a glycoprotein with a molecular weight of 34,000. Epo is an extensively glycosylated molecule (~50% carbohydrate). The gene is located on chromosome 7 and has been cloned. The production of Epo is responsive to changes in oxygen tension. Epo is produced in the kidneys, but the cells that it acts on are located in the bone marrow, and there is a deficiency of Epo in renal disease. Epo has been one of the most successful therapeutic agents to come from biotechnology and is extensively used for treatment of the anemia seen in renal disease (above). The target cells on which Epo acts are not known with certainty, but both the mouse and human receptors have been cloned, so its mode of action should be able to be studied.

Macrophage Colony-Stimulating Factor (M-CSF, CSF-1)

M-CSF was first purified from urine and from the conditioned medium of a pancreatic carcinoma cell line. It is a homodimer with molecular weight 45,000 to 90,000. The gene is located on chromosome 5, adjacent to the genes for GM-CSF and IL-3. M-CSF is produced by monocytes, as is G-CSF, but the two factors appear to be under independent regulation. Interferon induces M-CSF but not G-CSF, whereas endotoxin induces G-CSF but not M-CSF. Fungal and mycobacterial infection are associated with T-cell stimulation (interferon) and bacterial infections with the release of endotoxin; this might explain why monocytes are found in the former and granulocytes in the latter.

Granulocyte-Macrophage Colony-Stimulating Factor (GM-CSF)

GM-CSF is a multipotent growth factor originally purified from a cell line derived from hairy cell leukemia. It is a glycoprotein of molecular weight 35,000, and a wide variety of cells produce it. The gene is on chromosome 5.

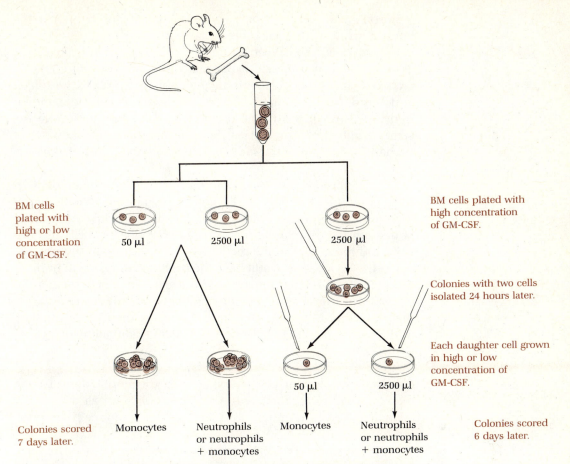

BM cells plated with high or low concentration of GM-CSF.

50 μl   2500 μl   2500 μl

BM cells plated with high concentration of GM-CSF.

Colonies with two cells isolated 24 hours later.

50 μl   2500 μl

Each daughter cell grown in high or low concentration of GM-CSF.

Colonies scored 7 days later.

Monocytes   Neutrophils or neutrophils + monocytes   Monocytes   Neutrophils or neutrophils + monocytes

Colonies scored 6 days later.

7   Effects of Concentration of Inducing Factor on Differentiation of Bone Marrow. Bone marrow (BM) cells are plated with either high or low concentrations of GM-CSF. On the left, bone marrow populations are used. On the right, individual colonies are examined. Low concentrations of GM-CSF result in monocytes; high levels result in neutrophils. [After Metcalf, 1980. *Proc. Natl. Acad. Sci. U.S.A.* 77: 5327]

Hemopoietic Inducing Microenvironments

Differentiation of myeloid cells such as erythrocytes and granulocytes from committed progenitors to mature end cells occurs primarily in the spleen and bone marrow. Because factors are needed to move the cells along the pathway of differentiation, we assume that these factors are found selectively in the sites of differentiation. With the exception of the thymus, as we will see in the next chapter, it has been very difficult to analyze the nature of the

HEMOPOIETIC INDUCING MICROENVIRONMENTS, or HIM. In the mouse the bone marrow produces more active granulocytes than erythrocytes, whereas the spleen gives rise to more erythrocytes than granulocytes. In a classic experiment in 1968, Wolf and Trentin grafted some bone marrow tissue into a discrete area of the spleen and found that the ratio of differentiating cell types was dependent upon the environment. The tissues could be shown to have the same number of progenitors, but the environment allowed (or perhaps more correctly, induced) the differentiation of one cell type.

The microenvironments supporting myeloid differentiation (Dexter cultures) and those supporting lymphoid differentiation (Whitlock-Witte cultures) have been cultured in vitro. As a result of this advance it may be possible to determine the cells responsible and the nature of the regulation they exert upon the progenitor cells. Of course, we still have the problem of the small number of stem cells and progenitors, and until someone devises a method for growing these cells in pure cultures, we must use indirect methods—mutant mice that have defects in their differentiation, or cloned tumor lines that mimic normal cells in some ways.

Mutant Mice and Cloned Tumor Lines

The low numbers of progenitor cells in the population of bone marrow cells make their study almost as difficult as that of the stem cell. However, mutant mice and cloned tumor cells are proving to be useful tools.

Mutant mice (Table 3) and certain disease states in humans have deficiencies that block differentiation in one or more of the progenitor cell types. By studying these blocks in differentiation, we can learn something about the normal process. The power of this type of analysis, using "experiments of nature," will be discussed in the section on human immunodeficiency diseases. The final proof of our understanding of the process of hemopoiesis will be our ability to cure the deficient state.

Work on the whole organism presents problems that in vitro studies do not have, and for the short term we will probably learn more about cellular differentiation by studying tumor cells in vitro. Many cultured tumor cells have been "trapped" at a certain state of differentiation but can still be induced to continue their differentiative pathway. Because tumor cells are able to grow clonally in the test tube, studies of homogeneous populations of cells are possible. However, experimenters must be aware of the possibility

Table 3   Some mouse mutants of hemopoietic development.

Mutation	Chromosomal location	Phenotype
HEMOPOIETIC SYSTEM		
W series (*W*)	5	Anemia due to intrinsic hemopoietic stem cell defect Pleiotropic effect on germ and pigment cells
Steel series (*Sl*)	10	Anemia due to defect in hemopoietic microenvironment Pleiotropic effect on germ and pigment cells
Hertwig's anemia (*an*)	4	Anemia due to intrinsic hemopoietic stem cell defect Germ-cell defect
ERYTHROID DEVELOPMENT		
Flexed-tail (*f*)	13	Hypochromic, microcytic anemia
Diminutive (*dm*)	2	Macrocytic anemia
Tail-short (*Ts*)	11	Prenatal anemia due to deficiency of blood islands in yolk sac
Sex-linked anemia (*sla*)	X	Hypochromic animals due to deficient intestinal iron transport
Jaundiced (*ja*)	—	Microcytic anemia
Hemolytic anemia (*ha*)	—	Neonatal hypochromic anemia, microcytosis; sterile
Spehocytosis (*sph*)	—	Hemolytic anemia
Microcytic anemia (*mk*)	15	Microcytic anemia due to defect in iron uptake from intestinal lumen to mucosa and plasma to erythroblasts
GRANULOCYTE DEVELOPMENT		
Beige (*bg*)	13	PMN granule defect; resembles Chediak-Higashi disease
Edematous (*oed*)	—	Increased granulocyte number
MACROPHAGE DEVELOPMENT		
Hepatitis virus susceptibility (*Hv*)	—	Resistance or susceptibility to hepatitis virus, associated with macrophage function
Myxovirus resistance (*mv*)	—	Resistance to infection with myxovirus, associated with macrophages
Tolerance to HGG (*Tol-1*)	—	Ease of immune tolerance induction, associated with macrophages
PLATELET DEVELOPMENT		
Beige (*bg*)	13	Serotonin granule defect
LYMPHOCYTE DEVELOPMENT		
Lipopolysaccharide response (*Lps*)	—	B-cell defect in mitogen response to lipopolysaccharide
X-linked immunodeficiency (*xid*)	—	B-cell response defect

of merely exchanging artifacts, because they are studying a regulatory process in a cell that, because it is a tumor, by definition has lost a significant part of its regulatory ability. Even with this caveat, however, to date a great deal has been learned about normal cell processes by studying cloned tumor cells.

Summary

1.   Hemopoiesis is the study of blood cell formation. All the cells of the blood are constantly being renewed in the adult animal and are derived from multipotent hemopoietic stem cells.

2.   The primordial stem cell gives rise to the colony-forming unit–spleen (CFU-S). Each colony is derived from a single cell. Spleen colonies contain several kinds of blood cells. Because each colony is derived from a single cell but contains different kinds of cells, we conclude that a single cell can give rise to several cell types.

3.   The process during which the stem cell establishes the lineage that it will follow during differentiation is called determination. Once a cell begins to differentiate along a pathway, it is called a committed cell. The earliest committed cells are called progenitor cells.

4.   A variety of inducing molecules, some of which are specific for a given lineage, have been identified.

Additional Readings

Burgess, A. and N. Nicola. 1983. *Growth Factors and Stem Cells*. Academic, Sydney.

Dexter, T. M., T. D. Allen and L. G. Lajtha. 1977. Conditions controlling the proliferation of hemopoietic stem cells *in vitro*. *Cell Physiol.* 91: 335.

Golub, E. S. 1982. In vitro approaches to hemopoiesis. *Cell* 28: 687.

Hall, A. K. 1983. Stem cell is a stem cell is a stem cell. *Cell* 33: 11.

Metcalf, D. 1984. *Clonal Culture of Hemopoietic Cells: Techniques and Application*. Elsevier, Amsterdam.

Metcalf, D. 1989. The molecular control of cell division, differentiation, commitment, and maturation in hemopoietic cells. *Nature* 339: 27.

Schrader, J. W. 1984. Bone marrow differentiation in vitro. *C.R.C. Crit. Rev. Immunol.* 4: 197.

Spangrude, G. J., S. Heimfeld and I. L. Weissman. 1988. Purification and characterization of mouse hematopoietic stem cells. *Science* 241: 58.

Visser, J. W. M. and P. de Vries. 1988. Isolation of spleen-colony forming cells (CFU-S) using wheat germ agglutinin and rhodamine-123 labeling. *Blood Cells* 14: 369.

Visser, J. W. M., J. G. J. Bauman, A. H. Mulder, J. F. Eliason and A. M. de Leeuw. 1984. Isolation of murine pluripotent hemopoietic stem cells. *J. Exp. Med.* 59: 1576.

Whitlock, N. A. and O. N. Witte. 1982. Long-term culture of B lymphocytes and their precursors from murine bone marrow. *Proc. Natl. Acad. Sci. U.S.A.* 79: 3608.

DIFFERENTIATION OF LYMPHOCYTES

Overview   Cellular immunology is essentially the study of the biology of lymphocytes, their interactions, and their products. In the last chapter we discussed the evidence for the multipotency of the hemopoietic stem cell and mentioned that lymphocytes are derived from this cell. In this chapter we will give some further data for that claim. We will also show that the lymphocytes differentiate in two distinct hemopoietic microenvironments, the thymus and the bone marrow, and that this leads to two very distinct functional kinds of lymphocytes: T cells and B cells. Since these cells cannot be distinguished by their morphology, we will discuss some of the surface properties, responses to mitogens, and, ultimately, functions that distinguish them.

This chapter, in addition to developing the evidence for the two paths of differentiation of lymphoid progenitor cells, will also describe and catalog many of the traits of the lymphocytes. This material will help the reader to understand the experiments that show how the cells in the immune response interact, the topic of much of this section.

Origin of Lymphocytes

Derivation of Lymphocytes from the Multipotent Stem Cell

Evidence that the lymphocytes are derived from multipotent stem cells comes from experiments very similar to those that showed that myeloid cells come from the CFU-S (Chapter 12). In the experiment diagrammed in Figure 1, unique chromosome markers were induced in +/+ mice by X irradiation and the bone marrow cells passaged into W/W^v mutant mice so that the number of cells with karyotype alterations could be increased. After several months the bone marrow and two organs known to contain lymphocytes—the thymus and the spleen—were removed from the W/W^v mice,

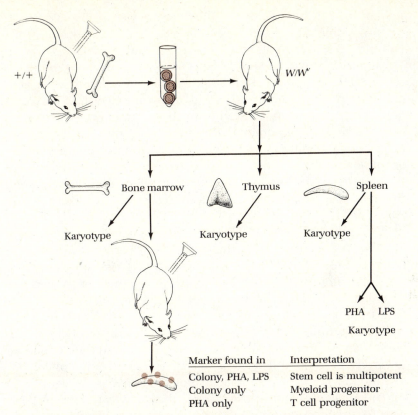

Karyotype marker induced in +/+ and grown in W/W^v.

Presence of marker established in lymphoid organs.

Presence of marker established in CFU-S and B and T cells.

Marker found in	Interpretation
Colony, PHA, LPS	Stem cell is multipotent
Colony only	Myeloid progenitor
PHA only	T cell progenitor

1   Determining the Common Lymphoid Progenitor. Karyotypic markers are introduced by X irradiation, and marked cells are expanded in W/W^v hosts. Bone marrow cells are injected into irradiated +/+ mice, and colonies are examined. Thymus cells and spleen cells are tested for karyotype, and spleen cells are tested for B cells and T cells by lipopolysaccharide (LPS) and phytohemagglutin (PHA). [After Abramson et al., 1971. *J. Exp. Med.* 145: 1567]

and those mice with a high percentage of cells carrying a unique chromosome marker were analyzed further. The bone marrow cells from these animals were injected into irradiated +/+ mice to ascertain whether the CFU-S had the marked cells. The spleen cells were treated with reagents that stimulate lymphocytes to enter mitosis (these will be discussed in detail later in this chapter), and the cells of the spleen and thymus were examined for the chromosome marker. In this way the presence of the marker in the CFU-S as well as in lymphocytes from the spleen and thymus could be correlated.

Three marker patterns were obtained: some mice had the

marker in both the CFU-S and the lymphocytes in the spleen and thymus; some had the marker in the myeloid cells but not in the lymphocytes; and some had the marker only in the lymphocytes. These results show several things. First, even though lymphocytes are not found in the spleen colonies, the multipotent stem cells give rise to lymphocytes as well as to myeloid cells. The second important thing to be learned from this experiment is that at an early stage of differentiation there are progenitor cells that are determined to differentiate along myeloid or lymphoid lineages (recall Figure 6 of Chapter 12). This experiment argues that one of the first "decisions" made in hemopoietic differentiation is between the lymphoid and the myeloid pathways.

Primary and Secondary Lymphoid Organs

We saw in the last chapter that myeloid differentiation occurs in hemopoietic inducing microenvironments (HIMs), sites in which the progenitor cells are acted upon by specific inducing molecules. The differentiation of lymphocytes also occurs in HIMs, in this case the bone marrow and the thymus. The thymus is an organ whose sole function appears to be lymphoid differentiation. The bone marrow, in contrast, is also a site of myeloid differentiation. In birds the bursa of Fabricius is a discrete site of lymphoid differentiation, and the mammalian bone marrow is thought of as the "bursal equivalent." Sites of differentiation of lymphoid progenitors to lymphocytes are called the PRIMARY LYMPHOID ORGANS.

After the lymphoid progenitor cells differentiate in the primary lymphoid organs, they migrate to such peripheral sites as the spleen and lymph nodes, which are called the SECONDARY LYMPHOID ORGANS. Figure 2 shows the locations of the primary and secondary lymphoid tissues. In Chapter 14 we will discuss the traffic of lymphocytes from the primary to the secondary organs and through the lymphatics, as well as the anatomy of the lymphoid organs.

Lymphocytes are the cells that carry out the immune function. However, very few of the lymphocytes in the bone marrow and thymus are functional. In contrast, the cells that are exported from these organs to the secondary lymphoid tissues are fully differentiated and functional. In addition, the ability of the thymus-derived lymphocytes to discriminate self from nonself—one of the most important functions of the immune system—is acquired during differentiation in the thymus.

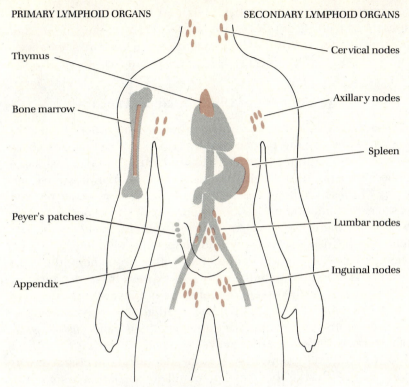

PRIMARY LYMPHOID ORGANS   SECONDARY LYMPHOID ORGANS

Thymus

Bone marrow

Peyer's patches

Appendix

Cervical nodes

Axillary nodes

Spleen

Lumbar nodes

Inguinal nodes

2   Location of Human Lymphoid Tissue.

B Cells and T Cells

The lymphocytes that differentiate in the bone marrow and the thymus are called B cells and T cells, respectively. B cells and T cells have similar morphology but differ in many fundamental ways.[1] The most important difference between them is functional. B cells are antibody-forming cells while T cells are not. But T cells act as helper cells, and as effector cells in cell-mediated responses. Thus the progeny of the cells that differentiate in each of the inducing microenvironments divide the labor of the immune

---

[1] To illustrate the lack of morphological difference between the cells, the late Richard Gershon would often begin a talk about functional subsets of T cells by showing a slide of a lymphocyte, which he told the audience was a helper T cell. After describing it, he would flash up another slide of the *same* cell, which he would call a cytotoxic T cell. He would then give the same description he had given for the previous slide. The audience quickly got the message: one cannot tell by sight alone what the function of the cell will be.

response (Chapter 16). Both B cells and the different functional subsets of T cells can also be distinguished by markers expressed on their surfaces and by their responses to certain substances, called mitogens, that induce cells to enter mitosis.

The Concept of Differentiation Markers

T cells and B cells can be distinguished by their totally different functions, but in the course of differentiation they acquire other sets of distinguishing characteristics, which in many cases seem to be independent of the cell's function. As we mentioned earlier, many of these characteristics are molecules expressed at the cell surface, and antibodies can be raised against them. Because antibodies are highly specific, they become potent, specific reagents that can be used to identify and detect the characteristic cell-surface markers. Used in conjunction with complement, they can also be used to eliminate the cells that express these markers.

Furthermore, the expression of some of these surface markers correlates with the stage of differentiation of the lymphocytes. Because of this correlation, they are sometimes called DIFFERENTIATION MARKERS. Differentiation markers on lymphocytes have proved to be exceptionally powerful tools for identification, characterization, and analysis. The concept of differentiation markers was derived from studies on lymphocytes by Lloyd Old and Edward Boyse at Sloan-Kettering in New York, but the idea has much greater applicability. We know, for example, that the developing embryo has stage-specific markers, and many other developing systems are being studied by utilizing the unique markers at certain stages of differentiation.

Differentiation Markers

In the bone marrow, the common lymphoid progenitor cell gives rise to progeny, called pre-T and pre-B cells, which then undergo differentiation in the proper microenvironment to become T cells or B cells. B-cell differentiation, as we said, occurs in the bone marrow. The fact that the stem cells, lymphoid progenitors, pre-B cells, and pre-T cells all are found in the bone marrow makes the study of B-cell differentiation rather difficult. In addition, myeloid progenitors are found in the bone marrow, and myeloid differentiation is going on in the same tissue. The study of T-cell differentiation, while not a walk in the park, is easier because the thymus is a discrete inducing microenvironment.

Pre-T cells leave the bone marrow and enter the thymus via the blood. In the thymus they begin to undergo differentiation and express differentiation markers that are characteristic of T cells. These markers are molecules not normally expressed on stem cells or pre-T cells.

Clusters of Differentiation

In humans we obviously cannot take advantage of any potential allelic differences in the differentiation markers by raising alloantisera.[2] For many years this made the task of identifying differentiation markers in humans very difficult. The advent of monoclonal antibodies, however, changed all that. In fact, we now know more about the surface markers at different stages of differentiation in humans than we do in the mouse.

As monoclonal antibodies against human T cell markers were generated, these were quite naturally named by each investigator as he or she produced them. Because several workers independently produced monoclonal antibody against the same determinant, a plethora of designations sprang up before it was possible to compare the specificities of the antibodies with each other. Manufacturers of these antibodies were reluctant to change their designation even after it was known that two or three separately designated antibodies were identifying the same marker. By common agreement the designation "T" followed by a number was adopted by many investigators. Thus, for example, we may see in the literature reference to T4 or T8 markers on human T cells.

In 1982 the First International Workshop on Human Leukocyte Differentiation Antigens was held in Paris. At that meeting 139 monoclonal antibodies were tested by immunofluorescence, and the antibodies were grouped into "clusters" on the basis of the results. At the Fifth International Congress of Immunology held in Kyoto, Japan in 1983, the Nomenclature Subcommittee officially adopted this scheme of nomenclature. The idea of the CLUSTER OF DIFFERENTIATION (CD) was to group all known antibodies that reacted with the same marker. From then on any investigator who pro-

---

[2] The antiserum that results after an antigen from one member of a species is injected into another member of the *same* species is called an ALLOANTISERUM, and the antigen is an ALLOANTIGEN. An antigen from one species injected into a member of a *different* species is called a XENOANTIGEN, and the antiserum is called a XENOANTISERUM. When tissue from an individual or inbred strain is injected into the *same* individual or member of the same strain, the antigen is called an ISOANTIGEN, and the antibody, if there should be one, is called an ISOANTIBODY. These terms will appear again in the chapter on transplantation.

duced a new monoclonal antibody against a human cell population could determine into which cluster group it fell or if it defined a new marker. Appendix 2 gives the CD grouping of human cells. As often as possible in this book we will use the CD designation. CD designations extend across species boundaries. When, for example, a mouse marker has been found to be homologous to a particular human marker, both markers receive the same CD designation.

Some Commonly Studied Differentiation Markers

Thy-1　The first T-cell differentiation marker was discovered in the mouse by Reiff and Allen, who found that all strains had an antigen on their thymic lymphocytes. This antigen was called *theta* (θ) and has been of great importance in experimental studies using mice. The name was later changed to THY-1. It was soon shown that in all mouse strains Thy-1 is not expressed on cells of the bone marrow, but it appears when pre-T cells differentiate into T cells in the thymus. Furthermore, it was soon shown that in the mouse Thy-1 continues to be expressed when the T cells leave the thymus and become part of the secondary lymphoid tissue (spleen and lymph nodes, see page 216).

Having a marker for cells of thymic origin allowed cellular immunologists to begin to dissect the cell interactions leading to an immune response. But Thy-1 was also found to be on other tissues of the mouse. For example, the brain is rich in Thy-1, and it is found on fibroblasts as well. Nevertheless, in the mouse it has been an invaluable marker for peripheral T cells.

In contrast, in humans Thy-1 is found on both early T cells and early B cells, as well as in the kidney and the brain but not on peripheral T cells. It clearly cannot serve as a marker for thymic-derived lymphocytes in humans. The rat has an expression pattern closer to that of the human than that of the mouse. In fact, Thy-1 expression in the brain tissue seems to be its most common feature among species, and, not surprisingly, anti-brain antiserum has anti-Thy-1 activity and was used as a source of this antiserum before the advent of monoclonal antibodies.

It has been possible to create transgenic mice that contain the human gene for Thy-1. These animals express the human gene in kidney cells. The cells expressing Thy-1 in an inappropriate site for the mouse become malignantly transformed, suggesting that Thy-1 may be a regulator of proliferation.

CD4 and CD8   We said above that Thy-1 was an important tool in the initial understanding of cellular interactions in the immune response in the mouse but not in humans. In contrast, two differentiation markers called CD4 and CD8 found in mouse, human, and other species have been crucial. Until quite recently human CD4 was called T4 and Leu3 and mouse CD4 was called L3T4. CD8 was called T8 and Leu2 in humans and Lyt2 in the mouse. They now are called CD4 and CD8 in all species (see the discussion of CDs above) and are probably the most common differentiation markers in experimental studies.

The reader will soon find that CD4 and CD8 are at the very heart of modern cellular immunology. In the chapters on cellular immunology, we will develop in great detail the facts that the subset of T cells that expresses CD4 is involved in class II MHC-restricted responses, and that the CD8 population is involved in class I MHC restriction.[3] CD4 has also been found to be the receptor for the AIDS virus.

Both CD4 and CD8 are members of the IG SUPERFAMILY. *CD4* is a 55-kilodalton (kd) glycoprotein consisting of a 372-amino acid extracellular domain composed of four tandem Ig-like VJ regions. There is a 23-amino acid transmembrane domain and a 38-amino acid cytoplasmic domain. The first VJ-like domain (V1) shares about 35% homology with κ L-chain V regions and is likely to fold in a manner analogous to an Ig V region.

Murine *CD8* exists as a *heterodimer* of two disulfide-linked subunits, α (38 kd) and β (30 kd). The human CD8 is composed of *homomultimers* of a single 34-kd subunit, the human homolog of the murine α subunit.

Induction of Lymphocyte Differentiation

Induction of T-Cell Differentiation

It is not known what cells in the thymus are responsible for causing the induction of lymphocyte differentiation in that organ. Epithelial cells, macrophages, and perhaps even the lymphocytes themselves may all play a role. Several soluble factors have been described, all of which are able to convert pre-T cells from the bone marrow into cells with surface markers associated with thy-

---

[3] This sentence may sound like complete nonsense but it will soon become a litany to the student of immunology. For the moment however, don't even worry about the MHC.

mic lymphocytes. Some of the factors are also able to induce functional differentiation. As in myeloid differentiation, it is assumed that the determined cell (in this case the pre-T cell) is expressing receptors for the proper inducing molecule.

THYMOSIN was the first of the factors to be described and was originally obtained from extracts of bovine thymus. Thymosin is actually a collection of molecules with different functions. One of these, thymosin fraction 5, causes the expression of Thy-1 on murine pre-T cells. It is a protein of molecular weight 12,000.

Another factor, THYMOPOIETIN, is a protein of molecular weight 7000 and induces the production of some differentiation markers. Fractionation of thymopoietin has produced a 12-amino acid peptide that contains the inducing activity. This peptide has been synthesized in vitro, which led to the discovery that the NH_2-terminal pentapeptide contains all the inducing activity.

THYMIC HUMORAL FACTOR (facteur humoral thymique) is a peptide that has both differentiation marker-inducing activity and, under appropriate conditions, function-inducing activity.

It is not known whether one of these molecules is the physiological inducing molecule in the thymus. Other candidates for factors having a possible role in thymic differentiation are IL-1, IL-2, IL-6, and IL-7. More information on these well characterized molecules will be provided in Chapter 27. The reader must be aware of the fact that just because a molecule is well characterized does not necessarily mean that its role has been defined, and we still know precious little about the physiologically important molecules involved in T-cell differentiation.

Induction of B-Cell Differentiation

As we stated earlier, there is no unique anatomical site for B-cell differentiation in mammals. In contrast, in the chicken, B cells develop in the bursa of Fabricius. The mammalian "bursal equivalent" seems to be distributed in the bone marrow, and it is reasonable to assume that there are epithelial and reticular cells in the bone marrow secreting molecules that induce the differentiation of the pre-B cells into functional B cells. Studying B-cell differentiation in mammals is difficult because of this lack of a discrete site, but in the last few years several growth factors have been associated with B-cell differentiation. These will be discussed in Chapter 27.

Mitogen Responses of T Cells and B Cells

B cells and T cells also differ rather dramatically in their responses to agents that induce cell proliferation. These substances are called MITOGENS because they induce the cells to enter mitosis. Because mitosis involves the synthesis of new DNA, the ability of an agent to act as a mitogen can easily be determined by adding tritiated thymidine to cultures of cells and quantifying the amount of the isotope incorporated into the newly synthesized DNA. When this is done with a wide array of agents, we find that some agents preferentially induce B cells and some induce T cells. Table 1 gives some of the more common B-cell and T-cell mitogens.

This peculiar property allows us to distinguish between cell populations, but as we will see in later chapters, mitogens are also of interest because they can act as surrogates for antigens. Such surrogates are useful because the frequency of any given antigen-specific cell is very low (about 10^{-6}). Because antigen will induce

Table 1   Some B and T cell mitogens

Mitogen	Inhibitor	Cell
Phytohemagglutinin (PHA)	N-acetyl-D-galactosamine	T cells (human and mouse)
Concanavalin A (ConA)	α-D-gluco and mannopyranosides	T cells (human and mouse); B cells if cross linked
Waxbean	—	T cells (human)
Pokeweed mitogen (PWM)	Di-N-acetylchitobiose	T and B (human and mouse but Pa-1 subunit acts only on B cells)
Lipopolysaccharide (LPS)	—	B cells (mouse, not human)
Aggregated tuberculin	—	B cells
Sodium periodate-reducing agents such as sodium borohydride (NaBH₄)	—	B cells
Dextran sulfate	—	Subset of B cells
Dextran polyvinylpyrrolidone	—	B cells
Trypsin, chymotrypsin	Leupeptin	B cells

such a small number of cells, it is often useful to study lymphocyte activation by mitogens, which induce large numbers of the cells with which they react to proliferate.

Summary

1.   Lymphocytes are derived from the pluripotent hemopoietic stem cell in the bone marrow. The lymphoid progenitor cells then undergo differentiation in either the thymus (for T cells) or the bone marrow (for B cells).

2.   As lymphocytes differentiate, they express markers that are restricted to either their stage of differentiation or their lineage. These are sometimes called differentiation markers.

3.   Differentiation markers are now identified as clusters of differentiation (CDs). Two of the most important of these on T cells are CD4 and CD8.

4.   Cells undergo differentiation in the thymus under the influence of the thymic epithelium and stromal cells. B cells differentiate in the bone marrow, which is the mammalian equivalent of the bursa in birds.

5.   B cells and T cells can be induced to proliferate by a variety of compounds called mitogens.

Additional Readings

Boyse, E. A. and L. J. Old. 1969. Some aspects of normal and abnormal surface genetics. *Annu. Rev. Genet.* 3: 269.

Fitch, F. W. 1986. Surface antigens on murine T cells. *Microbiol. Rev.* 50: 50.

Littman, D. R. 1987. The structure of the CD4 and CD8 genes. *Annu. Rev. Immunol.* 5: 561.

Scollay, R. and K. Shortman. 1983. Thymocyte subpopulations: An experimental review, including flow cytometry cross-correlations between the major murine thymocyte markers. *Thymus* 5: 245.

ORGANIZATION AND STRUCTURE OF LYMPHOID TISSUE

Overview We have learned that the cells of the immune system —lymphocytes and macrophages—arise from a common stem cell and undergo differentiation in specialized areas called hemopoietic inducing microenvironments. In addition, we have learned that the lymphocytes, both B cells and T cells, arise in the primary lymphoid organs, the bone marrow and the thymus, and are then exported to the secondary lymphoid organs, the spleen and the lymph nodes.

In this chapter we will examine the structure of the primary and secondary lymphoid organs and the circulation pattern of the lymphocytes. We will see that the lymphocytes circulate throughout the body by passing between the blood and lymphatic vascular systems. The passage points are at the lymph nodes, which are accumulations of lymphoid cells with an organized structure. At the point where a venule enters a lymph node, there is a specialized endothelium, called the high endothelial venule; lymphocytes have receptors for this structure. As the B and T lymphocytes enter the nodes and the spleen, they move to discrete areas of the organs.

Structure of Lymphoid Organs

Thymus

The thymus is a primary lymphatic organ. In humans it is located in the superior mediastinum, dorsal to the sternum. It is a bilaterally symmetrical organ divided into two LOBES. Each of the lobes is organized into broad, triangular LOBULES by connective tissue SEPTA that are continuous with the CAPSULE. The blood and lymphatic vessels run through the septa.

Lymphocytes and epithelial cells are the principal cells of the thymus. The lymphocytes are arranged in the lobules, forming a peripheral zone called the CORTEX and a central zone called the MEDULLA (Figure 1). Most proliferating lymphocytes in the thymus are found in the cortex. Although the medulla contains lymphocytes, it is relatively richer in epithelial cells than is the cortex. In addition, the medulla contains unique structures called HASSALL'S CORPUSCLES, which are concentric rings of tightly wound epithelial cells of unknown function. These are seen in Figure 2.

The thymus has no afferent lymphatic supply. Blood reaches the organ through branches of the subclavian artery that enter at

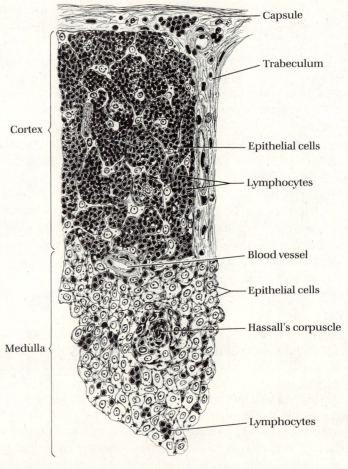

1 **Lobule of the Thymus.** A portion of a lobule in the human thymus. The cortex is rich in lymphocytes; the medulla is rich in epithelial cells; and the capsule and trabecula are rich in connective tissue and blood vessels. [From Weiss, 1972. *The Cells and Tissues of the Immune System*]

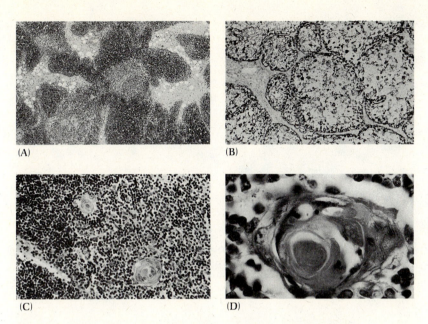

(A)

(B)

(C)

(D)

2 **Human Thymus.** (A) Sharp distinction between cortex (*dark areas*) and medulla. H&E stain ×400. (B) Epithelial cells stained with anti-cytokeratin B monoclonal antibody (*dark cells*). Immunoperoxidase stain ×100. (C) Cortico-medullary junction with two Hassall's bodies in the medulla. H&E stain ×250. (D) Hassall's body. H&E stain ×1000. [Courtesy of C. Baroni]

the medulla through the septa. The cortex is supplied by arterioles at the junction between the medulla and the cortex. The thymus connects to the lymphatic system by lymphatic vessels, which leave the medulla and drain into the mediastinal lymph nodes. Thus the traffic of pre-T cells to the thymus is via the blood, and the differentiated T cells leave through the efferent lymphatics or the venous drainage by the medullary vein. Lymphocytes can recirculate back into the thymus from the blood. Some factors involved in lymphocyte traffic will be discussed later in this chapter.

The thymus is large at birth and reaches its maximum size (~40 g in humans) at puberty, after which it begins to atrophy. As an animal ages, the parenchyma is replaced by fatty and fibrous tissue, but the organ remains functional (Figure 3). We will see that this is true because only a small percentage of cells in the thymus are functional; as the organ atrophies, the percentage of functional cells increases.

Cortical and Medullary Thymocytes The lymphocytes in the thy-

(A)   (B)

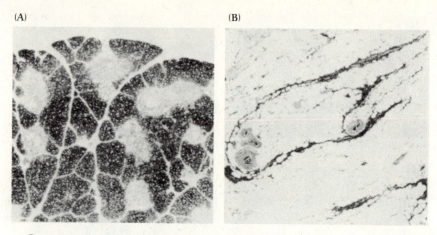

3 **Thymus Before and After Involution.** (A) Tissue from a 3-month-old human infant. (B) Tissue from a 72-year-old adult. The lobular pattern in the young thymus is not seen in the involuted adult thymus, which is filled with fat and fibrous tissue (×25). [From Weiss, 1983. *Histology: Cell and Tissue Biology*]

mus are distributed in both the cortex and the medulla. One of the enduring mysteries about the thymus concerns the fact that the vast majority of thymocytes (thymic lymphocytes) die in the thymus—only about 1% of the cells per day are exported to the periphery. The reason, if any, for the large, apparently nonfunctional population is not known, but the bulk of the literature shows that it is the cells in the medulla that are the maturing population destined to be exported to the peripheral tissues. Cortical and medullary populations differ in levels of MHC molecules (see next chapter) and other important cell-surface molecules, as well as in their ability to be agglutinated by the lectin peanut agglutinin (PNA). The most striking, and probably the most important, distribution of cells in the thymus is the distribution of $CD4^+$ and $CD8^+$ cells (Table 1). It appears from this distribution that the medullary cells are the "mature" cells and the cortical cells are "immature." One clue to the nature of the cells in the thymus comes from the following experiment. When a mouse is injected with cortisone, over 90% of its thymocytes die. The remaining cells, the CORTISONE-RESISTANT THYMOCYTES, or CRTs, are medullary cells. So we have come to equate the maturing functional cells with CRTs. In fact, when thymus cells are used in a variety of immunologic reactions, they show very low reactivity. But after cortisone treatment, all the immunologic activity of the thymus resides in the CRTs.

Table **1**   Distribution of CD4 and CD8 cells in the thymus.

CD4 profile	Percentage in thymus	Location
$CD4^+ CD8^+$ (double positives)	80–85	Majority in cortex
$CD4^- CD8^-$ (double negatives)	1–2	Under capsule of outer cortex
$CD4^+ CD8^-$ $CD4^- CD8^+$	10–15	Mostly in medulla

The generally held view of maturation in the thymus can be summarized as follows: cells enter as cortical cells, most of which die before maturing. A small number become medullary cells, acquire immunologic function, and are exported to the peripheral lymphoid tissue. It must be noted, however, that there is some evidence that this may be an oversimplification, and that a small subpopulation of cortical thymocytes also become functional cells and are exported without ever entering the medulla.

The Spleen

The spleen is the secondary lymphoid tissue used most often in cellular immunology experiments. It is a fascinating organ that has many functions other than those of the immune response. A fine description of the functions of the spleen is given by Leon Weiss:

> The spleen may be best understood as a discriminatory filter, consisting of specialized vascular spaces through which blood flows. The foundation of its structure and its filtration capacities is a reticular meshwork fashioned of reticular fibers. There is no element of the blood, cellular or plasmal, which the spleen may not affect. It monitors the red blood cells in the circulation and destroys or modifies imperfect ones. It removes other blood cells when damaged or aged. It sequesters monocytes from the blood and facilitates their transformation into macrophages and holds them as splenic macrophages which act in antibody formation and other splenic functions. It traps T and B cells from the blood and sorts them into compartments, permitting them to interact with macrophages and antigen in immune responses. It stores as many as a third of the platelets of the body in a ready reserve. In certain species, it can also function as a reservoir for erythrocytes and granulocytes, capable of delivering them rapidly to the blood when needed. [Leon Weiss, 1972. *The Cells and Tissues of the Immune System*]

This wondrous organ is enclosed by a CAPSULE of dense connective tissue and is divided into communicating compartments by a network of TRABECULAE that come from the capsular surface (Figure 4). The tissue enclosed by the capsule is called the SPLENIC PULP (a term that conjures up visions of old, dreary, smelly dissection laboratories). The pulp is mostly red, but it contains clusters of gray-white zones. These areas quite naturally are called the RED PULP and the WHITE PULP. The junction between red and white pulps is called the MARGINAL ZONE.

The red pulp is the site of storage of red blood cells (hence its color) and is composed of large, branching, thin-walled blood vessels called SPLENIC SINUSES. The tissue that lies between the sinuses is called the SPLENIC CORDS. The white pulp consists of cylinders surrounding the major arterial branches of the splenic pulp. These cylinders are called PERIARTERIAL LYMPHATIC SHEATHS, and within them are spherical clusters of lymphocytes called LYMPHATIC NODULES.

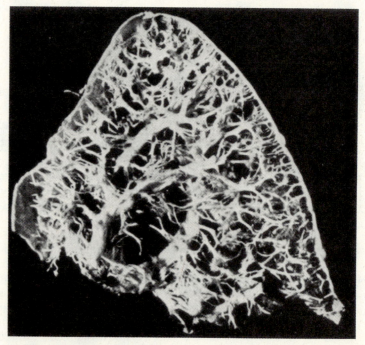

4   **Human Spleen.** In this spleen specimen (×4) the trabecular framework and capsule remain after the pulp has been digested by a solution of sodium carbonate. [From Weiss, 1983. *Histology: Cell and Tissue Biology*]

The white pulp, which contains the cells we will be most interested in, constitutes about 20% of the normal spleen and can be considered lymphoid tissue. It contains lymphocytes, macrophages, and other cells lying free in a reticular meshwork surrounding the arterial vessels. B cells and T cells are localized in the white pulp in what are known as T-dependent and B-dependent areas. The T-DEPENDENT AREAS of the spleen are primarily the lymphatic sheaths; the B-DEPENDENT AREAS are primarily the nodules.

Blood enters at the SPLENIC ARTERY through the hilus and branches into the trabeculae as TRABECULAR ARTERIES. These turn out of the trabeculae and enter the periarterial lymphatic sheaths; at this point they become CENTRAL ARTERIES. Lymphatic vessels are found within the trabeculae and in the white pulp closely associated with the central artery.

Lymphatic Vessels and Lymph Nodes

The lymphatic vessels, like the blood vessels, are a system of endothelium-lined tubes that transport cells and fluid. Unlike the blood vessels, the lymph vessels do not form a continuous, closed system. The lymphatic vessels carry their contents, called LYMPH, in only one direction—from connective tissue spaces toward the major lymphatic vessel (the THORACIC DUCT) and then into the venous system. The major function of the lymphatic vessels is to recover fluids that have escaped into the connective tissue spaces from the blood capillaries and venules and return them to the blood.

LYMPH NODES are structures along the path of the collecting lymphatic vessels. Because the cells of the lymph percolate through them, they are a major site of lymphocyte accumulation; it is in the lymph nodes that the exchange of material between blood and lymph occurs. Lymph nodes are surrounded by a CAPSULE (Figure 5). The afferent lymphatic vessels enter the node through the capsule at several sites and leave through a single site at the HILUS, an indentation on one surface. The blood vessels both enter and leave the node at the hilus. Figure 6 shows the organization of the lymph node in diagrammatic form.

Lymphocytes are the major cell type of the lymph node and lie in a fine meshwork called the RETICULUM. In the peripheral CORTEX, the lymphocytes are rather tightly packed; toward the hilus they are less dense and form the MEDULLA. Macrophages are found in the MEDULLARY SINUSES. At the periphery of the cortex are NODULES, or FOLLICLES, that are clearly discernible concentrations of lympho-

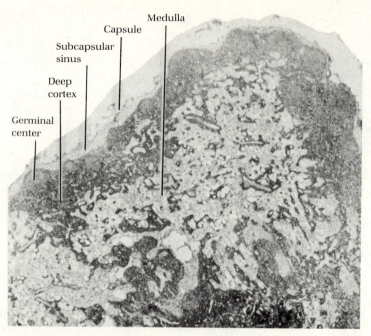

Germinal
center

Deep
cortex

Subcapsular
sinus

Capsule

Medulla

5 **Human Lymph Node.** A portion of the lymph node, showing the capsule, medulla, and cortex. Giemsa stain, ×30. [From Weiss, 1983. *Histology:
Cell and Tissue Biology*]

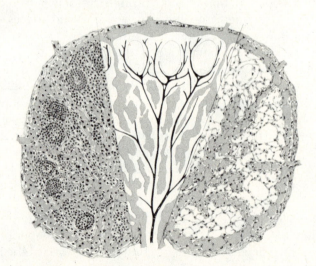

6 **Lymph Node.** Three diagrammatic views of a lymph node. (*Right*) Reticular cells. (*Center*) Distribution of veins. (*Left*) Distribution of lymphocytes.
[From Weiss, 1972. *The Cells and Tissues of the Immune System*]

cytes. PRIMARY NODULES are tightly packed and uniform and may contain a central zone of larger lymphocytes and macrophages. The central zone is called a GERMINAL CENTER. The deep part of the cortex between the nodules and the medulla is called the TERTIARY CORTEX. B cells are found in the primary nodules, and T cells are found in the tertiary cortex. Figure 7 shows these structured features in a human lymph node.

Circulation of Lymphocytes

As noted earlier, the lymphocytes circulate through the body, passing between the blood and lymphatic vascular systems at the lymph nodes. In the 1960s, J. L. Gowans and his co-workers carried out what are now considered classic studies on lymphocyte traffic. In these studies, lymphocytes collected from the thoracic duct were labeled with tritiated adenosine and then transfused into

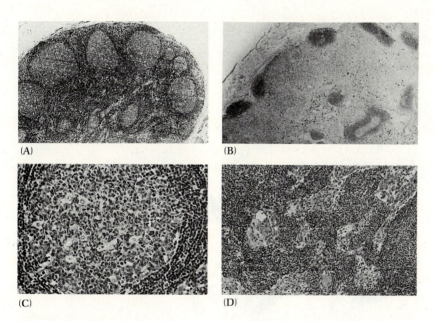

(A)   (B)   (C)   (D)

7   **Human Lymph Node.** (A) Secondary follicles with prominent germinal centers. H&E stain ×1000. (B) Follicles stained with Pan B monoclonal antibody. Follicles containing B cells are immunostained. Immunoperoxidase stain ×40. (C) Secondary follicle. Note the prominent and activated germinal center surrounded by the mantle zone. H&E stain ×400. (D) Medullary sinuses filled with macrophages. H&E stain ×250. [Courtesy of C. Baroni]

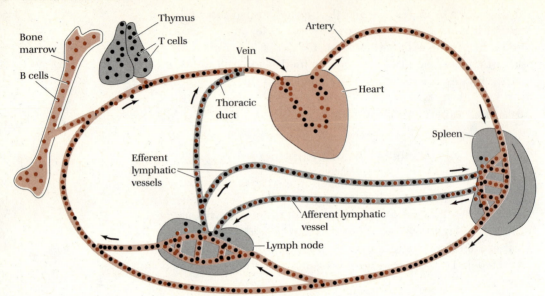

8 **Pathway of Lymphocyte Recirculation.** Lymphocytes enter the lymph nodes through the afferent lymphatics and enter the venous circulation via the thoracic duct. The arrows in the figure show the direction of movement of the lymphocytes.

normal animals. The fate of the transfused cells was determined by autoradiography at various time periods.

We now know that the lymphocytes move between the various organs of the body through the blood and lymphatic vessels (Figure 8). It can be seen in the figure that the lymphocytes enter the lymphatic circulation from the blood via the afferent lymphatics at the postcapillary venules. They re-enter the blood by way of the efferent lymphatics and then through the thoracic duct. From the thoracic duct they enter the circulation at the subclavian vein.

The lymphocytes leave the blood and enter the lymph nodes by passing across vessels. These specialized vessels are called HIGH ENDOTHELIAL VENULES (HEV), a name that describes the tall, plump shape of their lining cells (Figure 9). Because the emigration from blood into lymph nodes occurs only at HEVs and at no other endothelia, it was assumed that lymphocytes have receptors that recognize these structures. Recently a molecule on the surface of virtually all peripheral B and T cells has been identified by Irving

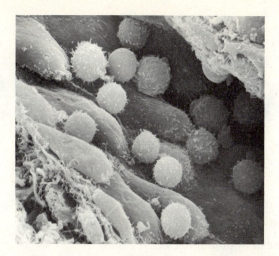

9   HEV in a Mouse Lymph Node. Scanning electron micrograph showing luminal surface of HEV in a mouse lymph node. Numerous lymphocytes are tightly bound to the plump endothelial cells. [Courtesy of E. C. Butcher and I. L. Weissman]

Weissman and his colleagues at Stanford; this molecule seems to be the one involved in recognition of the HEV. It is defined by a monoclonal antibody called MEL-14. The HEV-recognizing molecule is a glycoprotein with a molecular weight of approximately 80,000.

Preincubation of lymphocytes with the MEL-14 antibody in the absence of complement inhibits their binding to HEV in the in vitro test system. However, the ability of the MEL-14 antibody to block binding to HEV is seen only for cells in the peripheral lymph nodes and not for those in Peyer's patches. Cells that bind to Peyer's patch HEV can be shown to have reacted with the MEL-14 antibody even though they can still bind to the HEV. This argues for the existence of two means of recognition of endothelial surfaces: one in the peripheral nodes and one in the Peyer's patches.

B- and T-Cell Regions of Lymphoid Organs

After the lymphocytes cross the HEV and enter the lymph node or enter the white pulp of the spleen from the marginal zone, they become segregated into discrete areas. The B cells move to primary follicles in the lymph nodes, while the T cells remain diffused

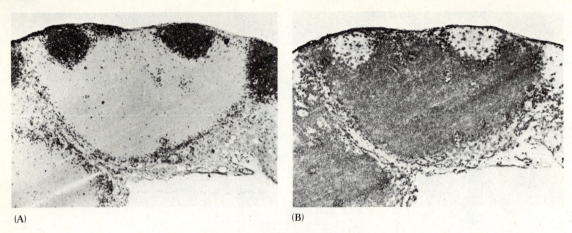

(A)

(B)

10   **Segregation of B and T Cells.** Immunoperoxidase staining of frozen sections of an unstimulated mouse lymph node, demonstrating the segregation of B and T lymphocytes into discrete domains. (A) Anti-IgD reveals the localization of B cells to discrete follicles in the outer cortex. (B) Anti-Thy-1 staining defines the paracortical T-cell region. [Courtesy of R. Reichert]

throughout the cortex of the lymph node (Figure 10) and the periarterial lymphatic sheath in the spleen.

The reason for this segregation by cell type is not known, but one reason currently being considered is based on the reticular cells found in the two areas. A cell called the INTERDIGITATING CELL (IDC) is found in the T-dependent areas. In contrast, the B-cell-rich areas have a reticular cell called the FOLLICULAR DENDRITIC CELL (FDC). It is not known, but has been predicted, that B cells and T cells interact preferentially with one or the other of these reticular cells. As we progress through the next chapters, we will be discussing B-cell and T-cell interactions and will see that many of the advances in cellular immunology have been made using dispersed cultures in vitro. The reader is urged to keep in mind at the end of those chapters that the time may now be right to go back to the animal, or at least to the lymphoid tissue in its actual in situ organization, to determine what happens in the animal.

Summary

1.   The thymus is a primary lymphoid organ composed of lymphocytes and epithelial cells. Pre-T cells enter the thymus via the blood and differentiate into thymic lymphocytes (or thymocytes). The thymocytes are found in both the cortex and the medulla.

2. The medullary thymocytes are the "mature" cells and differ from the cortical thymocytes in surface markers and cortisone sensitivity. The medullary cells are the cortisone-resistant thymocytes (CRTs), which are the functional cells of the thymus.

3. Lymphocytes circulate between the blood and the lymphatic vascular systems. They leave the venous circulation to enter the lymph nodes through vessels lined with specialized endothelia, called high endothelial venules (HEVs). Virtually all circulating B and T cells have a receptor for the HEV; this receptor is defined by a monoclonal antibody called MEL-14.

4. Lymphocytes are distributed in T- and B-dependent areas of the spleen and lymph nodes.

Additional Readings

Gallatin, M., T. P. St. John, M. Siegelman, R. Reichert, E. C. Butcher and I. L. Weissman. 1986. Lymphocyte homing receptors. *Cell* 44: 673.

Gowans, J.L. and E. J. Knight. 1964. The route of re-circulation of lymphocytes in the rat. *Proc. R. Soc. London B* 159: 257.

Weiss, L. 1972. *The Cells and Tissues of the Immune System*. Prentice-Hall, Englewood Cliffs, N.J.

THE MAJOR HISTOCOMPATIBILITY COMPLEX

<table>
<tr><td>

CHAPTER

15

</td></tr>
</table>

Overview We will see in the next few chapters that the products of a gene complex called the major histocompatibility complex (MHC) are involved in antigen presentation and cell interactions in the immune response. In the last decade the significance of the complex in many aspects of the immune response has been recognized. The MHC, called HLA in humans and H-2 in mice, is a multiallelic complex of genes that encodes surface molecules involved in many aspects of the immune response.

The genes of the MHC and their products are grouped into three classes. Class I genes encode surface molecules found on all cells of the body, and class II genes encode molecules found primarily on cells of the immune system. Class III genes encode serum proteins and complement components. We will see that the genes for the MHC products have been cloned and that modern technology is allowing us to rapidly gain an understanding of how these very important molecules function in the immune response.

Discovery of the Major Histocompatibility Complex

The development of our understanding of the major histocompatibility complex (MHC) is an instructive example of the merging of ideas and discoveries in many areas to produce the view we have at the present time. It is occasionally necessary, when we begin to feel very modern, to look at how we got to where we are today. By this exercise we are reminded that even though we work at the very edge of the known, we are really part of a continuum of developing scientific thought; today's discoveries are important not only for the solution of the problem as it is formulated today, but also as discoveries that will be used in a very different light further along the continuum.

The study of the MHC grew out of early work in cancer

research. When it was realized that the only way to propagate experimental tumors in mice was by using genetically homogeneous inbred strains, geneticists began to develop such strains. Because an inbred strain was either "susceptible" or "resistant" to a given tumor, a genetic theory of tumor susceptibility developed. All this was happening at the turn of the century when the germ theory of disease was being proved and the role of the immune system in defense against disease was the driving impetus of research. It was natural to link the two by predicting that the genes for resistance encoded structures that were important in immunity. But no immune theory of defense could explain why the tumors grew in the inbred strain in which they arose, because these mice should be able to respond to the tumor.

The great geneticist J. B. S. Haldane in 1933 introduced the contrary notion that the "immunity" was not directed against something unique to the tumor, but instead that the normal tissue molecules that served as antigens on the surface of the tumors, as with the blood group antigens, were what determined whether a tumor that arose in one strain would grow in another. In other words, he suggested that the immune response leading to rejection of the tumor would be directed against normal cellular antigens unique to *that* strain rather than against tumor-specific antigens unique to the tumor.

The testing of this hypothesis led to the search for tissue-specific antigens in mice. In the late 1930s Peter Gorer discovered four blood group antigens using the few inbred strains available at the time. He named these I, II, III, and IV. The growth or rejection of a tumor correlated with the expression of antigen II, and he found that C57BL mice that rejected a tumor of A-strain mice developed antibodies that reacted against antigen II on normal cells from strain A. The importance of this work cannot be overstated.

Gorer's early work established two important facts. First, it demonstrated that the genes for susceptibility to tumor transplants were identical with the genes coding for alloantigens. Second, it provided firm evidence for the immunological nature of resistance to tumor transplants by showing that rejection of a tumor is accompanied by production of alloantibodies. These two discoveries led Gorer to formulate the concept of tissue transplantation. According to Gorer, "normal and neoplastic tissues contain iso-antigenic factors which are genetically determined. Iso-antigenic factors present in the grafted tissue and absent in the host are capable of eliciting a response which results in the destruction of the graft." This immunological theory of transplantation represented one of the major advances in biological sciences of the twentieth century and marked the beginning of the era of transplantation immunology. Curiously, this fact was never formally recognized by prize-awarding committees, which often hailed discoveries of far less significance. [J. Klein, 1975. *Biology of the Mouse Histocompatibility-2 Complex*, p. 7]

While Gorer was carrying out his work in England, an equally remarkable investigator was examining the relationship between genetics and tumor susceptibility in the United States. George Snell joined the recently organized Jackson Laboratory in Bar Harbor, Maine, in 1935. The director of the laboratory was the great geneticist C. C. Little (called "Prexy" because he had been president of both the University of Michigan and the University of Maine). Snell took advantage of the inbred strains of mice available at Jackson to initiate a study of the formal genetics of the antigens responsible for tissue rejection. In 1948 he coined the term HISTOCOMPATIBILITY ANTIGENS (or H ANTIGENS).[1] The genes that coded for these antigens he termed HISTOCOMPATIBILITY GENES.

Using mice that differed only at the H locus, he found that the H genes were linked to a gene called *fused tail* (*Fu*) and that the gene coding for Gorer's antigen II was also linked to *Fu*.

Gorer and Snell began a lifelong friendship and collaboration in which Gorer spent his summers at the Jackson Lab (a tradition that many fortunate scientists have continued over the years). When they realized that the two systems were the same they combined the names, calling the antigens that were responsible for graft rejection H-2. This work was awarded the Nobel prize in 1980. Unfortunately, Gorer died in 1961 and could not share the prize, but his contributions are known and appreciated by all biologists interested in this area of work.[2]

Traits Controlled by the MHC

We noted earlier that the original reason for studying the MHC of both mouse and human was its clinical application to tumor

---

[1] In the early literature the molecules of the MHC were always referred to as "antigens" because they were detected by antibodies or other immune responses. We now refer to them as MHC "molecules," but the reader may still come across the older usage.

[2] A fairly detailed and highly readable history of the MHC can be found in J. Klein, 1975, *Biology of the Mouse Histocompatibility-2 Complex: Principles of Immunogenetics Applied to a Single System*, pp. 3–15.

growth and then graft rejection. But graft rejection is just one aspect of the response of the host to MHC molecules on foreign tissues. Graft rejection is a cell-mediated response brought about by effector T cells (Section II). Because, as we will see later, graft rejection is the archetypal cell-mediated response, the MHC molecules have been extensively studied as a means of understanding the mechanisms of cell-mediated responses.

As might be expected, the introduction of foreign tissue into a host also results in the production of antibodies against the MHC molecules. Of the two responses, the cell-mediated response is much more significant to the phenomenon of graft rejection. The reader should bear in mind, however, that the grafted individual responds to the foreign MHC molecules as it does to most other antigens by making both an antibody and a cell-mediated response.

Correlation of Structure and Function

During the course of research on the MHC, it gradually became clear that many other aspects of the immune response are also controlled by genes within the MHC. The traits controlled by the genes of the MHC are given in Table 1. What will become clear as we go along is that the MHC affects the entire range of the immune response and that two classes of molecules are the central players. These two classes of MHC molecules are called, with the usual erudition of immunologists, CLASS I and CLASS II. It can be seen in Table 1 that class I MHC molecules are associated with some of the functional traits and class II with others, and that the two classes have very different tissue distributions. The nature of these traits will become clear as the reader progresses through the chapters on cellular immunology, as will the significance of the different tissue distribution of the two classes of molecules.

Mapping the MHC Genes by Function and Gene Product

The MHC is a large gene complex, consisting of 1.5 recombination units in the mouse and 2 recombination units in humans. There is an appropriate assay for each of the traits in Table 1; thus the genetics of many of the functions was worked out. When the genes controlling these traits are mapped by standard genetic methods, it is found that they are all located as a gene complex on chromosome 17 in mice and on chromosome 6 in humans. The order of the genes as mapped by their *function* is seen in Figure 1. The various traits can be mapped to *regions*. Each region contains

Table 1 Traits controlled by the MHC.

	Class I	Class II
Mouse H-2	K, D, L	I-A, I-E
Human HLA	A, B, C, G	DR, DQ, DP
FUNCTIONAL TRAIT		
Graft rejection	Strong	Weak
MLR	Weak	Strong
CML	Strong	Weak
MHC restriction CD4	Weak	Strong
MHC restriction CD8	Strong	Weak
Ir genes	Weak	Strong
STRUCTURAL TRAIT		
Tissue distribution	Ubiquitous[a]	Macrophage Dendritic cells B cells
Polymorphic chains	1	2
Associated with β_2m	Yes	No
Domains per chain	2	3
Ig superfamily	Yes	Yes

[a] G is a newly described class I molecule found on the human trophoblast.

genes that encode the polymorphic chains of the MHC molecules (see next section), two for class II molecules and one for class I. Class III genes control the expression of some components of the complement system.[3]

Polymorphism of the MHC

MHC, Multigenic and Multiallelic

As work progressed on the MHC and as details of its organization and wide-ranging functions became known, some investigators argued that this may be the major system by which individuals distinguish *self* from *nonself*—one of the more profound problems

[3] The MHC is being introduced at this point in the book, in part because an understanding of the Class I and Class II molecules is needed to understand the cellular events in the immune response, which will be discussed in Section II. For that reason we will focus on these molecules and not discuss the class III genes or products.

1 MHC Regions and Loci of Human and Mouse. The position of the MHC locus on the *chromosome* is shown in the top row. Below that are shown the *regions* containing the MHC genes. Below that are the *products* of each of the genes shown above. The bottom row shows the location of the *class* of MHC.

in biology. Any system allowing an individual of the species to distinguish its tissues from the tissues of other members must be highly polymorphic; that is, there must be many forms of the molecules distributed among the various individual members of the population. The MHC is, in fact, one of the most highly polymorphic gene complexes known. Indeed, it is both *multiallelic* and *multigenic*.

Each of the genes in Figure 1 has many allelic forms (i.e., every member of the species has the gene, but different members have different forms of the gene), and this polymorphism is one of the most striking features of the MHC. It is difficult to give a definitive number to the allelic forms of the class I and class II genes. Part of the difficulty in accurately determining the number of allelic forms of the genes comes from the methods used. As newer and different techniques are used, new variants appear, and the use of DNA sequence and restriction site analysis has added to the numbers.

It must be emphasized that the polymorphism seen in MHC is not due to gene rearrangement of the kind seen in Igs.[4] It has

---

[4] Many students make this mistake. Class I and class II molecules are members of the Ig superfamily, but this does *not* mean that they rearrange. As the great Canadian immunologist-philosopher Thomas Wegman has said, "When you talk about MHC molecules, you go home with the one you brought to the dance, eh."

been suggested that one possible source of the polymorphism seen in the MHC is *micro-recombination* between class I genes. Stanley Nathenson and his colleagues at Albert Einstein College of Medicine in New York have shown that the sites of mutations in one of the murine class I genes (K^b, see nomenclature below) are clustered and consist of segments from parts of other class I genes (D and Qa). The Qa genes exhibit very little polymorphism and have no known function, and so the suggestion is that they may serve as a reservoir of genetic material that gets introduced into other class I genes resulting in their polymorphism. Again let us stress that this is not gene rearrangement as seen in Ig but rather classic gene conversion that occurs in the germ line.

The Notion of the Haplotype

The combination of linked alleles in a gene cluster is called the HAPLOTYPE. The term derives from *haploid genotype* and defines the entire constellation of alleles at individual linked regions that are inherited on a single chromosome. In the mouse the H-2 haplotype is denoted by a superscript, for example, $H\text{-}2^d$. This shorthand indicates the allelic form of each of the several genes in the MHC of that strain. In this case, all the alleles are called d. There are several mouse strains that have been termed TYPE STRAINS and serve as the arbitrarily chosen prototype for the haplotype. Some H-2 haplotypes of common strains are given in Table 2. Note that

Table 2   H-2 haplotypes of commonly used mouse strains and congenics.

H-2 haplotype	Alleles present in MHC regions					Strains with haplotype
	K	I-A	I-E	S	D	
$H\text{-}2^a$	k	k	d	d	d	A B10.A
$H\text{-}2^b$	b	b	b	b	b	B10 C57BL/6
$H\text{-}2^d$	d	d	d	d	d	DBA/2 BALB/c B10.D2
$H\text{-}2^k$	k	k	k	k	k	C3H CBA B10.BR

several strains can have the same H-2 haplotype. In other words, the allelic forms of all the H-2 genes in those strains are the same. But DBA, BALB/c, and B10.D2, for example, are different strains because their alleles for other genes are different.[5] Table 2 also shows that some strains are recombinants of two haplotypes; for example, strain A is a recombinant of the $H\text{-}2^k$ and the $H\text{-}2^d$ haplotypes.

In humans the class I HLA molecules are designated HLA-A, HLA-B, and HLA-C and the class II molecules as DR, DQ, and DP. The different alleles are numbered, so an individual can be A3, B27, and so forth.

wouldn't you have 1 A from each parent?

Public and Private Specificities

Until recently MHC alleles were defined by antibodies to the gene products. A given haplotype has unique, defined antigenic structures,[6] called PRIVATE SPECIFICITIES. Each haplotype has a private specificity, or determinant, that is unique to the haplotype. For example, all $H\text{-}2^k$ mice have the same antigens defined by antibody reactivity. There are many strains of mice with the $H\text{-}2^k$ haplotype, and they all contain these private specificity determinants.

In addition to the private specificities, there is a set of antigens called PUBLIC SPECIFICITIES, or public determinants. These antigens are not restricted to a given haplotype; one strain may have several of them, whereas another strain may have some of these as well as an array of other specificities. For example, some strains with the $H\text{-}2^k$ haplotype have an antigen specificity that is shared by virtually all haplotypes; it is therefore a public specificity antigen. As we will see, the MHC genes in many species have been identified, and we now discuss allelic differences at the genetic level. However, a discussion of public and private specificities is important because most human MHCs are still defined by antisera.

Congenic Mice

For experimental purposes, it is essential to have mice that differ in only one allele of the MHC. When mice differ at one locus but are the same at all other genetic loci, they are called CONGENIC. An example would be congenic B10 mice such as B10.A or B10.D2.

---

[5] As we go along it will seem to the reader that there are, in fact, no other genes than those that encode Igs and MHC. The reader should rest assured that there are many other genes known in both mouse and human, and some of them are even of some importance.

[6] See Footnote 1 on page 240.

These mice originally derive from C57BL/10 but have different H-2 haplotypes. They still have all the "background genes" of the original B10.[7]

For example, suppose we wanted to test the role of the H-2 complex on some aspect of the immune response. We would need mice that differ *only* at H-2 and not at any background genes— that is, mice with identical background genes but different H-2 genes. This arrangement would allow us to compare the response of B10 mice, which are $H\text{-}2^b$, with the response of mice with some other haplotype, say $H\text{-}2^a$. If there were a difference in the response being tested it could be attributed to a difference in H-2 genes and not to a difference in background genes. The mice that have B10 background genes and $H\text{-}2^k$ genes would be congenic for H-2.

Congenic strains are designated by the background strain, a dot, and then the donor of the differing gene. In the example used above, the background strain is B10. If the donor of the $H\text{-}2^a$ genes is strain A, then the congenic is designated B10.A (the term is spoken "B10 dot A"). It is essential not to confuse this notation with the designation of an F_1, which shows both strains within parentheses. An F_1 of B10 and A would be $(B10 \times A)F_1$.

Production of Congenic Mice

The production of mice that differ at only one specified gene requires some fancy genetic footwork. The genetic method of constructing congenic mice was worked out by George Snell. Suppose we have two strains, X and Y. A certain tumor is accepted (will grow) when injected into strain X but will be rejected (will not grow) by strain Y. The object is to introduce the genes of strain Y (the ability to reject this tumor) onto the genetic background of strain X so that we end up with an X.Y mouse in which the only Y trait present is the ability to reject the tumor.

The genetics involved are diagrammed in Figure 2. The procedure involves crossing an animal with the ability to reject the tumor (in this case, strain Y) with a member of the strain that does not (strain X). The offspring will have genes from both X and Y. These animals are then backcrossed to X, and the offspring of this backcross generation are screened for the ability to reject the tumor. If they do, they are assumed to be carrying this trait from strain Y. It is clear that in the backcross to X the Y genes have been diluted, but the mice are screened for only a single trait: Y. So even

---

[7] In the chauvinistic jargon of the MHC crowd, all genes in the mouse that are not MHC genes are referred to as background.

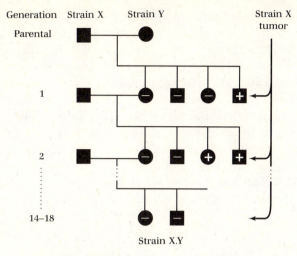

2   Production of Congenic Mice. The cross–intercross method of producing congenic lines of mice. Strain X mice accept the tumor and strain Y mice do not. They are mated and then intercrossed. The progeny that reject the tumor are then backcrossed to strain X. After 18 generations the background genes are from strain X but the genes involved with resistance to the tumor are from strain Y. The animal is an X.Y congenic. The method will work for any detectable and selectable trait. [After Snell, 1966. In Green, ed., *Biology of the Laboratory Mouse*]

though the general gene contribution of Y is reduced, the gene for tumor rejection has been enriched. Those animals that are able to reject the tumor are once again backcrossed to strain X and the offspring again screened for the Y trait. With each backcross there is further dilution of the Y genes, except for the genes determining the trait being selected. In contrast, there is a progressive enrichment of the X background genes. Somewhere around the eighteenth backcross generation the dilution is almost complete, and the result is a strain that has background genes of strain X and tumor rejection characteristics of strain Y; the new strain is now an X.Y congenic. In this example the rejection or growth of the tumor is a function of the MHC and so the congenic animals that result are in fact congenic for MHC. Because we now have monoclonal antibodies as reagents, we can now type the animals for the MHC for which we wish to select.

The example above is a scientific one, but an intuitive example may be of some use. Suppose you decide to systematically determine the amount of vermouth you want in your martini. You could start by adding to a chilled glass one jigger of vermouth, one jigger of gin, and an olive. After sipping it, you decide it should be drier, so you discard half the martini (retaining the olive) and add an equal volume of gin. Another sip tells you that this is still not dry enough, so you discard half the martini, retain the olive, and add an equal volume of gin. Another sip, another discard (not the olive, though) and another addition of equal volume follow. If you do this 10 times you will have a chilled glass that contains over 99% gin and the olive. Consider the gin to be the background and the olive to be the desired gene, and you have the notion of a congenic mouse.[8]

Structure of MHC Molecules

Class I Molecules

The molecules encoded by the class I genes are the classic transplantation antigens involved in graft rejection. Class I molecules are found on all cells of the body in various concentrations.

The class I molecules are composed of two chains, a variable chain called the α CHAIN and an invariant chain called β_2-MICRO-GLOBULIN (Figure 3A). β_2-microglobulin is not an MHC gene product, being encoded on a different chromosome. It is, however, a member of the Ig superfamily. The α chain has a molecular weight of 45,000, and β_2-microglobulin has a molecular weight of 12,000. The β_2-microglobulin is noncovalently linked to the α chain. All individuals of the species have the same β_2-microglobulin, no matter what their MHC haplotype.

The α chain of the class I molecules is composed of five distinct domains. There are three EXTERNAL DOMAINS (termed α_1, α_2, and α_3, each of approximately 90 residues); a TRANSMEMBRANE DOMAIN of 43 residues; and a CYTOPLASMIC DOMAIN. β_2-microglobulin associates with the α chain at the α_3 domain. The sites of extensive polymorphism are located on the α_1 and α_2 domains.

X-Ray Crystallographic Solution of Class I Structure

One of the most exciting and widely acclaimed advances in immunology was the X-ray crystallographic solution of the human class I MHC molecule by Pamela Bjorkman and colleagues at Harvard.

[8] We thank Jan Klein for this instructive illustration.

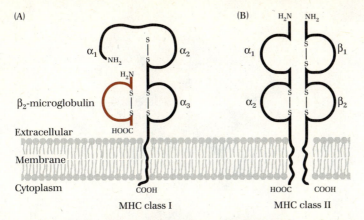

3   Schematic Representation of Class I and Class II MHC Molecules.
(A) Class I molecules consist of a heavy chain containing three extracellular domains, α_1, α_2, and α_3, plus a transmembrane and a cytoplasmic domain. Closely associated but noncovalently linked is the β_2-microglobulin chain. (B) Class II molecules consists of two chains, α and β. The α chain consists of two extracellular domains, α_1 and α_2. The β chain consists of two extracellular domains, β_1 and β_2. Each chain has a transmembrane and a cytoplasmic domain.

Bjorkman had begun the project as her Ph.D. problem in the lab of Donald Wiley and worked on it for over 8 years. The results had a dramatic effect on all of cellular immunology.

A human lymphoblast line that expressed HLA-A was used for this study. The external domains of the HLA and β_2-microglobulin were cleaved from purified cell membranes (i.e., no transmembrane or cytoplasmic domains) and the crystal structure resolved at 3.5 Å. As seen in Figure 4, the structure shows two pairs of similar domains. These correspond to the α_1/α_2 and $\alpha_3/\beta_2 m$ domains. The α_1/α_2 domains are on top and the $\alpha_3/\beta_2 m$ below. The α_1/α_2 domains have two α-HELICAL REGIONS that face outward (away from the cell membrane). The $\alpha_3/\beta_2 m$ domains also have helices similar but not identical to those of Ig (the homology between MHC, β_2-microglobulin, and Ig has been known for a long time; see the discussion of the Ig superfamily in Chapter 3).

All of this structural work would have been enough to make the work interesting and important, but the *functional* information that emerged from the structural data was the most exciting. As seen in Figure 4, there is a *groove* on the top of the molecule formed by the α-helical regions of the α_1 and α_2 domains. The importance of this groove will not only become apparent in the

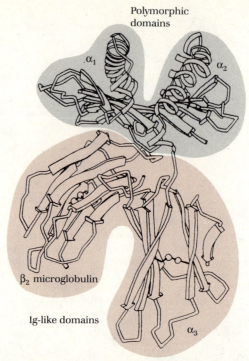

Polymorphic
domains

α_1 α_2

β_2 microglobulin

Ig-like domains

α_3

4   Schematic Representation of Class I MHC Molecule Based on X-Ray Crystallographic Solution. HLA-A1 molecule showing the four domains; the polymorphic domains α_1 and α_2 are at the top and the Ig-like domains α_3 and β_2m are at the bottom. Only the extracellular domains are shown. [After Bjorkman et al., 1987. *Nature* 329: 506. Courtesy of P. Bjorkman]

following chapters but will be seen as a central theme to this part of the book.

Another aspect of the role of the MHC in immune responses, the association of CD4 and CD8 molecules with MHC, will be discussed in later sections. At this point we will only mention that CD8 interacts with class I MHC molecules, and the site of the interaction on the MHC molecule has been determined by measuring the adhesion between CD8 and a large panel of point mutants of HLA-A. The binding was found to be located at three clusters of residues in α_3 and is illustrated in Figure 5.

Class II Molecules

The structure of class II molecules is shown in Figure 3B. Class II molecules are found on a limited array of cells, most of which are associated with the hemopoietic system (Chapter 12). This distri-

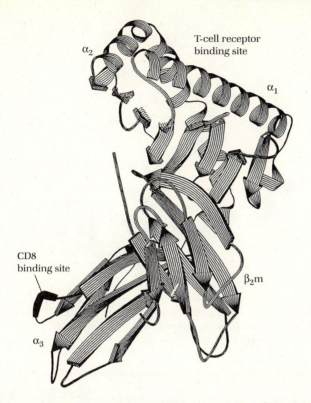

5 Binding Site of CD8 to Class I MHC. Accessibility of the CD8 binding site in the α_3 domain on a schematic representation of class I HLA structure is indicated. β-strands are shown as thick arrows and α-helixes as helical ribbons. [From Salter et al., 1990. *Nature* 345: 41. With permission]

bution is of very great importance in cell–cell interactions in the immune response (Chapters 16–20).

Class II molecules are composed of two chains, called α and β. Unlike class I molecules, in which the β_2-microglobulin chain is invariant, class II molecules have two variant chains both encoded within the MHC. The α chain has a molecular weight of 33,000 to 35,000, and the β chain has a molecular weight of 28,000 to 30,000.

There are several features about the class II molecules that suggest structural similarity with class I molecules. They have the same domain organization and similar COOH-terminal domain sequences, and the close association of the α_1 and α_2 domains in class II is similar to the α_1/β_2m domain association in class I. In fact, when the structural features in the groove at the top of the class I molecule (Figure 4) are compared with conserved and poly-

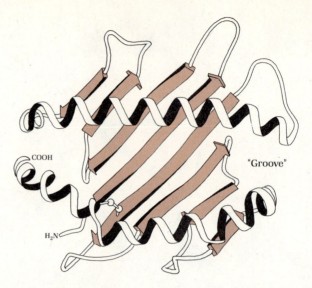

COOH

"Groove"

H₂N

6 **Hypothetical Model of the "Groove" of Class II MHC Molecule.** From sequence similarities, this hypothetical peptide-binding surface (groove) of the class II MHC has been proposed. In this model the tops of the class I and class II molecules are similar enough that they could each accommodate a peptide fragment. [After Brown et al., 1988. *Nature* 332: 845]

morphic amino acid residues in several class I and class II amino acid sequences, a hypothetical model for a similar groove in class II emerges (Figure 6). Although there has been no reported crystallographic solution to the structure of class II molecules, the calculated similarities have led most immunologists to assume that the structure of class II molecules includes a groove similar to that of class I.

Organization of the MHC Genes

Several class I and class II genes have been cloned and sequenced. The exon–intron relationship of MHC genes is shown in Figure 7. Note the precise correlation between the exons and the domains of the molecules discussed above.

Expression of MHC Molecules

The expression of class I molecules is coordinately controlled with β_2-microglobulin, which is on chromosome 2. A human Burkitt's lymphoma cell line called Daudi, for example, does not express cell surface HLA-A, HLA-B, or HLA-C, even though there are normal amounts of mRNA for the α chains from these genes in the cyto-

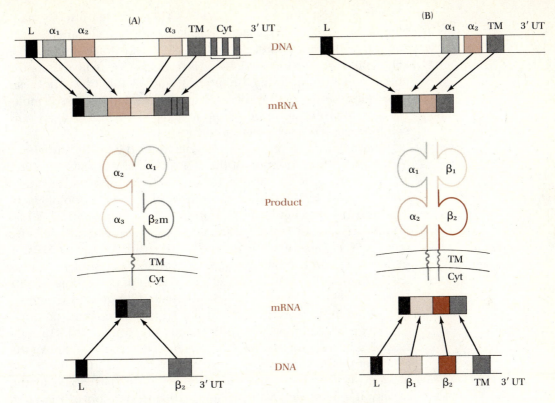

7   Organization of MHC Genes. The exons encoding the domains are shown. TM, transmembrane; Cyt, cytoplasmic. (A) Class I molecules and β_2-microglobulin (which is encoded by a non-MHC gene). (B) Class II molecules.

plasm. There is, however, no β_2-microglobulin protein or its mRNA. Similarly, the embryonic tumor ECC lines do not express cell surface class I molecules and also have no β_2-microglobulin. Thus, in some manner the expression of class I molecules depends upon the expression of β_2-microglobulin.

The expression of the two chains of class II molecules is also coordinately controlled. Some haplotypes, such as H-2^b, do not express I-E because they have defective promoter regions for Eβ, even though they have normal cytoplasmic levels of Eα. In normal cells the α and β chains are noncovalently associated with a 31,000-dalton invariant chain called Ii, which plays some role (though not a crucial one) in transporting the complex to the cell surface. Ii is present in those mice that do not express I-E, suggesting that the major coordinate control is at the α–β-chain complex level rather than at Ii.

We pointed out above that class II molecules are normally expressed primarily on macrophages, dendritic cells, and B cells. However, aberrant expression of class II MHC molecules in other cell types can be induced by γ INTERFERON. We will see in the chapter on autoimmunity (Chapters 35 and 36) that one hypothesis for autoimmunity is that the aberrant expression of class II molecules by thyroid cells, for example, can lead to self-antigen now being processed as if it were foreign.

The techniques of modern biology are now being brought to bear on the exact function of the MHC. It is now possible to carry out targeted gene disruption experiments in mice as had been done in yeast. In the first of these to be published, Rudolph Jaenisch and his colleagues at MIT and Oliver Smithies and his colleagues at Chapel Hill have created a β_2-microglobulin-negative mouse. Since, as we saw above, the expression of class I MHC is dependent upon the expression of β_2-microglobulin, they thus created a class I-negative mouse. The design of these experiments is seen in Figure 8. A normal β_2-microglobulin gene was altered by engineering it so that it could not be expressed, and then the altered gene was introduced into an embryonal stem cell. Through homologous recombination, the defective gene replaced one of the alleles of the normal gene in these cells. When introduced into the blastocyst of mice, embryonal stem cells can participate in the development of the animal. After such introduction of the stem cells, the disrupted β_2-microglobulin gene of these stem cells was transmitted along the germ line in a small number of the animals. Phenotypically, mice that are heterozygous for this gene are indistinguishable from normal mice, but when the heterozygotes are mated with each other, a proportion of the progeny are homozygous for the trait. In other words, they are β_2-microglobulin-negative and therefore class I MHC-negative as well.

The first important thing learned from this experiment was that class I molecules are evidently not needed in the normal development of the mouse. It had been speculated that these surface molecules might be important in cell trafficking, but the fact that the mice that developed without the gene product were normal is a strong argument against this idea.

From an immunologic point of view, the class I-negative animal had apparently normal levels of CD4$^+$8$^+$ and CD4$^+$8$^-$ T cells. However, they were defective for CD4$^-$8$^+$ cells. The immunologic significance of this finding will become apparent to the reader when we get to the study of the correlation of CD4 and CD8 with MHC class restriction (Chapter 19) and when we discuss positive

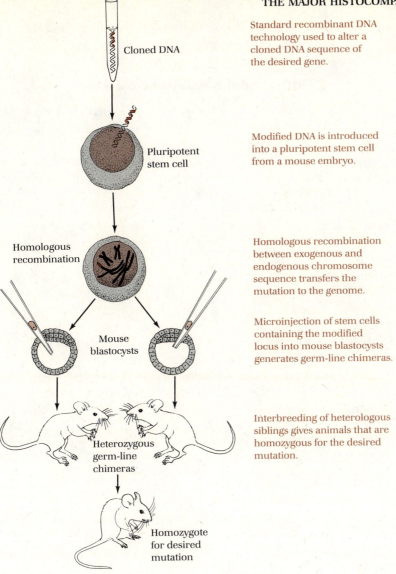

Standard recombinant DNA technology used to alter a cloned DNA sequence of the desired gene.

Modified DNA is introduced into a pluripotent stem cell from a mouse embryo.

Homologous recombination between exogenous and endogenous chromosome sequence transfers the mutation to the genome.

Microinjection of stem cells containing the modified locus into mouse blastocysts generates germ-line chimeras.

Interbreeding of heterologous siblings gives animals that are homozygous for the desired mutation.

8 Generation of Mice with a Desired Genetic Trait. A schematic presentation of the steps involved in introducing a desired gene into mice. The method involves introducing the desired cloned gene into a pluripotent embryonic stem cell. Homologous recombination occurs between the introduced gene and a gene in the stem cell, thus replacing the stem cell gene. The stem cell is then introduced into a mouse blastocyst and the embryos allowed to develop. Mice that are heterozygous for the trait of the introduced gene are mated to obtain mice that are homozygous for the trait. [After Capecchi, 1990. *Nature* 344: 105] and negative selection in the thymus (Chapters 24 and 25). The immune responses of these mice are now being tested.

MHC and the Immune Response

The primary reason that we have given so much detailed explanation of the MHC is because it is central in the immune response. Aside from their obvious role in transplantation, MHC products are involved in the generation and control of immune responses. This was first seen in a classic series of experiments carried out by Hugh McDevitt, now at Stanford, and Michael Sela. It had been known that there were strain differences between mice in their responses to some antigens. The experiments began with the observation (Figure 9) that C57BL/6 mice made vigorous antibody resonses to a polymer of a branched multichain amino acid copolymer of tyrosine–glutamic acid–alanine–lysine (TGAL).[9] However, CBA mice responded only weakly to this antigen. When the response of the F_1 mice was studied, it was found that they made an intermediate response.

In 1965, when these experiments were being carried out, there was evidence accumulating from the work of Benacerraf and his colleagues in New York and Biozzi and his colleagues in Paris that high and low responses may be under the control of a single gene. Reasoning from this premise, McDevitt and Sela did a series of backcrosses. If control was by a single gene, then the parental high responders (C57) could be thought of as having the genotype *HH* and the low responder (CBA) the genotype *LL*.

$$HH \times LL = HL$$

The F_1 would be *HL* and would give an intermediate response (the result obtained). The real test of the hypothesis would be by doing *backcrosses* of the F_1 to each of the parental strains. Under single gene control the backcross of the F_1 to the high responder would give

$$HL \times HH = HH + HL$$

and the backcross to the low responder would give

$$HL \times LL = HL + LL$$

As seen in Figure 9, the result showed that backcrossing the F_1 to the low responder gave a response that covered the range of

---

[9] This designation of the amino acids predates the single-letter amino acid code and therefore does not correspond to the current usage. In modern terminology, it would be YEAK.

low to intermediate (i.e., *LL* and *HL*). The backcross to the high resonder gave a pattern of responses that covered the range from intermediate to high (i.e., *HL* and *HH*).

By careful analysis McDevitt and Sela were able to show that the high–low antibody response phenomenon mapped into the MHC. At the time there were only three MHC genes known in the mouse, *K*, *S*, and *D*. This trait seemed to map between *K* and *S* and thus defined a new gene. Because it controlled the level of the immune response to antigens, it was called the *IR* GENE, and the designation was then changed to the I REGION. We now know that this is the region that encodes I-A and I-E.

The responses to many antigens are now known to be under *Ir* gene control (Table 3). But the reader now knows that the I region encodes the class II MHC molecules I-A and I-E. As the rest of the story of cellular interactions and MHC restriction in the immune response unfolds, we urge the reader to remember these seminal experiments and observe how so much of what we now know about the generation of immune responses can be traced back to these experiments.

(A) TGAL

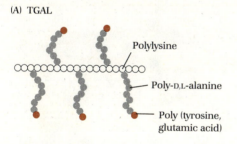

Polylysine

Poly-D,L-alanine

Poly (tyrosine, glutamic acid)

9   Genetics of the Response of Two Strains of Mice to TGAL. (A) TGAL. The branched, multichained amino acid copolymer contains a polylysine backbone with side chains of poly-D,L-alanine, and tyrosine and glutamic acid attached to the alanine side chains. (B) The top panel shows the antibody responses of CBA, the low responder (*LL*), and C57BL, the high responder (*HH*), to TGAL. The response of the F₁ is seen in the next panel and the responses of the F₁ backcrossed to each of the parents are seen in the bottom two. The theoretical genotypes if the response were under single-gene control are shown. [From McDevitt and Sela, 1985. *J. Exp. Med.* 122: 517]

(B) Response to TGAL

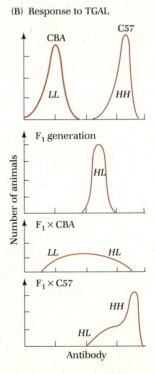

Number of animals

CBA   C57

LL   HH

F₁ generation

HL

F₁ × CBA

LL   HL

F₁ × C57

HH

HL

Antibody

Table **3** **Control of immune responses by Ir genes.**

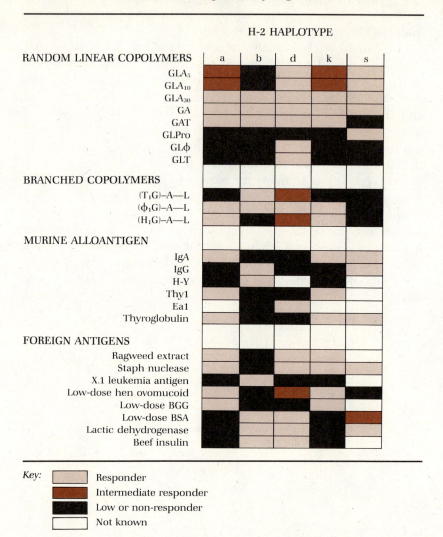

H-2 HAPLOTYPE

RANDOM LINEAR COPOLYMERS — a, b, d, k, s

GLA$_5$
GLA$_{10}$
GLA$_{30}$
GA
GAT
GLPro
GLϕ
GLT

BRANCHED COPOLYMERS

(T$_1$G)–A—L
(ϕ_1G)–A—L
(H$_1$G)–A—L

MURINE ALLOANTIGEN

IgA
IgG
H-Y
Thy1
Ea1
Thyroglobulin

FOREIGN ANTIGENS

Ragweed extract
Staph nuclease
X.1 leukemia antigen
Low-dose hen ovomucoid
Low-dose BGG
Low-dose BSA
Lactic dehydrogenase
Beef insulin

Key:
☐ Responder
☐ Intermediate responder
☐ Low or non-responder
☐ Not known

Summary

1.   The major histocompatibility complex (MHC) is a complex of genes that encodes molecules involved in various aspects of the immune response.

2.   The MHC gene products can be grouped into three classes, called I, II, and III. Class I products are found on all cells, class II products are found on cells of the immune system (Ia molecules), and class III

products are serum molecules, some of which are associated with the complement system.

3.   The MHC is one of the most highly polymorphic systems in biology. Each of the genes of the system has many alleles. The collection of the allelic forms expressed by an individual is called its haplotype.

4.   By selective backcrosses, mice can be bred to have the MHC genes of one haplotype and the background genes of another. These are called congenic mice.

5.   Class I molecules have a variant chain called α and an invariant chain called β_2-microglobulin. Class II molecules have two variable chains, α and β.

6.   The structure of the class I MHC molecule has been solved by X-ray crystallography.

7.   The magnitude of the immune response is controlled by class II genes. These are called *Ir* genes, and the region is called the I region.

Additional Readings

Bjorkman, P. J., M. A. Saper, B. Samraoui, W. S. Bennet, J. L. Strominger and D. C. Wiley. 1987. Structure of the human class I histocompatibility antigen, HLA-A2. *Nature* 329: 506.

Bjorkman, P. J., M. A. Saper, B. Samraoui, W. S. Bennet, J. L. Strominger and D. C. Wiley. 1987. The foreign antigen binding site and T cell recognition regions of class I histocompatibility antigens. *Nature* 329: 512.

Brown, J. H., T. Jardetzky, M. A. Saper, B. Samraoui, P. J. Bjorkman and D. C. Wiley. 1988. A hypothetical model of the foreign antigen binding site of class II histocompatibility molecules. *Nature* 332: 845.

Hood, L., M. Steinmetz and B. Malissen. 1983. Genes of the major histocompatibility complex of the mouse. *Annu. Rev. Immunol.* 1: 529.

Kappes, D. and J. L. Strominger. 1988. Human class II major histocompatibility complex genes and proteins. *Annu. Rev. Biochem.* 57: 591.

Mengle-Gaw, L., and H. O. McDevitt. 1985. Genetics and expression of murine Ia antigens. *Annu. Rev. Immunol.* 3: 367.

Parham, P. 1990. Some savage cuts in defence. *Nature* 344: 709.

Zijlstra, M., M. Bix, N. E. Simister, J. M. Loring, D. H. Raulet, and R. Jaenisch. 1990. β2-Microglobulin deficient mice lack CD4$^-$8$^+$ cytolytic T cells. *Nature* 344: 742.

CELLULAR INTERACTIONS

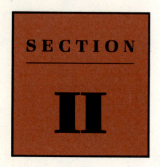

SECTION

II

If it aint complicated it dont matter whether it works or not because if it aint complicated up enough it aint right. So even if it works, dont believe it.

William Faulkner, *The Town*

In these five chapters we will discuss the cellular events that lead to an immune response, revealing the various layers of complexity of the cellular events in that response. The solution to the problem of cellular events in the immune response is a fascinating one that has taken many unexpected twists and turns. To understand that story and the current status of the problem, which involves B cells, various functional subsets of T cells, cell-surface marker phenotypes, and the role of the MHC (all of which were introduced in the previous section), it is necessary to follow the flow of discoveries that elucidated the role of each of these components. Furthermore, it will be necessary to understand the material in this section before the reader can fully comprehend the material in the next section, on receptors.

THE DIVISION OF LABOR

Overview   In this chapter we will see that there are two kinds of immune responses: humoral and cell-mediated. A division of labor is apparent among the cells that carry out the two kinds of responses; indeed, the responses are carried out by different sets of cells. The first clue that this division of labor existed came from experiments in which the thymus was removed from mice at birth; these neonatally thymectomized animals had impaired immune responses. A similar discovery was made with the avian bursa; it was found that neonatally bursectomized birds also had impaired responses to antigen. To complicate matters further, it was then found that removal of macrophages from in vitro cultures of spleen cells prevented the lymphocytes in these cultures from making immune responses. Together all these studies showed that there is a need for two kinds of lymphocytes—B cells and T cells—plus macrophages in the immune response.

CHAPTER
16

This chapter will develop the evidence for the division of labor. It will also introduce the reader to some of the methodology that will be needed to understand all cellular immunology experiments.

Humoral and Cell-Mediated Immune Responses

The Immunocompetent Cell

The introduction of antigen into an animal causes a complex series of events that result in a variety of responses. Because we almost always are interested in only one or a very few of these responses, we call the response to antigen *the immune response*, even though *the immune responses* is probably more appropriate.

It has been known since long before the modern era that the cells that carry out the immune response are LYMPHOCYTES. In 1958, Peter Medawar coined the term *immunologically competent cell* to define a cell that is "fully qualified to undertake an immunological response." Medawar later noted (1963) that he meant the term to indicate that the cells had the *potential* to carry out a response, and that to "describe an immunologically activated cell, a cell actually doing something, as immunologically competent strikes me as superogatory (*sic*), like describing an aircraft already overhead as competent to engage in flight."

The important point is that at the start of the Modern Era, circa 1960, the best immunological thinkers viewed the immune response as the domain of one kind of cell, the lymphocyte. It was known that there are large and small lymphocytes and that antibody is produced by a specialized lymphocyte called a PLASMA CELL, but there was little reason to think that there is a profound difference between lymphocytes.

Traditionally the immune response has been divided into the HUMORAL, or ANTIBODY RESPONSE, and the CELL-MEDIATED RESPONSES. The humoral response results in the production of antibody, so all of the effects that are observed or measured are the result of this *product* of lymphocytes. Cell-mediated responses, on the other hand, are reactions that are carried out *directly* by the cells themselves. These include the killing of tumor cells and cells infected with intracellular parasites. We now know that all lymphocytes are not the same and that different sets of lymphocytes are responsible for carrying out the humoral and cell-mediated responses.

Cell-Mediated Responses Defined[1]

The designation *cell-mediated response* is used to distinguish these reactions from immune reactions in which antibody is involved. Although many cell-mediated responses involve tissue destruction, other tissue-destroying reactions are caused by antibody. The reactions involving tissue damage are called *hypersensitivity reactions* and will be discussed in Chapter 34. Antibody-mediated hypersensitivity can be transferred to a normal animal with serum from an immune animal. Cell-mediated responses, however, can only be transferred to a normal animal by injecting the lymphoid cells of a sensitized animal. This result implies that the *product* of the B cell (antibody) is responsible for the humoral limb of the immune response, but that the cells themselves carry out the cell-mediated limb of the response.

[1] In Chapter 11 we discussed the methods used to describe and quantify the antibody and cell-mediated responses. At this point, before we examine some of the evidence concerning the mechanisms of cell-mediated responses, the reader may want to review that chapter.

Division of Labor among Cells in the Immune Response

One of the most important realizations in the development of our understanding of the nature of the immune response was that the notion of the immunocompetent cell is correct, but incomplete. In fact, as mentioned eariler, antibody and cell-mediated responses are carried out by different sets of cells; and even among these different populations there can be subpopulations of cells. Furthermore, in addition to the lymphocytes (which are responsible for the specificity of the immune response), accessory cells (macrophages) are also involved.

We will now begin to analyze the various levels of complexity of the cellular basis of the immune response. As you begin to see the beauty at any of these levels, remember that there is still another level to come. The whole process will be very much like peeling an onion; you uncover layer after layer and are often moved to tears during the process. If you like onions, the whole thing is worthwhile.

Effect of Neonatal Thymectomy

Lymphocytes arise from the pluripotent hemopoietic stem cell through the action of inducing factors in the lymphocyte-inducing microenvironments—the bone marrow and the thymus (Chapter 13). The Modern Era of the study of the cellular basis of the immune response can be looked upon as beginning with the simultaneous but independent observations on the role of the thymus by Robert A. Good in Minneapolis, J. F. A. P. Miller in London, and Byron Waksman in New Haven. Good, an immunologist and clinician, noted that in patients with thymomas (tumors of the thymus) there are often accompanying disorders of the immune system, especially acquired hypogammaglobulinemia (a severe reduction in the concentration of serum Igs). He and his colleagues carried out a very large series of experiments in which the thymus was removed from experimental animals and the effect of this THYMECTOMY on the immune response was studied. Miller, an Australian working in England, was studying lymphocytic leukemia in mice. Because the thymus was known to be the target organ of the disease, he asked what the effect of removal of the thymus would be. He showed that in the absence of the thymus the mice did not develop leukemia; but, perhaps of more importance, he also saw that the removal of the thymus had far-reaching effects on the immune response. Waksman was interested in the mechanism of cell-mediated tissue destruction, and he also found that the removal of the thymus at birth impaired the immune function of the adult.

These three investigators all found that removal of the thymus of mice within the first few days after birth (neonatal thymectomy) resulted in a severe *reduction* in immune potential. When the neonatally thymectomized mice reached several weeks of age, they either were given skin from mice of other strains to test their ability to reject grafts (a test of their cell-mediated response) or were inoculated with antigen to test their ability to produce antibody (the humoral response). The neonatally thymectomized mice failed to reject skin grafts, produce antibody, or give delayed skin reactions, whereas sham-thymectomized controls made normal responses.[2] If these neonatally thymectomized mice were repopulated with thymocytes when they reached several weeks of age, their ability to generate responses was restored. These results are shown in Figure 1.

These studies showed that the thymus plays a crucial role in the immune response. Furthermore, the data could be interpreted as showing that the thymus is both necessary and sufficient to allow an animal to carry out both kinds of immune responses. The thymus then seemed to be the source of the immunocompetent cell. Unfortunately, this reasonable assumption is wrong. Nevertheless, this pioneering work can be looked upon as the foundation of modern cellular immunology.

Effect of Bursectomy

The bursa of Fabricius is a lymphoid organ in the cloacal region of the chicken. Removal of this organ also leads to impaired immune function. This remarkable and important discovery was made in 1954 by Bruce Glick, then a graduate student at Ohio State University. He relates how he discovered the fact that the bursa plays a role in the immune response:

> Up to the summer of 1954, bursectomy experiments had failed to reveal a specific function for the bursa. At this time nine of my 6-month-old experimental birds were used by Timothy S. Chang, a fellow graduate student, in a class demonstration which consisted of injecting chickens with *Salmonella typhimurium* O antigen and then determining the antibody titer of

---

[2] In sham thymectomy, the animal is subjected to all aspects of the surgical procedure except the physical removal of the thymus. This control tests the effect of the stress of the thymectomy on the immune response.

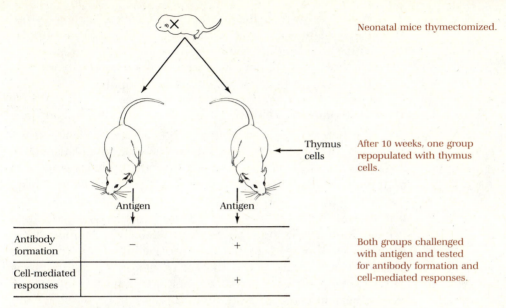

Neonatal mice thymectomized.

After 10 weeks, one group repopulated with thymus cells.

Thymus cells

Antigen   Antigen

Antibody formation	−	+
Cell-mediated responses	−	+

Both groups challenged with antigen and tested for antibody formation and cell-mediated responses.

1   Effect of Neonatal Thymectomy. Neonatal mice are thymectomized, and, after they mature, one group is injected with thymus cells. Both groups are then challenged with antigen, and assessed for antibody and cell-mediated immune responses. Only the group given thymus cells is capable of making immune responses. (There are, however, some "thymus-independent antigens" that will induce a primary antibody response in thymectomized mice.)

the serum. Six of the birds died immediately after the injection. Three survived, but to our surprise, their sera produced no agglutination when mixed with the homologous antigen. The wing-band numbers were checked with the record book, which revealed that all nine birds had previously been bursectomized. It appeared that the bursa was responsible for the result since the normal pen mates reacted to the injections by producing normal antibody titers. [B. Glick, 1964. *The Thymus in Immunobiology*, p. 348]

This rather startling result meant that both thymectomy and bursectomy could cause a severe depression of immune potential. It was soon found, however, that removal of the bursa did not impair the immune response in the same manner as did thymectomy. After neonatal thymectomy both graft rejection and antibody responses (cellular and humoral responses) were depressed. After neonatal bursectomy, however, antibody responses were depressed but skin graft rejection was normal. Indeed, bursectomized chickens rejected grafts as well as sham-operated controls.

These facts were a major piece of evidence leading to the insight that there is division of labor among lymphocyte populations. Other evidence indicated there is even further division of labor, because the lymphocytes must interact with accessory cells (e.g., macrophages) to generate an immune response.

The Role of the Macrophage[3]

The importance of a nonlymphoid cell—the MACROPHAGE—in the generation of immune responses in vivo had long been suspected, but it was not until the invention of in vitro methods for generating immune responses that more precise experiments could be carried out. Robert Mishell and Richard Dutton in La Jolla and John Marbrooke in Melbourne devised tissue culture methods for generating primary in vitro antibody responses in 1966. These methods were very quickly modified so that in vitro cell-mediated responses could also be carried out (see Chapter 11). One of the first problems to be explored using these new techniques was the role of the macrophage in generating immune responses.

Antibody Responses In Vitro: The Mosier Experiment

Cells from the mouse spleen can be separated into two functional populations by their differential ability to adhere to the surface of glass or plastic petri dishes. A few hours after introduction of cells to the containers, those cells not firmly attached to the surface are removed. The nonadherent cells are lymphocytes. The adherent cells are predominantly macrophages. When antigen is added to the unfractionated spleen cell population in vitro, antibody is produced. But when antigen is added to either the adherent or the nonadherent population, no antibody is produced. When these two populations are recombined, however, there is antibody production (Figure 2). This classic experiment, performed by Donald Mosier, was the first to show unequivocally that lymphocytes must interact with a nonlymphoid cell to be able to generate an antibody response.

Cytotoxic T Cells

Macrophages were soon found also to be required for the generation of cytotoxic lymphocytes (CTLs), as shown in Figure 3. In

---

[3] For historical reasons, we are considering only macrophages as the "accessory cells" required for the generation of antigen-specific responses. Later we'll see that many different cells can perform this function. These immunologically important cells are called, collectively, ANTIGEN-PRESENTING CELLS for reasons we'll go into in Chapter 20. The reader should be alert to the fact that at some point we will begin using the latter term.

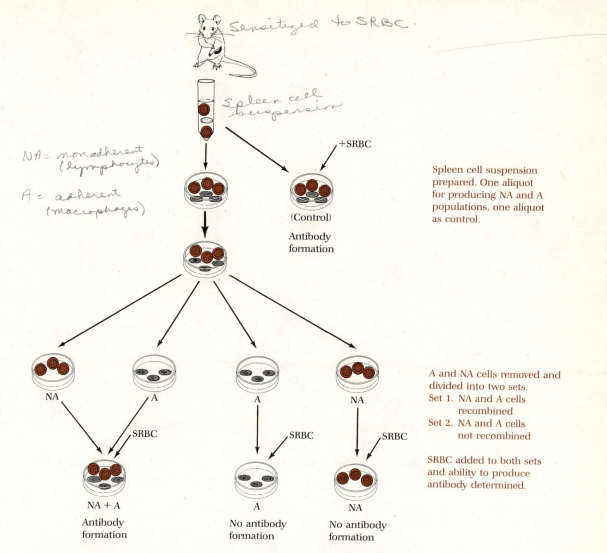

Sensitized to SRBC.

Spleen cell suspension

NA = nonadherent (lymphocytes)

A = adherent (macrophages)

+SRBC

(Control)

Antibody formation

Spleen cell suspension prepared. One aliquot for producing NA and A populations, one aliquot as control.

NA   A   A   NA

SRBC   SRBC   SRBC

NA + A   A   NA

Antibody formation

No antibody formation

No antibody formation

A and NA cells removed and divided into two sets.
Set 1. NA and A cells recombined
Set 2. NA and A cells not recombined

SRBC added to both sets and ability to produce antibody determined.

2   Nonadherent and Adherent Cells in Antibody Responses. Spleen cells are separated on the basis of adherence to glass or plastic, which enriches for the adherent (A) macrophages and the nonadherent (NA) lymphocytes. Neither population can respond to antigen in vitro by producing antibody, but a mixture of the two populations does respond. [After Mosier, 1967. *Science* 158: 1573]

this experiment, spleen cells from CBA ($H-2^k$) mice were immunized in vitro against cells from BALB/c ($H-2^d$) mice in the presence or absence of macrophages. Cytotoxic cell activity was determined by the release of ^{51}Cr from DBA/2 target cells. (DBA/2 mice are also

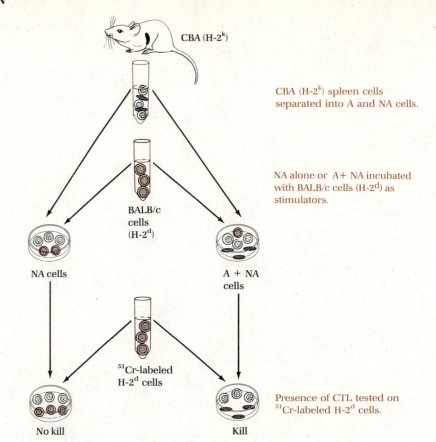

CBA (H-2^k)

CBA (H-2^k) spleen cells
separated into A and NA cells.

NA alone or A+ NA incubated
with BALB/c cells (H-2^d) as
stimulators.

BALB/c
cells
(H-2^d)

NA cells

A + NA
cells

^{51}Cr-labeled
H-2^d cells

No kill

Kill

Presence of CTL tested on
^{51}Cr-labeled H-2^d cells.

NA are lymphocytes
A are macrophages)

3 **Nonadherent and Adherent Cells in the Generation of CTL Effector Cells.** Spleen cells are separated as in Figure 2, but in this experiment the cells are stimulated with allogeneic cells to generate cytotoxic T cells (see Chapter 11). The nonadherent lymphocytes fail to generate CTLs in the absence of adherent macrophages. [After Wagner et al., 1972. *J. Exp. Med.* **136**: 331]

H-2^d.) It can be seen that in the absence of macrophages the numbers of cytotoxic cells generated were greatly reduced, showing the need for these cells in the generation of a CTL response.

All these experiments show that there are various forms of the immune response and that lymphocytes and macrophages must interact to generate them. This is another way of stating that there is a division of labor among the cells of the immune reponse.

Summary

1. The immune response consists of the humoral, or antibody, response and cell-mediated responses. Lymphocytes are responsible for both.

2. In the antibody response lymphocytes produce a product—antibody—that has immune function. In cell-mediated responses the lymphocytes themselves carry out the immune function.

3. Removal of the thymus at birth abolishes antibody and cell-mediated responses. Restoration of thymus cells restores the responses. Removal of the bursa of Fabricius from chickens at birth abolishes antibody but not cell-mediated responses.

4. Macrophages are required for the generation of antibody and for cytotoxic responses.

CELL COOPERATION IN ANTIBODY FORMATION

CHAPTER

17

Overview In the last chapter we saw that there is a division of labor among the cells of the immune response. In this chapter and the next, we will begin to see *how* the labor is divided. We will develop the evidence for the remarkable fact that there are cell interactions in both humoral and cell-mediated responses. These interactions take the form of cell cooperation in which some cells carry out the immune functions (these are called effector cells) and some cells act as helpers. Helper cells that participate in the generation of the effector cells in both humoral and cell-mediated responses are T cells. In this chapter we will examine evidence for cooperation in the production of antibody. B cells are the effector cells in antibody responses because they produce the antibodies; but they also require helper cells.

The next layer of complexity involves the means by which helper and effector cells interact with antigen. The reaction of helper T cells and effector B cells with different antigenic determinants (or epitopes) was discovered through the use of haptens and carriers. The explanation of what had been a rather mysterious phenomenon called the carrier effect allowed us to see that the helper cell (the T cell) reacts with the carrier portion of the antigen and the effector cell (the B cell) reacts with the haptenic determinant. This means that for a molecule to initiate an immune response (that is, to be an immunogen), it must have at least two kinds of determinants, helper and effector.

Evidence of Cooperating Cell Populations

In the early 1960s the picture that was emerging from the neonatal thymectomy and bursectomy studies showed that there is division of labor within the lymphocyte population. The bursa (or its equivalent in mammals) appeared to control some aspects of antibody formation, while the thymus appeared to be involved in both anti-body formation and graft rejection. The almost universal view of the thymectomy studies was that the thymus, a primary lymphoid organ, was both necessary and sufficient for the immune response and was seeding the secondary tissues with functional cells. This arrangement had been predicted at the turn of the century, as shown in the following quote, which was made at a time when people could be more certain about both science and nationalism.

> It has fallen to my lot to show that the first leucocytes arise in the thymus, from its epithelial cells, and that the thymus must be regarded as the parent source of all the lymphoid structures of the body. It does not cease to exist in later life no more than would the Anglo-Saxon race disappear, were the British Isles to sink beneath the waves. For just as the Anglo-Saxon stock has made its way from its original home into all parts of the world, and has there set up colonies for itself and for its increase, so the original leucocytes, starting from their birthplace and home in the thymus, have penetrated into almost every part of the body, and have there created new centres for growth, for increase and useful work for themselves and for the body. [J. Beard, 1899. The true function of the thymus. *Lancet* i: 144. Quoted by Defendi, 1964, in *The Thymus in Immunobiology*]

This comforting notion—that all immunocompetent cells come from the thymus—was shaken by experiments from at least two sources, which showed that the situation might not be this simple. Two groups, one in America and one in England, did experiments having different designs but addressing the same question and coming to the same conclusion. This kind of situation occurs over and over in science and should make us all aware that there are times when a question can be posed in such a manner that it can be answered, and the likelihood is that more than one creative person will realize this.

Bone Marrow–Thymus Reconstitution: The Claman Experiment

One set of experiments was carried out in Denver by Henry Claman and his co-workers, who X-irradiated mice to abolish their immune systems and then attempted to restore immune function with thymus cells. Given the view of the day, thymus cells should have restored the ability of the mice to produce antibody. In this experiment (Figure 1), the thymus and bone marrow of normal mice were removed and made into single-cell suspensions. An aliquot of each of the two cell populations was then injected into groups

*irradiation
kills lymphocytes
but not macrophages*

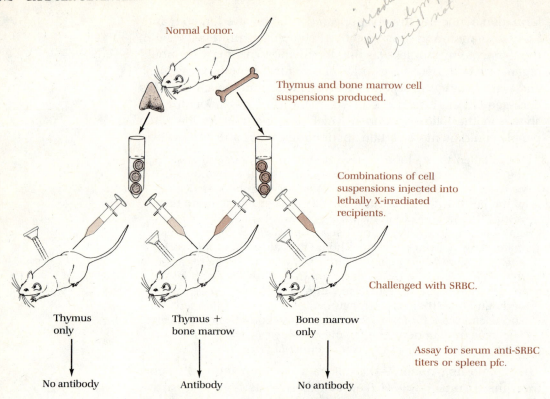

Normal donor.

Thymus and bone marrow cell
suspensions produced.

Combinations of cell
suspensions injected into
lethally X-irradiated
recipients.

Challenged with SRBC.

Thymus
only

Thymus +
bone marrow

Bone marrow
only

Assay for serum anti-SRBC
titers or spleen pfc.

No antibody

Antibody

No antibody

1   The Claman Experiment: Bone Marrow–Thymus Reconstitution.
Irradiated mice do not have their immune function restored if they are
repopulated with either bone marrow or thymus cells alone. The ability to
produce antibody in response to antigen (SRBC) is restored only by repopulating the irradiated mice with *both* bone marrow and thymus cells. [After
Claman et al., 1966. *Proc. Soc. Exp. Biol. Med.* 122: 1167]

of lethally X-irradiated, syngeneic recipients.[1] Marrow and thymus
were injected into one group, only thymus into another group,
and only marrow into a third group. In this way the experiment
had the necessary experimental and control groups to determine
whether either population alone produced antibody. The mice
were challenged with antigen (sheep red blood cells, SRBC), and
after an appropriate interval the amount of antibody produced
was determined.

   The results of the experiment in Figure 1 showed that repopulating irradiated mice with either marrow alone or thymus alone
was *not* sufficient to generate a significant titer of antibody. How-

---

[1] "Syngeneic" refers to genetically identical individuals. "Allogeneic" refers to genetically
different members of the same species.

ever, injection of cells from *both* the primary lymphoid organs resulted in restoration of the antibody response. This finding showed clearly that thymus cells alone are not able to reconstitute the antibody response and immediately questioned the view that the thymus exports all of the functional cells in the immune responses.

The second kind of experiment raising doubt that all immune function is due to the cells of the thymus was done by Anthony Davies and his co-workers in London using cells from animals bearing a chromosomal abnormality called T6. The T6 chromosome was used as a marker to identify cell populations that had been injected into animals. In these experiments, mice were lethally irradiated and repopulated with either bone marrow or thymus cells (one or the other bearing the T6 chromosome). By use of this marker it was possible to show that thymus cells proliferated in response to antigen but no antibody was made. When bone marrow cells were injected into irradiated recipients that then received antigen (but no thymus cells) they did not proliferate nor was antibody produced. But when bone marrow and thymus cells were injected together and the animals challenged with antigen, both populations proliferated and antibody was produced. So this experiment, like the one discussed above, shows that thymus cells alone do not restore to irradiated animals the ability to make antibody responses, but a combination of cells from the thymus and the bone marrow does.

These two experiments showed that there are at least two lymphocyte populations involved in antibody formation and that some form of *cellular cooperation* occurs between them. The inescapable conclusion from these experiments was that there is cellular cooperation between bone marrow and thymus cell populations and one or both of them are then able to produce antibody. The question then became: Which cell population is producing the antibody—the cells from the thymus or the cells derived from the bone marrow, or both?

Evidence for Effector and Helper Cells

Reconstitution after Neonatal Thymectomy: The Mitchell–Miller Experiment

Because repopulation of neonatally thymectomized mice with thymus cells reconstituted the ability of these mice to produce antibody, it was logical to assume that the thymus lymphocytes were the eventual antibody-forming cells. The bone marrow–thymus reconstitution experiments, however, suggested that cooperation was occurring between the thymus and bone marrow cells; and the experiments with chromosomally marked cells suggested that although the thymus-derived cells responded to antigen (by proliferating), they were unable to produce antibody. So it was crucial to determine definitively which cell was producing the antibody and what the other cell type was doing.

The experiment that gave the first clear answer to this question was performed by Graham Mitchell and Jacques Miller and is one of exceptional elegance. This experiment required readily identifiable markers for the cells of the thymus-derived population and another set of markers for the cells of the bone marrow-derived population. H-2 antigens served as perfect markers for this purpose. (At this point the reader should review Chapter 15 on the MHC, if needed.)

The idea of the Mitchell–Miller experiment (Figure 2) was to repopulate, at 8 weeks of age, neonatally thymectomized mice of one MHC haplotype with thymus cells from mice of another MHC haplotype. We already know that injecting thymus cells will restore the ability of the thymectomized animal to produce antibody-forming cells. The crucial part was to then determine which MHC molecules were on the surface of the antibody-producing cells. If they were the same as those of the injected thymus cells, then the thymus-derived cells were the cells that produce antibody. If they were not the same as those of the injected thymus cells but belonged to the haplotype of the thymectomized host, then a cell already present in the host was producing the antibody but was unable to do so until the thymus cells were present.[2]

Anti-H-2 antiserum was used to determine the MHC type of the antibody-forming cells in the following manner. Anti-H-2 antibody reacts with cells with the appropriate H-2 molecules on their surfaces and then allows complement to bind to the Ag-Ab complex. Thus these cells will be lysed in the presence of complement and will no longer be able to carry out any function. If these cells are antibody-forming cells, then the number of antibody-producing cells in the population will be drastically reduced. The appropriate controls for this experiment are to react the cells with an antiserum raised against an irrelevant MHC haplotype, and also with normal serum that contains no anti-H-2 antibodies.

[2] Virtually all the experiments discussed from now on in this chapter describe the quantification of the antibody-forming cells rather than the determination of the titer of antibody. The invention of a plaque-forming assay by Neils Jerne made this possible. The Jerne plaque assay was described in Chapter 11, and the reader may want to review this technique.

This experiment led to one of the great surprises in modern immunology and clearly showed the nature of the division of labor among lymphocytes. Figure 2 shows that there was no reduction in numbers of antibody-producing cells after treatment of the cells of the repopulated animals with antibodies directed against the

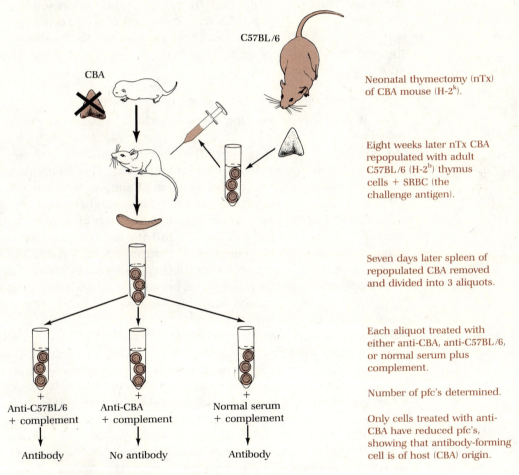

C57BL/6

CBA

Neonatal thymectomy (nTx) of CBA mouse (H-2^k).

Eight weeks later nTx CBA repopulated with adult C57BL/6 (H-2^b) thymus cells + SRBC (the challenge antigen).

Seven days later spleen of repopulated CBA removed and divided into 3 aliquots.

Each aliquot treated with either anti-CBA, anti-C57BL/6, or normal serum plus complement.

Number of pfc's determined.

Only cells treated with anti-CBA have reduced pfc's, showing that antibody-forming cell is of host (CBA) origin.

+	+	+
Anti-C57BL/6 + complement	Anti-CBA + complement	Normal serum + complement
↓	↓	↓
Antibody	No antibody	Antibody

2   The Mitchell–Miller Experiment. This experiment was designed to determine whether thymus cells become antibody-forming cells. Neonatally thymectomized CBA mice were repopulated with C57BL/6 thymus cells and challenged with antigen. Before the assay to determine the number of antibody-forming cells was carried out, aliquots of spleen cells were treated with anti-C57BL/6, anti-CBA, or normal serum, plus complement. Absence of antibody-forming cells after treatment with anti-CBA serum indicated that the cells producing antibody were from the thymectomized host and not from the injected thymus cells. [After Mitchell and Miller. 1968. *Proc. Natl. Acad. Sci. U.S.A.* 59: 296]

H-2 of the injected thymus cells. However, there was almost complete abolition of the antibody-forming cells after treatment with an antiserum directed against the cells of the neonatally thymectomized host. This experiment showed that the thymus cells do not become antibody-producing cells but do allow some cell type already present in the neonatally thymectomized mouse to become an antibody-forming cell. In other words, the presence of the thymus cell is required for the conversion of some other host cell to an antibody-forming cell. The thymus cell thus acts as a "helper" cell for some other cell that becomes an "effector" cell (i.e., an antibody-forming cell).

Thymus Cells Help Bone Marrow Cells Make Antibody

Once it was shown that the thymus-derived cells act as helper cells but do not become antibody-producing cells, the next logical step was to determine whether the effector cells—the antibody-producing cells—are cells from the other primary lymphoid organ, the bone marrow. The experiment seemed simple to do: merely carry out the marrow–thymus reconstitution experiment with bone marrow of one H-2 donor and thymus of another type and treat the antibody-forming cells with anti-H-2 antiserum—that is, carry out a combined Claman and Mitchell–Miller experiment. Surprisingly, when the first part of this experiment was attempted (the allogeneic reconstitution), it was found that no antibody-forming cells could be generated when bone marrow and thymus cells were of different H-2 haplotypes. In other words, attempts at allogeneic marrow–thymus interactions were unsuccessful. This is an important fact, and will be further emphasized later, but at the time the problem remained to determine whether the bone marrow cells are in fact the cells producing antibody.

Experimenters once again took advantage of markers, but this time of chromosomal markers, not cell-surface markers. And, once again, the T6 marker was used. T6 bone marrow and +/+ thymus were injected into irradiated +/+ mice. The antibody-forming cells were then examined and did indeed contain the T6 marker. This result showed that the bone marrow-derived cells produced the antibody. When the experiment was carried out in the other direction, that is, with thymus cells that had the marker and bone marrow cells that did not, none of the antibody-forming cells contained the T6 marker.

The results of this experiment showed that the bone marrow-derived cells produce antibody and thus are the *effector cells* in antibody formation, and that the cells of the thymus act as *helper cells*, because the bone marrow cells alone cannot be induced to produce antibody. Thus we see that there is B cell–T cell cooperation in the generation of an antibody response. It is also safe to conclude that in the thymectomy experiments, the cells of the thymectomized animal that were producing antibody were the bone marrow-derived lymphocytes.

However, the reader should keep in mind that although allogeneic thymus cells can reconstitute a neonatally thymectomized mouse, allogeneic bone marrow and thymus cells cannot cooperate in reconstituting an irradiated host. We will return to this point later and show that when this apparent contradiction was later studied in greater detail, it led to an understanding of a whole new level of complexity in cell cooperation.

Antigen Determinants and Cell Cooperation

We already know that the B cell is the effector cell and the T cell is the helper cell in antibody formation. Our understanding of helper and effector cell interactions in antibody formation came about through our understanding of the roles of *haptens* and *carriers*.

In Chapter 2 we saw that haptens were classically defined by Landsteiner as molecules that can react with antibody but cannot induce antibody formation (i.e., are antigenic but not immunogenic). However, a hapten can be made immunogenic by conjugating it to an immunogenic molecule, such as a foreign protein (the carrier). In this way, hapten–carrier conjugates (H-Cs) elicit anti-hapten and anti-carrier responses when injected into an animal. When a hapten such as DNP is conjugated to any of a variety of immunogenic proteins, the animal responds by producing anti-DNP antibodies as well as antibodies to the carrier. This finding naturally led to the idea that the carrier is only a passive vehicle, whose only function is to transport the hapten. The experiments below describe the *carrier effect* and show this idea to be an oversimplification.

The Carrier Effect

The carrier portion of the H-C has more than the mere transport role it was originally thought to play. An example of what came to be called the CARRIER EFFECT is shown in Figure 3. Dinitrophenol (DNP) is a hapten. When it is injected alone, it does not stimulate

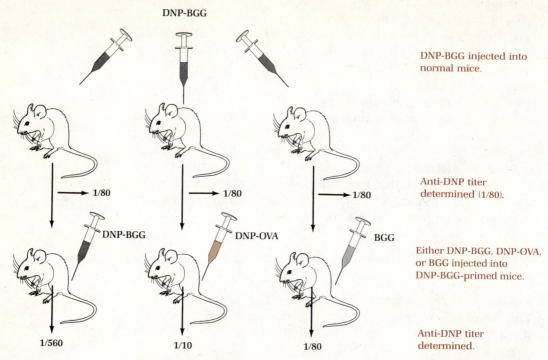

DNP-BGG

DNP-BGG injected into normal mice.

1/80   1/80   1/80

Anti-DNP titer determined (1/80).

DNP-BGG   DNP-OVA   BGG

Either DNP-BGG, DNP-OVA, or BGG injected into DNP-BGG-primed mice.

1/560   1/10   1/80

Anti-DNP titer determined.

3   **The Carrier Effect.** A secondary anti-hapten response is obtained only when the hapten is on the same carrier in both the primary and the secondary injections. This is true even though the mice have made comparable primary anti-hapten responses. [After Ovary and Benaceraff, 1963. *Proc. Soc. Exp. Biol. Med.* 114: 72]

antibody formation. Bovine γ-globulin (BGG) is a carrier. When it is injected alone, it stimulates anti-BGG antibody production. In the experiment shown in Figure 3, animals were immunized with DNP conjugated to BGG (DNP-BGG). After suitable intervals, the serum of the animals was assayed for anti-DNP antibody. As shown in Figure 3, all of the animals made a low anti-DNP response.[3] This response to the first exposure to antigen is called a PRIMARY RESPONSE. The animals were then reinjected with either DNP-BGG (the homologous H-C), DNP-ovalbumin (DNP-OVA) (the same hapten on a different carrier protein), or BGG (the original carrier without hapten). This was to see if they had made a heightened SECONDARY RESPONSE. This response, a characteristic of immunologic

[3] Recall from Chapter 11 that antibody titer, as used in this experiment, is a measurement of specific antibody concentration.

memory, is greatly enhanced over that of the primary response (the dynamics of the antibody response are discussed in detail in Chapter 21). Only the animals that received a second injection of DNP-BGG made a good secondary response to DNP. Thus, even though all the animals had received a first injection of DNP (were *primed* to DNP), they made a secondary response to the second confrontation of DNP only when it was conjugated to the *same* carrier used in the initial injection. This experiment shows that even though an animal is injected with the same hapten for both the primary and the secondary responses, it will make a secondary, or augmented, response to the second injection of hapten only when the hapten is on the same carrier for both injections. In other words, the carrier molecule plays more than a passive role.

Adoptive Transfer of the Carrier Effect

To analyze the cellular events responsible for this surprising result (the carrier effect), N. Avrion Mitchison and his co-workers in London carried out a series of experiments using *adoptive transfer* of the carrier effect. The idea of these experiments was to use an irradiated mouse as a biological test tube. Various spleen cell populations were injected into the irradiated mouse; in this manner the experimenter could determine the role played by a particular cell population in the cellular interactions leading to antibody formation. The beauty of this system was that a variety of experimental manipulations could be made on the spleen cells before transfer. By use of this experimental design the carrier effect could be transferred adoptively, as diagrammed in Figure 4.

In these adoptive transfer experiments mice were lethally irradiated and injected with spleen cells from syngeneic mice. The donor mice had usually been primed to either of two H-Cs that we will call hapten–carrier I (H-CI) and hapten–carrier II (H-CII). Unprimed donor mice were used as a source of control cells. After repopulation with the primed cells, the recipients were challenged with H-CI. Figure 4 shows that only the recipients that were primed with H-CI made a secondary anti-hapten response. Thus, the carrier effect can be adoptively transferred to unprimed, irradiated recipients with spleen cells from H-C-immunized donors.

Overcoming the Carrier Effect by Carrier Priming

The carrier effect can be overcome (that is, a secondary response to H-CII can be obtained) if the recipient mice in the adoptive transfer are repopulated with H-CI-primed cells *plus* cells from

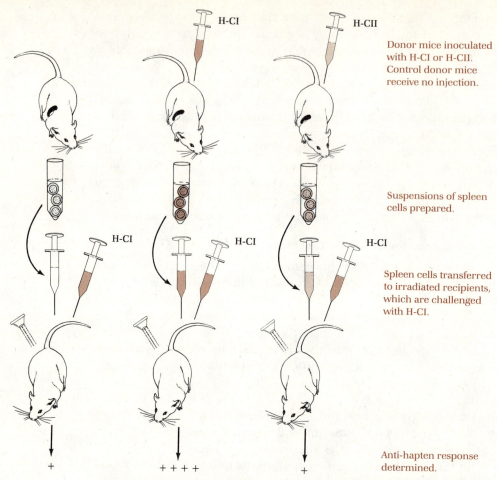

H-CI   H-CII

Donor mice inoculated
with H-CI or H-CII.
Control donor mice
receive no injection.

Suspensions of spleen
cells prepared.

H-CI   H-CI   H-CI

Spleen cells transferred
to irradiated recipients,
which are challenged
with H-CI.

Anti-hapten response
determined.

+   + + + +   +

4   Adoptive Transfer of the Carrier Effect. Mice are immunized with
either H-CI or H-CII and their spleen cells transferred to syngeneic, irradiated
recipients. The recipients are challenged with H-CI. The carrier effect is seen
in the new hosts, in that only those that received spleen cells from H-CI-
immunized donors can give a secondary response to H-CI.

mice *primed to the heterologous carrier alone* (CII). This experiment is diagrammed in Figure 5.

Part A of this experiment was a repeat of the adoptive transfer
of the carrier effect. In part B there were two groups of donors,
one primed to H-CI and one primed only to the heterologous
carrier, CII. The irradiated recipients received primed cells from
each set of donors and were then challenged with hapten conjugated with the heterologous carrier (H-CII). The amount of anti-
hapten antibody produced by these recipients was comparable to

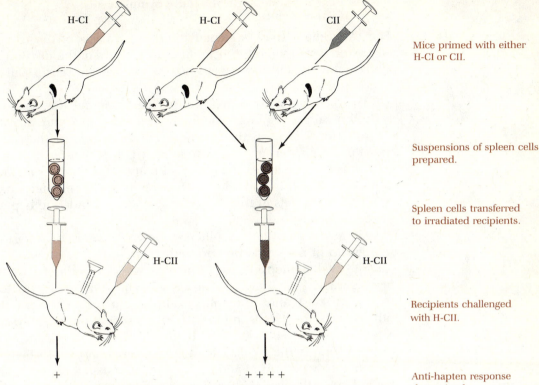

Mice primed with either H-CI or CII.

Suspensions of spleen cells prepared.

Spleen cells transferred to irradiated recipients.

Recipients challenged with H-CII.

Anti-hapten response determined.

5   Overcoming the Carrier Effect. Carrier priming overcomes the carrier effect in an adoptive transfer experiment. Irradiated recipients that received a mixture of spleen cells from mice primed with H-CI and mice primed with CII (with no conjugated hapten) produce a secondary response to H-CII.

that in the mice in Figure 4 that received homologous H-C (H-CI). This result means that the presence of the CII-primed cells over-came the carrier effect. The CII-primed spleen cells could not be contributing the extra anti-hapten antibody because they were not primed to the hapten, but it is clear that they were necessary for the production of a response by the anti-hapten-producing cells.

This experiment shows some form of *cooperation* between the hapten-primed and the carrier-primed populations. It appears that when one set of cells is primed to hapten (H-CI) and one to carrier (CII), they interact to produce a secondary response to the hapten even though it is conjugated to the heterologous carrier. Thus if we can understand the cellular basis of the carrier effect, we will be on the path to understanding the nature of the cell cooperation in the generation of an antibody response.

Hapten-Reactive and Carrier-Reactive Lymphocytes: The Raff Experiment

The experiment that explained the cellular basis of the carrier effect and gave the first indication of the nature of the division of labor among B cells and T cells was carried out by Martin Raff in London in 1970.

The plan of the experiment was elegantly simple. It was essentially the carrier-priming experiment described in Figure 5, with the additional step of treating the primed cells with either anti-Thy-1 or normal serum, plus complement, before transferring them to irradiated recipients. Treatment with anti-Thy-1 antiserum and complement will lyse T cells; in this way it could be determined whether the T cells in the primed mice had responded to hapten or to carrier.

The experiment and results are shown in Figure 6. In part A, one group of mice was primed with H-CI and another with CII. After a suitable interval (approximately 1 week) the adoptive transfer was carried out. However, the carrier-primed cells were treated with anti-Thy-1 antiserum plus complement before transfer. In other words, the T cells in the CII-primed suspension were lysed. The hapten-primed cells were treated with normal serum plus complement, so the T cells in this group were unaffected. The two populations were mixed and injected into irradiated hosts, which were then challenged with hapten conjugated to carrier II (H-CII). We see in Figure 6 that treating the CII-primed population with anti-Thy-1 resulted in a poor anti-hapten response. That is, the carrier effect was *not* overcome. This means that removal of T cells from the CII-primed population abolished the ability to overcome the carrier effect.

In contrast (part B), when the hapten-primed spleen cells were treated with anti-Thy-1 antiserum plus complement and the CII-primed cells were treated with normal serum, the carrier effect *was* overcome. This result shows that killing the T cells had no effect on the hapten-primed population. We know that antibody-producing cells are B cells and that antibody was being produced against the hapten. Therefore this experiment dramatically showed that helper T cells respond to the carrier.

The results of this experiment show that the effector cells and the helper cells in antibody formation each react with a different part of the immunogen. It also shows that we can think of an immunogen as being composed of helper determinants and effector determinants. The different antigenic determinants that interact with T or B cells are called the "epitopes" of the antigen.

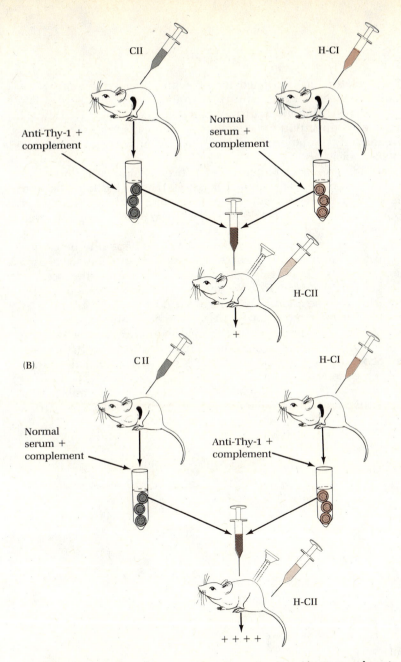

CII

H-CI

Mice primed with CII or H-CI.

Anti-Thy-1 +
complement

Normal
serum +
complement

Suspensions of spleen cells
prepared. CII-primed cells
treated with anti-Thy -1 +
complement. H-CI-primed
cells treated with normal
serum + complement.

Suspensions mixed and injected
into irradiated recipients.

Recipients challenged with
H-CII.

H-CII

Anti-hapten response
determined.

+

(B)

C II

H-CI

Mice primed with CII or H-CI.

Normal
serum +
complement

Anti-Thy-1 +
complement

Suspensions of spleen cells
prepared. CII-primed cells
treated with normal serum +
complement. H-CI-primed
cells treated with anti-Thy-1
+ complement.

Suspensions mixed and injected
into irradiated recipients.

Recipients challenged with H-CII.

H-CII

Anti-hapten response
determined.

+ + +

6   The Raff Experiment: T Cells Recognize Carrier Determinants. This
experiment demonstrates that carrier-primed cells are T cells, because when
cells from CII-immunized mice are treated with anti-Thy-1 plus complement
(to remove T cells), the remaining cells fail to overcome the carrier effect
when mixed with H-CI primed cells. In contrast, there is no effect of treating
the hapten-immunized cells with anti-Thy-1. [After Raff, 1970. *Nature* 226:
1257]

Summary

1.   Repopulating an irradiated mouse with either bone marrow *or* thymus cells does not reconstitute its antibody response. Repopulating the mouse with bone marrow *and* thymus cells does. This shows there is cell cooperation in generating antibody responses.

2.   In antibody formation, B cells are the effector cells and T cells are the helper cells.

3.   The nature of the cell interactions between helper cells and effector cells in antibody formation can be studied using haptens and carriers. Haptens are molecules that do not induce the production of antibody by themselves but do when conjugated to an immunogenic molecule called a carrier.

4.   The carrier effect is the requirement for the hapten to be conjugated to the same carrier in both the primary and the secondary challenge. Hapten conjugated to a second carrier for the second challenge does not lead to a secondary anti-hapten response. The carrier effect can be adoptively transferred.

5.   Priming with heterologous carrier overcomes the carrier effect. When carrier-primed cells are pretreated with anti-Thy-1 and complement and are transferred along with cells primed to hapten on heterologous carrier, the carrier effect is not overcome. This shows that T helper cells are primed to carrier.

6.   Antigen can be thought of as having at least two determinants or epitopes: haptenic determinants that react with B cells and carrier determinants that react with T cells.

CELL COOPERATION IN CELL-MEDIATED IMMUNITY

CHAPTER

18

Overview In the last chapter we saw that in antibody formation, one set of cells acts as effector cells and the other acts as helper cells, and that helper and effector cells interact with different parts of the antigen. As we examine the cellular interactions involved in cell-mediated responses, we will once again see the same basic pattern. The reaction of helper T cells and effector B cells with different antigenic determinants (or epitopes) was discovered through the use of haptens and carriers. This showed that the helper cell (the T cell) reacts with the carrier portion of the antigen and the effector cell (the B cell) reacts with the haptenic determinant. In cell-mediated responses, the same pattern of reaction by the helper and effector cells is seen. The reader should keep in mind the symmetry that is beginning to emerge in humoral and cell-mediated responses. Both use the strategy of helper cell and effector cell, each of which reacts with helper determinants and effector determinants, respectively.

Cell-Mediated versus Humoral Immunity

We saw in the previous chapter that antibodies are formed by cells. It has probably occurred to the reader to ask, "What distinguishes the humoral response from cell-mediated responses, since cells are involved in both?" The difference between humoral and cell-mediated responses is really at the level of the *effector* phase. Antibodies are able to carry out their effects (Chapter 7) in the absence of the cells that made them. In contrast, the effector functions in cell-mediated responses are carried out by the cells themselves. This was shown in the 1940s in a series of classic experiments by Landsteiner (whose fundamental work on the nature of antigens was discussed in Chapter 2) and his student Merrill Chase (who went on to make many important contributions to our understanding of cell-mediated responses).

In these experiments, allergies to drugs, tuberculin, and contact sensitizing agents were induced in guinea pigs. These allergies were of the delayed type (Chapter 11; see also Chapter 34), that is, exposure to the antigen resulted in a response approximately 24 hours later. Landsteiner and Chase then asked if they could get the effect (delayed reaction to antigen) in normal guinea pigs that had received either serum (containing antibody) or cells from the sensitized animals. The animals were challenged with the antigen immediately after transfer of serum or cells, and the responses were checked over the next 24 hours. They found that only the immune cells were able to give the effect, indicating that cells, and not antibodies, were directly responsible.

Varied Nature of Cell-Mediated Responses

The experiments described in the last chapter reveal the flow of discoveries leading to the idea that there are helper cells and effector cells in antibody formation. We will now look at some of the experiments showing that there are also helper cells and effector cells in cell-mediated responses.

Delayed hypersensitivity reactions had been studied for many years. When allograft rejection came to be investigated as a means of studying skin and organ transplantation, it was soon realized that allograft and delayed hypersensitivity reactions are similar because both are cell-mediated responses. With the discovery that the graft-versus-host (GVH) reaction was a form of rejection phenomenon, it made sense to unify all the cell-mediated reactions and to think of them as being roughly equivalent. When in vitro reactions such as the mixed lymphocyte response were found to be cell-mediated reactions, there was initial jubilation because it appeared that more precise and quantitative means of measuring cell-mediated reactions would be available. But, as with most initial unifying notions in science, more and more exceptions were found, until it became clear that all cell-mediated responses are not merely manifestations of the same phenomenon measured in different ways. In fact, the various cell-mediated reactions often measure separate effector and helper functions.

Just as the rapid advances in helper and effector cell cooperation in antibody formation came to dominate so much of immunologic thought in the late 1960s, helper and effector cell cooperation in cell-mediated responses came to dominate much thought in the 1970s. We will see in later chapters that the role of the MHC in these reactions came to dominate cellular immunologic thought in the 1980s.

Helper and Effector Cells in Cell-Mediated Immunity

T Cells Are Required for Cell-Mediated Responses

In antibody formation, the T cell acts as a helper cell and the B cell is the effector cell. Figure 1 shows the results of experiments designed to determine whether the effector cells in cell-mediated responses are B cells or T cells. To carry out these experiments, cell-mediated responses were generated in which the responding

Reaction	Stimulator cell	Responder cell	Reaction	Effect of anti-Thy-1 treatment of responder cell		
				Normal serum	Anti-Thy-1	Percentage reduction
MLR	BALB/c (X-irradiated)	B10	Proliferation as incorporation of [^{3}H]TdR (cpm)	8249	331	94
CTL	BALB/c (mitomycin-treated)	CBA	Release of ^{51}Cr (percentage lysis)	100	4	96
GVH	CBA × C57BL/6 host	CBA graft	Spleen index	1.32	0.91	

1   T Cells Are Required for Cell-Mediated Responses. Removal of T cells from the responder cells in the mixed lymphocyte response (MLR), the generation of cytotoxic cells (CTLs), or the induction of graft-versus-host (GVH) reaction abolishes the response. T cells are removed by treatment of the responder cells with anti-Thy-1 plus complement. The genetic differences in MHC that stimulate each type of response are illustrated by a *square* (H-2^d), *triangle* (H-2^b), or *circle* (H-2^k) on the surface of each cell.

population was treated with anti-Thy-1 (or normal serum) plus complement. The MLR, CTL, and GVH reactions[1] are all abolished by treatment with anti-Thy-1 and complement. In contrast, removal of B cells in similar experiments did not affect the responses. This shows that the cells responsible for these cell-mediated responses are T cells.

A mutation in mice, called "nude," also helped to elucidate the cells responsible for cell-mediated immunity. Mice that are homozygous for this mutation (*nu/nu*) have an epithelial cell defect, which not only makes them hairless (or nude) but also renders them athymic. Since they don't have a thymus, these mutant mice also don't have T cells.[2] These mice also fail to develop cell-mediated immunity, such as delayed-type hypersensitivity and graft rejection. If they are injected with Thy-1$^+$ cells from syngeneic +/+ or *nu/+* animals, their cell-mediated responses return.

Cell Cooperation in GVH Reaction

Cell cooperation in cell-mediated responses was first shown in 1970 by Richard Asofsky and his colleagues at NIH, using the GVH reaction. The recipients were newborn (BALB/c × C57BL/6)F$_1$ mice. Various numbers of parental thymus *or* peripheral blood cells were injected into the F$_1$, and the spleen index for each concentration of injected cells was noted. A third group of F$_1$ recipients was inoculated with both thymus cells *and* peripheral blood cells. The resulting spleen index was greater than the sum of the two reactions to each of the cell types alone. The important point demonstrated by the data (Figure 2) is that by varying the number of cells injected, one can obtain a titration curve relating the spleen index to the number of cells injected. From this titration curve the number of thymus or peripheral blood cells required to give a positive spleen index of 1.3 can easily be determined. In the experiment in Figure 2, an index of 1.3 was achieved with 5×10^6 thymus cells or with 2×10^5 peripheral blood cells. When thymus and peripheral blood cells were injected together, a synergistic reaction occurred, because mixing 5×10^6 thymus with as few as 3×10^4 peripheral blood cells gave an index *greater* than 1.3. Because it required 2×10^5 peripheral blood lymphocytes alone to give an index of 1.3, this result showed that the thymus cells and periph-

See p. 185

---

[1] You should refer back to Chapters 11 and 16 if these terms are unfamiliar.

[2] Nude mice lack conventional, thymus-dependent T cells. We'll see later that they do have a related population of T cells that don't mature in the thymus (the γδ T cells), but the function of this population is still not known.

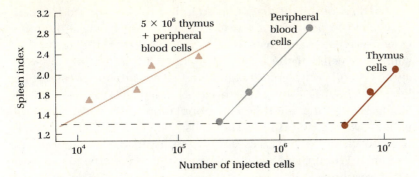

2   Cell Cooperation in the GVH Reaction. Irradiated F_1 mice are injected with varying numbers of parent-strain thymus and/or peripheral blood cells to induce a GVH reaction, measured by spleen index. A mixture of peripheral blood cells and thymus cells produces much greater GVH reaction than the sum of the effects of each population alone. [After Asofsky et al., 1971. *Prog. Immunol.* 1: 369]

eral blood cells together are over *10 times* more effective than they would be if the response were additive. This experiment also showed that in cell-mediated responses, as in antibody formation, there is some sort of cell cooperation going on.

Evidence for Cell Cooperation in the Generation of CTLs

We saw above that the effector cell in cell-mediated responses is a T cell. In this section we will present evidence that the helper cell in these reactions is also a T cell, indicating T cell–T cell cooperation in cell-mediated responses. In these reactions, one T cell is the helper and another the effector. We will also see that there are distinct subpopulations of T cells, which can be identified by surface markers.

The experiments described in the preceding section showing that the cells involved in cell-mediated reactions are T cells required the use of a marker (Thy-1) that distinguishes T cells from B cells. The experiments described in this section showed T cell–T cell interactions in the generation of a CTL response and required a marker that distinguishes different subpopulations of T cells. Such markers exist as a series of surface molecules, called cluster of differentiation (CD) markers (see Chapter 13). Fortunately, there were two well-studied markers, CD5 and CD8, that could be used to delineate T-cell subpopulations (anti-CD4 antibodies were not available at the time, but helped to confirm the results discussed below).

In the experiment diagrammed in Figure 3, lymph node T cells were used to generate an in vitro CTL response. These lymphocytes were pretreated with various antisera *before* the addition of stimulator cells, in the following manner. Treatment of cells with anti-CD5 and complement eliminated all cells that expressed high levels of CD5 (CD5^{hi}) on their surfaces but left cells expressing CD8. Similarly, treating another cell population with anti-CD8 eliminated CD8$^+$ cells and left CD5^{hi} cells.[3] When the CD5^{hi} cells were used to generate the CTLs, they were incapable of generating a response. When CD8$^+$ cells were used, they were able to carry out a CTL response at only 30% of the control value. This result shows that the situation is rather complicated and signals that cell cooperation is probably occurring. When the two (CD5^{hi} and CD8$^+$) populations were combined, however, control levels of CTLs were generated. This result shows that there are two populations of T lymphocytes that interact synergistically in CTL responses. One of these is the effector cell, but it needs the helper cell to fully generate its cytotoxic capacity.

Helper and Effector Cells in Cell-Mediated Responses

To determine which cells were the helpers and which the effectors, another experiment was done (Figure 4). CTLs were generated with lymph node T cells that were *not* treated with any antiserum. After the response had developed, however, and before the cells were assayed for their ability to cause ^{51}Cr release, they were treated with either anti-CD5 or anti-CD8 antiserum and complement. The cells remaining after this treatment were then tested for their

---

[3] Subsequently, it was realized that all T cells (and, in fact, some B cells) carry at least some CD5 molecules on their surface. Cells with *high* CD5 are more susceptible to killing with anti-CD5 antibody, and these are the T cells with helper function. First in studies using human T cells, then with mouse cells, it was found that the best marker for the helper cells was actually *CD4*.

3 Cell Cooperation in the Generation of CTL. (A) Normal spleen cells ▶ are treated with either normal serum (as control), anti-CD5, or anti-CD8 (plus complement in all cases). T cells remaining after each treatment are shown. (B) Each population or mixture is cultured with mitomycin-treated stimulator cells, then assessed for CTL response. Control T cells give a response of 100%. In contrast, CD8$^+$ T cells give a response of 30%, and CD4$^+$,CD5^{hi} T cells give a response of only 5%. Combining the CD8$^+$ and CD4$^+$ populations, however, restores the response to almost control levels, demonstrating cell cooperation in the generation of a CTL response. [After Cantor and Boyse, 1975. *J. Exp. Med.* 141: 1376 and 1390]

(A)

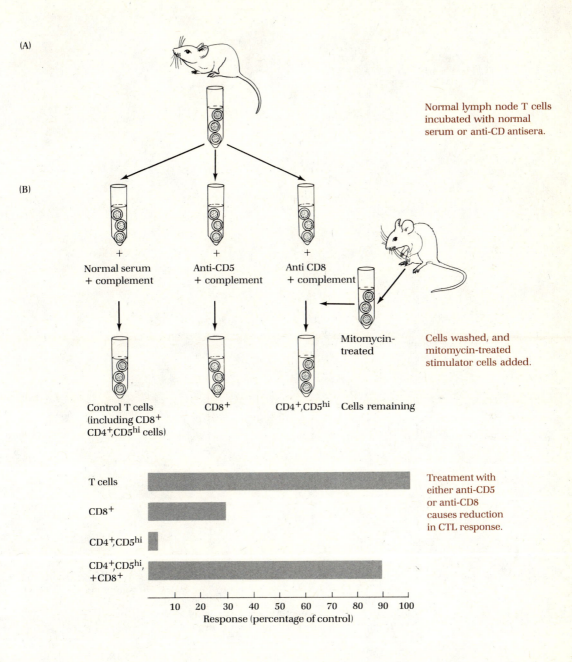

Normal lymph node T cells incubated with normal serum or anti-CD antisera.

(B)

+
Normal serum
+ complement

+
Anti-CD5
+ complement

+
Anti CD8
+ complement

Mitomycin-
treated

Cells washed, and mitomycin-treated stimulator cells added.

Control T cells
(including CD8$^+$
CD4$^+$,CD5^{hi} cells)

CD8$^+$

CD4$^+$,CD5^{hi} Cells remaining

T cells

CD8$^+$

CD4$^+$,CD5^{hi}

CD4$^+$,CD5^{hi},
+CD8$^+$

Treatment with either anti-CD5 or anti-CD8 causes reduction in CTL response.

10 20 30 40 50 60 70 80 90 100
Response (percentage of control)

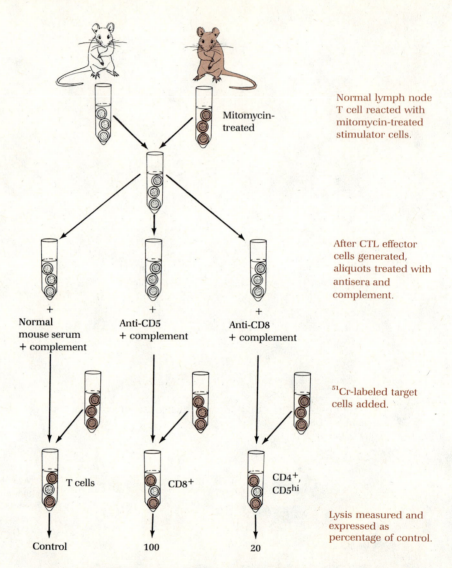

Normal lymph node T cell reacted with mitomycin-treated stimulator cells.

Mitomycin-treated

After CTL effector cells generated, aliquots treated with antisera and complement.

+
Normal mouse serum + complement

+
Anti-CD5 + complement

+
Anti-CD8 + complement

^{51}Cr-labeled target cells added.

T cells

CD8$^+$

CD4$^+$, CD5^{hi}

Lysis measured and expressed as percentage of control.

Control

100

20

4   CD Profile of CTL Effector Cells. CTLs are generated by culturing normal lymph node T cells with mitomycin-treated stimulator cells. Following culture, the cells are treated with antisera plus complement and then assessed for CTL by reaction with ^{51}Cr-labeled targets. Treatment with anti-CD5 (leaving CD8$^+$ T cells) does not reduce the CTL function (measured as percentage lysis), but treatment with anti-CD8 does. Thus, the CTL effector in this system is CD8$^+$. [After Cantor and Boyse, 1975. *J. Exp. Med.* 141: 1376] ability to act as effector cells in a CTL response. In this way it was possible to determine the CD phenotype of the *effector* population. It was found that only treatment with anti-CD8 and complement abolished the ability of the cells to carry out lysis of the target cells. This result shows that the $CD8^+$ cells are the *effector* cells and that the $CD5^{hi}$ cells act as *helper* cells. Today, we know that a better marker for helper T cells in these kinds of experiments is CD4, but the general conclusions remain the same.

Cell-Mediated Responses

In the above experiments, neither the $CD5^{hi}$ nor the $CD8^+$ T cells alone were able to generate large numbers of CTL effector cells. Combining the $CD5^{hi}$ and the $CD8^+$ populations, however, restored CTL activity to levels comparable to those of the untreated cells. By treating cells with antisera *after* CTLs had been generated, it was shown that the effector cell was the $CD8^+$ cell and the helper cell the $CD5^{hi}$ cell. More recent experiments, using monoclonal anti-CD antibodies, have confirmed that, in general, the helper cells for generation of a CTL response are $CD4^+$ and $CD5^{hi}$, and the effector cells are $CD8^+$. This has been demonstrated in humans, mice, rats, and a number of other animals. In later chapters we will see that there can be exceptions to this rule, but for now this conclusion is useful as a first approximation.

MLR and CTL Responses and MHC Molecules

An important series of experiments by Fritz Bach and his co-workers in Madison showed that there are separate *subpopulations* of T cells, which react with different molecules of the MHC complex.[4] The general plan of these experiments was to test the ability of cells to stimulate an MLR by using cells from strains of mice with known differences in the MHC. By choosing the proper congenic strains, it was possible to test the contribution to the MLR of a difference in only one region of the MHC. To test the role of the molecules of the D region, for example, one could choose as responder a strain that is *bbbb* ($K^b I^b S^b D^b$). The stimulator cell (which is treated with mitomycin C so that it cannot proliferate)

---

[4] In the rest of this chapter we will be discussing the generation of cytotoxic T lymphocytes (CTLs), the mixed lymphocyte response (MLR), and the major histocompatibility complex (MHC). It will be necessary to lapse into "immunologese" at times. The reader is urged to review CTL and MLR in Chapters 11 and 16 and MHC in Chapter 15 before proceeding.

could then be *bbbk*. In this case the only difference is in the D region of the H-2 complex: *b* in one case, *k* in the other. Similar combinations could be set up for the K region (class I MHC, like the D region) or the I region (class II MHC). The results of MLR stimulation studies are expressed as a stimulation index (SI), which is calculated as

$$SI = \frac{\text{Incorporation of } [^3H]Tdr \text{ in experimental}}{\text{Incorporation of } [^3H]Tdr \text{ in control}}$$

If the incorporation in the experimental group is the same as that in the control group, the SI is 1.0. If the experimental value is six times that of the control, the SI is 6.0, and so on.

When a large number of combinations were examined, a pattern emerged (Table 1). The greatest stimulation of the MLR came from differences in the class II MHC (the I region of H-2). Similar kinds of experiments were also carried out in the generation of CTLs, the idea being to vary only one region of the MHC and examine the effect on the CTL response. Differences in class II MHC gave little or no CTL response, while differences in class I MHC regions gave good stimulation. Thus we see that the MLR is associated with class II molecules and the CTL response with class I molecules.

The "Three-Cell Experiment"

The most dramatic results of this series of experiments came from Bach's three-cell experiment. Now we know that cells that differ in class II MHC give the best MLR and cells that differ in class I MHC give a good CTL response. If the MLR and CTL responses

Table 1   Effect of various regions of the MHC on the generation of mixed lymphocyte responses (MLRs) and cytotoxic T cells (CTLs).

Difference between responder and stimulator cells	MLR	CTL response
Class I MHC	Poor	Good
Class II MHC	Very good	Poor
Class III MHC	Poor	Poor
Class I and Class II MHC	—	Very good

are manifestations of helper and effector cell stimulation, respectively, then combining the cells with the differences seen in Table 1 should give strong MLRs and even stronger CTL responses. Figure 5 shows that this is exactly the result obtained. Although differences at class I MHC gave good CTL responses and differences at class II MHC gave poor CTL responses, the combination

MLR (proliferation, as cpm [^{3}H]thymidine)	Stimulator cells	Responder cells	CTL (cytotoxicity, as percentage of maximum ^{51}Cr release)
10,000	Stimulator and responder cells differ only at class II		0
3000	Stimulator and responder cells differ only at class I.		15
10,000	Mixture of stimulators differs at class I and class II		50

5   The Three-Cell Experiment. This experiment shows that there is a collaboration between class I and class II MHC differences in the generation of a CTL response. When stimulator and responder cells differ only at class II MHC, an MLR is generated, but not a CTL response. A difference only at class I MHC results in a relatively low MLR with some CTLs generated. A mixture of the two types of stimulator cells, however, results in both MLR and strong CTL responses. [After Schendel et al., 1976. *Nature* 259: 273] of differences at class I and class II gave the best response. It turned out, though, that these MHC differences need not be on the same stimulator cell. Optimal responses were also obtained when two stimulator cell populations, one differing at class I and one at class II MHC, were added to the responding cells (hence three cells).

Related experiments showed that the targets of the CD8$^+$ cytotoxic T cells have to bear the class I MHC difference used to stimulate the CTL response. Thus, the effector cells of the CTL response recognize class I MHC.

Other experiments carried out at about this time showed that the MLR reactive cell is a CD4$^+$,CD5^{hi} cell. This finding leads to the conclusion that in the generation of CTLs the cells reactive with class II MHC molecules are the *helper* cells and cells reactive with class I MHC determinants are the *effector* cells. Thus in cell-mediated responses, just as in antibody responses, there are helper cells and effector cells, each of which reacts with unique determinants on the antigen. The association of CD4$^+$ helper cells with recognition of class II MHC and CD8$^+$ effector cells with recognition of class I MHC will be a recurring theme in the following chapters.

Cellular Cooperation in Delayed-Type Hypersensitivity

In Chapter 11, we introduced another variety of cell-mediated immunity, the delayed-type hypersensitive (DTH) response. In this response, immune individuals respond to antigen by an influx of cells into the area, resulting in a swelling of the tissues after approximately 24 hours. Like other forms of cell-mediated immunity, the DTH response can be adoptively transferred by T cells. The T cells that transfer DTH are CD4$^+$, which suggested to some investigators that these are helper cells for the response. What, then, are the effector cells?

It turns out that the effector cells in this response are myeloid cells, usually macrophages (but sometimes basophils). These cells are not antigen-specific, and all the specificity of the response comes from the helper T cells. In response to specific antigen the helper cells release substances that lead to the recruitment and activation of the nonspecific effector cells, which then mediate the effects of the immunity. Thus, in this response, the principle of cell cooperation is upheld, even though one of the interacting cell populations (the effectors) is not, itself, antigen-specific.

Summary

1. In cell-mediated immune responses, T cells can act as either helper or effector cells.

2. Experiments in which T-cell populations were treated with anti-CD antibodies and complement showed that CD4$^+$,CD5^{hi} T cells and CD8$^+$ T cells cooperate in the generation of cytotoxic T cells.

3. In the cytotoxic T-cell responses, CD8$^+$ T cells are usually the effector cells and CD4$^+$,CD5^{hi} T cells are usually the helper cells.

4. Cells which respond in the MLR and cells which act as helper cells for the generation of CTL usually react with Class II MHC determinants. CTL effector cells usually react with class I MHC determinants.

5. In delayed-type hypersensitive responses, CD4$^+$ helper cells are antigen-specific; however, they stimulate antigen-nonspecific effector cells, which are usually macrophages.

MHC RESTRICTION

Overview We have been dropping tantalizing hints that the MHC plays a central role in generating immune responses. In this chapter we will present some of the evidence showing that this is the case. The first inkling of the importance of the MHC in the generation of immune responses came when we saw that the high versus low responder trait mapped to the MHC and, in fact, defined the I region, encoding class II MHC molecules (Chapter 15) . We will see in this chapter that the next important realization came when it was found that cell cooperation apparently can occur only between cells with the same MHC, a phenomenon called MHC RESTRICTION. One of the more surprising results we will see (in this and in subsequent chapters) is the finding of ADAPTIVE DIFFERENTIATION, in which MHC restriction can be acquired or learned. Thus, there is yet another level of complexity of cell interactions. The picture that will emerge is one of the foundations of modern immunology.

MHC Restriction in Antibody Formation

We have suggested that the MHC plays an important role in cellular cooperation. In this chapter (and the next), we will see that T cells are capable of responding to an antigen only when it is "presented" to the T cell together with the appropriate MHC molecule. This is referred to as MHC-RESTRICTED ANTIGEN RECOGNITION. We begin with the studies that suggested that MHC restriction is a real phenomenon. In the next chapter, we'll move on to the developments that gave us a picture of what causes MHC restriction. This involves the processing and presentation of antigen by a macrophage (or other antigen-presenting cell) to a T cell.

Mitchell–Miller Revisited: The Need for Syngeneic Cells

The Mitchell–Miller experiment (Chapter 17) was one of the crucial experiments in the development of the idea of cell cooperation in the immune response. In that experiment, neonatally thymecto-mized mice of one MHC haplotype were repopulated with thymus cells from mice of another haplotype (allogeneic thymus cells) to determine whether the thymus-derived lymphocytes were the antibody-producing cells. The haplotype of the antibody-forming cells was shown to be that of the host rather than that of the donor of the thymus cells, proving that the thymus cells did not produce antibody, but only acted as helper cells for a cell already present in the thymectomized mouse. However, a difficulty devel-oped when the approach of using different MHC haplotypes as markers could not be used in a Claman-type experiment of bone marrow–thymus reconstitution of irradiated mice. In that experi-ment, allogeneic bone marrow and thymus cells failed to cooperate in an irradiated host. This inability to cooperate across an MHC barrier was thought to be merely a technical nuisance. As we will now see, the "nuisance" became a profound observation. There is undoubtedly some great lesson of social significance to be learned from this.

[handwritten margin note: ? Didn't they cooperate in 1st expt ??]

[handwritten margin note: No – Bone M. has both T & B cell precursors]

Repopulation Failure in Nude Mice

The inability of allogeneic bone marrow and thymus cells to coop-erate was seen again in some very important experiments carried out by Bernice Kindred and Donald Shreffler. They found that nude mice (which are congenitally athymic) could have their im-mune response restored only transiently with allogeneic thymus cells. In these studies, BALB/c nudes were repopulated with thy-mus cells from syngeneic BALB/c mice (H-2^d) or with allogenic thymus cells of CBA (H-2^k) or C57BL/6 (H-2^b) mice. If the animals were challenged with antigen and assayed for antibody within a few days after reconstitution, they produced a good antibody response, whether reconstituted with syngeneic or allogeneic thy-mus cells. But if there was an interval of several days between repopulating with thymus cells and challenge with antigen, only the animals reconstituted with the syngeneic thymus cells responded. The lack of response by the animals repopulated with allogeneic thymus cells was not due to the disappearance of the allogeneic cells or to reaction by the host against them, but was, rather, a reflection of an inability to cooperate with cells in the host.

Kindred went on to do a large series of experiments with thymus grafts and was able to show clearly that the responses of nude mice were restored much more efficiently with syngeneic than with allogeneic grafts. It is now safe to assume that the transient restoration seen using allogeneic cells was caused by a different phenomenon. The irony is that this also means that the Mitchell–Miller experiment—the crucial experiment showing helper and effector cells, upon which so much followed—probably gave "correct" results for the wrong reason. The B cells that were activated in these experiments were almost certainly activated by an ALLOGENEIC EFFECT (see below), in which helper T cells were activated by the allogeneic MHC and, in turn, stimulated the B cells.

Overcoming the Carrier Effect with Allogeneic Cells: The Allogeneic Effect

We saw in Chapter 17 that it is possible to overcome the carrier effect with carrier priming and that this second effect is the result of a reaction between helper T cells and carrier determinants on the antigen. David Katz and his co-workers, first at NIH and then in Boston, found that it is possible to overcome the carrier effect in another, quite different way. They observed that the injection of *allogeneic cells* could also allow the animals to respond to H-CII with a secondary anti-hapten response (see Chapter 17).

As shown in Figure 1, an H-CI-primed animal makes a secondary anti-hapten response to H-CII when allogeneic cells are injected. This is an apparent paradox. In one set of circumstances (the Claman experiment), allogeneic cells fail to cooperate to produce an immune response. Under slightly different circumstances (the Mitchell–Miller experiment), not only do the allogeneic cells cooperate, but they even bypass the need for carrier priming (the Katz experiment). What's going on here? Is MHC compatibility required for cellular cooperation, or not? The experiments that unfold in the next few chapters will go a long way toward putting this puzzle together.[1]

---

[1] We are aware that to a student approaching a field for the first time, this kind of thing is nearly intolerable. However, to a scientist confronting such problems, there is a comfort and excitement in the realization that when the problem is solved, important insights are to be gained. Our goal is to minimize the discomfort while attempting to share some of the excitement that comes with the resolution of the paradox. So, stick with us on this.

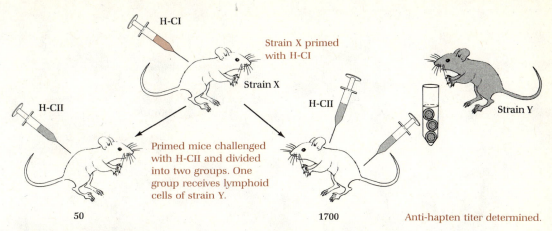

H-CI

Strain X primed
with H-CI

Strain X

H-CII

H-CII

Strain Y

Primed mice challenged
with H-CII and divided
into two groups. One
group receives lymphoid
cells of strain Y.

50

1700

Anti-hapten titer determined.

1   The Allogeneic Effect. Mice of one strain are immunized with hapten–carrier I and their spleen cells are transferred to syngeneic, irradiated recipients. Some animals are also injected with spleen cells from unimmunized mice of another strain. The recipients are then challenged with hapten–carrier II. A good anti-hapten antibody response develops (i.e., the carrier effect is overcome) if the animals also received allogeneic (MHC different) spleen cells.

Claman Revisited: The Need for I Region (Class II) MHC Identity

The examples of the inability of bone marrow- and thymus-derived cells to cooperate across MHC barriers were studied extensively by Katz and his co-workers, who showed that a fundamental principle in the immune response was involved. Using a reconstitution system that was designed to *minimize the allogeneic effect*, they primed T cells to carrier (CI) in one strain of mice (B10.A) and primed B cells to hapten (H-CII) in mice of homologous (B10.A) and heterologous (A.A.By) strains.[2] The system, which is a variation of the original Claman experiment, is diagrammed in Figure 2. These primed populations were then allowed to cooperate in an irradiated F_1 of the two parental strains. The recipient was then challenged with hapten (H-CI), and the anti-hapten response was tested. In this way, the researchers were able to determine whether carrier-primed T cells could cooperate with B cells of any MHC haplotype, or whether there was genetic restriction in the interaction of T cells and B cells. Figure 2 shows that when both cell populations were from the same strain (group I), there was good cooperation—as expected. When the cells were from strains that were allogeneic at both background and MHC (group II), there was

---

[2] Many experiments in this and the next chapter will use congenic mice; the reader may want to review Chapter 15. A thorough understanding of the carrier effect (Chapter 17) is also needed at this point.

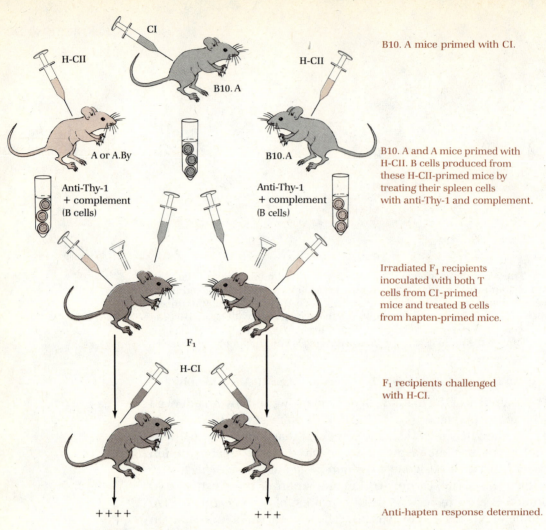

CI

H-CII

B10.A

H-CII

B10. A mice primed with CI.

A or A.By

B10.A

Anti-Thy-1
+ complement
(B cells)

Anti-Thy-1
+ complement
(B cells)

B10. A and A mice primed with
H-CII. B cells produced from
these H-CII-primed mice by
treating their spleen cells
with anti-Thy-1 and complement.

F_1

Irradiated F_1 recipients
inoculated with both T
cells from CI-primed
mice and treated B cells
from hapten-primed mice.

H-CI

F_1 recipients challenged
with H-CI.

++++

+++

Anti-hapten response determined.

	T cells (K, I-A, I-E, D)	B cells (K, I-A, I-E, D)	Genetic difference	Anti-hapten antibody produced
I	B10.A (kkdd)	B10.A (kkdd)	H-2 same, background same	
II	B10.A (kkdd)	A.By (bbbb)	H-2 different, background different	
III	B10.A (kkdd)	A (kkdd)	H-2 same, background different	
IV	B10.A (kkdd)	B10 (bbbb)	H-2 different, background same	

poor cooperation. The crucial groups here are groups III and IV. In group III, the MHC regions are identical ($H\text{-}2^a$), but the backgrounds are different (B10 and A). Nevertheless, there is good cooperation, indicating that any barrier to cooperation is not found in the background but in MHC. In group IV, the backgrounds are identical (B10 and B10.A), but the MHC is different. This arrangement results in poor cooperation. From this experiment, Katz concluded that identity at MHC is required for B cell–T cell cooperation.

The results in Figure 2 show that there can be cooperation of populations when background genes are different, but no cooperation unless the MHC genes are identical. But these results do not show *which* region of MHC must be shared. Experiments of similar design using other recombinant strains showed that the crucial differences in the MHC complex are localized in the I region (class II MHC).

MHC Restriction in Cell-Mediated Responses

Shortly after Katz showed that there was MHC restriction in the generation of an antibody response, two groups working independently showed that there is also MHC restriction in the generation of cell-mediated responses.

The Zinkernagel–Doherty–Shearer Phenomenon

The generation of cytotoxic T cells is also MHC-restricted.[3] This phenomenon was demonstrated for viruses and haptens by Rolf Zinkernagel and Peter Doherty in Australia and Eugene Shearer at NIH. It was soon extended to minor histocompatibility antigens (non-MHC molecules that cause a slow rejection response) and

---

[3] When CTLs are generated against allogeneic MHC, the effect is specific for the foreign MHC molecule and is therefore *not* restricted to self-MHC (by definition). We will return to the special problem of allogeneic responses in Chapter 20.

---

2   MHC Restriction in Antibody Responses. Mice of different strains are immunized with carrier I or with hapten–carrier II. Spleen cells from mice primed with the latter are treated with anti-Thy-1 plus complement (leaving hapten-primed B cells). The carrier-primed spleen cells and the hapten-primed B cells are then injected into irradiated F_1 recipients, which are then challenged with hapten–carrier I. The anti-hapten antibody response is assessed as an indication of cell cooperation between hapten- and carrier-primed cells.

the male H-Y antigen.[4] It is now seen as one of the basic rules of the immune response.

The basis of the phenomenon is shown in Figure 3. Mice of one strain are immunized with antigen to generate CTLs. After an appropriate interval their spleen cells are added to ^{51}Cr-labeled target cells of the same or a different strain. When the antigen (virus, TNP, minor H, or H-Y) is on a target cell of the same MHC haplotype as that of the immunized mouse, killing of the target cells occurs (group A). The following controls show that the spleen cells contain cytotoxic cells specific for *both* the antigen and the MHC molecules on the target cells. When the sensitized spleen cells are added to cells of the same MHC haplotype that have no antigen (group B) or an inappropriate antigen (group C), no killing occurs. This result shows that the injection of antigen has resulted in antigen-specific cytotoxic cells. The important group is group D, in which the specific antigen is on target cells of another MHC haplotype. In this group, no killing occurs. This means that even though antigen-specific cytotoxic cells were generated, they could only kill target cells displaying the appropriate antigen when the target cells were also of the same MHC haplotype. Thus, there is MHC restriction in the function of cytotoxic T cells, just as there is in antibody formation.

The Site of MHC Restriction

The MHC restriction in antibody formation was localized to the I region, that is, the region coding for class II MHC antigens. When a similar analysis was done for CD8$^+$ cytotoxic T cells, it was found that the restriction is exerted not in the I region, but in the K and D regions (class I). This is shown in Table 1. We thus have a situation in which the generation of helper cells is restricted at the I region (class II) and the generation of cytotoxic effector cells is restricted in the K/D regions (class I). This tendency is found in rodents, humans, and many other species.

Compatibility between Responder and Stimulator

The data in Figure 3 could be interpreted to mean that there is MHC restriction between the cytotoxic cell and the target (that is, in the effector, or killing, phase of the CTL reaction), or it could indicate MHC restriction in the generation of the cytotoxic cells.

[4] H-Y is a minor histocompatibility antigen expressed in male but not female mice. Though its precise nature (or physiological function) is not known, it has been useful in some important immunologic studies (see Chapters 24 and 25).

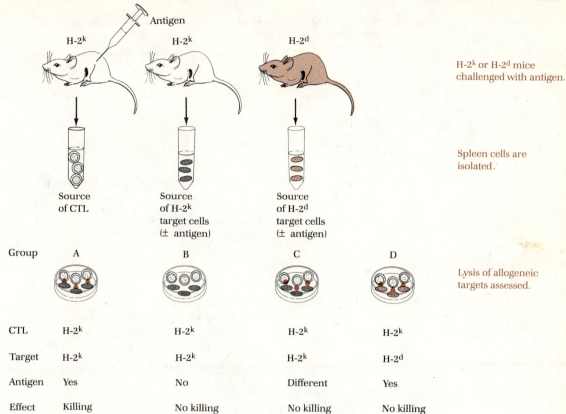

Group	A	B	C	D
CTL	H-2^k	H-2^k	H-2^k	H-2^k
Target	H-2^k	H-2^k	H-2^k	H-2^d
Antigen	Yes	No	Different	Yes
Effect	Killing	No killing	No killing	No killing

3 **MHC Restriction in Cell-Mediated Responses.** Mice are challenged with antigen, which can be virus [Zinkernagel and Doherty, 1974. *Nature* 248: 701]; TNP-modified syngeneic cells [Shearer, 1974. *Eur. J. Immunol.* 4: 527]; minor histocompatibility antigens [Bevan, 1975. *J. Exp. Med.* 142: 1347]; or H-Y antigens [Gordon et al., 1975. *J. Exp. Med.* 142: 1108]. Spleen cells from these mice are then assessed for their ability to lyse syngeneic versus allogeneic targets, with or without antigen. The results show that cytotoxic T cells kill target cells in an MHC-restricted manner.

To distinguish between these possibilities, several groups did the following experiment (Figure 4) in each of the model systems described above. (A × B)F$_1$ animals were challenged with antigen that was associated with cells of either parent A or parent B. The spleen cells were then tested for killing on antigen-coated targets from parent A and parent B. If the MHC restriction is only between effector and target, then the (A × B)F$_1$ cells should kill both A and B targets, because the F$_1$ effector has both MHC haplotypes. If, however, the MHC restriction is between the responding precursor

Table 1   Effect of various regions of the H-2 complex on the generation of MLRs and CTLs.

Difference between responder and stimulator cells	MHC	MLR	CTL
K	Class I	Poor	Good
I	Class II	Very good	Poor
S	Class III	Poor	Poor
D	Class I	Poor	Good
K or D plus I	—	—	Very good

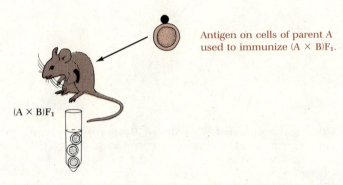

Antigen on cells of parent A used to immunize (A × B)F₁.

(A × B)F₁

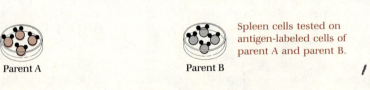

Spleen cells tested on antigen-labeled cells of parent A and parent B.

Parent A   Parent B

Kill   No kill   Only parent A targets are killed.

4   MHC Restriction in the Generation of Cytotoxic T Cells. F₁ mice are challenged with antigen on cells of one parental type. Spleen cells are recovered and then assessed for their ability to lyse cells (with antigen) from either parent. Only target cells with the MHC of the cells used in the initial immunization are killed. This result shows that MHC restriction is dictated during the generation of the cytotoxic effector cells.

cell and the stimulating cell in the generation of the cytotoxic cell, an (A × B)F$_1$ challenged with antigen on the cells of parent A should lyse only A targets because only A MHC was present at the initiation of the response. Conversely, challenge of the F$_1$ with antigen-coated cells of B would lead to killing of B but not A targets. As shown in Figure 4, the killing was restricted to the parental haplotype used for immunization, indicating that MHC restriction occurs during the generation of the cytotoxic cells and not only during the effector phase.

relate to paper ?

SYNTHESIS
CD Phenotype and Recognition of MHC Class

So far we have seen that CD4$^+$ cells are helper cells in both cell-mediated responses and antibody formation, and that helper cells are restricted to class II antigens. Alternatively, CD8$^+$ cytotoxic cells are restricted to class I (this chapter). The same correlations are seen in mouse, rat, human, and other species (using the genetically homologous markers). In addition, investigators quickly found that anti-CD4 and anti-CD8 antibodies, in the absence of complement, have the ability to *block* the activation and functions of the cells bearing these molecules.

These facts led originally to the conclusion that the CD4/8 phenotype of a T cell correlates with the *functional* subclass of the cell. It seemed logical to assume that these CD antigens are obligate markers for the subclasses, but we know now that this is *not* the case. Rather, *the phenotype correlates with the class of MHC antigen that the cell recognizes*. In other words, T cells that are restricted to class I molecules are CD8$^+$ and those that are restricted to class II molecules are CD4$^+$. This very important fact comes from experiments using cells bearing the "wrong" phenotype for their function. For example, Susan Swain and her co-workers in La Jolla found that under the appropriate conditions they could generate helper T cells against class I MHC, and that the cells that carry out this helper function express *CD8* (rather than the CD4 found on conventional, class II MHC-restricted, helper cells). In addition, if these cells are treated with anti-CD8 antibody in the absence of complement so that the CD8 molecules are blocked, their helper activity is blocked. Treating with the antibody before challenge with antigen blocks the induction of functional cells. Conversely, under conditions in which cytotoxic cells are generated against class II MHC molecules, the effector cells express and utilize CD4. Thus, while there is a *tendency* for CD4$^+$ T cells to be helper cells and CD8$^+$ T cells to be cytotoxic cells, there is a much stronger correlation between these markers and the MHC class recognized by the T cell.

Many other groups have produced results similar to this, in mice and humans, and there is now general agreement that the class of MHC molecule to which the cell exhibits restriction is correlated with the CD4/8 phenotype. The ability of anti-CD4 and anti-CD8 antibodies to block, respectively, anti-class II and anti-class I responses tells us that these molecules on the cell surface are functionally involved in recognizing MHC. In fact, there is a general belief that the CD4 and CD8 molecules, themselves, can distinguish between (and probably bind to) class I or class II MHC, respectively. CD4 and CD8 are members of the Ig superfamily, making this idea easier to swallow. In Chapter 15, we mentioned the binding of CD8 to the α_3 domain of a class I MHC molecule, and this binding site has been shown to be important for interaction with CD8$^+$ T cells.

We will have to wait until Chapter 25 to see how this correlation between MHC specificity and CD4/8 expression comes about. For now, however, the fact that this strong correlation exists should be kept in mind.

Studies Using Chimeras

As so often happens in science, further advances required the introduction of another experimental model to open new ways of examining the means by which cells interact in an MHC-restricted manner. This system was the use of the CHIMERIC MOUSE. The original chimera in Greek mythology was a fire-breathing monster, usually represented as a composite of a lion, a goat, and a serpent. Chimeric mice are more gentle creatures. They are animals containing tissues that have developed from two genetically distinct parents; the tissues exist side by side in the same animal. This is in contrast to an F_1 animal, in which the characteristics of each of the parents are expressed in each cell. Chimeras provide the opportunity, if they can be constructed, of having cells of two different genotypes maturing and functioning in the same animal.

Bone Marrow Chimeras

BONE MARROW CHIMERAS are adult animals that are lethally irradiated and then repopulated with bone marrow cells from other strains.

Because lymphocytes differentiate from stem cells in the bone marrow, the animals eventually contain lymphocytes derived from the donor strain, but all other tissues are from the irradiated recipient. This point will become important later.

The chimeras can be made by injecting parental bone marrow cells (P) into an F_1, F_1 into a parent, or one strain into another. The nomenclature for chimeras is as follows:

- $P_1 \rightarrow F_1$ indicates injection of bone marrow from one parent into an F_1 of that parent and another parental strain.
- $F_1 \rightarrow P_1$ indicates injection of bone marrow from an F_1 into one of the parental strains.
- $P_1 + P_2 \rightarrow F_1$ indicates injection of bone marrow from each parent into an F_1.
- $A \rightarrow B$ indicates injection of bone marrow from one strain into another.

Any recirculated T cells in the bone marrow are killed before injection so that the chance of GVH reaction is lessened. The method used by Harald von Boehmer and Jonathan Sprent for making bone marrow chimeras is illustrated in Figure 5.

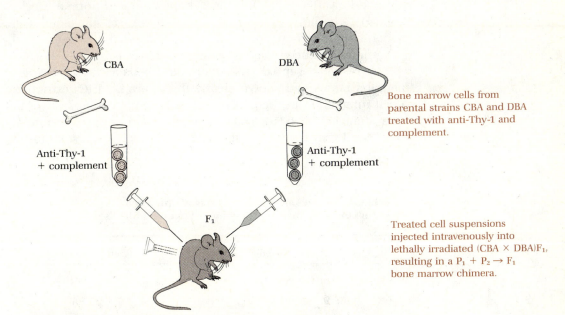

Bone marrow cells from parental strains CBA and DBA treated with anti-Thy-1 and complement.

Treated cell suspensions injected intravenously into lethally irradiated (CBA × DBA)F_1, resulting in a $P_1 + P_2 \rightarrow F_1$ bone marrow chimera.

5   Production of Bone Marrow Chimeras. Bone marrow is treated with anti-Thy-1 and complement (to remove any mature, recirculated T cells) and injected into an irradiated recipient. The production of $P_1 + P_2 \rightarrow F_1$ chimeras is illustrated. [After von Boehmer et al., 1975. *J. Exp. Med.* 141: 322]

Experiments Using $P_1 + P_2 \rightarrow F_1$: Evidence for Histoincompatible Cooperation

The first experiments that used chimeras to determine whether B cells of one parental MHC could cooperate with T cells of another are diagrammed in Figures 5 and 6. In this experiment, the bone marrows of two parental types (CBA and DBA) were injected into irradiated (CBA × DBA)F_1 mice; that is, $P_1 + P_2 \rightarrow F_1$ chimeras were produced (Figure 5). Several months later, cells from the lymph nodes of these chimeras were obtained and passed over an anti-Ig column to remove B cells. The T cells were a mixture of cells of the two parental haplotypes; half the cells expressed $H\text{-}2^d$ (from the DBA parent) and half the cells expressed $H\text{-}2^k$ (from the CBA parent). The DBA cells were then eliminated by treating the population with anti-$H\text{-}2^d$ antiserum plus complement, and the dead cells were removed, thus leaving a population of CBA ($H\text{-}2^k$) T cells. These CBA T cells from the chimera were then injected into irradiated F_1 mice along with B cells of the same or different haplotype, and the recipients were challenged with antigen. The number of antibody-forming cells was then determined. It can be seen from the data in Table 2 that there was cooperation between chimera-derived T cells of the $H\text{-}2^k$ haplotype and normal B cells of the $H\text{-}2^d$ haplotype. In other words, there was allogeneic cell cooperation, which would not have occurred if a conventional $H\text{-}2^k$ animal had been used as a source of T cells.

This result presented a real dilemma. The data in several experimental systems had shown clearly that there is MHC restriction in cell interaction in the generation of immune responses, yet in this system, in which $H\text{-}2^k$ cells differentiated in an F_1 environment, it appeared that there was no such restriction. The resolution of this dilemma revealed another previously unthought of layer of

Table 2 T cells from bone marrow chimeras act as helper cells for syngeneic and allogeneic B cells.

Cells transferred	Plaque-forming cells
CBA chimeric T cells alone	964
CBA chimeric T cells + CBA B cells	35,107
CBA chimeric T cells + DBA B cells	17,763

Source: From von Boehmer et al., 1975. *J. Exp. Med.* 142: 989.

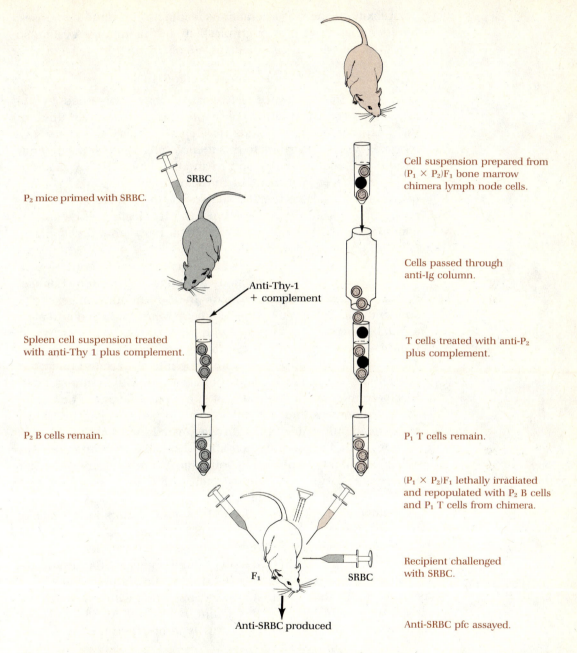

SRBC

P_2 mice primed with SRBC.

Cell suspension prepared from $(P_1 \times P_2)F_1$ bone marrow chimera lymph node cells.

Cells passed through anti-Ig column.

Anti-Thy-1 + complement

Spleen cell suspension treated with anti-Thy 1 plus complement.

T cells treated with anti-P_2 plus complement.

P_2 B cells remain.

P_1 T cells remain.

$(P_1 \times P_2)F_1$ lethally irradiated and repopulated with P_2 B cells and P_1 T cells from chimera.

Recipient challenged with SRBC.

F_1

SRBC

Anti-SRBC produced

Anti-SRBC pfc assayed.

6 **Cooperation of Allogeneic T and B Cells.** Lymph nodes from a P_1 + $P_2 \rightarrow F_1$ chimera are passed through an anti-Ig column to remove B cells. The remaining T cells are treated with anti-P_2 plus complement, leaving only the P_1 T cells.

complexity in the cell interactions leading to immune responses: the idea that there is enough plasticity in the immune system so that MHC restriction can be changed, or "learned."

Experiments Using F$_1$ → P$_1$: Adaptive Differentiation

To explain the difference between the results obtained in the allogeneic reconstitution experiments and the results in the chimera experiments, David Katz developed a theory called ADAPTIVE DIFFERENTIATION. According to this theory, cells can in some manner "adaptively" acquire restriction to an allogeneic MHC by differentiation in the environment of the allogeneic haplotype. Thus, if developing T cells of the H-2^k haplotype can differentiate in the environment of the H-2^d haplotype, the H-2^k cells will be able to cooperate with the H-2^d cells. They will have "adaptively" differentiated the ability to interact.

Experiments using F$_1$ → P$_1$ chimeras were carried out by Katz and his co-workers in an antibody-forming system and by Michael Bevan in a cell-mediated system. In the antibody experiment, shown in Figure 7, the F$_1$ → P$_1$ chimeras were produced and after a suitable interval were primed with carrier. Their spleen or lymph node cells were then used as a source of carrier-primed T cells. These carrier-primed T cells from the chimera were then injected into lethally irradiated F$_1$ recipient mice along with hapten-primed B cells from conventional mice of either parental strain or the F$_1$. The recipient was then challenged with hapten and carrier. In this manner adaptive differentiation was tested by asking if the F$_1$ T cells from the chimera (which should be able to cooperate with either parental type of B cell) would "adapt" to being able to react preferentially with only one parental haplotype.

As an example, parental strains P$_1$ and P$_2$ serve as irradiated recipients for bone marrow from (P$_1$ × P$_2$)F$_1$ donors in forming F$_1$ → P$_1$ or F$_1$ → P$_2$ chimeras. (F$_1$ → F$_1$ animals serve as controls.) The T cells from the F$_1$ will differentiate in the environment of either one of the parental MHC haplotypes. If the idea of adaptive differentiation is correct, these F$_1$ cells should show a preference (or a restriction) in their interaction by cooperating with B cells of the haplotype of the strain of the parent in which they differentiated. Figure 7 shows an example of this type of experiment in which this is the result obtained.

In the results shown in Figure 7, the controls show that F$_1$ bone marrow cells differentiating in an F$_1$ environment (F$_1$ → F$_1$) are able to cooperate well with B cells of the F$_1$ and of each of the

(A)

Conventional (P_1, P_2, or F_1) mouse primed with H-CII.

$F_1 \rightarrow P_1$ or $F_1 \rightarrow F_1$ bone marrow chimera primed with CI.

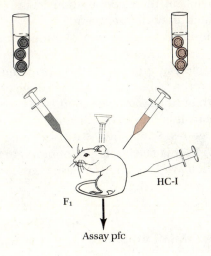

Primed B cells prepared from spleen cells treated with anti-Thy-1 plus complement.

Primed T cells prepared from spleen cells.

T cells from carrier-primed chimera and B cells from hapten-primed conventional mouse injected into irradiated, conventional F_1 recipient.

HC-I

F_1

Recipient (F_1) challenged with H-CI.

Assay pfc

Anti-hapten pfc's assayed.

(B)

Source of chimeric T cells	Source of conventional B cells	Response	Interpretation
$F_1 \rightarrow F_1$	P_1		Chimeric $F_1 \rightarrow F_1$ T cells cooperate with F_1 and both parental B cells.
	P_2		
	$(P_1 \times P_2)F_1$		
$F_1 \rightarrow P_1$	P_1		Chimeric $F_1 \rightarrow P_1$ T cells cooperate with F_1 T cells and T cells of the strain in which they differentiated.
	P_2		
	$(P_1 \times P_2)F_1$		

7 Adaptive Differentiation. T cells from an $F_1 \rightarrow P_1$ bone marrow chimera primed with CI are injected into an irradiated recipient along with H-CII-primed conventional B cells. If there is adaptive differentiation, then the F_1 T cells should cooperate preferentially with P_1 B cells. $F_1 \rightarrow P_1$ T cells cooperate with P_1 cells but not P_2 cells. [After Katz et al., 1978. *J. Exp. Med.* 148: 727]

parental strains. In the experimental group, we see that T cells from an $F_1 \rightarrow P_1$ cooperate preferentially with B cells of the parental type in which they differentiated but not with the other parental type. This result indicates that F_1 cells that have undergone differentiation in an F_1 environment can cooperate with either parental type (the controls); but when differentiation occurs in one of the parental types, there is cooperation only with that parental type of cells (the experimental groups). Thus, even though the primed T cells should have the genetic potential to cooperate with B cells of both parental types because they are of F_1 origin, they are restricted in their cooperation to the B cells of the parental type in which they differentiated.

Similar results were obtained in cell-mediated responses. When F_1 cells were allowed to differentiate in the environment of only one parental type, they preferentially lysed targets of that MHC rather than those of the other haplotype. We see then that in both antibody and cell-mediated responses there is MHC restriction, but it is more complicated than just the sharing of the same MHC genes. Somehow MHC restriction can be "learned." We will return to this fascinating phenomenon in a later chapter (Chapter 25) once we've gained a better grasp of how T cells recognize antigen plus MHC.

SYNTHESIS
MHC and Antigen Form the Ligand for the T-Cell Receptor

In this chapter we have discussed some of the experiments that showed that lymphocytes can interact in an MHC-restricted manner. One possible explanation for this was the idea that cells interact via their MHC molecules in a "like–like" interaction (that is, that an MHC molecule can recognize and bind to an identical MHC molecule). Experiments showing phenomena such as adaptive differentiation, however, argued against this idea and led to a completely different concept: T cells bear receptors that specifically recognize both antigen *and* an MHC molecule. Somehow, the MHC molecule and antigen combine to form the ligand that is recognized by the T cell. As we'll see in the next chapter, this is the case. For convenience, immunologists refer to this ligand as a combination of MHC and antigen, or MHC–antigen complex.

The combination of MHC and antigen to form a ligand that is recognized by T cells accounts for MHC restriction in the immune system, as well as the phenomena surrounding immune response genes (discussed in Chapter 15). As far as we know, T cells are the only cells that "see" antigen in this way. The nature of the T-cell receptor and that of the ligand for the T-cell receptor have formed the basis for much of modern immunology and have given us important clues to how the immune system works. How T cells "learn" to recognize self-MHC (plus antigen) will be discussed in a later chapter (Chapter 25).

Thus, the idea is that MHC restriction is a consequence of the interaction of a particular MHC molecule (plus antigen) with a specific T-cell receptor. One prediction of this idea is that in an F_1 mouse, some T cells should be restricted to the MHC molecules of one parental haplotype, and some to the other. A further prediction is that a single T cell will recognize only *one* of the MHC molecules expressed by its host. For example, a CD4$^+$ T cell in a (H-2^d × H-2^k)F_1 mouse will recognize only one of the many MHC molecules that are present (e.g., I-A^d but not I-E^d, I-A^k, or I-E^k). These predictions have all held true.

MHC molecules are codominantly expressed, that is, all the MHC molecules that can be expressed by a single cell are expressed. A single T cell, however, will recognize antigen together with only one of these MHC molecules.[5] In the next chapter, we'll see how cells "present" antigen to these extremely fussy T cells.

Summary

1.   The immune response of nude mice can be restored with syngeneic but not allogeneic thymus cells, and the immune response of irradiated mice can be restored only with bone marrow and thymus cells that are syngeneic at the class II region of MHC.

2.   CD8$^+$ cytotoxic T cells (other than alloreactive CTL) can lyse only targets that have the appropriate antigen (e.g., virus, hapten, or minor histocompatibility antigen) and express the same class I MHC as the CTL.

3.   CD phenotype strongly correlates with MHC class restriction (and less strongly with function). CD4$^+$ T cells are reactive with class II MHC and CD8$^+$ T cells are reactive with class I MHC.

4.   Studies using bone marrow chimeras have shown that the T helper cell must recognize the self MHC on the host cells. By a phenomenon called "adaptive differentiation," the self-MHC can be learned.

---

[5] This is sometimes a tricky point (partly because of our tendency to use "cartoons" to illustrate ideas). Antigen-presenting cells express the entire available array of class I and class II molecules (other cells express the entire available set of class I molecules). That is, they express all the alleles present on the two MHC complexes (one complex from each parent). The T cell, on the other hand, expresses receptors that are specific for only *one* MHC molecule (plus antigen).

Additional Readings

Carbone, F. R. and M. J. Bevan. 1989. Major histocompatibility complex control of T cell recognition. In Paul, W., ed., *Fundamental Immunology*, 2nd ed. Raven, New York, p. 541.

Golub, E. S. 1980. Know thyself: autoreactivity in the immune response. *Cell* 21: 603.

Swain, S. L. 1981. Significance of Lyt phenotypes: Lyt 2 antibodies block activities of T cells that recognize Class I major histocompatibility complex antigens regardless of their function. *Proc. Natl. Acad. Sci. U.S.A.*, 78: 7101.

ANTIGEN PROCESSING AND PRESENTATION

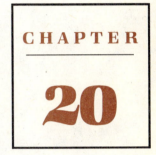

CHAPTER

20

Overview So far, we've considered antigen presentation from the point of view of the T cell that recognizes the MHC molecule plus antigen. There is also the point of view of the antigen-presenting cell, which often must "process" the antigen into a form that can be recognized by the T cell. This antigen processing and presentation is a crucial step in the generation of an immune response. In a sense it is remarkable that when the immune system is activated to destroy a foreign invader, it is not the rampaging pathogen (e.g., bacterium or virus) that triggers the response, but rather a fragment from an already-destroyed sampling. Thus, the processed fragment becomes a signal to the immune system.

The story of antigen processing and presentation began with the realization that antigen-presenting cells are required for the activation of T cells. It quickly became apparent, however, that like most things in the immune system, antigen presentation is a fairly complex affair. We'll begin with the processing and presentation of antigen plus class II MHC molecules to CD4$^+$ T cells, which turns out to be different from the presentation of antigen plus class I MHC molecules to CD8$^+$ T cells.

The idea that antigen-presenting cells "process" antigens before presenting them was based on a number of observations. We knew, for example, that T cells recognize (predominantly) protein antigens, and that unlike B cells, T cells can recognize denatured antigen. This was a hint that, perhaps, antigen is being denatured (at least) before being recognized by T cells. We'll consider several other observations that have led to the elucidation of what we now know of the mechanisms of antigen processing and presentation.

MHC Restriction and Antigen-Presenting Cells

We saw in Chapter 16 that macrophages or other accessory cells are necessary for many immune functions. We will now develop this idea in detail for T-cell activation; that is, we will examine the evidence that shows that MHC restriction is between antigen-presenting cells (such as macrophages) and T cells. The designation *antigen-presenting cell* (or APC) is meant to indicate any cell that has the capacity to participate in the stimulation of T cells by antigen. In the course of the next several pages, we will more rigorously define this capacity. As we will see (and you might already suspect), an APC has at least one critical characteristic: it expresses class II MHC molecules.

While we will concentrate on macrophages and B cells as APCs (because most of the development of the field concentrated on these cells), it is important to realize that many other cells in the body have this ability. Some of these are listed in Table 1.

APCs and T-Cell Activation

A population of resting T cells exhibits the capacity to carry out functions only after antigenic stimulation. This response is termed

Table 1   Some of the different APCs of the body.[a]

Organ	APC	Function
Skin	Langerhans cell	Normal defense
	Dermal fibroblast	Inflammatory disease?
Liver	Kupfer cell	Normal defense
Kidney	Mesangial cell	Normal defense?
Lung	Alveolar macrophage	Normal defense?
		Inflammatory disease?
Spleen	Splenic dendritic cell	Normal defense
Thymus	Thymic dendritic cell	T-cell selection (Chapter 24)
Thymus	Thymic epithelial cell	T-cell selection (Chapter 25)
Thyroid	Thyroid epithelial cell	Inflammatory disease?
Brain	Astrocyte	Inflammatory disease?

[a]This table represents only a partial list of the many types of APCs in the body. Some of these cells we've listed as participating in inflammatory diseases because (1) they do not normally have the capability to present antigen *unless* inflammation is occurring, and/or (2) they are situated in sites to which T cells do not normally have access unless there is inflammation.

ANTIGENIC ACTIVATION. One of the most dramatic aspects of activation is the induction of proliferation of the antigen-specific cells (this process is one of the basic tenets of clonal selection).

An experiment by Allan Rosenthal and Ethan Shevach (Figure 1) showed that APCs are required for the activation of T cells. In this experiment, peritoneal exudate cells (PECs), which are 75 to 85% macrophages, were harvested from guinea pigs and allowed to adhere to glass for several hours. The nonadherent cells were then removed and discarded. This procedure produces a population of cells that contain over 98% macrophages. The adherent cells were then incubated with antigen (a process called ANTIGEN PULSING). T cells obtained from lymph nodes were then added to the antigen-pulsed macrophages, and after a suitable interval, the amount of T-cell proliferation was determined by adding tritiated thymidine. Figure 1 shows that proliferation of the T cells occurred only when both antigen and macrophages were present. This result indicates that one of the crucial initial steps in the generation of the immune response—the activation of T-cell proliferation by antigen—is a step that requires the presence of an APC. This observation basically accounts for the macrophage requirement for in vitro immune responses discussed in Chapter 16. Here, however, we are getting closer to the idea of what the macrophage's role is (i.e., antigen presentation).

Role of MHC Haplotype of APCs and T Cells

The experimental system in Figure 1 was used to test the role of the MHC in the activation of T cells by antigen and macrophages. Guinea pig macrophages of one MHC haplotype were pulsed with antigen, and then T cells from animals of another MHC haplotype were added. The amount of T-cell proliferation was determined (Table 2). When macrophages from strain 2 guinea pigs were pulsed with antigen and added to T cells of strain 2, strain 13, or a $(2 \times 13)F_1$, there was proliferation only with strain 2 or the $(2 \times 13)F_1$ macrophages. Similarly, the antigen-pulsed macrophages from strain 13 were able to activate only strain 13 or the F_1 T cells. This experiment shows that even though APCs are required for the induction of antigen-specific T-cell proliferation, the macrophages and T cells must have the same MHC haplotype. In other words, T-cell activation by antigen and macrophage is MHC-restricted.

Ronald Schwartz and others followed up on these experiments, using congenic mice rather than guinea pigs. In the guinea pig experiments the two strains differed not only in MHC but in other

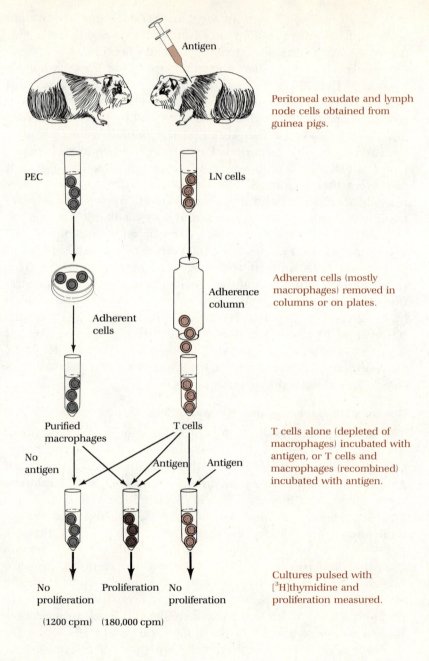

Antigen

Peritoneal exudate and lymph node cells obtained from guinea pigs.

PEC

LN cells

Adherent cells (mostly macrophages) removed in columns or on plates.

Adherence column

Adherent cells

Purified macrophages

T cells

No antigen

Antigen

Antigen

T cells alone (depleted of macrophages) incubated with antigen, or T cells and macrophages (recombined) incubated with antigen.

No proliferation

Proliferation

No proliferation

Cultures pulsed with [^{3}H]thymidine and proliferation measured.

(1200 cpm)

(180,000 cpm)

◄ **1 Macrophages Are Required for Antigen-Induced T-Cell Proliferation.** Cells were prepared from the lymph nodes of immunized guinea pigs and were treated to remove macrophages. Meanwhile, cells from nonimmune animals were collected from the peritoneum after injection of an irritating substance (this causes a cellular exudate into the peritoneum, which at the appropriate time is predominantly macrophages). Plastic adherent peritoneal macrophages and immune T cells were mixed in the presence or absence of antigen, and proliferation of the T cells was assessed several days later. Using this system, it was possible to examine the genetic restriction between macrophages and T cells (see Table 2). [After Rosenthal and Shevach, 1974. *J. Exp. Med.* 138: 1194]

genes as well. It will be recalled, however, that MHC congenic mice differ *only* in MHC (Chapter 15). Experiments using congenic mouse strains confirmed that restriction between APCs and T cells is indeed due to MHC and further showed that this restriction maps to class II MHC. We now know that in all species examined, including humans, there is MHC restriction between APCs and T cells.

The Use of T-Cell Clones

One of the difficulties in doing research on T cells is that the number of cells with specific receptors for a given antigen–MHC molecule combination is very low. The antibody problem was solved by using myeloma cells, which secrete large amounts of Ig. It had not been possible to grow antigen-specific functional T cells until the discovery of T-cell growth factor (or IL-2; see Chapter 27). Long-term maintenance of T-cell clones (from mouse, rat, human,

Table 2   Genetic restriction in T-cell activation.[a]

| | Source of T cells | | |
Macrophage	Strain 2	Strain 13	$(2 \times 13)F_1$
2	25.4	2.9	5.3
13	0	18.2	6.0
$(2 \times 13)F_1$	10.5	7.6	11.00

Source: Data from Rosenthal and Shevach, 1974. *J. Exp. Med.* 138: 1194.

[a]The system shown in Figure 1 was employed, using two different strains of guinea pigs (or F_1 animals) as sources of immune T cells or macrophages. Although this system did not map the genetic restriction to MHC, studies in other animals showed that this was the controlling genetic region.

and other species) has been carried out by maintaining the cells with growth factors and antigenic stimulation. This development means that one can now have a large supply of cells bearing a single specificity.

Another advance was the production of ANTIGEN-SPECIFIC T-CELL HYBRIDOMAS. These cells are produced by using a technology similar to that used for production of monoclonal antibody: fusing an antigen-specific T cell with a tumor. In this case, the tumors are T-cell tumors rather than the B-cell tumors used in producing monoclonal antibodies. These T-cell hybridomas are able to grow in continuous culture in the *absence* of added growth factors. By immunizing a mouse with an antigen of choice, growing the cells in vitro with growth factors, fusing them to a T-cell tumor, and selecting fused cells of the desired specificity, one can get clones of antigen-specific T cells growing in continuous culture. In other words, the problem of not having enough cells to work with is solved. The requirements for antigen-specific activation of T-cell hybridomas can then be assessed by measuring the release of growth factors from these cells after stimulation. (The release of growth factors from stimulated T cells will be discussed in more detail in Chapter 27.)

When such T-cell clones and hybridomas were used, it quickly became clear that antigen-specific T cells are specific for both a particular antigen and a particular MHC molecule. Thus, not only is an F_1 T cell restricted to the MHC haplotype of only one of the parents, but it is restricted to only one of the molecules. For example, in mice, where there are two class II MHC loci (I-A and I-E), some of the T cells are restricted to I-A and some to I-E. (If this is still confusing, go back and reread the end of Chapter 19—the concept is very important.)

Problems of alloreactivity (the response of a population of T cells to allogeneic MHC, e.g., an MLR response) are relatively easy to avoid with the use of T-cell clones or hybridomas (see below), and the study of T-cell specificity with such cells has been greatly facilitated.

Antibody and B Cells in Antigen Presentation

Like macrophages, B cells bear class II MHC molecules on their surfaces, and can serve as APCs. With B cells, however, the presentation is most efficient when the antigen binds to the Ig on the B-cell surface. Thus, if antigen binds to a B cell with receptors for the antigen, it is then taken up and presented to antigen-specific

T cells. As we'll see, this may be an important mechanism of cell–cell cooperation.

Investigators have also learned that, like macrophages, some B-cell lymphoma lines are capable of presenting *any* antigen, as long as it is present in sufficient quantities. This provides a useful model to study antigen presentation by a uniform cell population. Some of the experiments described later in this chapter utilized such APC lines.

For many years it was known that specific antibody can enhance immune responses. We now know that one way in which this works involves antigen presentation by macrophages and other APCs that bear receptors (FcR) for the Fc portion of the antibody. Although specific antibody is not required for antigen presentation by such cells, when the antibody binds to the APC it can increase the uptake of specific antigen, thus improving presentation. B cells focus antigen via their surface Ig, as discussed above. The difference, of course, is that B cells make the antibody on their surface, while FcR$^+$ APCs passively acquire this facility. As we will see later in this chapter, the antigen is then taken up by the cell and converted to a form that can be recognized by the T cell.

SYNTHESIS
"Self-Restriction" and Cell–Cell Interactions

From the work we've outlined (above and Chapter 19), it is apparent that T-cell activation requires recognition of antigen together with self-MHC molecules. The CD4$^+$ helper T cells recognize antigen only together with class II MHC molecules, following which the cells become activated and proceed to proliferate and help immune responses. Similarly CD8$^+$ cytotoxic cells recognize antigen plus self-class I MHC molecules, for their activation and also for the delivery of their lethal "hit." Each T cell is restricted to only one self-MHC molecule and to one antigen (i.e., it is MHC- and antigen-specific). In a later chapter, we'll consider how it happens that all of an individual's T cells come to be specific for a self-MHC molecule, but for now it is sufficient to note that this is the case.

Why has this complex situation evolved? What does MHC restriction actually *do* for the immune system? This is perhaps easiest to understand in the case of cytotoxic T cells killing a virally infected target. Because of the requirement that the cytotoxic T cell must recognize both a class I MHC molecule and viral antigen on the infected cell, there is no chance that the cytotoxic mechanism will "fire" in response to shed viral proteins. That is, cytotoxicity is activated only upon cell contact.

The same reasoning applies to helper T cells. When a helper T cell contacts class II MHC molecules plus specific antigen, it is stimulated to release growth and differentiation factors (or LYMPHOKINES, see Chapter 27), which, in turn, stimulate other cells. If the MHC molecule and antigen are presented by a macrophage, the factors released by the helper T cell can stimulate the macrophage, as in many cell-mediated immune responses. Alternatively, recognition of an MHC molecule and antigen on a B cell results in B-cell activation by such lymphokines. Thus, not only is the T cell activated to proliferate, but the effector cells (B cell or macrophage) that presented the antigen are stimulated in turn. This is discussed in more detail in Chapters 26 and 27 when we consider the mechanisms of lymphocyte activation.

Besides stimulation of effector cells, activation of helper T cells also serves the important function of selection and expansion of the specific helper T-cell clone. If a particular response is going to result in antibody formation, however, do we even need macrophages (since B cells can present antigen plus class II MHC molecules)? A logical (and possibly even correct) answer to this question involves imagining the first time a specific antigen enters the body (Figure 2). Macrophages or similar APCs that present antigen can do so for any antigen, and therefore a T cell that is specific for this antigen (plus class II MHC molecule) has a very good chance of recognizing the antigen on a macrophage. The T cell then proliferates, and the cells of the expanded clone await further activation. B cells are very effective at presenting the antigens that bind to their surface Ig (see above), but those specific for the antigen in question will be at low numbers (which is why the antigen-specific T cells didn't see them at first). Now the expanded clone of T cells has a much better chance of finding the appropriate B cell, and, upon recognizing antigen plus class II MHC molecules on the B cell, stimulating it.

What it all comes down to is this: MHC restriction of T-cell function forces the occurrence of the cellular interactions that are necessary for immune responses.

The Paradox of T-Cell Alloreactivity

We now know that T cells recognize specific antigen only when it is presented with the appropriate (usually syngeneic) MHC. On

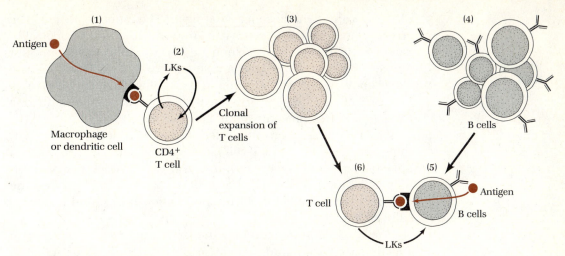

2 A Model for the Roles of Antigen Presentation by Macrophages versus B Cells during a Primary Antibody Reponse. (1) Antigen enters the system and is processed and presented by macrophages or dendritic cells. (2) Antigen-specific CD4$^+$ T cells respond to the presented antigen plus class II MHC by producing lymphokines (LKs) that stimulate the T cell to proliferate. The cells in the expanded clone of T cells (3) are now more likely to contact a relatively rare antigen-specific B cell (4), which has taken up and processed the antigen after specific binding to cell-surface Igs (5). The specific T cell finds the B cell (relatively easily because the T cell now has many copies) and responds to the processed antigen (plus class II MHC) presented by the B cell by releasing LKs (6), which stimulate clonal expansion and differentiation of the specific B cell. Note that this model requires that the carrier and hapten be linked in order for the expanded T cell to contact the appropriate B cell, and that the LKs act only at short range.

the other hand, we have also seen that T cells make strong responses to allogeneic MHC (without a requirement for antigen), which accounts for the MLR response in vitro and for graft rejection in vivo. It has been known for a long time that the frequency of alloreactive cells is much higher than the frequency of T cells responding to a particular antigen. On the surface, these facts appear to be inconsistent: how can T cells respond to allogeneic MHC *and* be restricted to self-MHC?

In order to understand this apparent contradiction, it is important to think of the response of a *single* T cell (or a T-cell clone). First Harald von Boehmer, and then many other investigators, showed that a T-cell clone can have *two* specificities: it will respond to antigen plus the appropriate self-MHC molecule *and* it may respond to one or a few allogeneic MHC molecules (but not others), even in the absence of antigen. The latter represents the ALLOSPECIFICITY of the T cell. With APCs bearing the "wrong" allogeneic MHC molecule, the clone fails to respond, with or without antigen. Results of this kind are shown in Table 3. Thus, a single T cell may respond to specific antigen plus one MHC molecule and not others (MHC restriction) but will *also* respond to one allogeneic MHC molecule alone (allospecificity).

Several investigators attempted to relate the antigen plus MHC molecule specificity of a T-cell clone with its alloreactivity, but no obvious correlations were found. When we consider a population of T cells, the effect of all the different allospecificities of all the cells results in the ability of the population to respond to practically any allogeneic MHC.

We can see, therefore, that the high frequency of alloreactive T cells isn't very paradoxical when looked at this way. What *is* puzzling, however, is why T cells very often have these two specificities (antigen plus MHC molecule and allospecificity).[1] There are no clear-cut answers to this question at present, and this may be the real paradox of alloreactivity. So far, it's just something that immunologists have had to live with, but there is probably something very significant lurking beneath this annoying puzzle.

[1] No doubt it has occurred to the reader that in the normal, physiological situation, antigen is *always* presented with self-MHC molecules (almost by definition). In getting to the point where we could understand antigen presentation (and other phenomena), however, manipulated model systems with allogeneic MHC molecules had to be used. Translation from models back to the natural situation is one of the real challenges of immunology.

Table 3 Allorecognition by antigen-specific, MHC-restricted T-cell clones.[a]

Class II MHC haplotype	Clone K22		Clone 5	
	− antigen	+ antigen	− antigen	+ antigen
b	300	28,900	233	nd
k	500	500	180	39,200
d	71,400	nd	410	nd
s	nd	nd	36,300	nd

Source: Data from Sredni and Schwartz, 1980. *Nature* 287: 855; and Finnegan et al., 1985. *J. Immunol.* 134: 2960.

[a]Cloned T-cell lines were cultured with or without antigen plus APC of the indicated MHC haplotype. Antigen-specific, MHC-restricted response is shaded gray. Allospecific response, in the absence of added antigen, is shaded in color. nd, Not determined.

Immune Response Genes and MHC Restriction

In Chapter 15, we mentioned important observations that showed that the haplotype of MHC, especially class II MHC, appears to control the ability to make an immune response to a particular antigen. This mapping of immune responsiveness to the MHC I region (for "immune response") gave us the concept of immune response (*Ir*) genes. With what we've discussed in this chapter, we can now begin to make some sense out of this phenomenon.

From what we've seen, it was reasonable to conclude that T cells somehow specifically recognize a complex, on the APC, of an MHC molecule and antigen, and that this complex forms the ligand that interacts with the antigen receptor on the T cell. There are, therefore, three components to the recognition: the antigen, the MHC molecule, and the T-cell receptor. (The nature of the T-cell receptor is discussed in detail in Chapter 22.) These three components all interact with each other, forming a TRIMOLECULAR COMPLEX.

MHC molecules are therefore critical for the specific interaction of T cells with antigen. *Ir* gene effects may occur, therefore, because not all MHC molecules can present all antigens to all populations of T cells. If none of the available MHC molecules in an individual are capable of interacting with an antigen, the antigen-specific T cell has nothing to see, and no response occurs. This idea, called DETERMINANT SELECTION, is one explanation for *Ir* gene phenomena, as we'll see below. Another possibility is that the MHC molecule and the antigen *do* combine, but that there are no T cells with receptors that recognize this complex. This idea is called the HOLE IN THE REPERTOIRE, and it, too, explains some *Ir* gene phenomena (as we'll see in Chapter 24). For now, however, it is only necessary to realize that MHC haplotypes control immune responsiveness, simply because a particular T cell only recognizes antigen when it is complexed with a particular MHC molecule.

The Processing and Presentation of Antigen

Requirements for APC Function

In the preceding sections, we've described the T-cell recognition of MHC molecule and antigen. We will now develop the idea that it is not the whole antigen, but rather only fragments of it that are associated with MHC molecules to form the ligand recognized by the T-cell receptor. The first step towards this realization was the observation that antigen must often be PROCESSED before it can be presented. At first, processing was seen as "something" that an APC had to do with the antigen for a time before presentation. As we'll see, the concept of processing was considerably refined as research continued.

Kirk Zeigler and Emil Unanue performed a number of experiments illustrating that *Listeria* bacteria are processed by macrophages for presentation to immune cells. Based on these experiments, Robert Chestnut and Howard Grey examined the response of antigen-specific T-cell hybridomas (see above) to protein antigens. They used a B-cell lymphoma as an APC and incubated these cells with antigen for varying periods of time before treating them with paraformaldehyde. Paraformaldehyde (or a similar agent) effectively "fixes" the cells at the point of their treatment. The fixed APCs were then tested for their ability to present the antigen to the T cells. As shown in Figure 3, the APCs had to be incubated with the antigen (at 37°C) for at least 45 minutes prior to fixing to be able to present the antigen. They also examined peritoneal macrophages as APCs and obtained similar results. This suggests that the APCs need time to process the antigen to a "presentable" form.

Since macrophages were known to be able to degrade antigens by the action of proteases and other lysosomal enzymes (present in the lysosomes of the cell), it was possible that other APCs do

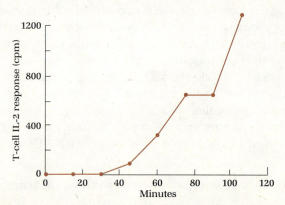

3   Requirement for Antigen Processing for Presentation to T Cells. A B-cell lymphoma line was used as a source of APCs. Antigen was added for various periods of time to the APCs, which were then washed and fixed with paraformaldehyde. The fixed APCs were then added to antigen-specific T-hybridoma cells and cultured for 24 hours. The supernatants were collected and assessed for the production of a growth factor (IL2) from the T cells (see Chapter 27) as a measurement of T-cell activation by the antigen plus APC. Activation only occurred if the APCs were incubated with the antigen for more than 45 minutes. [Data from Chestnut et al., 1982. *J. Immunol.* 129: 2382]

this as well, and that this plays some role in processing the antigen. Again, based on experiments by Zeigler and Unanue, Chestnut and Grey radiolabeled protein antigens and added these to APCs. As expected, the proteins were degraded over time. If, however, the APCs were treated with either ammonium chloride or chloroquine (both of which inactivate many lysosomal functions), this degradation did not occur. More importantly, neither did antigen processing. On the other hand, these substances had no effect on antigen presentation *after* the antigen had been processed for 60 minutes. Thus, the enzymes in the lysosome play an important role in antigen processing before the antigen can be presented.

Proteases and Antigen Processing

The next step in understanding this phenomenon involved artificially processing antigens by treatment with proteases. As mentioned above, fixed APCs (that have not been previously incubated with antigen) do not present most antigens to T cells. Grey and colleagues now showed, however, that trypsin treatment of ovalbumin yields peptide fragments that are fully capable of being presented by a fixed APC to a T-cell hybridoma. This finding led to a more detailed analysis of the effects of proteases and protease inhibitors on antigen processing and presentation.

Jay Berzofsky and his colleagues then examined the responses of three T-cell clones specific for different portions of sperm whale myoglobin.[2] They found that a number of protease inhibitors prevented the processing of this antigen for presentation to any of the T cells. All these inhibitors held in common the ability to inhibit a particular protease, cathepsin B. When the antigen was treated with cathepsin B, the fragments produced were precisely those that the T cells recognized. Thus, it is likely that cathepsin B in the lysosome is responsible for processing this antigen (at least for presentation to these T cells).

When Joseph Puri and Yfat Factorovich examined a number of different T cells with specificities for different class II MHC molecules and different antigens, they found that the effects of protease inhibitors were much more difficult to predict. It seems likely, therefore, that a *number* of different proteases play a role in the processing of antigen within an APC.

[2] This antigen once evoked images of immunologists sailing off to unknown ports, but has steadily lost popularity as our responsibility for preserving this endangered animal matured. Given the universe of antigens, it is as hard to rationalize using this one as it would be to rationalize using whooping crane ovalbumin (which, fortunately, never became fashionable).

Association of Antigen Peptides and Class II MHC

It was beginning to look as though antigen processing involves breaking down a protein antigen into peptide fragments that then become associated with class II MHC molecules. If this is really the case, then it should be possible to identify the minimal antigenic peptide for a particular T cell. The strategy to test this would involve identifying a proteolytic fragment that would stimulate the cell (when presented by fixed APCs). One would then test an array of synthetic peptides corresponding to different parts of the active fragment. Once identified, the minimal peptide could then be "mapped" to determine which amino acids at which positions are critical for antigenicity.

This was done for a number of T-cell clones and hybridomas. Antigens were proteolytically cleaved into fragments, and these peptide fragments were tested for their ability to be presented to T cells. This was done under conditions in which no further processing of the antigen could occur (e.g., fixed APCs). In all cases, the identified peptides could be presented to T cells in the absence of any requirement for processing. Thus, it was possible to separate the two functions of the APC, processing and presentation.

Antigenic Peptides Can Compete for Association with Class II MHC Molecules on the Surface of an APC

If these ideas are correct, then the antigenic peptides that do not require processing are probably capable of directly interacting with class II MHC molecules. This interaction results in the formation of the complex ligand for the T-cell receptor. This idea led to the development of another, more easily tested idea: maybe there are only a limited number of sites on a class II MHC molecule with which antigenic peptides associate. One way to test *this* idea was to attempt to compete for the binding of a peptide (antigenic for one T cell) with another peptide (antigenic for a different T cell). This type of experiment is described in Table 4. Indeed, excess amounts of one antigenic peptide were often capable of interfering with the ability of a second peptide to be presented. Other peptides were incapable of competing with the antigen peptide. In general, peptides that can be presented by a particular MHC molecule can compete with each other. Peptides that are never presented with that MHC molecule do not compete with those that are. These observations provided not only a nice demonstration that the peptides were probably binding directly to some limiting site on the

Table 4   Competition between peptides for binding to I-A^d MHC molecules.[a]

Inhibitory peptide	Restriction	Concentration (μM) of inhibitor required for 75% inhibition of T cell plus OVA (323-339)
Ha (130–142)	I-A^d	8
λ repr (12–26)	I-A^d, I-E^k	370
HEL (46–61)	I-A^k	>1000
HEL (74–86)	I-A^k	30
Ha (81–96)	I-E^d	>1000
Myo (132–153)	I-E^d	>1000
HSV (8–23)	I-E^d, I-E^k	>1000

Source: From Buus et al., 1987. *Science* 235: 1353.

[a]Fixed H-2^d APCs are cultured for 2 hours with different peptides to which the T-cell hybridoma does *not* respond, plus a suboptimal dose of the antigenic peptide (normally capable of stimulating the T cell) and washed. The APCs and responding T cell hybridoma are placed in culture, and the ability of the first peptide to compete for binding to the MHC molecule is assessed in terms of its ability to prevent the T cell from recognizing the MHC molecule plus appropriate antigen. Note that because *peptides* are being used, there is no requirement for processing. The concentration of competitor necessary for 75% inhibition of antigen presentation is shown (therefore, lower numbers indicate better competition). The T-cell hybridoma normally recognizes a fragment of ovalbumin (323-339) plus I-A^d. Class II molecules that normally present the other antigen fragments are listed under *Restriction*. Note that peptides that are normally presented with I-A molecules tend to be better inhibitors than those normally presented with I-E.

APC (probably class II MHC molecules), but also provided a convenient way to determine the residues on a peptide that are required for binding to this site. Thus, a peptide could be "mapped" for (1) those residues required for antigenicity in general and (2) those residues required for binding to the site on the MHC molecule.

Antigenic Peptides Can Directly Bind to Class II MHC Molecules

The logical prediction from the studies above was that antigenic peptides physically bind to class II MHC molecules. The laboratories of Unanue and Grey set out to directly test this prediction. They purified class II MHC molecules from the surface of APCs and mixed them with a radiolabeled antigenic peptide under conditions of equilibrium dialysis (see Chapter 10). In the experiments outlined in Figure 4, they found that the peptide and the MHC molecules did, indeed, bind with a low affinity. The question then became: Is this binding physiologically relevant?

To answer this question, they made an assumption. As we've discussed, poor immune responses are made to some antigen–class II MHC molecule combinations, a phenomenon related to

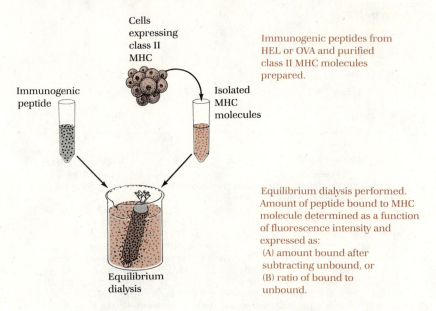

Cells expressing class II MHC

Immunogenic peptide

Isolated MHC molecules

Immunogenic peptides from HEL or OVA and purified class II MHC molecules prepared.

Equilibrium dialysis

Equilibrium dialysis performed. Amount of peptide bound to MHC molecule determined as a function of fluorescence intensity and expressed as:
(A) amount bound after subtracting unbound, or
(B) ratio of bound to unbound.

(A) Hen egg lysozyme peptide

Class II	Fluorescence intensity
I-A^k	250
I-A^d	0

(B) Ovalbumin peptide

Class II	Ratio of bound/unbound
I-A^d	128
I-E^d	101
Control	100

4 Antigenic Peptides Bind to Isolated MHC Molecules. Antigenic peptides of hen egg lysozyme (HEL) and ovalbumin (OVA) were identified and synthesized. Class II MHC molecules (I-A^k, I-A^d, and I-E^d) were purified from APC membranes. Equilibrium dialysis (see Chapter 10) was performed, and the amount of peptide bound to each class II molecule was determined. Binding is expressed as (A) fluorescent intensity of bound minus unbound or as (B) the ratio of bound to unbound. (A value of 100 in (B) indicates no binding.) Thus, HEL binds to I-A^k but not I-A^d, while OVA binds to I-A^d but not I-E^d. Previous studies have shown that T cells can recognize HEL plus I-A^k but not I-A^d, or OVA plus I-A^d but not I-E^d. [Data from (A) Bobbitt et al., 1985. *Nature* 317: 359; and (B) Buss et al., 1986. *Proc. Natl. Acad. Sci. U.S.A.* 83: 3586] the *Ir* genes (see Chapter 15). One explanation for this could be that some antigenic peptides simply fail to bind to some class II MHC molecules. If so, then this failure to bind should also be observable by equilibrium dialysis. When a class II MHC molecule that did not efficiently present the fragment was used, they found that the peptide bound with a 10-fold-lower affinity. Thus, it looked as if they had demonstrated not only that antigenic peptides bind to class II MHC molecules, but also that lack of this binding explains one type of *Ir* gene defect.[3]

SYNTHESIS
Processing and Presentation of Antigen with Class II MHC Molecules to CD4[+] T Cells

It was now very likely that the ligand for the T-cell receptor had been found: a complex of an antigenic peptide (produced by proteolytic cleavage within an APC) and a class II MHC molecule.

The idea that there might be some specificity in the interaction between a particular peptide and a particular MHC molecule may not be surprising when we consider the likelihood that MHC molecules and antigen receptors on B and T cells probably evolved from a common primordial gene. In the case of MHC molecule–peptide interactions, differences in binding affinities might well determine whether an immune response will occur.

Putting together the observations we've discussed so far leads to a scheme of antigen processing and presentation by APCs. This scheme is shown in Figure 5. Antigen is taken up by the APC (in the case of B cells, this is most efficiently done following binding to the surface Ig). The antigen is then cleaved by proteases, and the antigenic fragments associate with class II MHC molecules within the cell. The complexes of MHC and antigen fragment are then brought to the cell surface, where they can be recognized by a CD4[+] T cell, specific for the MHC molecule–antigen complex.

Raff's Riddle and the Binding of Self-Peptides

Martin Raff is a developmental neurobiologist who has the annoying habit of making important contributions to immunology. Before much of the above story had been worked out, he introduced a

[3] The laboratories of Unanue and Grey, and the colleagues who have left to form their own labs, comprise two of the great dynasties of antigen presentation. In the spirit of dynasties of old, they were symbolically merged when Marie Unanue married Harry Grey in 1988.

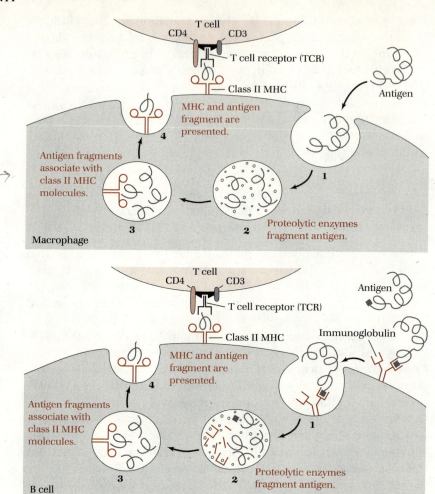

Class II MHC molec. mfg. in ER

5 Processing and Presentation of Antigen with Class II MHC Molecules to CD4$^+$ T Cells. Antigen is taken up by an APC (in the case of B cells, this can be via specific binding to the surface Ig). The antigen is endocytosed into vesicles within the cytoplasm, which then fuse with vesicles containing proteolytic enzymes. The enzymes fragment the antigen, and the fragments now associate with class II MHC molecules. The antigen–MHC molecule complex is then transported to the surface of the cell for presentation to CD4$^+$ T cells.

problem that still requires some explanation. It is this: How can an antigen be processed and presented when it is only available at low concentrations relative to endogenous proteins?

Some answers to this question have been proposed, but there are problems with all of them. The first possibility is that APCs (or even MHC molecules themselves) have the ability to discriminate self from nonself. This idea was popular for some time and received much discussion, until it was proved wrong.

Proofs came from (at least) three laboratories. Using the strategy of antigen peptide competition for presentation by fixed APCs, Luciano Adorini and colleagues showed that proteolytic fragments of an endogenous protein (mouse serum albumin) would compete for binding and presentation with peptides antigenic for a T-cell hybridoma. Thus, the MHC molecules didn't discriminate between self and nonself, and self-proteins could well yield peptides that prevent presentation of "foreign" peptides.

The second proof made matters even more interesting. Paul Allen and his colleagues demonstrated that at least one self-protein is normally both processed and presented by many different APCs of the body. To show this, it was necessary to obtain a T cell that could recognize this presented "self" antigen. (Normal individuals don't generally make detectable immune responses to their own antigens.) They took advantage of a genetic polymorphism in murine hemoglobin and generated T-cell hybridomas capable of recognizing one form of this protein. They then simply examined APCs from animals carrying this form of hemoglobin for their ability, straight out of the animal, to stimulate these T-cell hybridomas (the animals from which the T cells and the APCs were derived bore the same MHC haplotype). They found that APCs from several different organs all stimulated these T-cell hybridomas. Thus, hemoglobin, a "self" protein, is routinely processed and presented by APCs in the body. (The fact that the immune system does not normally respond to these presented self-antigens is discussed in Chapters 24, 31, 35, and 36.)

The third line of investigation was even more to the point. Grey and colleagues purified class II MHC molecules from murine APCs (again, "straight out of the animal") and treated the MHC molecules with low pH, a treatment that they had previously found would release bound antigenic peptides. They recovered a wide array of bound peptides, many of which, based on the above experiments, were presumably derived from "self" proteins. They then showed that these peptides were capable of competing with specific antigenic peptides for presentation by class II MHC molecules on fixed APCs. In addition, they found an interesting tendency. Peptides eluted from I-A molecules were better competitors for I-A interactions than for I-E interactions, and those from I-E molecules were better for I-E competition.

Thus, it is clear that the answer to Raff's riddle does not lie in self–nonself discrimination by APCs. Other possibilities suggest that the answer might lie in a role for preexisting antibody to facilitate antigen presentation (which doesn't really solve the problem) or perhaps a requirement for nonspecific activation of APC function. The latter is a feature of ADJUVANTS, substances that nonspecifically enhance immune responses. Some have suggested that adjuvants facilitate specific immune responses precisely because they allow APCs to preferentially process a particular foreign antigen. This certainly is not the whole key, since, while adjuvants enhance immune responses, they are not necessarily required, which is why (for example) some unfortunate hemophiliac patients make immune responses to injected clotting factor VIII.

For now, it seems that Raff's riddle will be with us for a while longer. If nothing else, it will keep us humble until Marty Raff thinks of something else.

Presentation of Class I MHC Molecules plus Antigen to CD8[+] T cells

Throughout much of the time during which the above processes were being worked out, there was an annoying disquiet about CD8[+] cytotoxic T cells. For one thing, it was easy to demonstrate the generation, effect, and MHC restriction of these cells against virally infected targets and tumor cells, as well as against haptenated cells. On the other hand, it wasn't possible to generate cytotoxic cells against soluble protein antigens. Is processing and presentation of antigen plus class I MHC molecules fundamentally different from that of antigen plus class II MHC? The answer, like so many in biology, is. "well, . . . yes and no."

CD8[+] T Cells Respond to Intracellularly Synthesized Antigen plus Class I MHC Molecules

A number of investigators studying the cytotoxic T-cell response to virally infected targets took a cue from the antigenic peptide studies described above. They found that proteolytic fragments of viral proteins, added to cultures of cells with the appropriate class I MHC haplotype, could make these cells targets for virus-specific cytotoxic T cells. However, if the viral proteins were not artificially cleaved, they generally failed to show this effect.

One of the most elegant studies that explained the solution to this problem was performed by Mark Moore, Francis Carbone, and Michael Bevan. They reasoned (as did many others) that the fun-

Table 5   A cell line expressing an ovalbumin gene induces antigen-specific, class I MHC-restricted CTL reaction.[a]

Mice immunized with	^{51}Cr-labeled targets	Percent lysis	Notes
	EL-4 + peptide	1	In vitro culture, alone, does not induce CTL reaction
OVA-EL-4	EL-4	9	Control targets
OVA-EL-4	OVA-EL-4	70	Specific CTL
OVA-EL-4	EL-4 + peptide	65	CTLs recognize OVA peptide
OVA-EL-4	EL-4 + OVA	5	Extracellular OVA not presented to CTLs
OVA-EL-4	L cell + peptide	5	L cells fail to present peptide to CTLs
OVA-EL-4	L/K^b + peptide	56	K^b-transfected L cells present peptide to CTLs
OVA	EL-4 + peptide	1	OVA, in vivo, does not prime CTLs

Source: Data from Moore et al., 1988. *Cell* 54: 777.

[a]EL-4 cells were transfected with the gene for chicken ovalbumin (OVA) to make the OVA-EL-4 line. Mice were immunized with the transfected cells, and then T cells from the immunized mice were cultured with OVA-EL-4 for 5 days. The cultured cells were recovered and assayed for CTL activity using ^{51}Cr-labeled targets. Targets were cultured with a peptide fragment of OVA, which associated with the class I MHC without a requirement for processing. Significant lysis of targets is indicated in color.

damental difference between presenting antigen with class I and class II MHC molecules might be that class I processing requires that the antigen be present in the *cytoplasm* of the cell. They demonstrated that this was the case by two different methods.

First, they transfected a murine lymphoma cell, called EL-4, with the gene encoding chicken ovalbumin. This engineered cell (which we'll call OVA-EL-4) synthesized ovalbumin. When the cell was injected into syngeneic mice (H-2^b) the animals generated CD8$^+$ cytotoxic T cells specific for ovalbumin plus H-2K^b (see Table 5). That is, the cytotoxic T cells would kill OVA-EL-4 but not EL-4 cells. Further, the cells killed other H-2K^b targets that were cultured with peptide fragments of ovalbumin, but not those cultured with intact ovalbumin.

They then did a clever trick to place intact ovalbumin molecules within various target cells. By culturing cells plus ovalbumin in a hypertonic solution, they were able to make the antigen enter the cells via pinocytosis (like endocytosis, only involving much smaller vesicles). The cells were then cultured briefly in a hypotonic medium, which caused the intracellular vesicles to lyse, releasing the antigen into the cytoplasm. These cells were then shown to be very good targets for the ovalbumin-specific cytotoxic T cells. Thus, the cytotoxic T cells recognized target cells that had been pulsed with ovalbumin "from the inside." Target cells exposed to exogenous ovalbumin were not recognized unless the ovalbumin was in the form of peptide fragments. Since peptides added to the outside of the cell generated effective targets, the difference between targets exposed to intact ovalbumin on the inside versus the outside must have been due to processing.

SYNTHESIS
Two Pathways of Antigen Processing

Based on these and other experiments, it is now clear that there are two general pathways of antigen processing and presentation (Figure 6). One involves endogenous antigens that are degraded within the cytoplasm and associate with class I MHC molecules. The other pathway involves exogenous antigens that are taken up and processed by an endosomal degradation mechanism and presented with class II MHC molecules.

The recognition that there are these two distinct processing pathways has important implications for the development of vaccines. If we wish to induce the generation of cytotoxic T cells, we must find a way to ensure that a vaccine will enter the class I processing pathway.

The Structure of the MHC Molecule–Antigenic Peptide Ligand for the T-Cell Receptor

As discussed in Chapter 15, the X-ray crystal structure of a human class I MHC molecule has been elucidated. Neither the structure of class II MHC molecule alone nor the structure of any MHC molecule with its associated antigen peptide has yet been ascertained, but this hasn't stopped the development of models. There are good reasons, though, why these models are probably correct.

You should recall that the structure of the class I MHC molecule includes a "groove" in the region of the molecule farthest from

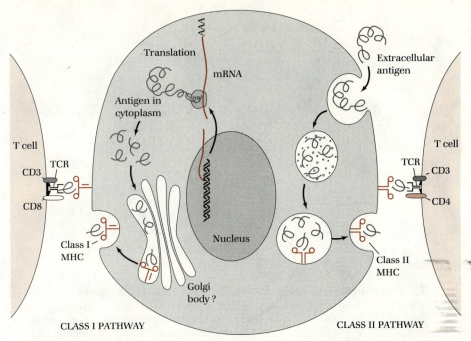

6 **Two Pathways of Antigen Processing and Presentation.** The location of antigen within a cell appears to determine whether the processed antigen will be presented with class I or class II MHC molecules. Antigens present in the cytoplasm (normally as a consequence of having been synthesized within the cell) are processed and presented with class I MHC molecules. Those antigens that enter the cell from the outside are generally processed and presented with class II MHC molecules.

the portion that is anchored in the membrane. This groove was found to contain an electron-dense material that is not an integral part of the MHC molecule itself (see Plate 20-1). Given the evidence we've discussed, this was very exciting because it was consistent with the idea that this density represents a number of antigen peptides bound into the groove of the purified class I molecules. If the groove contains different peptides, as is likely, it would explain why one specific peptide was not elucidated in the analysis. Further evidence that this groove is, indeed, responsible for binding and presenting antigen is based on MHC polymorphism. First, the most polymorphic residues in class I MHC molecules are those that line this groove (see Figure 7). Second, amino acid substitutions that render the molecule unable to present a particular antigen peptide also line this groove.

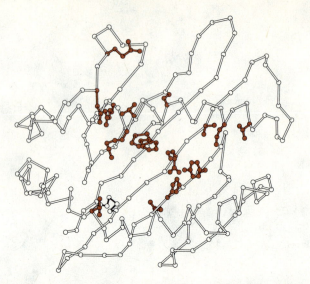

7 **Polymorphic Residues on Related Class I MHC Molecules Lie In and Around the Groove.** A number of HLA-A alleles have been sequenced, and their predicted amino acid sequences reveal polymorphism at particular residues, as represented in this figure. The majority of the polymorphic residues lie within or around the groove. [From Bjorkman et al., 1987. *Nature* 329: 512]

Class II MHC molecules may have a similar structure (which we now think is likely, though not proved). In these molecules the α helices that form the sides of the groove are thought to be formed by the α_2 and β_2 domains, while the β-pleated sheet that forms the base of the groove is thought to be formed by the α_1 and β_1 domains. It is interesting that if, indeed, such a structure forms, then the polymorphic residues (as well as those that are critical for presenting antigen) predominantly lie within and around the groove.

Agretopes, Epitopes, and the Mapping of Antigenic Peptides

In this section of the book, we've described many of the experiments leading to our current models of antigen presentation. To put it all together, it will be useful to present Ronald Schwartz's model (and terminology) for peptide–MHC molecule interactions. We can think of the combination of an MHC molecule and its associated antigen fragment as the ligand for the T-cell receptor. There are, then, four sites on this ligand that we should consider, and each of these has its own name (Figure 8). Two of these describe the way in which the MHC molecule and the antigen peptide fragment interact. The amino acids on the MHC molecule that are critical for effective association with an antigen fragment compose the DESETOPE, while the critical amino acids in the antigen that are required for association with the MHC molecule make up the AGRETOPE. The other two sites describe the interaction with the T-cell receptor. Those amino acids in the MHC molecule that are critical for recognition by a particular T cell form the HISTOTOPE, and the critical amino acids in the antigen that are required for recognition by a particular T cell make up the EPITOPE.

The critical sites on an antigenic fragment (agretope and epitope) are usually studied by synthesizing antigenic peptides that differ by one or a few amino acids, and then assessing their ability to stimulate a T cell. Mapping an antigen in this way reveals the critical amino acid residues but doesn't tell us which site they belong to. The agretope can then be mapped by examining the ability of the synthetic peptides to bind to a purified MHC molecule, by examining the ability of the peptides to compete with the original peptide for presentation by fixed APCs, and/or by examining which of the peptides can stimulate *any* T cells when presented with the appropriate MHC. Once the agretope is mapped, the epitope is assumed to be composed of the remaining critical amino acid residues. Until direct interaction with the T-cell receptor can be assessed, this seems to be the best we can do.

Mapping regions on an MHC molecule is a little trickier. In general, this is done by SITE-DIRECTED MUTAGENESIS of an MHC gene, in which the codons for specific amino acids in the molecule are specifically mutated. The gene is then transfected into a cell such as a fibroblast, which is then used to present antigen to a T cell. Although such analyses have not been exhaustively performed, we should expect that the histotopes and desetopes will tend to map into the regions facing and/or surrounding the MHC molecule groove. The critical residues that have, so far, been mapped in this

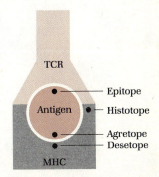

8   The Components of the Trimolecular Complex of Antigen, MHC Molecule, and the T-Cell Receptor. A cartoon representation of the T-cell receptor binding its ligand is shown. The *epitope* is the site on the antigen recognized by the T-cell receptor, while the *agretope* is the site on the antigen that binds to the MHC molecule. The *histotope* is the site on the MHC molecule recognized by the T-cell receptor, while the *desetope* is the site on the MHC molecule that binds to the antigen fragment. Although the precise structure of the interaction is not yet known, these terms are useful in discussing this complex receptor–ligand recognition.

way, although we don't know whether they compose the histotope, desetope, or both, fit this pattern.

A better understanding of the ways in which antigenic peptides interact with MHC molecules will help in the eventual design of vaccines capable of stimulating T cells (and thus producing immunity to the whole antigen). At present, the "rules" that determine which peptide will interact with which MHC molecule are not yet delineated; all we have are hints. One such hint is that immunogenic peptides appear to be AMPHIPATHIC. That is, they contain a mixture of hydrophobic and hydrophilic amino acids such that one face of the peptide can be hydrophilic and another face hydrophobic. There appears to be a tendency for the hydrophobic residues to interact with the MHC molecule, and for the hydrophilic residues to interact with the T-cell receptor. Computer programs that search amino acid sequences for such amphipathic regions have had some success in predicting which peptides will be immunogenic.

Summary

1. Antigen-presenting cells (APCs) are required for the activation of T cells by antigen. The APCs and T cells must be of the same MHC haplotype, indicating that this is the site of MHC restriction.
2. Antigen processing for presentation with class II MHC molecules involves the uptake of antigen into endosome vesicles, followed by cleavage of the antigen into fragments. These antigenic fragments are bound by class II MHC molecules and are then presented to $CD4^+$ T cells.
3. Antigen processing for presentation with class I MHC molecules requires that the antigen be present in the cytoplasm of the cell (most often because it is made by the cell). The antigen is cleaved into fragments and associates with class I MHC molecules and is exported to the surface for presentation to $CD8^+$ T cells.
4. The best current explanation of MHC restriction is that the ligand for the T-cell receptor is a fragment of antigen bound into the "groove" of an MHC molecule. The T-cell receptor recognizes parts of both the antigen fragment and the MHC molecule.

Additional Readings

Berzofsky, J. A., S. J. Brett, H. Z. Streicher and H. Takahashi. 1988. Antigen processing for presentation to T lymphocytes. *Immunol. Rev.* 106: 5.

Lorenz, R. G. and P. M. Allen. 1988. Processing and presentation of self proteins. *Immunol. Rev.* 106: 115.

Townsend, A. and H. Bodmer. 1989. Antigen recognition by class I–restricted T lymphocytes. *Annu. Rev. Immunol.* 7: 601.

Unanue, E. R. 1989. Macrophages, antigen-presenting cells, and the phenomenon of antigen handling and presentation. In Paul, W., ed. *Fundamental Immunology*, 2nd ed. Raven, New York, p. 95.

Werdelin, O., S. Mouritsen, B. L. Petersen, A. Sette and S. Buus. 1988. Facts on the fragmentation of antigens in presenting cells, on the association of antigen fragments with MHC molecules in cell free systems, and speculation on the cell biology of antigen processing. *Immunol. Rev.* 106: 181.

RECEPTORS

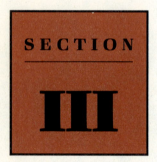

SECTION

III

But there is trouble in store for anyone who surrenders to the temptation of mistaking an elegant hypothesis for a certainty.

Primo Levi, *The Periodic Table*

In these three chapters we will examine the nature of the antigen-specific receptors used by B and T cells to recognize and react with antigen. We will also examine the nature of the molecules that the cells synthesize as a result of these reactions.

We already know that B cells can react with free antigen but that T cells react with foreign antigen only in the context of self-MHC. An understanding of the nature of the receptors and the consequences of cell activation through these receptors is crucial to understanding how the immune system is regulated—the topic to be covered in Section IV.

ANTIGEN-SPECIFIC RECEPTORS ON B CELLS AND THE DYNAMICS OF THE ANTIBODY RESPONSE

<table>
<tr><td>

CHAPTER

21
</td></tr>
</table>

Overview Clonal selection requires that antigen react with a cell that has rearranged its genes and is expressing an antibody molecule of a given specificity. The B cell has abundant Ig on its surface, and it is known that this Ig acts as the cell-surface receptor. Thus we have the situation that a B cell rearranges its Ig genes and uses the message both for the exported product (the antibody) and as a receptor for antigen at the cell surface. In this chapter we will discuss the nature of the antigen-specific receptor on the surface of the B cell. It will be seen that there are two isotypes of Ig on the surface, μ and δ, and that these membrane forms are derived from differential splicing of the same piece of mRNA.

We will also examine the dynamics of the immune response. We will see that the character of the response changes during the course of antigen-driven activation of B cells. Not only is there a switch of isotype from IgM to IgG, but the affinity of the antibodies also changes. Finally, we will discuss the nature of immunological memory.

CHAPTER 21

The B-Cell Receptor

Surface Antigen Receptors on B Cells

One of the few things that all immunologists agree on is that the Ig molecules found at the surface of B cells act as receptors for antigen.

In a now-classic series of experiments, Sell and Gell showed in 1965 that anti-Ig antiserum raised against secreted Ig could to some extent mimic the action of antigen by causing B cells to undergo blastogenesis. This is indirect evidence that the receptor on the B cell is Ig, since it assumes that the anti-Ig is activating the cell via the surface Ig (sIg) in a manner similar to that occurring

345

when antigen binds to the combining site. More direct studies soon followed, and these showed that free antigen binds to the surface of the B cell and that this binding can be competitively inhibited by anti-Ig. This finding argues that the antigen is binding to an Ig molecule on the surface of the B cell.

The assumption from clonal selection is that the specificity of the Ig that a B cell displays on its surface is the same as the specificity of the Ig secreted by the cell. To test this, several variations of the following experiment have been carried out. Spleen or lymph node cells (containing both B cells and T cells) are passed over a column of immobilized antigen. Only a very small fraction of the cells are retained on the column, that is, have reacted with the antigen on the column. We know that these cells are B cells (they are Ig$^+$) and that they react *specifically* with the antigen, because when the cells are eluted from the column and stimulated with antigen, they respond only to the specific antigen and not to other antigens.

B cells express the same Ig idiotype on their surface as that of the secreted Ig. Furthermore, anti-idiotype (antibody against the antigen-combining site) can stimulate B cells to proliferate in a manner similar to that of antigen. This also is a very strong argument that the surface and secreted molecules have the same specificity.

Isotype and Idiotype of Surface Ig

Although there is general agreement that the sIg molecules on B cells act as antigen-specific receptors, we are only beginning to understand how their reaction with antigen transduces the signal to the cell to proliferate and secrete Ig. Some of the current notions about signal transduction in general and B cells in particular will be discussed in Chapter 26.

The lymphoid stem cell and the early precursors of B cells do not express Ig on their surfaces. However, it can be shown that gene rearrangement is occurring in the early lineage precursors and that there is *internal* μ chain in the pre-B cell population. It can be seen in Figure 1 that the first Ig expressed on the surface is IgM (sIgM). This sIgM is an 8 S monomer, in contrast to the secreted IgM, which is a 19 S pentamer. As B cells mature, they begin to express another isotype of Ig on their surfaces, IgD. The monomeric membrane forms of Ig all have slightly higher molecular weights than the monomers of the secreted forms, because

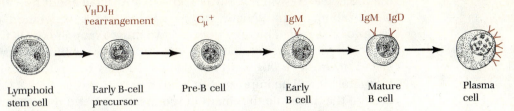

1   Development of Surface Ig Expression in B Cells. The earliest B-cell precursor rearranges the genes for the μ chain, and the first intracellular μ chain is expressed at the pre-B cell stage. The B cell goes through a maturation process in which it first expresses surface IgM but no IgD (early, large B cell), and then both IgM and IgD (mature, small B cell). After antigenic stimulation, the B cell matures to a terminally differentiated, Ig-secreting cell called the plasma cell.

the membrane molecules contain a hydrophobic region that is used to anchor them in the membrane.

Recall from Chapter 6 that IgD is an isotype found in vanishingly small amounts in the serum. The general consensus is that this isotype in some way plays a role as antigen-specific receptor. The mechanism of this dual isotype expression was discussed in Chapter 6. The fact that the sIgM and sIgD both have the same antigen specificity and idiotype is a point in favor of their acting as receptors. Other Ig isotypes (IgG, IgA, and IgE) are also found on B cells after they have undergone the class switch after antigenic stimulation. In contrast, IgM and IgD appear on resting cells, which argues that they are receptor molecules that are used at the initiation of an antibody response.

Taken together, all this points to the fact that the resting B cell displays molecules of two isotypes, IgM and IgD, but one idiotype at the cell surface. These molecules act as receptors to transduce the signal to proliferate and differentiate into antibody-secreting cells after antigenic stimulation. At that time the cell begins to secrete IgM but not IgD. After stimulation, some of the B cells undergo class switching and then express another isotype (with the original idiotype) at the cell surface. This will be the same isotype and idiotype as the secreted antibody.

Organization of Receptor Genes in B Cells

Because the B-cell antigen-specific receptor is an Ig molecule with structural properties very similar to those of the secreted form of the molecule, we will not have to go into any detail about how the organization of the genetic material leads to the generation of receptor diversity. The only question we must examine now is the nature of the differences between the surface, or membrane-associated, form of Ig (sIg) and the secreted forms of the molecule. Ultimately it will be important to know the features that allow one form of the molecule to remain in the membrane and the other to be secreted.

Synthesis of Surface and Secreted IgM

Two groups of researchers have independently concluded that the membrane form and the secreted form of μ chain are encoded from the same gene. The difference between the two forms is achieved during the processing of the mRNA. Frederick Alt and his colleagues isolated mRNA from two different B-cell lines. One of these lines produced equal amounts of secreted and membrane forms of IgM, and one produced almost exclusively membrane form. The mRNA from the line producing both forms of μ chain encoded two proteins, one with a molecular weight of 64,000 and one with a molecular weight of 67,000. The less mature line, which did not produce secreted form, had only mRNA encoding the 67,000-dalton protein. This suggested that one mRNA was encoding secreted forms and one encoding membrane forms of μ chain. When fetal liver (which is a site of embryonic B-cell development) was examined, it was found that the only mRNA present was identical to that thought to encode the membrane form. The developing B cells in the fetal liver do not secrete any Ig, but they do have surface IgM.

Then cDNA was prepared from the two forms of mRNA, and it was found that the sequences are identical through the 3' end of the fourth constant region $(C_\mu 4)$; that is, the two forms of μ chain use the same gene. They differ only in untranslated segments at the COOH terminus. Thus the secreted and membrane forms are produced from transcripts of a single gene that are alternatively spliced. The membrane form is generated by two extra mRNA splices, resulting in the association of the M segment with $C_\mu 4$. The mechanism for the alternative mRNA splicing is not known. This is seen diagrammatically in Figure 2.

Splicing of the μ–δ Transcript

It will be recalled that the genes for μ and δ are adjacent (located within 2.3 kb of each other). It is known that there is no class

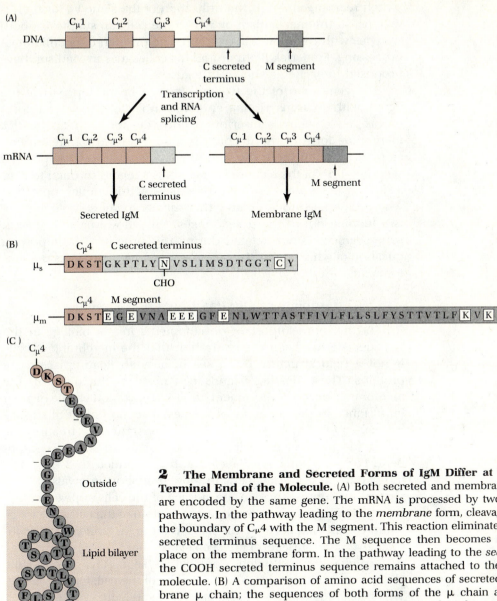

2   The Membrane and Secreted Forms of IgM Differ at the COOH-Terminal End of the Molecule. (A) Both secreted and membrane μ chains are encoded by the same gene. The mRNA is processed by two alternative pathways. In the pathway leading to the *membrane* form, cleavage occurs at the boundary of $C_\mu 4$ with the M segment. This reaction eliminates the COOH secreted terminus sequence. The M sequence then becomes spliced into place on the membrane form. In the pathway leading to the *secreted* form, the COOH secreted terminus sequence remains attached to the rest of the molecule. (B) A comparison of amino acid sequences of secreted and membrane μ chain; the sequences of both forms of the μ chain are identical through $C_\mu 4$. The COOH terminus of the membrane form has many charged residues and a long hydrophobic sequence that is the transmembrane component. The charged residues are boxed, and the long hydrophobic sequence is underlined. (C) The amino acid sequence of the membrane form of IgM seen in B as it might be in the membrane. Note that the long hydrophobic sequence underlined in B is folded into the lipid bilayer. [Redrawn from Rogers et al., 1980. *Cell* 20: 303; and from Early et al., 1980. *Cell* 20: 313]

switch rearrangement in the utilization of the same V_H for both C regions, so the mechanism by which the cell can synthesize both isotypes with the same idiotype must be through differential RNA processing. Frederick Blattner and his colleagues in Madison have proposed the scheme shown in Figure 3.

The gene map of the H chain is seen in the top part of the figure, with six transcription end sites indicated. A secreted form (μ_s) is made when transcription ends at site 1. In contrast, a membrane form of the μ chain is made when the transcription stops at site 2. If the transcription goes through to sites 3 or 4, a secreted form of the δ chain is made, but if it goes through to sites 5 or 6, a membrane form of δ results. In this model, note that when the read-through is to either membrane or soluble δ, there is a looping out of the μ sequences. Note, however, that the Cμ gene segment is not deleted during this process. The important question of what causes the use of each of these end sites remains to be answered.

Mobility of sIg: Patching and Capping

One of the more important developments in cell biology in the past decade has been the realization that the membrane of cells is not a rigid structure but a sea of oil with floating islands of proteins. These floating islands can move in the plane of the membrane, and their movement and reorganization can be of great importance in the economy of the cell. The movement of surface molecules of lymphocytes can be demonstrated by treating the cells with fluorescein-labeled antibody against a surface component. For example, when labeled anti-Ig is added to B cells and the pattern of fluorescence is examined at short intervals, a "ring pattern" of fluorescence on the surface of the cells appears immediately. Through the microscope, the outline of the cell appears as a fluorescent ring because the labeled anti-Ig is uniformly distributed over the surface of the cell. Very soon, however, the ring pattern changes and patches of label are seen. After a short time all the patches of label move to one pole of the cell, forming a cap. This process is called PATCHING AND CAPPING (Figure 4).

Although the significance of patching and capping is not completely understood, it is thought that the reorganization of the Ig molecules (i.e., the receptors) in the membrane is important for signal transduction from the surface of the cell to the nucleus (see Chapter 26). It is likely that this leads to the internalization of the

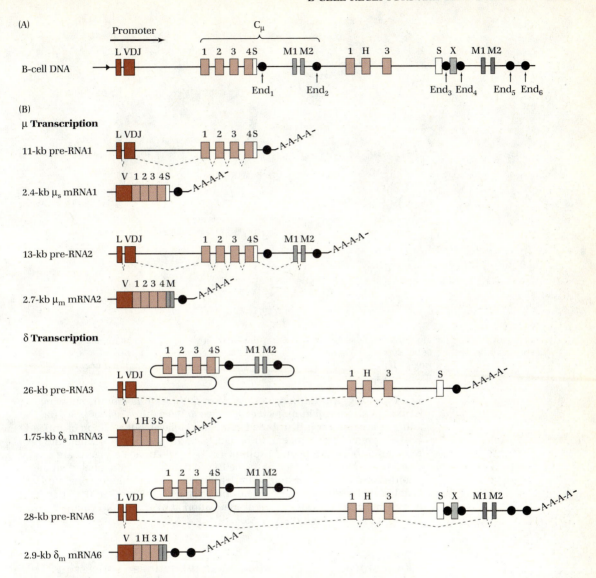

3 **Hypothetical Splicing Pattern of the μ–δ Transcript.** (A) The gene map of the H chain. In the C_μ and the C_δ regions, there are six sites for termination of transcription (marked END). (B) Pre-RNA and mRNA for the membrane and secreted forms of both μ and δ chains. For secreted μ, the termination of transcription is at END_1, and for membrane-bound μ, the termination is at END_2. This results in transcripts of different lengths and the two different forms of the molecule. For the δ chain, termination is at $END_{3,4}$ for the secreted form, and at $END_{5,6}$ for the membrane-bound form. [From Blattner and Tucker, 1984. *Nature* 307: 417. With permission]

(A)

(B)

(C)

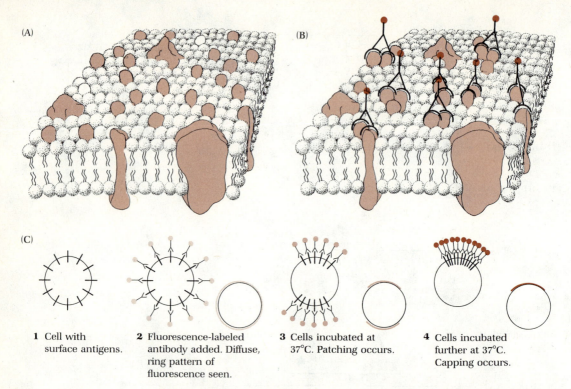

1 Cell with surface antigens.

2 Fluorescence-labeled antibody added. Diffuse, ring pattern of fluorescence seen.

3 Cells incubated at 37°C. Patching occurs.

4 Cells incubated further at 37°C. Capping occurs.

4   Patching and Capping. (A) Diagram of the cell membrane showing the islands of glycoprotein molecules (surface antigens) in a sea of lipid. (B) The antigens are randomly distributed in the lipid bilayer, but addition of antibody causes some of the antigens to be clustered in patches. (C) Schematic representation of patching and capping. (1) The cell-surface antigens are evenly distributed over the surface of the cell. (2) When fluorescein-labeled antibody is added and the cells examined under the fluorescence microscope, a diffuse staining pattern is visible. (3) When the cells are incubated at 37°C, patching of the antigens occurs. (4) Further incubation at 37°C leads to capping. [After Taylor et al., 1971. *Nature, New Biology* 233: 225]

bound antigen, which is the first step in antigen processing. This could explain why an individual B cell most efficiently processes and presents antigen for which it is specific.

Dynamics of the Antibody Response

According to clonal selection there must be a means of specifically activating the B cells that have rearranged their antibody gene segments in a manner that results in an antibody of a given specificity. So far in this chapter we have established the fact that it is the surface Ig on the B cell that acts as this receptor for antigen. In the previous chapters we have also examined the cellular events leading to the production of antibody. We will now briefly consider the *dynamics* of the B cell in the antibody response.

Primary and Secondary Antibody Responses

Kinetics of the Antibody Response.   The receptors of resting B cells are sIgM. It should therefore come as no surprise to the reader at this stage of our narrative that the first antibodies that appear in the serum of an animal after stimulation with antigen are IgM.

Figure 5 shows the KINETICS of a typical antibody response. After the introduction of antigen there is a period of time in which no antibody to the antigen is found in the serum nor are new antibody-forming cells present in spleen or lymph nodes. This

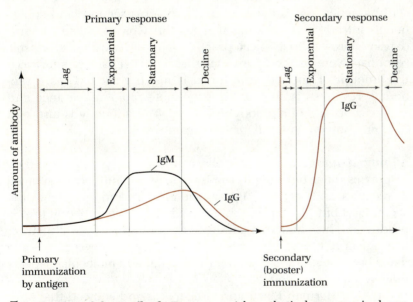

5   Kinetics of the Antibody Response. A hypothetical response is shown. After primary immunization there is a long lag period, an exponential increase in the amount of antibody, and a stationary and decline phase. Most of the antibody produced in the primary response is IgM, but there can be detectable IgG. Upon secondary (booster) immunization, the lag phase is shorter and the exponential phase reaches a plateau at a much higher concentration of antibody. The antibody in the secondary response is IgG. Not indicated in the figure is the fact that the affinity of the antibody increases during the course of the immunization.

period is called the LAG or LATENT PHASE. The lag phase is followed by the rapid appearance of antibody-forming cells in secondary lymphoid organs and of circulating antibody in the serum. In fact the rate of increase is often exponential, and this phase is called the EXPONENTIAL PHASE. This is followed by a leveling off of the rate of antibody production that is called the STATIONARY PHASE and then the decline in the rate of production and appearance in the serum called the DECLINE PHASE.

Note in the figure that the response to this first confrontation with the antigen is called the PRIMARY RESPONSE, and the first antibody that appears is IgM. But as the primary response proceeds, some antibody of other isotypes begins to appear. In the figure, for the sake of clarity, we use IgG as the second isotype. Thus we see that the primary response is characterized by a delay in the onset of appearance of antibody, and the isotype of the antibody that is produced is initially IgM.

The introduction of antigen a second time leads to a different set of kinetics and isotypes of antibody. This second (and subsequent) introduction of antigen results in what is called the SECONDARY RESPONSE. In clinical practice it is often called a *booster* response. Note in the figure that the lag phase is very short and the amount of antibody produced is much greater. Thus a secondary response is characterized by more rapid appearance and greater amounts of antibody produced. The antibody is also of a different isotype; in the figure we again use IgG.

Affinity Maturation. The B cells in the primary and secondary responses differ not only in the isotype of the antibody displayed as receptor and secreted (IgM in the primary and IgG, etc. in the secondary) but also in the binding affinity of the antibody that is produced. This change in affinity is a very important and instructive aspect of the immune response, and we will cover it in some detail because it brings together the cellular and molecular aspects that we have been covering.

In 1964 Herman Eisen and Gregory Siskind showed that after rabbits were immunized with DNP conjugated to an appropriate carrier, the *affinity* of the antibody in the serum increased with time. They showed that the antibodies obtained at 6 weeks after immunization had at least 100-fold greater affinity than the antibodies obtained 2 weeks after immunization. The use of high concentrations of antigen to immunize the animals, however, prevented this change. In 1969 Norman Klinman showed that the increased affinity is clonal, that is, some clones of cells produce antibody of high affinity and some clones produce antibody of low affinity.

Putting these data together into a unified theory, Siskind and Baruj Benaceraff proposed the ANTIGEN SELECTION HYPOTHESIS. This theory assumed that the binding properties of an antibody are the same as the antigen-binding properties of the receptor on the cell that will produce the antibody. Thus they proposed that a cell that makes high-affinity antibody will have high-affinity receptors and therefore will have a better chance of reacting with antigen when that antigen is in limiting amounts. When the antigen is in high concentration, there is no competition between the receptors of high and low affinity for the antigen, and so the theory also explained the lack of affinity maturation in the presence of high concentrations of immunizing antigen. But as the antigen is cleared and the concentration declines, those cells with high-affinity receptors are preferentially activated. The whole idea was consistent with clonal selection and very appealing.

With the application of the tools of molecular biology, however, it was found that affinity maturation is apparently not due to selection alone, but rather to a combination of *mutation* and selection. Several groups have shown that during the response to antigen there is *hypermutation* in restricted parts of the rearranged Ig genes. This mutation can result in new specificities, but it is now thought that the greatest effect is on affinity.

As an example, Claudia Berek and Cesar Milstein carried out the experiment illustrated in Figure 6. Mice were given a primary or secondary immunization with a hapten coupled to an appropriate carrier. They were sacrificed and their spleen cells fused to form hybridomas at various times, either after the first injection (primary response) or after a second or even third injection (secondary and tertiary responses) at later times. The sequences of the genes encoding the anti-hapten were then compared at each of these times.

It was already known that most of the antibodies produced by mice to the hapten that was used (phOx) preferentially use germ-line V segments called V_H *Ox-1* or V_κ *Ox-1*. As seen in Figure 7, all the hybridomas made 7 days after primary immunization used the V_H *Ox-1* gene H-chain and all but one the V_κ *Ox-1* L-chain gene. At 14 days into the primary response, the same *Ox-1* H- and L-chain germ-line genes were still being used but the number of mutations seen in both was large. These mutations seem to cluster

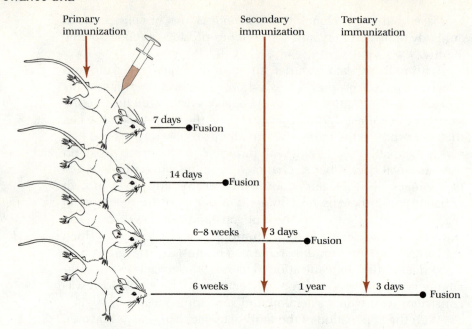

Primary immunization

Secondary immunization

Tertiary immunization

7 days → Fusion

14 days → Fusion

6–8 weeks | 3 days → Fusion

6 weeks | 1 year | 3 days → Fusion

6   Protocol for Affinity Maturation Experiment. Mice were immunized with hapten (phOx) conjugated to carrier on day 0 (the primary immunization). Two groups received a secondary immunization at 6 to 8 weeks, and a third received a tertiary immunization over 1 year later. Fusions of spleen cells were made at indicated times, and hybridoma lines were established. [After Berek and Milstein, 1987. *Immunol. Rev.* 96: 23]

around the CDR2 of the H chain and the CDR1 of the L chain. The affinity of the antibodies can also be seen to have increased during the intervening 7 days.

When the animals were given a second injection of antigen 6 to 8 weeks later and hybridomas made a few days later, it is clear that there were more mutations, especially in the L-chain genes. Even more striking is the fact that many of the H-chain genes are

7   Comparison of Gene Sequences from phOx-Specific Hybridomas. The hybridomas generated in Figure 6 were analyzed to determine if they used the *Ox-1* gene, the number of mutations, and the affinity of the antibody secreted. Solid lines represent the *Ox-1* gene. Dashed lines are other germ line genes that were not analyzed for mutations. Each dot represents a mutation. Note the increase in mutations during the course of the immunization and the correlation with affinity. [After Berek and Milstein, 1987. *Immunol. Rev.* 96: 23. Courtesy of C. Berek]

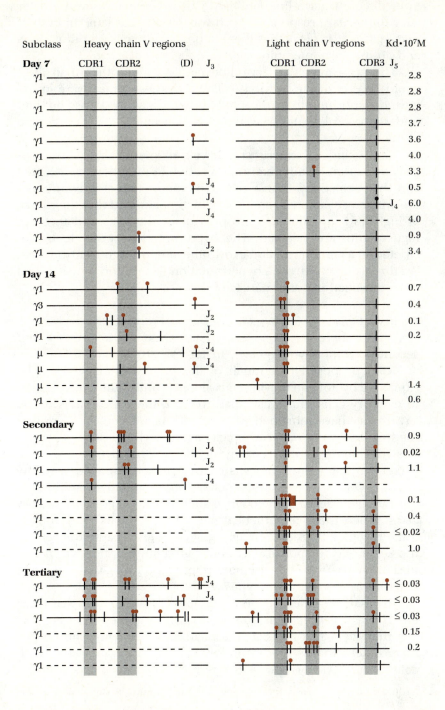

from different germ-line families. This difference is even greater after the tertiary response, which was over 1 year later. In both of these cases it is clear that there is both an increase in mutations and an increase in affinity.

The appearance of germ-line family genes other than *Ox-1* could be due to the fact that cells using these genes were in too low concentration to be detected in the primary response but had undergone proliferation (i.e., they were selected) during the course of the response.[1]

These kinds of experiments have now made most immunologists think that affinity maturation is due to mutation in the CDRs and then selection of these mutated clones. This is in contrast to the antigen selection hypothesis, which postulated that the clones of high and low affinities are present at the start and those of high affinity are selected. The hypermutation seems to be restricted to a certain rather narrow time after antigen is introduced. We do not know why the hypermutation begins and why it seems to be localized in certain areas of the molecule.

Memory Cells or Memory Populations. From all the above it is clear that there are very great differences in the primary and secondary antibody responses. In 1968 Vera Byers and Eli Sercarz at UCLA proposed that much of the phenomenology could be explained by antigen moving cells along a continuum from primary to memory cells (this was called the XYZ theory). Variants of the XYZ theory have remained with us and have taken the form that there is *unequal division* of B cells after reaction with antigen. In this idea some of the progeny of the original B cells go on to become antibody-forming cells in the primary response (IgM, low affinity). Others, however, do not become antibody-forming cells but rather undergo some change such that they are now MEMORY CELLS. When these hypothetical memory cells react with antigen (via a receptor that is no longer IgM), they give rise to the cells of the secondary response (IgG and high-affinity antibody). In this idea, then, there is one precursor population that gives rise to two different functional B-cell types.

Norman Klinman has proposed another alternative: that there are in fact two precursor populations. His argument relies on the fact that there is a marker present in high concentration on primary B cells that is present in low concentration in secondary B cells. This marker is a cell-surface molecule that reacts with the

[1] In the experiment shown, the mutations were not studied in any other germ-line gene family than *Ox-1*.

monoclonal antibody called J11D, and the marker is therefore called J11D. Phyllis Linton and colleagues in Klinman's lab separated unprimed spleen cells from mice in a cell sorter based on their expression of J11D. When J11D^{hi} cells were cultured with helper T cells and antigen, they gave rise in vitro to a vigorous primary response but were unable to give a secondary response. In contrast, the J11D^{lo} cells gave little or no primary response under the same culture conditions but did give a vigorous secondary response. This is consistent with there being two separate precursor populations. Recall from the experiments discussed above that in the secondary and tertiary responses some of the cells were using a germ-line gene other than the one seen in the primary response. One explanation for this is that the population of cells in the primary response that were using other germ-line V-gene segments were in too low concentration to see, but their numbers increased through selection. From what we have just seen, though, one must consider the possibility that the cells using these genes are from a population of separate precursors that did not participate in the primary response.

(handwritten margin note: – B cell & B memory cell)

SYNTHESIS
Primary and Secondary Antibody Responses

The introduction of antigen initiates a complex series of events. If we focus on the B cell in antibody formation for a moment, we see that the first requisite of clonal selection, that the cell have an antigen-specific receptor, is met. Resting B cells express Ig molecules of the IgM and IgD isotypes on their surfaces. With T-cell help, the cells whose receptors have reacted with antigen begin to proliferate. This accounts for the increase in antibody after immunization. But we have now seen that other events also occur. Gene rearrangement leading to the expression and secretion of antibody of a new isotype occurs (class switch), and a series of mutations occurs that is associated with the increase in affinity of the antibody that is produced. The individual that is making the antibody response thus ends up with many cells producing antibody of high affinity.

Summary

1. Antigen binds directly to B-cell receptors, which are surface Ig molecules.
2. The B cell has two surface isotypes that act as antigen-specific

receptors: sIgM and sIgD. These molecules share idiotypic and antigenic specificity.

3.   During B-cell development, sIgM is the first isotype expressed at the cell surface, but as B cells develop they also begin to express surface IgD.

4.   The membrane-bound form of IgM and the secreted form are encoded from the same gene. The differences between the two forms are achieved during mRNA processing.

5.   The sIg antigen-specific receptors on B cells are mobile within the membrane and can be "patched" and "capped." This may be of importance in signal transduction by antigen.

6.   The first introduction of antigen results in a primary response which is characterized by a long lag period and IgM antibody. Subsequent injection results in the secondary response, which is characterized by a shorter lag period, higher concentration of antibody that is of a new isotype, and higher affinity.

7.   Affinity maturation is thought to be due to mutations during the response, although a separate precursor subpopulation of B cells cannot be ruled out.

Additional Readings

Alt, F. W., A. L. M. Bothwell, M. Knapp, E. Siden, E. Mather, M. Koshland and D. Baltimore. 1980. Synthesis of secreted and membrane-bound μ heavy chains is directed by mRNAs that differ at their 3' ends. *Cell* 20: 293.

Berek, C. and C. Milstein. 1987. Mutation drift and repertoire shift in the maturation of the immune response. *Immunol. Rev.* 96: 23.

Blattner, F. R. and P. W. Tucker. 1984. The molecular biology of immunoglobulin D. *Nature* 307: 417.

Linton, P-J., D. J. Decker and N. R. Klinman. 1989. Primary antibody-forming cells and secondary B cells are generated from separate precursor cell subpopulations. *Cell* 59: 1049.

Unanue, E. R. and M. J. Karnovsky. 1973. Redistribution and fate of Ig complexes on surface of B lymphocytes: Functional implications and mechanisms. *Transplant. Rev.* 14: 184

THE T-CELL RECEPTOR

Overview   Until a few years ago the T-cell receptor was the major enigma in cellular immunology. It was known that T cells do not react with free antigen, only with antigen in association with the MHC molecule. In this chapter we will develop the evidence that has led us to our current understanding of the nature of the T-cell receptor. The bottom line is that it is a two-chain molecule with constant and variable regions. But to know this without the reasoning that led to its discovery is to miss out on a great scientific adventure. Our discussion is intended to leave the reader in the position of being prepared for the next phases of the research on the receptor (and the surprises that no doubt will come with them).

Until a few years ago, our lack of real understanding of the structure and function of the T-cell receptor was a roadblock to further understanding of the regulation of the immune response. The great progress toward the solution to the T-cell receptor problem has allowed us to begin to understand the mechanism of MHC restriction and antigen presentation (Chapters 19 and 20).

Initially there were technical difficulties that accounted for some of the lack of insight (the Ig molecule is secreted in large quantities and could be studied, for example, but the T-cell receptor is not). But the real difficulty was theoretical because any solution had to address the problem of MHC restriction. When it was discovered that some of the regulation of the immune response is controlled by genes coding for MHC molecules (the *Ir* genes), there was a movement to implicate the MHC products as the T-cell receptor. This was the first explanation that tried to join the recognition of antigen by the T-cell receptor and MHC restriction. This idea did not survive and after much controversy and gnashing of teeth it was also concluded that T cells do not have surface Ig. Thus, the search was on for a unique molecule.

Models for the T-Cell Receptor

So far we have focused on the mechanisms by which antigen is processed and by which a peptide fragment is associated with the MHC molecule by antigen-presenting cells for presentation to the T cell. In this chapter we will focus on the nature of the receptor on the T cell.

Single Receptor versus Dual Recognition

When MHC restriction was first discovered, Rolf Zinkernagel and Peter Doherty proposed two alternative models. The first was known as the DUAL RECOGNITION MODEL and postulated a receptor for antigen and another receptor for self-MHC molecules. Binding of one of these receptors with the appropriate ligand (antigen or self-MHC molecule) was thought to be insufficient to trigger the cell; only when *both* receptors were occupied would an activation signal get transduced from the membrane to the cell interior. The other alternative was called the NEOANTIGENIC DETERMINANT MODEL. This model postulated that there is a receptor, *not* for antigen *or* for self-MHC molecules, but rather for the *combination* of the two. This complex of antigen and MHC molecule on the surface of the antigen-presenting cell was thought to be seen by the T cell as a new antigen (hence the term *neoantigenic determinant*). These possibilities are diagrammed in their most simplistic form in Figure 1.

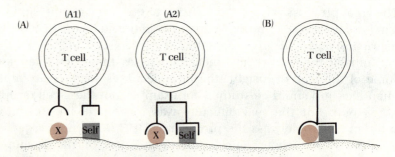

1 Models of the T-Cell Receptor. (A) A1 and A2 are *dual recognition* models. In these models the T cell has a receptor for foreign antigen (X) and a receptor for self-MHC molecule (self). These receptors can exist as separate molecules in the membrane (A1), or can be joined to a common structure and have one chain reactive with X and one with self (A2). (B) The *neoantigenic determinant* model in which the T cell has a receptor that is specific neither for antigen nor for self but rather for a unique determinant that is formed by the association of antigen and self-MHC molecule. [After Zinkernagel, 1978. *Immunol. Rev.* 42: 224]

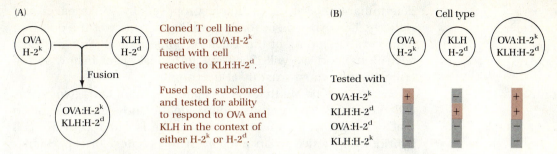

2 Test of Dual-Receptor or Single-Receptor Models of the T-Cell Receptor. When cells reactive to an antigen in the context of one H-2 molecule are fused with cells reactive to a different antigen in the context of another H-2 molecule, and the fused cell tested with all combinations of antigen and H-2 molecules, it is found that the fused cell is reactive to the two antigens, but only in the context of the orignal H-2. This finding argues that if there are separate receptors for antigen and H-2 molecules, they function as a single unit. [After Kappler et al., 1981. *J. Exp. Med.* 153: 1198]

Ruling Out the Two-Independent-Receptors Model

To test the model of two independent receptors, one of which recognizes antigen and the other self-MHC molecules, John Kappler and Phillipa Marrack and their co-workers in Denver carried out the experiment outlined in Figure 2. They used a cloned, antigen-specific, T-cell hybridoma that reacted to ovalbumin presented in the context of MHC molecules (OVA/I-A^k). These hybridoma cells were *fused* with normal activated T cells (called blasts) that responded to an antigen, keyhole limpet hemocyanin (KLH) in the context of another MHC molecule (KLH/I-A^d). The fused cells were shown to respond when presented with the antigen/MHC combination with which each fusion partner reacted (KLH/I-A^d and OVA/I-A^k). It was then asked if the restriction elements of the receptor are joined or separate, that is, can this multispecific cell respond to KLH only in the context of I-A^d or can it also respond in the context of I-A^k? In other words, can the antigen specificity of one of the parent cells be mixed with the MHC restriction of the other? The answer is no. The cells respond only when the antigen and MHC molecule are presented coordinately (Figure 2B). This elegant experiment argues against two *independent* receptors, one for MHC molecule alone and one for antigen alone.

Evidence for a Single Receptor for MHC and Antigen

The data that we have discussed up to now rule out the dual receptor model. The alternative, of course, was the neoantigenic determinant model as originally proposed by Zinkernagel and Doherty. The experiment that would begin to answer the question required the cloning of the T-cell receptor gene(s). This has now been done, and we will discuss it in logical order below, so the critical reader must trust us at this point.

We will see below that the T-cell receptor contains two chains called α and β. Two groups independently and elegantly showed that when genes for these two chains are isolated from a T-cell hybridoma reactive to an antigen in the context of a particular MHC and transfected into a cell with completely different specificities, the cell acquires the specificity and MHC restriction of the transfected genes. This is diagrammed in Figure 3. In this case the genes for the α and β chains of a cytotoxic T cell specific for fluorescein (FL) in the context of H-2D^d were transfected into a T-cell hybridoma specific for the hapten SP [3-(p-sulphophenyldiazo)-4-hydroxyphenylacetic acid] in the context of H-2K^k. The resulting clone was found to express both the transfected and endogenous receptors and, most importantly, was found to be specific for both SP/K^k and FL/D^d. In this case the cell was a class I-restricted CTL, but the same kind of experiment was done with a class II-restricted helper cell.

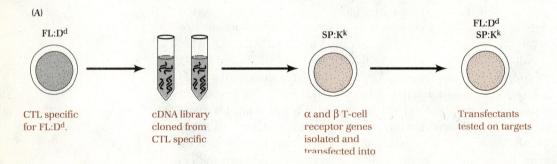

(A)

FL:D^d → CTL specific for FL:D^d.

cDNA library cloned from CTL specific

SP:K^k → α and β T-cell receptor genes isolated and transfected into

FL:D^d SP:K^k → Transfectants tested on targets

(B)

	Cell type		
Tested with	FL/D^d	SP/K^k	FL/D^d SP/K^k
SP:K^k	–	+	+
SP:D^d	–	–	–
FL:K^k	–	–	+
FL:D^d	+	–	–

3   Test of One-Receptor Hypothesis. (A) When the α and β T-cell receptor genes from a CTL specific for fluorescein (FL) restricted to H-2D^d (D^d) are transfected into another CTL specific for 3(p-sulphophenyldiazo)-4-hydroxyphenylacetic acid (SP) restricted to H-2K^k (K^k) and the cells are tested with all combinations of antigen and H-2, it is found (B) that transfectants have acquired the ability to react with FL only in the context of D^d. This finding argues that a single T-cell receptor is responsible for MHC restriction, that is, the specificity for antigen in the context of MHC. [After Dembic et al., 1986. *Nature* 320: 232]

These experiments show decisively that the two properties of the T-cell receptor, antigen recognition and MHC restriction, are carried out by the same molecule: the two-chained T-cell receptor.

SYNTHESIS
One T-Cell Receptor for MHC and Antigen

One of the great mysteries of the immune system was the way the T cell recognized antigen. It had no Ig on its surface, yet was clearly specific. It did not bind free antigen but was certainly antigen-reactive. The discovery that it reacts with antigen only in association with an MHC molecule was surprising, but gave the answer. We have seen so far that the T cell has a single receptor that reacts with specificity for a ligand of peptide in the MHC groove. Thus there is a single ligand composed of two parts (antigen and MHC). The question now becomes: Are there two *sites* on the receptor (one for antigen and one for the MHC molecule) or only one site that recognizes a determinant formed by the combination? Transfection experiments have not yet clearly discriminated between these possiblities, and we see that the alternatives as originally proposed by Zinkernagel and Doherty have not yet been completely resolved.

The Nature of the T-Cell Receptor

We saw above that a single T-cell receptor is responsible for MHC-restricted recognition of antigen. We will now address the nature of the receptor.

An Immunologic Approach to the Nature of the T-Cell Receptor

Anti-Idiotypic Antibody against the Receptor: The Classical Approach.   Just as every sailor knows that if it doesn't move you paint it, and every hunter knows that if it does move you shoot it, every immunologist knows that when in doubt, you make an antibody against it. The Middle Ages of the saga of the quest for the T-cell receptor began in the 1970s with experiments of Ramsier and Lindemann, who made antibodies against the T-cell receptor. These investigators used a unique variation on the usual theme of making antibody against everything—a clever plan. They reasoned that, because parental cells (P) are not recognized as foreign when injected into an F_1 but can themselves recognize the host as foreign (the basis of the GVH reaction), then the P cells must have *receptors* for the antigens of the other parental strain in the $(P_1 \times P_2)F_1$. The F_1, to be sure, does not recognize MHC antigens on the P_1 cells; but, they reasoned, there is no reason why it should not recognize the *receptors* as foreign. With a little luck, the F_1 should even produce antibody against the receptors, and this anti-receptor antibody might be a useful tool for studying the receptors.

When this experiment was carried out (Figure 4), the F_1 did produce antibody against the receptor molecules on the parental cells. This antibody, when radiolabeled, was found to bind to cells of the P_1 but not the P_2. More important, the antibody could specifically inhibit the reaction of P_1 against P_2, but it did not have an effect on any other reactions that the P_1 cells can carry out. These results are consistent with the idea that the antibody is directed against the receptor on the T cell for a specific antigen.

A variety of experiments then followed, some of great complexity, and all pointing to the conclusion that even though one could not demonstrate Ig on the surface of the T cell, the antibody against the receptor behaved like an ANTI-IDIOTYPE ANTIBODY—that is, like an antibody against an antigen-binding site. The next phase required two technical advances: the use of T-cell clones and of monoclonal antibodies.

Monoclonal Antibody against the Receptor: The Modern Approach. With the availability of antigen-specific T-cell clones and hybridomas, several groups independently set about to raise monoclonal antibodies to the receptor. The same basic experiment was carried out successfully with mouse and human T cells. The principle in each case was to immunize a host with the cloned T cells and select monoclonal antibodies directed against a determinant unique to the clone (Figure 5). This CLONOTYPIC DETERMINANT would be a strong candidate for the antigen-specific receptor. The cloned cell used as immunogen differed in each of the experiments, ranging from an antigen-specific, MHC-restricted helper cell to a tumor-specific cytotoxic cell to an alloreactive clone of cytotoxic cells. But in each case an antibody directed against the receptor was produced. Of course, other antibodies directed against other components of the cells used as immunogens were also obtained, and in each case very careful specificity controls had to be carried out to ensure that the antibody was indeed against the T-cell receptor—that is, that it was directed against the clonotypic determinant. The most crucial result of these experiments was the demonstration that addition of the anti-receptor antibody blocked antigen-specific recognition.

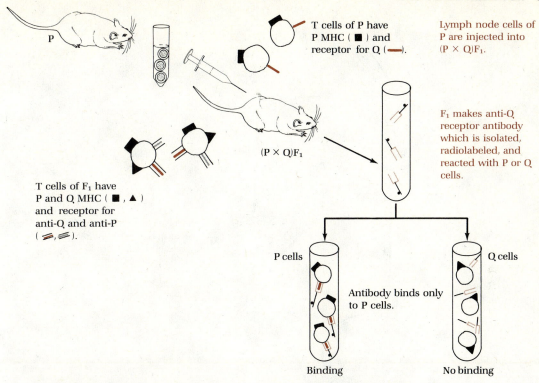

T cells of P have
P MHC (■) and
receptor for Q (━).

Lymph node cells of
P are injected into
(P × Q)F₁.

F_1 makes anti-Q
receptor antibody
which is isolated,
radiolabeled, and
reacted with P or Q
cells.

(P × Q)F₁

T cells of F_1 have
P and Q MHC (■ , ▲)
and receptor for
anti-Q and anti-P
(▰ , ▰).

P cells

Q cells

Antibody binds only
to P cells.

Binding

No binding

4   Generation of Anti–T-Cell Receptor Antibody: The Classical Approach. The principle of the experiment is that a (P × Q)F₁, which has P and Q MHC molecules, will not have T cells that respond to P or Q. Since T cells from strain P mice will respond to strain Q stimulator cells, these responding T cells must bear anti-Q receptors. T cells with anti-Q receptors (or anti-P receptors) are not found in the F₁, and therefore the F₁ immune system should recognize such receptors as novel molecules. By immunizing the F₁ with T cells from the P strain, antibodies against the anti-Q receptor were generated. [After Ramsier and Lindemann, 1972. *Transplant Rev.* 10: 57; and Binz and Wigzell, 1972. *J. Exp. Med.* 136: 872]

Once it was certain that the antibody was directed against the receptor on the cells, it was possible to use the antibody as a specific reagent to *isolate* the receptor molecule using the method of IMMUNOPRECIPITATION. To do this, all the surface membrane proteins are labeled with ^{125}I. The cells are then lysed and the radiolabeled lysate is incubated with the monoclonal anti-receptor antibody. In this manner the labeled receptor is bound to the antibody in an antigen–antibody complex. These complexes are then isolated by adsorbing them to Staph A (which binds antibody molecules) or anti-Ig and analyzed by sodium dodecyl sulfate

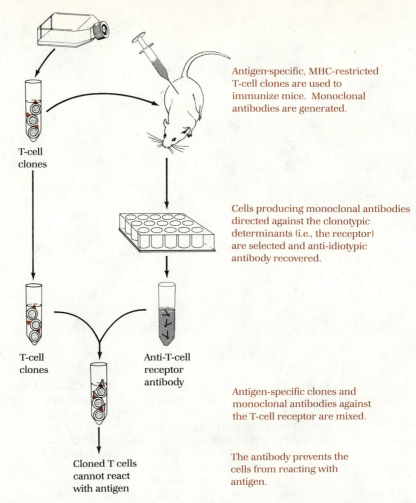

Antigen-specific, MHC-restricted T-cell clones are used to immunize mice. Monoclonal antibodies are generated.

Cells producing monoclonal antibodies directed against the clonotypic determinants (i.e., the receptor) are selected and anti-idiotypic antibody recovered.

T-cell clones

T-cell clones

Anti-T-cell receptor antibody

Antigen-specific clones and monoclonal antibodies against the T-cell receptor are mixed.

Cloned T cells cannot react with antigen

The antibody prevents the cells from reacting with antigen.

5 **Generation of Monoclonal Anti–T-Cell Receptor Antibody: The Modern Approach.** The figure shows the steps in producing monoclonal antibody to the receptors on antigen-specific, MHC-restricted clones of T cells. When the antibody is mixed with the cloned cells, they lose their ability to react with antigen, showing that the antibody has reacted with the receptor. Specificity controls are carried out to show that the antibody is specific for the antigen–MHC combination.

polyacrylamide gel electrophoresis (SDS-PAGE). Because the receptor is labelled, it can be visualized by autoradiography.

A typical result of such an experiment is shown in Figure 6. When the gel is run under *reducing* conditions in which interchain disulfide bonds are cleaved (lane 1), molecules of molecular weight

6 **Immunoprecipitation of T-Cell Receptor.** T-cell hybridomas were surface labeled with ^{125}I and the membranes separated by electrophoresis in SDS-PAGE gels. Lanes 1 and 2 were run under reducing conditions, and lanes 3 and 4 were run under nonreducing conditions. Lanes 1 and 3 are from the sepcific cells; lanes 2 and 4 are from cells of another specificity and serve as controls. Under nonreducing conditions a molecule of ~80,000 is precipitated by the anti-receptor antibody. [From Haskins et al., 1983. *J. Exp. Med.* 157: 1149; with permission]

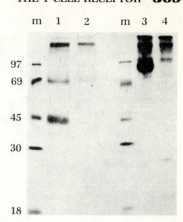

40,000 to 45,000 are seen. Under *nonreducing* conditions (disulfide bonds remain intact), there is a band at molecular weight around 80,000 (lane 3). In the figure, lanes 1 and 3 contain the membranes of the specific cells and lanes 2 and 4 are from a clone of another specificity.

Two-Chained T-Cell Receptor. The fact that the molecular weight of the unreduced molecule was about 80,000 whereas that of the reduced molecule was 40,000 suggests that the 40,000-dalton material really consists of subunits joined together in the intact molecule by disulfide bonds. These subunits were resolved by isoelectric focusing. As shown in Figure 7, there was clear evidence

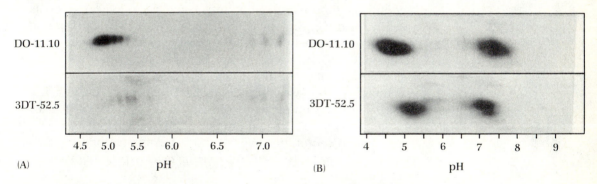

7 **Subunits of the T-Cell Receptor.** (A) Isoelectric focusing of surface-labeled proteins of two T-cell hybridomas after immunoprecipitation. (B) Nonequilibrium pH gradient electrophoresis of the same preparations. Under these conditions two molecules can be discerned. [From Kappler et al., 1983. *Cell* 34: 727]

of a molecule with a pI of about 5; but there was also a more basic molecule with a pI of about 7. This second band was further analyzed by a technique using nonequilibrium pH gradient electrophoresis in one dimension and SDS-PAGE in the second.

Together all these manipulations show that the antigen-specific T-cell receptor is a heterodimer of molecular weight 85,000 to 90,000, which consists of two polypeptide chains (each of molecular weight 40,000 to 43,000) linked by disulfide bonds. The two chains were named α and β.

The T-Cell Receptor Complex: TCR:CD3

We saw that when monoclonal antibodies against the T-cell receptor were used to immunoprecipitate the receptor from membrane preparations, the α and β chains were found. In these experiments, nonionic detergents were used to solubilize the membranes. When other detergents (digitonin or Triton X-100) were used, several other proteins were found in addition to the α and β chains (Figure 8). These proteins were called γ, δ, ϵ and ζ, and were collectively termed T3. It later was changed to CD3 when the surface molecules were grouped according to clusters of differentiation (see Chapter 13). The fact that these molecules coprecipitate with the T-cell receptor indicates that they are intimately associated in the membrane. More recently an additional chain called η (eta) has been added to the collection.

There is other evidence to indicate that the proteins of CD3 form a complex with the T-cell receptor. For example, if the T-cell receptor is modulated with anti–T-cell receptor antibody (see patching and capping (page 350), the CD3 molecules are *comodulated*, indicating that they are very closely associated. Furthermore, CD3 and the T-cell receptor can be cross-linked by bifunctional reagents. Also, if a cell line is mutagenized so that it loses its T-cell receptor, it ceases to express CD3, and conversely, if it expresses T-cell receptor genes but not those of CD3, no T-cell receptor appears on the cell surface. Thus a cell that is $CD3^+$ is also T-cell receptor–positive (TCR^+). The appearance of CD3 is therefore a very convenient marker for cells expressing the T-cell receptor.

The current model of how the chains of CD3 are associated with the T-cell receptor is seen in Figure 9.

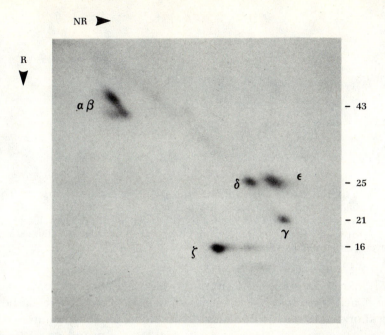

8 Two-Dimensional SDS-PAGE Analysis of the T-Cell Receptor Complex. The T cells were surface-labeled with radioiodine and solubilized membrane proteins were immunoprecipitated with a monoclonal antibody against the T-cell receptor. The precipitate was then run in the first dimension, a nonreducing gel of 10% polyacrylamide. After electrophoresis, the gel was equilibrated with reducing agents, and electrophoresis in a 12.5% polyacrylamide gel was performed. This analysis resolves the components on the basis of their molecular weight. Note the antigen receptors (α and β) and the associated peptides of the CD3 complex, $\gamma,\delta,\epsilon,\zeta$. NR, nonreducing; R, reducing. [From Samelson et al., 1985. *Cell* 43: 223. With permission. Photo courtesy of L. Samelson]

T-Cell Interactions with the Antigen–MHC Complex

In Chapter 20 we saw that processed antigenic peptides become associated with the MHC and that this complex is the ligand for the T-cell receptor. The discovery that the peptide probably sits in the groove at the top of the MHC molecule has been a dramatic confirmation of the idea. We still do not know how the ligand interacts and is "seen" by the T-cell receptor, but sequence homology to the antigen-binding sites of Ig has led to a proposed structure for the ligand-binding site of the T-cell receptor.

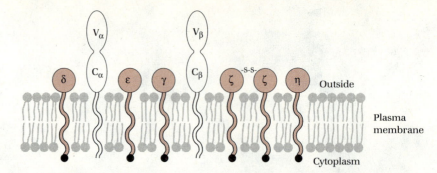

9   Schematic Representation of the T-Cell Receptor Complex. The seven chains of the complex are shown. The T-cell receptor α and β chains are shown in white. The CD3 chains, δ,ε,γ,ζ, and η are shown in color. [After Samelson et al., 1985. *Cell* 43: 223; and Terhorst et al., 1989. In Hames and Glover, eds., *Molecular Immunology*]

Plate 22-1A shows the proposed Ig-like ligand-binding site of the T-cell receptor. In this view, seen from above, the α-carbon backbone of the areas homologous to the V_H and V_L in Ig are seen in red. The van der Waals surfaces of the three proposed CDRs of each domain are seen in blue (CDR1), pink (CDR2), and yellow (CDR3). Plate 20-1 shows the now-famous groove at the top of the MHC molecule with the hypothetical peptide. Plate 22-1B is a model of the interaction between the T-cell receptor and the peptide–MHC complex. The T-cell receptor is on top and the MHC molecule is below. In this alignment it can be proposed that the CDRs of the receptor can bind in different registers along the MHC α helices, depending on the nature of the peptide in the groove. While we must remind the reader that the model is speculative, it does provide a reasonable view of how the two chains of the T-cell receptor combine to form an MHC- and antigen-specific receptor.

Summary

1.   The recognition of MHC–antigen complex by T cells is via a single T-cell receptor.
2.   The receptor is composed of two chains, α and β, that dictate both the antigen and MHC specificity of the receptor.
3.   Immunoprecipitation studies using anti-clonotypic antibodies (i.e., antibodies against the T-cell receptor) reveal a disulfide-linked heterodimer with chains of 40 to 45 kd.

4.   The T-cell receptor is associated with a set of nonpolymorphic molecules collectively called CD3. There is coordinate expression of CD3 and the T-cell receptor.

Additional Reading

Allison, J. P., B. W. McIntyre and D. Bloch. 1982. Tumor-specific antigen of murine T lymphoma defined with monoclonal antibody. *J. Immunol.* 129: 2293.

Davis, M. M. and P. J. Bjorkman. 1988. T-cell antigen receptor genes and T-cell recognition. *Nature* 334: 395.

Dembic, Z., W. Haas, S. Weiss, J. McCubrey, H. Kiefer, H. von Boehmer and M. Steinmetz. 1986. Transfer of specificity by murine α and β T-cell receptor genes. *Nature* 320: 232.

Haskins, K., R. Kubo, J. White, M. Pigeon, J. Kappler and P. Marrack. 1983. The major histocompatibility complex-restricted antigen receptor on T cells. I. Isolation with a monoclonal antibody. *J. Exp. Med.* 157: 1149.

Meure, S. C., K. A. Fitzgerald, R. E. Hussey, J. C. Hodgdon, S. F. Schlossman and E. L. Reinherz. 1983. Clonotypic structures involved in antigen specific human T cell function: Relationship to the Tc molecular complex. *J. Exp. Med.* 157: 705.

Saito, T., A. Weiss, J. Miller, M. A. Norcross and R. N. Germain. 1987. Specific antigen-Ia activation of transfected human T cells expressing Ti αβ-human T3 receptor complexes. *Nature* 325: 125.

Samelson, L. E., H. B. Harford, and R. D. Klausner. 1985. Identification of the components of the murine T cell antigen receptor complex. *Cell* 43: 223.

Terhorst, C., B. Alarcon, J. de Vries, and H. Spits. 1989. T lymphocyte recognition and activation. In Hames, B. D., and D. M. Glover, eds. *Molecular Immunology*. IRL, Oxford, p. 145.

ORGANIZATION OF THE T-CELL RECEPTOR GENES

CHAPTER

23

Overview   In the last chapter we followed the evidence pointing to the fact that the antigen-specific, MHC-restricted receptor on T cells is a two-chain molecule that is expressed in association with CD3 on the surface of T cells. In this chapter we will examine the genetic organization of the molecules that make up the T-cell receptor. Just as the use of cloned lines of functional T cells and monoclonal antibodies made the isolation of the receptor protein possible, so also were they crucial for the cloning of the T-cell receptor gene. This was an event that was awaited with great anticipation by immunologists and one that has lived up to the expectations. We will see that many of the same mechanisms used for generating diversity in the Ig genes are used in the T-cell receptor genes. We will also see that in addition to genes for the α and β chains discussed in the last chapter, two other genes that encode another T-cell receptor have been discovered. The function of this γ δ T-cell receptor is not well understood.

Cloning of the T-Cell Receptor Genes

We have been emphasizing that the question of how the T-cell receptor works is complicated, because we must explain not only how diversity is generated in the 90-kd heterodimer but also how antigen is recognized by T cells in an MHC-restricted manner.[1] The cloning of the genes that encode the two chains was crucial toward our start on understanding this fundamental question.

---

[1] If by chance the reader has entered the narrative at this point for a quick fix on the T-cell receptor, be advised that there are no free lunches. To really understand the organization of the T-cell receptor genes and what that organization means to the function of the T cell, you must go back and read (at least) the previous chapter.

Isolation of cDNA Clones: The Subtraction Method

Complementary DNA clones for the T-cell receptor were isolated simultaneously and independently by Stephen Hedrick, Mark Davis, and their co-workers at NIH who worked with a murine system, and by Tak Mak and his co-workers in Toronto who worked with human cells. The strategies differed slightly, but we will describe only the "subtractive method" of Hedrick and Davis in detail. The basis of the approach was to isolate the genes that encode the T-cell receptor from antigen-specific, MHC-restricted T-cell hybridomas. In the original work a T helper clone was used, but since that time cytotoxic T clones have also been used.

Several assumptions were made at the outset of the work. *First*, it was assumed that the genes being sought must be expressed in T cells but not in B cells. This means that the mRNA encoding the T-cell receptor will not be found in B cells. *Second*, the mRNA for the protein should be found on membrane-bound polysomes and attached to the endoplasmic reticulum by a signal sequence. This notion derives from the extensive work of Gunther Blobel and his colleagues, who have proposed the *signal hypothesis* to account for the means by which proteins are transported into and across membranes. Because the T-cell receptor is a membrane-associated protein, it was assumed that it would follow this pattern of behavior. *Third*, the T-cell receptor genes will be rearranged. This assumes that there will be a similarity between the structures used for recognition of antigen by B cells and T cells. If the T-cell receptor is formed by rearranged genes, then the diversity of the receptor should be generated in a manner similar to the generation of diversity in Ig—that is, there should be variable, constant, and joining regions.

Having made these assumptions, the researchers then used the strategy in Figure 1 to clone the T-cell receptor. The basis of the cloning strategy was basically this: starting from an antigen-specific, MHC-restricted T cell (in this case a helper cell), isolate RNA and rid it of all RNA that is shared with B cells. This same source of RNA then can serve as both the source of the cDNA LIBRARY of genes that will contain the T-cell receptor and the labeled cDNA to probe the library.

The library is produced by extracting poly (A)$^+$ cytoplasmic RNA and, with reverse transcriptase, making a cDNA from it. This

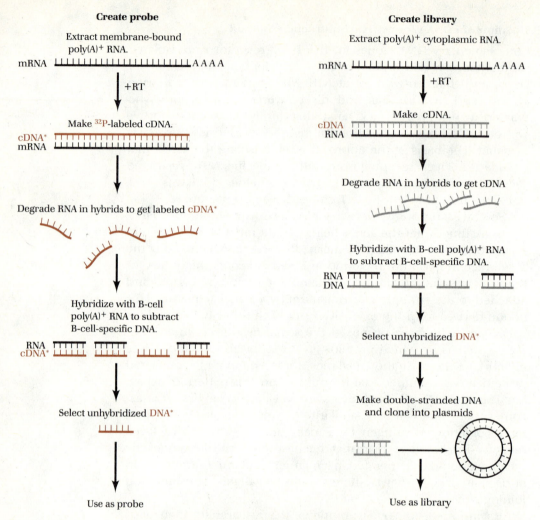

Create probe

Extract membrane-bound poly(A)+ RNA.

mRNA └┴┴┴┴┴┴┴┴┴┴┴┴┴┴┴┴┴┴┴┴┴┘AAAA

+RT

Make ^{32}P-labeled cDNA.

cDNA*
mRNA

Degrade RNA in hybrids to get labeled cDNA*

Hybridize with B-cell poly(A)+ RNA to subtract B-cell-specific DNA.

RNA
cDNA*

Select unhybridized DNA*

Use as probe

Create library

Extract poly(A)+ cytoplasmic RNA.

mRNA └┴┴┴┴┴┴┴┴┴┴┴┴┴┴┴┴┴┴┴┴┴┘AAAA

+RT

Make cDNA.

cDNA
RNA

Degrade RNA in hybrids to get cDNA

Hybridize with B-cell poly(A)+ RNA to subtract B-cell-specific DNA.

RNA
DNA

Select unhybridized DNA*

Make double-stranded DNA and clone into plasmids

Use as library

1   The Subtractive Method of Cloning the T-Cell Receptor. RNA from a cloned antigen-specific, MHC-restricted helper T-cell line is used to create a library of T cell-specific genes, and the labeled probe is used to identify the T-cell receptor gene. By hybridizing the T-cell DNA with B-cell RNA, one can "subtract" all B-cell specificities from the probe and the library. [After Hedrick et al., 1984. *Nature* 308: 149]

cDNA is then reacted with RNA from B cells so that any B-cell cDNA will be bound (hybridized) to the RNA. This leaves T cell-specific cDNA as single-stranded molecules that are isolated and converted to double stranded DNA with DNA polymerase I. This DNA is then cloned into plasmids to become the cDNA library that will be probed.

The PROBE is made by a similar strategy, but, of course, these molecules must have a label so that the reaction with the DNA in the library can be detected. This limb of the reaction starts with membrane-bound poly(A)$^+$ mRNA. A cDNA that is labeled with ^{32}P is made using reverse transcriptase. This labeled cDNA (DNA$^{\cdot}$) is then hybridized with poly(A)$^+$ RNA from B cells. By discarding all the DNA–RNA hybrids, one can "subtract" the DNA shared with B cells. Now the remaining DNA$^{\cdot}$ can be used as a probe for the T cell-specific library created above.

The problem now becomes to identify those genes that are for the T-cell receptor from among the other T cell-specific genes in the library. The only way to identify them was based on assumption 3, that is, to look for *rearranged* T cell-specific genes. When this was done it was found that a few of the clones that they had selected were in fact rearranged. This is seen in Figure 2. Because all the B cell-specific genes had been "subtracted," it followed that these were clones encoding the T-cell receptor and not rearranged antibody genes. The final proof of this came when the amino acid sequence of the isolated T-cell receptor was compared with the

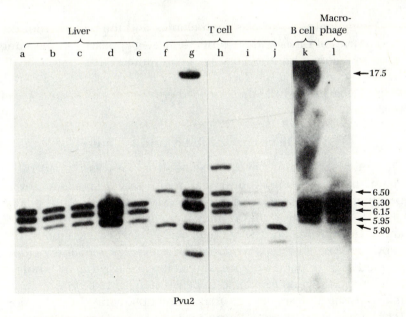

2   Gene Rearrangement in the T-Cell Receptor. Genomic DNA was prepared from T-cell lines, B cells, macrophages, and liver cells. After digestion with the restriction enzyme *Pvu*II, Southern blot analysis was carried out using probes prepared by the method diagrammed in Figure 1. [From Davis et al., 1984. *Immunol. Rev.* 81: 235; with permission]

predicted amino acid sequence from the nucleotide sequences of the T cell-specific cDNA clones. They found that they had indeed cloned the β chain of the T-cell receptor.

V, D, J, and C Regions in the β Chain

It was also assumed that the T-cell receptor genes would have V, D, and J regions similar to those in the Ig genes. Having already shown that the gene for the β chain is rearranged, Davis and his co-workers screened a thymocyte cDNA library, looking for evidence of these regions. When DNA from thymus-derived clones was sequenced and the data bank of known protein sequences searched for similar sequences, it was found there were similarities in V, D, J, and C regions of Ig and T-cell receptor genes. Subsequent work has fully confirmed the similarities between Ig and T-cell receptor gene organization.

After the β chain was cloned in 1984, another chain that seemed to meet the criteria for the α chain was cloned. However, it was known that α chains are glycosylated, and from the deduced protein sequence for the new chain it was found that there are no glycosylation sites. This meant that the gene could not be encoding the α chain.

The actual α chain was soon cloned, and the papers from the laboratories of Davis and Susumu Tonegawa appeared in the same issue of *Nature*. Immunology was confronted with a strange dilemma: after seeking the T-cell receptor as if it were the Holy Grail, immunologists found that now there were too many T-cell receptors!

The Discovery of the γ and δ Chains

The "mystery" chain that we discussed above was named the γ chain. In 1986 it was found that there was a small subset of peripheral T cells that did not express either the α or the β chains of the T-cell receptor, that is, they were $(\alpha\beta)^-$, but expressed CD3 and a heterodimer of the γ chain with a second heretofore unknown chain. This second chain did not react with monoclonal antibodies to α, β, or γ chains, and so it was clear that yet another T-cell receptor gene remained to be isolated. In 1987, while studying unusual rearrangements that occur upstream of the J_α gene, Davis and his co-workers found novel C, J, and D gene segments. Protein sequencing showed that this was the δ gene.[2]

---

[2] The story of the discovery of the γδ genes, which reads very much like a detective story, is admirably told in a model of review writing by David Raulet (Raulet, 1989. *Annu. Rev. Immunol.* 7: 175).

T-Cell Receptor Genes and Proteins

Figure 3 shows the genetic organization of the T-cell receptor genes and the principal structural features of the proteins that they encode. A very striking feature of the organization of the δ gene is that it occurs in the middle of the α-gene region (between the V_α and the J_α segments). The α and γ chains are composed of V, J, and C regions (no D) while the β and δ chains are composed of V, D, J, and C regions. These form αβ and γδ heterodimers that, very much like Igs, have two disulfide-linked chains composed of VDJC and one of VJC.

Chromosome Locations of T-Cell Receptor Genes

The chromosome locations of the *human* α and β genes have been determined by in situ hybridization. The α gene is found on chromosome 14 in a position proximal to the H-chain gene of Ig. The gene is found on a region of the chromosome (14q11-q12) known to be involved in translocations and inversions in human T-cell leukemias and lymphomas. It has been suggested that the locus for the α chain may participate in oncogene activation of T-cell tumors, but, of course, we do not know if this is really the case. Since the δ gene is located within the α gene, it has the same chromosomal location.

The human β-chain gene has been localized to the long arm of chromosome 7 at band q35. The terminal segment of 7q (as well as 7p and 14q) is a "hot spot" for chromosome rearrangements. The human γ gene is located on chromosome 7 at band p15.

The *mouse* T-cell receptor α-chain and δ-chain genes are located on chromosome 14, and the β gene is located on chromosome 6. The γ-chain gene is on chromosome 13.

Generation of Diversity in T-Cell Receptor Genes

It should not have escaped the reader's notice that the organization of the T-cell receptor genes and the proteins they encode has great similarity to that of the Igs. The αβ and γδ heterodimers each have one molecule that is encoded from VDJ and one from VJ regions (both have C regions). Thus it should come as no surprise that the diversity of the T-cell receptor is achieved in almost the same manner as is the diversity of Igs, that is, recombinatorial diversity and combinatorial associations. The great exceptions are that there is no junctional site diversity or somatic mutation. The genetic elements that we saw in Igs that allow recombinatorial

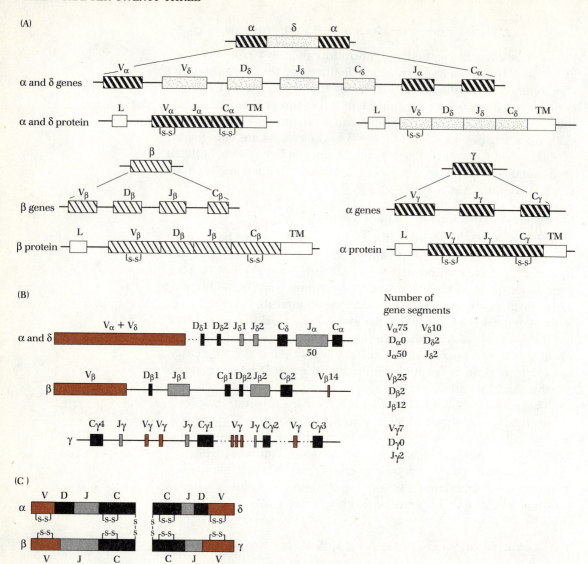

3 **Organization of T-Cell Receptor Genes and Proteins.** (A) Simplified and stylized view showing the location of the major elements and the proteins that they encode. Note that the δ genes and α genes are interspersed. (B) A more detailed view of the genes showing their relative positions (not to true scale). The numbers of gene segments are listed. [Data from Davis, 1989. In Hanes and Glover, eds., *Molecular Immunology*] (C) The organization of the T-cell receptor heterodimers showing that αβ and γδ associate. Note that the organization resembles Ig H- and L-chain organization with one VDJC and one VJC chain in each disulfide-linked unit.

diversity, the RSS's (heptamer–nonamer and 12/23 base pairs) are present in the T-cell receptor genes.

Recombinatorial diversity is achieved by the joining of VDJ and VJ segments. The pool of gene segments available for these rearrangements is seen in Table 1. From these numbers, it is clear that the $\alpha\beta$ dimer combinations are of the same order of magnitude as those in Ig genes. The $\gamma\delta$ numbers are lower, but it has been argued that there may be as much, if not greater, potential diversity in these genes as in the others. For example, the rearrangement of the δ genes can occur with two D segments. There appears to be some overlap in the V-gene usage between α and δ. This is not unexpected, since the D_δ, J_δ, and C_δ segments lie between V_α and J_α. The mechanism that allows preferential usage of V_α or V_δ by the respective D regions is not known. There is, however, no class switching in T cells, so a cell that is using δ does not then use α.

Another significant difference in the generation of diversity between the Igs and T-cell receptors is in somatic mutation. It will be recalled that during the immune response there are areas of the Ig gene that undergo a high rate of mutation. The T-cell receptor does not undergo this hypermutation. We saw in Chapter 5 that the recombinases that mediate Ig gene segment rearrangement in B cells are being elucidated (RAG-1 and RAG-2). We saw then that these same recombinases occur in T cells, so their discovery holds the promise of our having a clear understanding of this remarkable process in both cell lineages.[3]

Functions of the $\gamma\delta$ Genes

The $\gamma\delta$ genes of the T-cell receptor are one of the most intensively studied topics in immunology today, but we still do not have a clear idea about their functions or their relationship to the $\alpha\beta$ receptors. It is clear, however, that the $\gamma\delta$ cells do not routinely carry out the functions that we have ascribed to T cells up to now.

Developmental Expression

Because T cells differentiate in the thymus, it is logical to assume that the gene rearrangements will occur in this organ. The first

---

[3] The authors want the readers to know that they disagree on how much difference we should predict will be found between the B-cell and T-cell systems. ESG thinks that the enzymes will be only similar, DRG thinks they will be the same. A pair of box seat tickets to a Cubs–Padres game or rinkside seats to an Oilers–Kings game is on the line.

Table 1 **Diversity by recombination of gene segments of the T-cell receptor.**

	V	D	J
α	75	0	50
β	25	2	12
γ	7	0	2
δ	10	2	2

Combinations: α–β $3750 \times 600 = 2.2 \times 10^6$
γ–δ $14 \times 40 = 5.6 \times 10^2$

Source: After Davis, 1989. In B. D. Hames and D. M. Glover, eds. *Molecular Immunology.*

lymphoid migration into the fetal thymus occurs on day 11 or 12 in the mouse. Thy-1 is expressed by days 13 to 14, and immunocompetent cells can be found by days 18 to 19. The first rearranged T-cell receptor gene to be found in the fetal mouse thymus is the γ gene by day 13. In fact, this gene can be found in the rearranged form in the fetal liver, the source of the pre-T cells in the embryo. The δ gene also rearranges before the α or β undergo their rearrangements. Neither α nor β genes are rearranged in fetal liver or the 14-day thymus. The β gene is rearranged in the thymus by day 15, and the α gene by day 16 or 17. Therefore, while αβ gene rearrangement is dependent on thymic maturation, it seems that some γδ rearrangement is not. In fact thymus-deficient mice have large numbers of γδ-bearing T cells.

Cellular Distribution

In humans, between 0.5 and 10% of the peripheral T cells are double-negative (CD4⁻CD8⁻) γδ T cells. In the mouse, these cells make up about 3% of the peripheral T cells but are the predominant type of T cell found in the epidermis, the dendritic epidermal cells (DEC). In addition, the γδ T cell is prominent in the epithelium of the gut of both mice and humans. This prevalence in epithelial tissues has led Charles Janeway to propose that a primary function of these cells may be as a first line of defense against pathogens that penetrate the epithelium.

While the role of these cells and their relative importance is not known, what has emerged is that there is selective use of V, J, and D segments in different tissues. For example, the epidermal γδ T cells use a receptor composed of V$_\gamma$3-J$_\gamma$1 and V$_\delta$1-D$_\delta$-J$_\delta$2. In contrast, the cells in the intestinal epithelium commonly express a V$_\gamma$5-J$_\gamma$1. It is not known if this reflects different functions at different anatomical sites.

Summary

1.   The genes for four T-cell receptor chains have been identified. Two sets are for the α and β chains that encode the receptors found on functional T cells. An additional set of genes that encode the γ and δ chains are expressed on a small subset of T cells of unknown function.
2.   The T-cell receptor genes for the α and β chains were isolated by the "subtractive" method.
3.   The genes for the T-cell receptor exhibit gene segment rearrangements similar to those seen in Ig genes to generate diversity. The α and δ genes have V, D, and J segments, and the β and γ genes have V and J segments. The rearranged V regions are associated with C regions.
4.   The γ and δ genes are the first T-cell receptor genes to become rearranged during development. This is followed by the rearrangement of the β and then the α genes. These define two distinct T-cell lineages.

Additional Readings

Chien, Y., N. Gascoigne, J. Kavaler, N. Lee and M. Davis. 1984. Somatic recombination in a murine T-cell receptor gene. *Nature* 309: 322.

Chieu, Y.-H., D. M. Becker, T. Lindsten, M. Okamura, D. J. Cohen and M. Davis. 1984. Third type of murine T-cell receptor gene. *Nature* 312: 31.

Davis, M. M. 1989. T cell antigen receptor genes. In Hames, B. D., and D. M. Glover, eds. *Molecular Immunology*. IRL, Oxford, p. 61.

Hayday, A. C., H. Saito, S. D. Gillies, D. M. Kranz, G. Tanigawa, H. N. Eisen and S. Tonegawa. 1985. Structure, organization and somatic rearrangements of T cell γ genes. *Cell* 40: 259.

Hedrick, S., D. Cohen, E. Nielsen, and M. Davis. 1984. Isolation of cDNA clones encoding T cell–specific membrane-associated proteins. *Nature* 308: 149.

Raulet, D. H. 1989. The structure, function and molecular genetics of the γδ T-cell receptor. *Annu. Rev. Immunol.* 7: 175.

Toyonaga, B. and T. W. Mak. 1987. Genes of the T-cell antigen receptor in normal and malignant T cells. *Annu. Rev. Immunol.* 5: 585.

Yanagi, Y., Y. Yoshika, K. Leggett, S. Clark, I. Aleksander and T. Mak. 1984. A human T cell-specific cDNA clone encodes a protein having extensive homology to immunoglobulin chains. *Nature* 308: 145.

SELECTION AND ACTIVATION OF LYMPHOCYTES

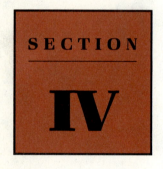

SECTION

IV

Marco Polo describes a bridge, stone by stone.

"But which is the stone that supports the bridge?" Kublai Khan asks.

"The bridge is not supported by one stone or another," Marco Polo answers, "but by the line of the arch they form."

Kublai Khan remains silent, reflecting. Then he adds, "Why do you speak of stones? It is only the arch that matters to me."

Polo answers: "Without stones there is no arch."

Italo Calvino, *Invisible Cities*

In these five chapters we will begin to get down to mechanisms: how some of the elements actually *work* (or at least how we *think* they might work). The first two chapters refer exclusively to the development of T lymphocytes, but, more importantly, to the selection of developing T cells on the basis of the specificity of their T-cell receptors. In the following two chapters, we will begin to unravel the complexities of lymphocyte activation and the molecules responsible for intercellular communication. Finally, we will examine the basis for cell-mediated cytotoxicity, one of the important effector mechanisms of the immune system. In a sense, these chapters deal with issues that are as much a part of developmental and cell biology as they are of immunology, and because they cross these established borders, they are among the "hottest" areas currently being studied. Unfortunately, this means that the information in these areas is rapidly changing, and, therefore, some of the ideas we will promote will also have to change.

DEVELOPMENT AND SELECTION OF THE T-CELL RECEPTOR REPERTOIRE I
Negative Selection

Overview   We have seen that most immune responses, regardless of the effector mechanisms used, depend upon the activation of helper T cells. Further, the activation of these cells is complicated by the requirement for antigen processing by an APC and presentation of antigenic peptides in the groove of a class II MHC molecule. Why does the system operate in this complex way? Since the discovery of MHC restriction, we've had a notion that this arrangement might contribute to self–nonself discrimination in some way.

This question gets right to the soul of the immune system. To begin to address it, immunologists have focused on T-cell development, and some of the answers have been found in the interactions of developing T cells and the other resident cells of the thymus. For the first time we think that we are getting a glimmer of how the immune system performs the trick of distinguishing self from nonself, and part of the key is in the workings of the thymus.

The Thymus Is a Site of Selection of the T-Cell Receptor Repertoire

In this chapter and the next we will be developing the evidence for the idea that the fate of a developing T cell (maturation or death) depends on the interaction of the molecules on the surface of the cell with the molecules of the thymic environment. To begin, we will consider the maturation of T cells in the thymus and some of the changes they undergo. As T lymphocytes develop from bone marrow stem cells, they migrate to the thymus, where they rearrange the genes for the T-cell receptor α and β chains (see Chapter 22). These randomly generated receptors are then expressed on the surface of the developing thymocytes. At this point, a remarkable event occurs: cells die if they bear receptors that recognize

385

and react to "self" (self-MHC and ubiquitous molecules). This culling of self-reactive cells is termed NEGATIVE SELECTION. One outcome of this event, acting through most of the life of the individual, is the development of a T-cell receptor repertoire (represented by the population of mature of T cells) that lacks reactivity to self but is capable of responding to nonself. This chapter will focus on this negative selection event, while another selection event (positive selection) is the subject of the next.

Changes in Surface Markers during T-Cell Development

As discussed in Chapter 13, T cells develop from a stem cell arising in the bone marrow and migrating to the thymus. In the thymus, these thymocytes proliferate and differentiate in several stages before becoming mature T cells. Using the strategies outlined in Figure 1, Roland Scollay, Irving Weissman, and others have identified several of these stages in T-cell development in the thymus. Developing T cells in the thymus were sorted into populations on the basis of staining with different antibodies directed to cell-surface molecules on the cells (this involves the use of a fluorescence-activated cell sorter (FACS; see Chapter 11). The separated populations were then injected into the thymuses of irradiated mice. Because of the irradiation, the thymuses were devoid of resident developing T cells. At various times, the thymuses were removed and the cells were reanalyzed for their expression of surface markers. In this way, it was possible to determine which developmental stages (defined by surface markers) give rise to later stages. While many cell-surface molecules have been studied, we will concentrate on CD4, CD8, and the T-cell receptor.

Figure 2 gives a likely scheme of T-cell development arrived at from these experiments. It is important to remember that this process begins with the embryonic development of the thymus and continues at least into adolescence (and maybe through adulthood, albeit to a lesser degree).

Many T Cells Die during Development in the Thymus

Cells that leave the thymus represent only a very small percentage of those going in. The cells of the thymus have one of the highest proliferation rates of any organ in the body, but the number of cells that mature and leave the thymus is relatively small. Somehow, a large number of developing T cells are lost during maturation. Neils Jerne noticed this fact and suggested in 1971 that a selection process was occurring.

We now know that some of this loss occurs during T-cell

receptor rearrangement; if the rearrangement is defective, it is likely that the cell will die. The cells that successfully rearrange and express T-cell receptor genes are then subjected to the selection processes that we will discuss. The selection events depend on the cell-surface expression of a functional T-cell receptor and probably occur at the stage in which the cells bear both CD4 and CD8 molecules (see Figure 2). These CD4$^+$CD8$^+$ thymocytes are called, for convenience, DOUBLE-POSITIVE thymocytes. Double-positive thymocytes represent the majority of lymphoid cells in the thymus, and both the CD4$^+$CD8$^-$ T cells and the CD4$^-$CD8$^+$ T cells (so-called SINGLE-POSITIVE thymocytes) derive from them.

We begin our discussion of thymocyte selection with a consideration of negative selection. Presently, we do not know whether

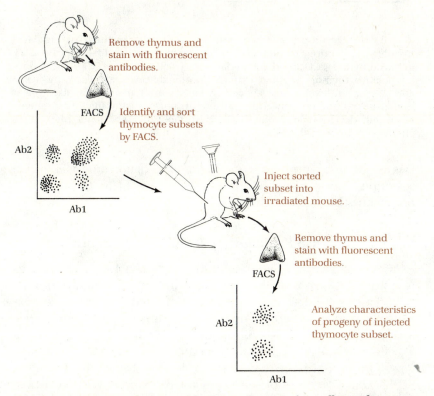

Remove thymus and stain with fluorescent antibodies.

FACS

Identify and sort thymocyte subsets by FACS.

Ab2

Ab1

Inject sorted subset into irradiated mouse.

Remove thymus and stain with fluorescent antibodies.

FACS

Ab2

Analyze characteristics of progeny of injected thymocyte subset.

Ab1

1   An Approach to Determining the Pathways of T-Cell Development. Thymocytes are separated on the basis of cell-surface markers and then injected into lethally irradiated animals. The injected population continues its maturation, and the cell-surface phenotypes of its progeny are then assessed. By studying a number of different thymocyte subpopulations, one can determine a pathway of development.

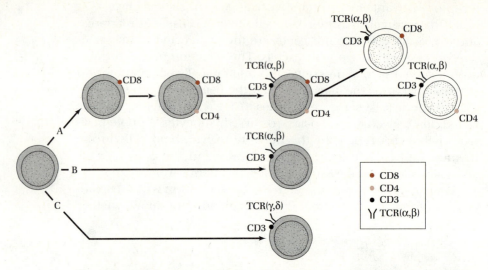

2 **T Cells Develop via Three Different Pathways in the Thymus.** Most thymocytes mature via pathway A, in which the cells first express CD8, followed by CD4, CD3, and cell-surface αβ T-cell receptor (TCR). These double-positive thymocytes then mature into single-positive cells. Pathways B and C exist but involve very few cells. T cells bearing the γδ TCR also appear to mature extra-thymically. This figure represents a highly simplified scheme of T-cell development—many other surface markers (and phenotypic changes) have been described.

this selection occurs before or after (or at the same time as) positive selection, and in discussing it first we do not mean to imply that one occurs before the other.

Negative Selection in T-Cell Development

As a general rule, T cells that could react against our own tissues (self-antigens) are functionally absent in normal, healthy individuals. This "self-tolerance" is the topic of later chapters. One possible mechanism whereby this could occur is for such self-reactive T cells simply not to exist normally. That is, a T cell (or a clone of T cells) that bears a particular receptor that reacts with self-antigens plus self-MHC may be lost, or deleted during development. Such CLONAL DELETION of self-reactive lymphocytes had been postulated by Sir Macfarlane Burnett in the 1950s, but a convincing demonstration of this process required technical advances that only became available in the 1980s. One such advance was the development of techniques for the generation of TRANSGENIC MICE: animals that have been genetically engineered to express certain defined genes. Another advance was the generation of monoclonal antibodies that detect potentially self-reactive T-cell receptors. We will separately consider the studies that utilize these techniques, beginning with the transgenic mouse experiments.

Studies with T-Cell Receptor–Transgenic Mice

One approach to studying the selection of the T-cell receptor repertoire is to engineer a system in which all (or most) of the T cells that develop in an animal express the same T-cell receptor. The impact of the thymic environment on how the T cells mature can then be addressed by doing the experiment in different strains of mice.

Michael Steinmetz and his colleagues constructed transgenic mice using T-cell receptor α- and β-chain genes from a cytotoxic T-cell clone. This CD8$^+$ T-cell clone had the capability of recognizing H-2D^b plus an antigen called H-Y, which is expressed in male, but not female, mice.

The scheme for the construction of the transgenic mice is shown in Figure 3. The T-cell receptor α- and β-chain genes were cloned into vectors designed for in vivo expression. These were then mixed and injected into mouse embryos to produce transgenic mice for these genes. When these transgenic animals were successfully generated, they were mated with normal mice, and the TRANSGENES behaved like a Mendelian locus: that is, approximately 50% of the offspring carried the transgenic TCR. (In other cases, the two TCR transgenes behave as independent loci.) The offspring that carry both the α and the β T-cell receptor transgenes and express them in their T cells are referred to as DOUBLE TRANSGENICS. Remember that most of the T cells of these animals now had the same T-cell receptor, specific for H-Y plus H-2D^b.

The next step was relatively simple: von Boehmer and his colleagues compared the maturation of thymocytes in male versus female H-2^b double-transgenic mice (remember that only the male expresses H-Y). The results were striking (see Figure 4). In female H-2^b mice, CD8 single-positive T cells developed normally. However, in male H-2^b animals, in which H-Y is a self-antigen, few thymocytes matured beyond the double-positive stage[1]. This experiment elegantly established that thymocytes that display T-cell receptors with anti-self activity are effectively deleted during

---

[1] Those thymocytes that did mature were found to be lacking in one or the other chain of the transgenic TCR (expressing an endogenous chain instead) or to be lacking in the CD8 molecule needed for cell activation. Thus, though these few cells were not removed, they were also not reactive to the self-antigen.

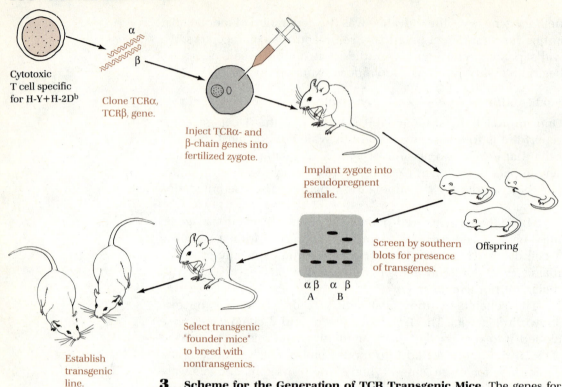

Cytotoxic
T cell specific
for H-Y+H-2D^b

Clone TCRα,
TCRβ, gene.

Inject TCRα- and
β-chain genes into
fertilized zygote.

Implant zygote into
pseudopregnant
female.

Screen by southern
blots for presence
of transgenes.

αβ   α β
A   B

Offspring

Select transgenic
"founder mice"
to breed with
nontransgenics.

Establish
transgenic
line.

3   Scheme for the Generation of TCR Transgenic Mice. The genes for
the TCR α and β chains were obtained from a CD8$^+$ T cell specific for H-2D^b
plus the male antigen H-Y. These were cloned into a vector for in vivo expression, and injected into 1-day-old embryos. The embryos were then implanted
into foster mothers, and the offspring were tested for presence of the transgenes. Male mice carrying both transgenes ("founders") were then mated to
normal females, and their offspring were again examined for the transgenes.
Continued matings produced lines of animals expressing the TCR transgenes
[for a review, see von Boehmer et al., 1989. *Immunol. Today.* 10: 57]. Transgenic
mice carrying other TCR genes have also been generated.

their maturation. Other studies using TCR transgenes that recognize other self-antigens have now been performed, and these studies generally confirm these conclusions.

These animals were also utilized for additional studies on the
role of MHC in thymocyte maturation. We will consider these
studies later in the next chapter, which discusses positive selection.

Thus, T cells bearing a defined receptor recognizing a self-
antigen (plus self-MHC) are eliminated from the developing T-cell
pool. This is negative selection. Of course, these transgenic mice
are not normal for the same reason that they are useful—most of
their T cells express engineered TCR transgenes. Independent

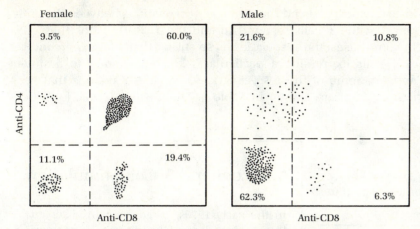

4 **Negative Selection of Double-Positive Thymocytes in TCR Transgenic Mice.** Mice were made transgenic for the TCR of a T cell specific for H-2D^b plus H-Y (male specific antigen). Thymocytes were stained with anti-CD4 and anti-CD8 and analyzed by FACS (see Chapter 11). The double-positive thymocytes present in transgenic female H-2^b mice (60%) are depleted in transgenic males (10.8%). [Adapted from Kisielow et al., 1988. *Nature* 333: 742]

demonstrations of negative selection in normal mice are discussed below.

Antibodies to T-Cell Receptor V Regions in the Study of Negative Selection

Another line of evidence for the existence of negative selection does not rely on the use of transgenic animals. Instead, it takes advantage of a type of antigen (often, a self-molecule in some animals) for which a large proportion of T cells bearing a particular T-cell receptor V region respond. As we'll see, antibodies to these V regions can trace the fate of such T cells during thymic development.

Some T-Cell Receptor V Regions Are Associated with Recognition of Potential "Self"-Antigens

In Chapter 22, we described how monoclonal antibodies to the unique T-cell receptor of a T-cell clone were originally used to identify the T-cell receptor proteins. Many of these anticlonotypic antibodies actually recognize only one specific V region (either α or β) and, as such, can be used to assess whether a particular T cell uses a particular TCR V region. In the process of screening large numbers of T-cell clones and hybrids in this way, several investigators observed that there are correlations between the antigen that the T cells respond to and the TCR V regions they use. In some cases, the association is so strong that a large percentage of T cells expressing a particular V region respond to a single antigen. Some of these SUPERANTIGENS and the V regions that recognize them are shown in Table 1. Thus, when T cells from one

Table 1   Some "superantigens" and their recognition by CD4$^+$ cells bearing specific TCR V$_\beta$.

Superantigen[a]	TCR V$_\beta$	Notes
Mls-1^a	6, 8.1	See Box 1
Mls-2^a	3	See Box 1
I-E	17	Probably I-E plus an uncharacterized self-antigen
Staphylococcus enterotoxin A	3, 11	
Staphylococcus enterotoxin B	3, 8	

[a]An antigen is a superantigen if the majority of T cells bearing a particular TCR V$_\beta$ will respond to it. Because of this, such antigens will induce significant T-cell proliferation in unprimed populations. Mice carry 11–12 different V$_\beta$ genes, and these are each given a number. Closely related genes fall into "families" and are denoted by a decimal (e.g., V$_{\beta 8.1}$). For the superantigens shown, the responding T cells are CD4$^+$CD8$^+$ single positive T cells, even if they bear the appropriate V$_\beta$, do not respond to these antigens in this manner.

Mls Loci and T-Cell Stimulation

In the early 1970s, H. Festenstein observed that murine mixed lymphocyte responses (see Chapter 11) could be generated in some strain combinations, even when the MHC of the responder and the stimulator were matched. This effect was attributed to genetic differences at a locus distinct from MHC that is called MLS ("Minor lymphocyte stimulatory"). It is now known that there are at least two Mls loci (Mls-1 and Mls-2) that are allelic in that they express the stimulation capacity (*a* allele) or they don't (*b* allele). This accounts for the first property of Mls responses: they are unidirectional. For example, cells from an animal that bears Mls-1^a (such as DBA/2) stimulate proliferation in T cells from an Mls-1^b animal (such as BALB/c), but not vice versa.

The realization that there are two different Mls loci (rather than one, as originally proposed) required that the nomenclature be redone, which, as usual, introduces a degree of confusion into the literature. In the table below, the old and new nomenclatures (proposed by Charles Janeway) are listed, as well as some typical strains. In this book, we use only the new nomenclature.

The products of the Mls genes are not known, nor is it known why they so potently stimulate T-cell responses. The frequency of cells that respond to Mls is very high, 3 to 5 mouse strain recognize foreign antigens presented on cells from another mouse strain, the cells that respond may use a limited number of V-region genes in constructing their T-cell receptors. For example, T cells that are capable of recognizing an unusual antigen called Mls-1^a (see Box 1) predominantly express either V$_{\beta 8.1}$ or V$_{\beta 6}$. If a T cell is simply selected by the criterion that it express

---

BOX 1

Old nomenclature	New nomenclature	Typical strains
Mls^a	Mls-1^a, Mls-2^b	AKR, DBA/2
Mls^b	Mls-1^b, Mls-2^b	C57BL/10
Mls^c	Mls-1^b, Mls-2^a	C3H/He, A, BALB/c
Mls^d	Mls-1^a, Mls-2^a	CBA
Mls^x	Mls-1^b, Mls-2?	PL

times higher than that of cells that respond to allogeneic MHC. A number of clues to the nature of Mls, though, make this a very interesting phenomenon for the understanding of the immune system.

The cells that respond to Mls are CD4$^+$, and these responses are inhibited by antibodies to class II MHC, CD4, or T-cell receptor. So far, this looks like a typical, antigen-specific T-cell response. However, three features of the response make it very atypical. First, the response of T-cell clones to Mls is influenced by, but not restricted to, MHC. Such MHC-*unrestricted* Mls reactivity is often observed in T-cell clones that also respond to other antigens in the normal, MHC-restricted way. Thus, a T cell can have two different specificities: (1) response to Mls that requires class II MHC of nearly any

haplotype, and (2) response to antigen plus a particular class II MHC. Even though we don't understand how Mls responses come about, such observations tell us that the class II MHC molecule probably performs more than one function in T-cell activation.

The second feature of Mls reactivity that makes it especially interesting is the fact that Mls appears to be recognized by only the β chain of the TCR. This was elegantly demonstrated by Jonathan Kaye and Stephan Hedrick, who transfected an Mls-nonresponsive T-cell clone with the *TCR* β gene from an Mls-responsive T cell, and in so doing transferred Mls responsiveness. This property of Mls recognition may account for the third feature of Mls reactivity: the vast majority of T cells that bear particular TCR V$_\beta$ regions respond to particular Mls differences (Table 1). Because of this feature, T cells bearing such TCR V$_\beta$ regions are negatively selected in animals expressing the appropriate Mls allele. This phenomenon has helped shape our understanding of negative selection and self–nonself discrimination, as discussed in the text. Although we do not yet fully understand the nature of Mls, or how it stimulates some T cells, its study is bound to reveal more interesting information about the function of the immune system (see Appendix 3).

5 **One Scheme for Analysis of Negative Selection in Normal Mice.** ▶
Animals that are known to carry a *TCR* V_β gene whose product (TCR V_β)
recognizes a self-antigen (see Table 1) are bred to mice that express the self-
antigen. The F_1 therefore carries both the TCR V_β and the antigen it recognizes.
T cells from these animals are then examined for expression of the specific
V_β, using monoclonal anti-TCR V-region antibodies. Results of two such experiments are shown in Table 2.

either of these V_β regions (and a large number of T cells in some
strains of mice do), then it is very likely to respond to Mls-1^a. The
experiments that follow use some of these superantigens in order
to follow the process of negative selection, but the conclusions are
believed to apply to *any* antigen in the body.

Self-Reactive T Cells Are Lost During T-Cell Development

Because there is sometimes a correlation between use of a particular V_β by a T cell and response to a certain antigen (such as Mls),
the question quickly arose as to what would happen if a T cell
bearing such a T-cell receptor matured in the thymus of an animal
that carried the antigen. The strategy of the experiments is shown
in Figure 5. A mouse from a strain known to express a particular
T-cell receptor V-region gene in some of its mature T cells is mated
with an animal that expresses a self-molecule recognized by the V
region. The offspring are then examined for the expression of the
relevant V region on mature T cells. In these F_1 offspring, there
will be developing T cells bearing the V_β from one parent that
recognize the superantigen from the other parent. If negative selection occurs, then these T cells will be eliminated and the V_β
will not be found on mature T cells.

As shown in Figure 5 and Table 2, thymocytes carrying a potentially self-reactive T-cell receptor simply fail to mature in the thymus, that is, there is negative selection of this population of T
cells.

Negative Selection Occurs Mostly in Immature, Double-Positive (CD4$^+$CD8$^+$) Developing T Cells

To find out where the negative selection event actually occurs, H.
Robson MacDonald and his colleagues stained histologic sections
of thymuses with an antibody to $V_{\beta6}$. A majority of T cells expressing this V region respond to Mls-1^a. In animals in which thymocytes bearing $V_{\beta6}$ were not deleted (i.e., animals that do not express

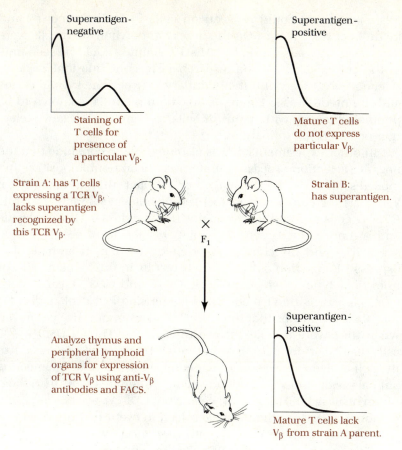

Superantigen-negative

Staining of
T cells for
presence of
a particular V_β.

Superantigen-positive

Mature T cells
do not express
particular V_β.

Strain A: has T cells
expressing a TCR V_β,
lacks superantigen
recognized by
this TCR V_β.

Strain B:
has superantigen.

$\times$

F_1

Analyze thymus and
peripheral lymphoid
organs for expression
of TCR V_β using anti-V_β
antibodies and FACS.

Superantigen-positive

Mature T cells lack
V_β from strain A parent.

Table 2   Negative selection in normal F₁ mice.[a]

Strain A	V_β	Strain B	Superantigen	Percentage of T cells expressing appropriate V_β	
				Strain A	(A × B)F₁
SJA	17	BALB/c	I-E (plus self)	9.4	0.2
BALB/c	6	DBA/2	Mls-1[a]	11	0.4

Source: Data from Kappler et al., 1987. *Cell* 49: 273; and MacDonald et al., 1988. *Nature* 332: 40.

[a]The protocol for this experiment is shown in Figure 5. T cells were obtained from lymph nodes in both cases.

Mls-1^a), staining could be seen on cells in both the cortex and medulla of the thymus. On the other hand, when such cells were deleted (in animals expressing Mls-1^a), staining could be seen only in the cortex. This led the researchers to conclude that negative selection occurs around the boundary between the thymic cortex and the medulla (see Figure 6). Since the medulla is known to be populated mainly with mature T cells, it seems that negative selection occurs *prior* to maturation.

In other experiments, it was also possible to conclude that the negative selection process operates mainly on double-positive thymocytes. This took advantage of the fact that a majority of $V_{\beta 17}^+ CD4^+$ T cells respond to I-E molecules (see Table 1), while $CD8^+$ T cells expressing $V_{\beta 17}$ do not. (I-E is a class II MHC molecule and is therefore not recognized by $CD8^+$ T cells.) Nevertheless, B. J. Fowlkes and his colleagues pointed out that in animals that express I-E, deletion of $V_{\beta 17}^+$ T cells results in this V_β being absent from *both* types of single-positive ($CD4^+$ and $CD8^+$)T cells. Since $CD8^+{}_{v\beta 17}^+$ cells don't recognize I-E, the simplest explanation for this observation was that the $V_{\beta 17}^+$ T cells were negatively selected when they were double-positive thymocytes. Thus, $CD8^+ V_{\beta 17}^+$ T cells also failed to mature, even though they would not recognize the self-antigen. The researchers confirmed this idea by injecting animals with anti-CD4 antibody, which interferes with the recognition of class II MHC by $CD4^+$cells. Now, $CD8^+ V_{\beta 17}^+$ cells matured, demonstrating that the negative selection event had to have been at a time when the cells bore both CD4 and CD8.

This finding, that negative selection appears to occur in the double-positive thymocyte population, has been made by several laboratories, though there is some suggestion that negative selection can also occur in the single-positive (especially $CD4^+ CD8^-$) population.

SYNTHESIS
Why Doesn't Negative Selection Prevent Immune Responses to All Antigens?

If negative selection has such a powerful effect on the TCR repertoire, how do we ever get immune responses? It might seem as though an antigen should enter the system, induce negative selection, and thereby avoid being recognized.

To understand why this usually doesn't occur, we have to remember that T cells constantly mature, especially in early life. Negative selection ensures that any T cell that responds to any

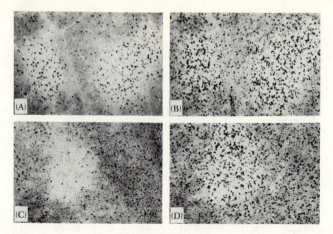

6 **Negative Selection Occurs at the Corticomedullary Boundary.** Thymus sections were stained with antibodies to $V_{\beta6}$ (*a* and *c*) or $V_{\beta8}$ (*b* and *d*). Thymuses were from $H\text{-}2^d$, $Mls\text{-}1^b$ BALB/c mice (*a* and *b*) or $H\text{-}2^d$, $Mls\text{-}1^a$ DBA/2 mice (*c* and *d*). Staining, which appears as black spots, can be seen in the darker cortical regions in all the photographs but is absent from the lighter medullary region in *c*. Since negative selection of T cells bearing $V_{\beta6}$ is known to occur in animals expressing $Mls\text{-}1^a$ (see text), this indicates that the negative selection occurs somewhere between the transition of cells from the cortex to the medulla. [From Hengartner et al., 1988. *Nature* 336: 388, with permission]

antigen that is present at the time of maturation will be removed. Thus, if an antigen persists throughout our lives (a "self" antigen), there will be no mature T cells in the system that recognize it. If a novel antigen enters the system, it could, conceivably, induce negative selection (if it makes its way to the thymus), but since it is novel, there will already be mature T cells present in the system that recognize it, and an immune response will occur. Therefore, the effect of negative selection on a constantly developing population of cells results in that *population's* having the ability to discriminate self from nonself. It might be more accurate, in this view, to say that the immune system discriminates between persistent (= self) and transient (= nonself) antigens.

Self–nonself discrimination is therefore not a property of an individual cell, but rather a property of the receptor repertoire of the entire population. The system regards "self" as anything present throughout the maturation of the population, and "nonself" as anything present only periodically or not at all. For the first time (in this book) we've got a clue as to how the immune system manages its remarkable discrimination. Other processes also contribute to this, and these will be discussed in later chapters.

The Process of Negative Selection

The Role of Nonlymphoid Cells in the Thymus during Negative Selection

So far, we have discussed the phenomenon of negative selection mainly from the point of view of the developing T cell and its response to the thymic environment. Now we'll focus on the stimulus, that is, the cells that present antigen to these developing T cells to induce negative selection. The cells responsible for the presentation, however, originate in the bone marrow and appear to be myeloid. Two lines of evidence support this assertion.

We saw previously that F_1 bone marrow cells maturing in a parental type (P_1) thymus produce T cells that recognize antigen together with only the P_1 MHC (Chapter 19; we'll consider this in more detail later in the next chapter). Even though the cells become restricted to the MHC of the thymus in which they matured, they fail to respond to the MHC of the other parent (P_2) —i.e., they are tolerant. Since the only source of the P_2 MHC was from the injected F_1 bone marrow, a likely explanation for this finding is that cells from the bone marrow (bearing both parental MHC haplotypes) directed the negative selection of potentially reactive T cells in the thymus.

To test this idea, John Kappler and Philippa Marrack took advantage of the anti–I-E response of $V_{\beta 17}^+$ T cells (see Table 1). Animals lacking I-E served as hosts for bone marrow cells from an I-E$^+$ donor. When the donor thymocytes matured, those thymocytes bearing $V_{\beta 17}$ were negatively selected. The only source of I-E$^+$ cells was the injected bone marrow. This strongly suggested that the signal (I-E) for the negative selection of $V_{\beta 17}^+$ T cells was provided by the cells derived from the bone marrow, which were now resident in the thymus.

Thymic Dendritic Cells and the Induction of Negative Selection

It seems remarkable that negative selection in the thymus can be efficient enough to eliminate any cell with anti–self-reactivity. Can't some self-reactive cells escape just by failing to contact the appropriate APC? While this is possible in principle, the cells most likely to be involved in antigen presentation for negative selection seem to be situated so as to contact the largest number of thymocytes. These class II MHC$^+$ bone marrow-derived cells, called THYMIC DENDRITIC CELLS, extend vast membrane sheets and branches among the thymocytes (see Figure 7). In this way, nearly every thymocyte can be "tested" for self-reactivity and negatively selected.

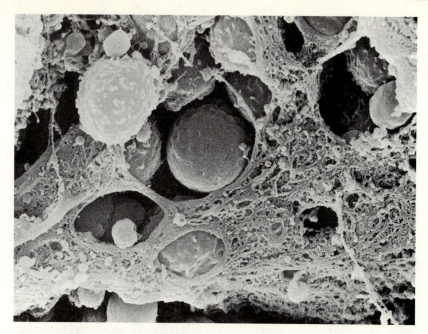

7 **Scanning Electron Micrograph of the Thymus.** Cortical thymocytes can be seen within a "mesh" of other cell types in the thymus. These include epithelial cells and dendritic cells. Note that there is extensive contact with the thymocytes. [Courtesy of Yufang Shi. Similar photographs appear in van Ewijk, 1988. *Lab. Invest.* 59: 577]

In Chapter 20, experiments were described that demonstrate that self-antigens are processed and presented by APCs. In the studies performed by Paul Allen, we saw that APCs from normal mice contain processed self-antigen that can stimulate T-cell hybridomas. Using this strategy, Allen went on to demonstrate similarly that APCs in the *thymus* are actively presenting self-antigen. Such thymic APCs provide a stimulus for the negative selection of T cells reactive with self-molecules.

It now should not be surprising that although all APCs appear to process and present self-antigen, the appropriate mature T cells are generally not around to recognize them. We call this a HOLE IN THE T-CELL RECEPTOR REPERTOIRE, and negative selection is one way this hole is punched.

Possible Mechanisms of Negative Selection

Negative selection, as we've considered it, seems to involve presentation of self-antigens by a bone marrow-derived thymic dendritic cell to a double-positive thymocyte. If the thymocyte responds to the presented antigen, it dies. Why? We will see in Chapters 26 and 27 that upon recognition of presented antigen, mature T cells become activated, release lymphokines, express lymphokine receptors, and proliferate. What is special about antigen presentation in the thymus that results in the death of the cells?

It was suggested that the APCs (the thymic dendritic cells) have the ability to kill any thymocyte when the thymocyte recognizes the MHC (plus processed antigen) on the dendritic cell surface. This would then be analogous to the action of cells called VETO CELLS that appear to have just this type of activity (see Chapter 31). However, it has now been shown that thymic dendritic cells are very good APCs for mature T cells, appearing to lack any special killing or inhibitory activity. In experiments by Polly Matzinger, different thymic APCs were tested for their ability to induce negative selection in thymocytes developing in thymic organ cultures. The same populations were tested for their ability to stimulate mature T cells. Dendritic cells appeared to be very good at *both* inducing negative selection and stimulating mature T cells. Thus, it doesn't appear as though there is specialized APC with a "search and destroy" mission.

An alternative view suggests that it is not the APC but the immature thymocyte that is "special." Eric Jenkinson and his colleagues have shown that activation of developing thymocytes in organ culture causes them to die. This cell death resembles a form of developmental cell death called APOPTOSIS in which the DNA of the cell fragments into pieces that are multiples of approximately 200 base pairs, the size of a nucleosome. Unlike cell death by injury (necrosis), apoptosis in thymocytes requires the participation of the cell, in that inhibition of RNA synthesis blocks the cell death. Similar observations have now been made in vivo by Yufang Shi and colleagues, by simply injecting antibodies to the T-cell receptor that are capable of activating T cells. In these experiments, when antibody was injected, DNA from the thymus showed the fragmentation of apoptosis, but DNA from other lymphoid organs did not. The effect in both the in vitro and in vivo systems appeared to be predominantly on the double-positive (CD4$^+$CD8$^+$) thymocytes. Thus, it seems as though activation of a double-positive thymocyte causes the cell to "commit suicide." More recently, Dennis Loh and colleagues have shown that injection of specific antigen into TCR-double transgenic mice similarly induces apoptosis in the immature thymocytes.

This is a description and not really an explanation. It now remains to determine precisely what the mechanism of suicide is. The answer is not known, but it may be linked to another phenomenon. It has been known for many years that some thymocytes are killed by corticosteroids while others are resistant. It now appears that double-positive thymocytes, when exposed to corticosteroids, undergo apoptosis, but upon maturation, thymocytes become resistant to this effect. We know that under conditions of stress, when corticosteroid levels become elevated, there is a dramatic loss of cells from the thymus. The relationship between corticosteroid sensitivity and susceptibility to negative selection is not entirely understood but may hold keys to understanding T-cell maturation.

The Fate of Negatively Selected Cells

Thus far, we have seen that developing T cells apparently die if they fail to successfully rearrange and express T-cell receptor genes, if their T-cell receptors react with self-antigens plus MHC in the thymus, or, as we'll see in the next chapter, if their T-cell receptors are not restricted to MHC alleles in the thymus. This cell death probably accounts for the discrepancy between the numbers of cells that enter the thymus and the numbers that finally mature. If greater than 95% of thymocytes die during development as a result of these processes, however, where do they all go? When we look at a normal thymus histologically, there is no accumulation of dead cells, so there must be a mechanism by which they are removed.

At the boundary between the cortex and the medulla of the thymus (the cortico-medullary boundary) there are large numbers of macrophages. When examined by transmission electron microscopy, these cells contain dense debris, which might represent apoptosed cells. This is likely, since a number of investigators have observed that thymocytes undergoing apoptosis (for example, following glucocorticoid treatment) become adherent to macrophages and are readily engulfed.

Therefore, as cells move through the selection processes, they may die at any of several points, but upon undergoing apoptosis they are rapidly cleared by active phagocytic macrophages. Since both apoptosis and phagocytosis are relatively rapid processes (taking only a few hours relative to several days for development), large numbers of dead thymocytes do not accumulate.

Consequences of Negative Selection: Holes in the T-Cell Repertoire

Clearly, negative selection must play a major role in the development of self–nonself discrimination by removing developing T cells that have the potential for responding to self-antigens (together with self-MHC). We will consider this role further in Chapter 31 when we discuss the phenomenon of tolerance. There is an additional effect, however, of negative selection that is highly relevant to our discussion of the T-cell repertoire. When the selection process removes T cells bearing certain T-cell receptor V regions, it naturally alters the overall repertoire. Suppose, for example, that the response of T cells to a particular foreign antigen relies upon the use of a T-cell receptor V region that is deleted by negative selection. The result may be a failure to respond, or an altered response, to this antigen. That is, there is a hole in the repertoire affecting the response to the antigen.

In Chapter 15, we introduced the problem of the immune response (*Ir*) genes, MHC alleles that control the ability to respond to certain antigens. In Chapter 20, we discussed how some peptides fail to associate with some MHC molecules, which can account for how some *Ir* genes work (the *determinant selection* model). We now have another possibility. Negative selection, due to a combination of certain self-molecules and self-MHC alleles, might remove T cells capable of responding to a particular foreign antigen. This hole in the T-cell repertoire due to negative selection might appear to be due to the MHC allele, since other alleles could lead to negative selection of a different set of T cells.

Polly Matzinger and her colleagues in Basel found that this was the case for *Ir* gene control of the immune response to a synthetic antigen. They found that a self-antigen expressed on B cells in some mouse strains, when presented with a particular MHC allele, led to negative selection of the T cells capable of responding to the synthetic antigen. Given the extent of negative selection induced by some of the self-antigens we've discussed (such as Mls), it is likely that more examples of this phenomenon will be found.

Such holes in the TCR repertoire may be more or less important, depending on the antigen, and may even be beneficial in some cases. It has been suggested, for example, that the holes induced by Mls antigens result in diminished responsiveness to staphylococcal enterotoxins (see Table 1), and thus a reduction in the pathologic T-cell responses induced by these toxins. Therefore, the shaping of the TCR repertoire by negative selection can have consequences beyond self-tolerance.

Summary

1. T cells develop in the thymus from bone marrow-derived stem cells. The developing T cells express the $\alpha\beta$ T-cell receptor and both CD4 and CD8 (*double-positive* thymocytes). As they mature, they lose either CD4 or CD8 to become *single-positive* cells. A small number of T cells that bear either the $\alpha\beta$ or $\gamma\delta$ TCR with neither CD4 nor CD8 (*double-negative* thymocytes) apparently mature via other pathways.
2. The double-positive thymocytes undergo negative selection during development. If the T-cell receptor of one of these cells recognizes its ligand in the thymus, the thymocyte dies, probably by the activation of apoptosis, or programmed cell death. The dead cell is then rapidly cleared by phagocytes.
3. The phenomenon of negative selection has been shown by two approaches. One involves the use of transgenic mice, in which every T cell expresses the TCR α and β chains from a T cell of known specificity. The presence of the ligand for this TCR results in the loss of double-positive thymocytes as they mature.
4. The second approach depends upon the phenomenon of *superantigens*. Such antigens stimulate almost any T cell bearing a particular TCR V_β. If the superantigen is present in the thymus, then developing T cells bearing this TCR V_β are lost via negative selection.
5. The APC responsible for inducing negative selection is of bone marrow origin, most likely the thymic dendritic cell.

Additional Reading

Janeway, C. A., J. Yagi, P. J. Conrad, M. E. Katz, B. Jones, S. Vroegop and S. Buxser. 1989. T cell responses to Mls and to bacterial proteins that mimic its behavior. *Immunol. Rev.*, 107: 61.

McDonald, H. R., A. L. Glasebrook, R. Schneider, R. K. Lees, H. Pircher, T. Pedrazzini, O. Kanagawa, J.-F. Nicolas, R. C. Howe, R. M. Zinkernagel and H. Hengartner. 1989. T cell reactivity and tolerance to Mls[a] encoded antigens *Immunol. Rev.* 107: 89.

Pullen, A. M., J. W. Kappler and P. Marrack. 1989. Tolerance to self antigens shapes the T cell repertoire. *Immunol. Rev.* 107: 125.

Scollay, R., P. Bartlett and K. Shortman. 1984. T cell development in the adult murine thymus. *Immunol. Rev.* 82: 79.

von Boehmer, H., H.-S. Teh, and P. Kisielow. 1989. The thymus selects the useful, neglects the useless, and destroys the harmful. *Immunol. Today.* 10: 57.

DEVELOPMENT AND SELECTION OF THE T-CELL RECEPTOR REPERTOIRE II
Positive Selection

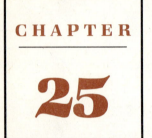

CHAPTER

25

Overview In the last chapter we discussed a critically important process in T-cell development: the removal of potentially self-reactive T cells during maturation in the thymus. We saw how negative selection shapes the T-cell receptor repertoire expressed on mature T cells. A second selection process also operates during T-cell development, and this is the subject of this chapter.

In Chapters 19 and 20, we discussed experiments that showed that the MHC restriction of T cells is for MHC antigens on APCs of the host in which the T cell developed, rather than the MHC haplotype of the T cell itself. As with negative selection, the thymus came to mind as a logical site for the acquisition of this MHC restriction. As we'll see in this section, interactions between the T-cell receptor on developing thymocytes and the MHC of the thymus result not only in the selection of self-MHC-restricted T cells but also in the pairing of the CD4 accessory molecule with class II MHC-restricted T-cell receptors and CD8 with class I MHC-restricted receptors.

Immature T cells are moved along the T-cell developmental pathway and mature if they are able to recognize self-MHC. This has been termed *positive selection*. Remember, however, that these cells must also pass the test of negative selection and will die if they respond strongly to self. The positively selected cells therefore fail to respond to MHC alone, but would probably respond to MHC plus some foreign peptide. Any other unselected developing cell seems to die from lack of attention. From the outset we must warn the reader that while positive selection has been clearly demonstrated, the mechanisms of this process are obscure. Nevertheless, the outcome of the negative- and positive-selection events is the development of a repertoire of T-cell receptors on mature T cells in the immune system.

The Evidence For Positive Selection: Studies with Thymus Chimeras

In Chapter 19 we described experiments showing adaptive differentiation in which developing T cells appear to "learn" MHC restriction. We now know that this apparent education is actually the result of positive selection—only those T cells that are restricted to the MHC of the thymus are allowed to mature.

One of the first approaches to determining whether the thymus is indeed the site of acquisition of MHC restriction was to produce bone marrow chimeras that have no thymus and then implant into them a thymus of any desired MHC haplotype. In this way the pre-T cell from the donor bone marrow of one haplotype can mature in a thymus from a mouse of another haplotype. This is accomplished by thymectomizing mice shortly before irradiation and bone marrow repopulation (Figure 1). After a suitable interval, the mice are implanted with several lobes of irradiated thymus so that these animals become both bone marrow and thymus chimeras. The MHC restriction they display after immunization can

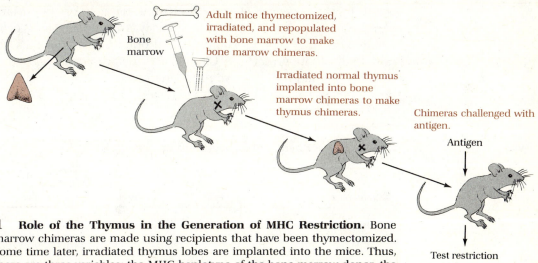

1 Role of the Thymus in the Generation of MHC Restriction. Bone marrow chimeras are made using recipients that have been thymectomized. Some time later, irradiated thymus lobes are implanted into the mice. Thus, there are three variables: the MHC haplotype of the bone marrow donor, the MHC haplotype of the thymus donor, and the MHC haplotype of the recipient. These animals are then infected with virus to prime CTLs. T cells are removed, cultured for 5 days with virally infected F_1 cells, and then tested for specificity on virally infected targets of different MHC haplotypes. [After Zinkernagel et al., 1978. *J. Exp. Med.* 147: 882]

thus be used to determine the role that the thymus plays in the acquisition of that restriction.

Rolf Zinkernagel and his co-workers did the first series of experiments using thymus chimeras. Table 1 shows the results of an experiment in which F_1 bone marrow develops in F_1 recipients with transplanted thymuses from one or the other of the parental types: the restriction is for the haplotype of the *thymus*. It will strike the reader that this experiment gives the same result as the $F_1 \rightarrow P_1$ experiment, which was used as the test of the adaptive differentiation hypothesis (see Chapter 19). The conclusion seems to be that the thymus is the site of adaptive differentiation, which is really another way of saying that the thymus is the site of acquisition of MHC restriction.

These experiments suggested that in the thymus, developing T cells that have a preference for recognizing host MHC antigens are positively selected in some way. Presumably, these developing thymocytes, and not others, are permitted to mature. The critical concept, to which we'll return, is that the T cells that mature following positive selection respond to "self" (or host) MHC only when the MHC molecule presents foreign antigenic peptides, and not to the MHC molecule alone. How this positive selection can occur in the *absence* of such foreign antigen is an important paradox. One solution to this paradox was the idea that T cells use two receptors, one for antigen and one for MHC, an idea we now know is incorrect (see Chapter 22). Before considering this paradox further, however, we must first consider whether the evidence in favor of positive selection is really unequivocal. Following

Table 1   **Influence of transplanted thymus on MHC restriction.**[a]

Bone marrow donor	Thymectomized recipient	Thymus	Restriction
(BALB/c × A)F_1	(BALB/c × A)F_1	(BALB/c × A)F_1	BALB/c and A
(BALB/c × A)F_1	(BALB/c × A)F_1	BALB/c	BALB/c only
(BALB/c × A)F_1	(BALB/c × A)F_1	A	A only
BALB/c	BALB/c	(BALB/c × A)F_1	BALB/c and A

Source: Data from Zinkernagel et al., 1978. *J. Exp. Med.* 147: 882.

[a]The design of this experiment is given in the legend to Figure 1. "Restriction" refers to the virally infected target cells that CTLs from the animals will kill.

the experiments of Zinkernagel and co-workers, a number of groups brought up evidence that contradicts these results or that strengthens them.

Experiments with Nude Mice

Another experimental approach to test the possible role of the thymus in conferring MHC restriction involves the use of nude mice. Because these mice are congenitally athymic, they have no environment in which T cells can differentiate into functional, immunocompetent cells. However, they do have normal pre-T cells, so if they are provided with a thymus, these pre-T cells can differentiate into functional T cells. Therefore, if the thymus from a mouse with an MHC haplotype that differs from that of a nude mouse is implanted into the nude mouse, the pre-T cells will mature in this thymus. But because the T cells are derived from host stem cells, they will be of host origin, even though they will have matured in a thymus with a different haplotype. The question now is: Will these host T cells show restriction for the host MHC or for the MHC of the donor thymus?

Experiments from Alfred Singer's group, using antibody formation as the test system, yielded a result similar to that of Zinkernagel's group, described above. These studies used the T cells of thymus-implanted nude mice in a manner similar to that shown in Figure 1. The T cells were incubated with B cells and macrophages in vitro, and their ability to provide help was assessed by the number of antibody-forming cells generated. As shown in Table 2, T cells from $H-2^d$ nude mice implanted with $H-2^b$ thymus gave antibody responses only with B cells and macrophages from $H-2^b$ mice, the haplotype of the implanted thymus. Thus, the T cells that developed in the mouse were apparently restricted to the MHC of the thymus in which they matured.

Unresponsiveness in $P_1 \rightarrow P_2$ Chimeras

Two of the observations we have discussed now come together as we try to make sense out of the flow of discoveries. The $F_1 \rightarrow P_1$ chimera experiments show that the T cells of an F_1 cooperate preferentially with P_1 cells over P_2 cells. An elegant and important series of experiments by Singer and his co-workers at NIH offered the start of the possible explanation.

First, these investigators constructed bone marrow chimeras in all possible combinations (Table 3). The spleen cells of these chimeras were challenged with antigen in vitro and the number

Table 2   MHC restriction of antibody formation in nude mice with grafted allogeneic thymus.[a]

T cells from nu/nu	Implanted thymus	B cells plus macrophages	Antibody response (pfc/culture)
H-2^d	H-2^a	H-2^d	<10
H-2^d	H-2^a	H-2^a	300
H-2^d	H-2^b	H-2^d	<10
H-2^d	H-2^b	H-2^b	1000

Source: Data from Singer et al., 1982. *J. Exp. Med.* 155: 339.

[a]H-2^d nude mice were grafted with an H-2^a or H-2^b thymus, and some time later, mature T cells were recovered from the spleens of the animals. These T cells were mixed with B cells plus macrophages from normal animals of the indicated MHC haplotype. Antigen was added and the generation of antibody-producing cells (plaque-forming cells) was assessed as a measure of antibody response. Responses were made only when the MHC haplotype of the B cells plus macrophages matched that of the grafted thymus.

of antibody-forming cells determined. This experiment tested the ability of the cells of one MHC that have developed in different MHC environments to cooperate. The controls are homologous reconstitutions, for example, $P_1 \rightarrow P_1$.

It was found that all the combinations except the completely allogeneic $P_1 \rightarrow P_2$ and $P_2 \rightarrow P_1$ spleen cells were able to give responses equivalent to the controls. One of the conclusions from this experiment is something that we already know: that under appropriate circumstances allogeneic cells can cooperate. The intriguing group is the $P_1 \rightarrow P_2$ (and vice versa) that were not able to respond. If allogeneic cells can cooperate, at least under some circumstances, why are the cells in these chimeras apparently unresponsive? For example, recall that P_1 T cells from $P_1 + P_2 \rightarrow F_1$ chimeras can cooperate with P_2 B cells when both are transferred into irradiated F_1 animals (see Chapter 19). In the F_1 animals, however, the APCs are of both parental types. One possibility, therefore, was that, in the $P_1 \rightarrow P_2$ chimera, the T cells become restricted to P_2 MHC, but the APCs (derived from P_1 bone marrow) bear only P_1 MHC. Thus, there is no cellular cooperation and the T cells fail to respond.

Table 3   Antibody responses of spleen cells from bone marrow chimeras.[a]

Reconstitution type	Strains used	Antibody response (pfc/culture)
CONTROLS		
$P_1 \rightarrow P_1$	B10	184
$P_2 \rightarrow P_2$	B10.A	118
$F_1 \rightarrow F_1$	(B10 × B10.A)	175
CHIMERAS		
$P \rightarrow F_1$	B10 → (B10 × B10.A)	102
	B10.A → (B10 × B10.A)	126
$F_1 \rightarrow P$	(B10 × B10.A) → B10	252
	(B10 × B10.A) → B10.A	143
$P_1 \rightarrow P_2$	B10 → B10.A	1
$P_2 \rightarrow P_1$	B10.A → B10	1
MIXING EXPERIMENT		
—	B10 + B10.A → B10	90
—	(B10 → B10.A) + (B10.A → B10)	327

Source: Data from Singer et al., 1981. *J. Exp. Med.* 153: 1286.

[a]The various chimeras shown in the table were generated and their spleen cells assessed for responsiveness to antigen in vivo. The generation of antibody-forming cells (plaque-forming cells) in response to antigen was used as a measure of responsiveness. Only the $P_1 \rightarrow P_2$ and $P_2 \rightarrow P_1$ combinations failed to respond. In the "mixing experiments," cells from $P_1 + P_2 \rightarrow P_1$ responded, as did a mixture of cells from $P_1 \rightarrow P_2$ and $P_2 \rightarrow P_1$ mice.

To test this idea, spleen cells from $P_1 \rightarrow P_2$ chimeras were fractionated into T lymphocytes, and macrophages plus B cells (Figure 2). We know from the Mosier experiment done in the Dark Ages of cellular immunology (Chapter 16) that the lymphocytes will not react unless macrophages are present. When P_1 or P_2 macrophages were added to the chimeric lymphocytes, the results in Table 4 were obtained. The lymphocytes from $P_1 \rightarrow F_1$ chimeras were able to cooperate with both P_1 and P_2 macrophages. This means that the P_1 T cells maturing in an F_1 environment had acquired the ability to react with macrophages of both parental types. The lymphocytes from $F_1 \rightarrow P_1$ chimeras, in contrast, could cooperate only with P_1 and not with P_2 cells. This result shows that even though there are two populations of T cells in the F_1,

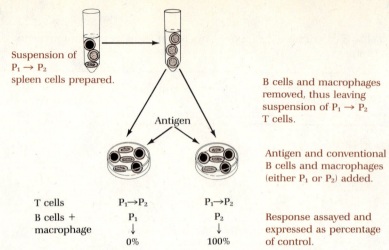

Suspension of
$P_1 \rightarrow P_2$
spleen cells prepared.

B cells and macrophages
removed, thus leaving
suspension of $P_1 \rightarrow P_2$
T cells.

Antigen

Antigen and conventional
B cells and macrophages
(either P_1 or P_2) added.

T cells	$P_1 \rightarrow P_2$	$P_1 \rightarrow P_2$
B cells +	P_1	P_2
macrophage	↓	↓
	0%	100%

Response assayed and
expressed as percentage
of control.

2   Unresponsiveness in $P_1 \rightarrow P_2$ Chimeras is Due to Lack of P_2 APCs.
T cells are prepared from $P_1 \rightarrow P_2$ chimeras and incubated with macrophages
and B cells from conventional P_1 or P_2 mice. Antigen is added and the number
of antibody-forming cells determined. In this way, it was shown that the
unresponsiveness in $P_1 \rightarrow P_2$ chimeras was because the T cells were restricted
to P_2 cells, but that only bone marrow-derived, P_1 APCs were present in the
animal. Results from other chimeras are summarized in Table 3. [After Singer
et al., 1981. *J. Exp. Med.* 153: 1286]

**Table 4   MHC restriction of antibody
responses in chimeric mice.[a]**

Chimera (T cells)	APC and B cells	Antibody response
$P_1 \rightarrow F_1$	P_1	+++
	P_2	+++
$F_1 \rightarrow P_1$	P_1	+++
	P_2	0
$F_1 \rightarrow P_2$	P_1	0
	P_2	+++
$P_1 \rightarrow P_2$	P_1	0
	P_2	+++
$P_2 \rightarrow P_1$	P_1	+++
	P_2	0

Source: After Singer et al., 1981. *J. Exp. Med.* 153:
1286.

[a]The basic design of the experiment is described
in the legend to Figure 2.

the environment in which the cells mature determines their MHC restriction. The $P_1 \rightarrow P_2$ cells that did not respond when unfractionated (Table 3) cooperated fully with macrophages from the P_2 host but not with those from the P_1 donor. This shows that the P_1 T cells can react *only* with macrophages having the same MHC haplotype as that of the cells among which they matured. Similarly, $P_2 \rightarrow P_1$ T cells can cooperate only with P_1 macrophages.

Clearly, then, the MHC haplotype of the cells in the environment in which the T cell differentiates determines the MHC haplotype of the accessory cell with which it can react.

Not all experiments were so clear-cut. Many investigators, including Zinkernagel's and Singer's groups, showed that in some situations there was no acquisition of restriction to the host's MHC, or that the restriction was incomplete. While positive selection seemed possible, it also seemed to be untestable, and for several years the concept became extremely unpopular.[1]

SYNTHESIS
Selection versus Education of MHC Restriction

From the experiments discussed so far in this chapter (and previous chapters) we can already draw several conclusions regarding the acquisition of MHC restriction. First, it is clear that it is the MHC of the *thymus*, not that of the T cell, that is important in this process. Given our understanding of the T-cell receptor and its ligand (MHC plus antigen), this conclusion should not surprise us. This is noteworthy, though, because this conclusion was reached *before* immunologists had a clear picture of either of these elements. There are other conclusions, however, that are less obvious.

We know that the specificity of the T-cell receptor is generated by a random process (Chapter 23) and that, once generated, it does not undergo further change. Thus, the interaction of the T-cell receptor with an MHC molecule in the thymus does not alter the receptor. In other words, no education process occurs. The alternative is that this interaction results in a selection event. While this idea is certainly consistent with the facts and fits in well with

---

[1] This lack of popularity is pointed out in a 1988 meeting report in which it is described how the concept of positive selection was greeted with "vociferous heckling from the floor." In retrospect, it is ironic that the meeting (and the report) occurred just prior to the publication of several very convincing studies on positive selection, which effectively shifted the phenomenon back into fashion. Often the movie cliché of the scientist being laughed at by his or her peers until being proved correct seems more like Hollywood fantasy than real life, but it is unfortunately part of the scientific process.

other selection processes in the immune system, the mechanisms of this particular selection event still remain obscure.

In the last chapter, we discussed the evidence that if a developing T cell responds to its ligand in the thymus it dies, that is, is negatively selected. The results discussed so far in this chapter (and below) suggest that there is a process that selects developing T cells that are restricted to the MHC of the thymus. This is positive selection. The existence of these two selection processes implies that somehow the T-cell receptor transmits two completely different signals to the cell: negative selection if the receptor contacts its ligand (MHC plus antigen) or positive selection if the receptor contacts the appropriate MHC (without antigen). We will return to this difficult point later in the chapter, but we will not resolve it.

Experiments were designed to directly demonstrate the positive selection event, without resorting to restriction studies. These experiments were dependent upon a new technique that we have already seen: TCR-transgenic mice. We consider these experiments next.

The Evidence For Positive Selection: Experiments with T-Cell Receptor–Transgenic Mice

In our discussion of negative selection in the last chapter, we described animals that are double-transgenic for the T-cell receptor α and β genes from a cytotoxic T cell specific for H-Y plus H-2D^b. We considered the case of H-2D^b male animals (which express H-Y) versus H-2D^b female animals (which lack H-Y). T cells mature in the female animals, whereas they are eliminated by negative selection during maturation in the males.

What happens to the maturation of the double-transgenic T cells (T cells in animals expressing both transgenic T-cell receptor genes) in female mice that carry a different MHC haplotype? The original cytotoxic T-cell clone used as the source of T-cell receptor genes recognized H-Y plus H-2D^b. By producing double-transgenic animals differing at the class I and class II loci, researchers were able to determine the role of the MHC in the maturation of the transgenic T cells (in the absence of the H-Y antigen). These T cells simply did not mature in female animals lacking H-2D^b. It seemed, therefore, that the H-2D^b molecule had an effect on the maturation of these T cells, *even in the complete absence of specific antigen.* In other words, the T cells were positively selected to mature only if the right MHC molecule was present.

The double-transgenic T cells that matured in female H-2D^b

mice, however, were all CD8$^+$, like the cytotoxic T-cell clone from which the T-cell receptor genes were derived. This was most strikingly seen when an ingenious step was added to the design of the transgenic mice. The transgenes were bred into mice with a genetic defect called SCIDS in which neither T-cell receptor nor Ig gene rearrangements occur (resulting in a severe immunodeficiency). Therefore, the only T-cell receptors that could be expressed were those that derived from the transgenes. In the double-transgenic animals, all the mature T cells were CD8$^+$ (Figure 3A). It was as though the transgenic T-cell receptor directed the double-positive thymocytes to become CD8$^+$ single-positive T cells. As mentioned above, this maturation of CD8$^+$ T cells was dependent upon the presence of the appropriate MHC molecule (H-2D^b) in the thymus.

Similar experiments have now been done by Mark Davis and his colleagues using transgenic mice carrying T-cell receptors specific for antigen plus class II MHC. In these mice, double-transgenic T cells mature only in the presence of the appropriate class II MHC molecule. The developing T cells, however, all mature into CD4$^+$ single-positive T cells (Figure 3B).

Thus, in these experiments T cells matured only if the MHC restriction of the T-cell receptor matched one of the MHC alleles expressed in the thymus. Further, this interaction also appeared to determine whether a mature T cell would be CD4 or CD8 single-positive. When the T-cell receptor was restricted to class I MHC, only CD8$^+$ T cells matured, and when the receptor was restricted to class II MHC, only CD4$^+$ T cells matured.

SYNTHESIS
Making Sense of Positive Selection

We can now start to put the pieces of the positive-selection puzzle together. T-cell receptors become expressed on the surface of CD4$^+$CD8$^+$ thymocytes, and if the cells are not negatively selected, they have the potential to mature into single-positive T cells. This maturation depends on the MHC restriction of the T-cell receptor on the cell. If the thymus in which the T cell is developing lacks the MHC allele to which the T-cell receptor is restricted, then the thymocyte does not mature (i.e., it is not positively selected). If the T-cell receptor is restricted to a class I MHC allele present in the thymus, then the CD4$^+$CD8$^+$ thymocyte matures into a CD8$^+$ T cell. If the restriction is to a class II MHC allele, then the cell becomes CD4$^+$.

This has two effects. First, developing T cells are selected to

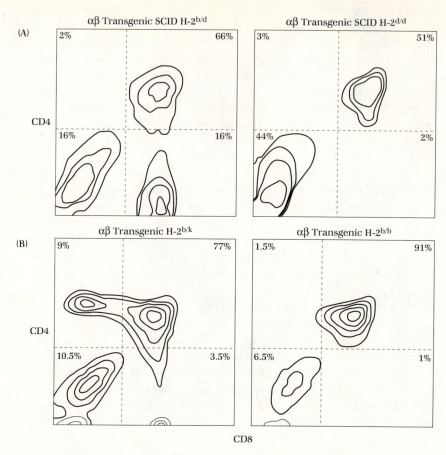

3 **Thymocyte Subpopulations in TCR α-β Transgenic Mice.** (A) The TCR α and β genes from a CD8$^+$ T cell specific for H-Y plus H-2D^b were used to generate transgenic mice (see Chapter 24, Figure 3). The TCR transgenes were bred into animals bearing the SCID mutation, which prevents rearrangement of endogenous TCR genes. Animals were either homozygous for H-2^d or heterozygous H-2$^{b/d}$. Thymuses from female mice (which lack H-Y) were examined by FACS after staining cells with anti-CD4 and anti-CD8. As shown, no single-positive cells matured in the H-2^d mice. CD8 single-positive cells matured in the H-2$^{b/d}$ mice, but CD4 single-positive cells did not. [From Scott et al., 1989. *Nature* 338: 591] (B) The TCR α and β genes from a CD4$^+$ T cell specific for pigeon cytochrome *c* plus I-E^k were used to generate transgenic mice. A thymus from a TCR-transgenic, homozygous H-2^b mouse revealed no mature single-positive thymocytes. CD4 single-positive cells matured in the TCR-transgenic heterozygous H-2$^{b/k}$ thymus, but CD8 single-positive cells did not. [From Berg, et al., 1989. *Cell* 58: 1035] These experiments strongly support the idea that MHC specificity of the TCR influences the maturation of thymocytes in the absence of antigen.

be restricted to the MHC of the thymus, that is, they seem to acquire MHC restriction. The second effect results in mature $CD4^+$ T cells bearing class II MHC-restricted T-cell receptors, and $CD8^+$ T cells bearing class I MHC-restricted T-cell receptors. Although we don't yet know the mechanism, it is during positive selection that the MHC restriction of the T-cell receptor dictates the maturation of the $CD4^+CD8^+$ thymocytes into the appropriate single-positive subsets.

Something more, though, is probably happening to the cells during the positive selection process. As we discussed in Chapter 19, $CD4^+$ and $CD8^+$ T cells have a number of functional differences, including a tendency to function as helper and cytotoxic cells, respectively. It seems likely, therefore, that when the T-cell receptor directs a cell to become single-positive, this also tends to favor the expression of a functional program (i.e., one that will cause the cell to act like a helper versus a cytotoxic cell). We say *tends* because the association of CD4 or CD8 with function is not complete (see Chapter 19). It will be interesting to discover how these functional programs come about following selection. However it occurs, though, it may well be the restriction of the T-cell receptor during positive selection that directs the acquisition of a T cell's function.

The Process of Positive Selection

Directed versus Stochastic Loss of CD4 or CD8 during Positive Selection

So far, we have suggested that the recognition of an MHC molecule by a TCR directs the developing, double-positive T cell to lose the inappropriate CD molecule (CD4 or CD8). In this way, class II-restricted T cells would lose CD8 and become CD4 single-positive cells. According to this idea, the TCR signal generated by the recognition of MHC (in the absence of antigen) instructs the cell to turn off the inappropriate gene.

There is, however, another possibility. It may be that the maturation of a $CD4^+CD8^+$ T cell into a single-positive cell is random— that is, a cell spontaneously loses either CD4 or CD8 without any regard for the MHC restriction of its TCR. Once this occurs, however, only those cells that have the expression of CD4 or CD8 appropriate for the TCR on the cell will survive. This STOCHASTIC MODEL predicts that in transgenic mice bearing TCR restricted to class I MHC, CD4 single-positive cells are generated, but these die before they can be detected.

While the stochastic model does not get around the problem of how a TCR that is restricted for MHC plus antigen can somehow "see" MHC alone (see below), it does get around a second problem: how the T cell can somehow know which CD molecule to lose. This theory says that the loss is random, but that subsequent survival of the cell will depend on whether or not the right choice was made. Although we don't yet know if the stochastic model is correct, it has the flavor of some of the other processes we have already seen in the immune system (e.g., clonal selection).

How Can Positive Selection Happen?

We don't really understand what exactly the T-cell receptor recognizes during the positive selection event, or how this recognition advances (or protects) the thymocyte maturation process. From the experiments we've discussed, it is certain that at least part of what is being recognized is MHC. It is also reasonably certain that specific antigen is not involved. (If the antigen *were* present, the cells would probably have been negatively selected.)

In Chapter 22, we described the early controversies surrounding the T-cell receptor—whether there is a single receptor that recognizes MHC plus antigen (which is the case) or two receptors, one for antigen and one for MHC (the two-independent-receptor model). Positive selection would be relatively easy to understand if the two-receptor model had turned out to be right. It wasn't, and we are left trying to figure out how the T-cell receptor functions in positive selection for MHC in the absence of antigen.

First, let's consider which cells in the thymus seem to be involved in presenting the MHC to the developing thymocyte. From the original chimera experiments, it is apparent that the responsible cells are likely to be in the thymus and not derived from the bone marrow. Most experiments have confirmed this and point to the thymic epithelial cells. Thus, while negative selection appears to be directed by the bone marrow-derived, thymic dendritic cells (Chapter 24), positive selection appears to be bone marrow-independent, being directed, probably, by the thymic epithelial cells.

John Kappler and Phillipa Marrack, in attempting to explain how MHC on a thymic epithelial cell could direct positive selection in the absence of antigen, suggested that perhaps thymic epithelial cells present a specialized, "sticky" peptide with their class I and class II MHC, such that any T-cell receptor restricted to the presented MHC will be bound by the peptide. In this way, the affinity of the interaction will be increased sufficiently to lead to thymocyte activation, which then presumably plays a role in positive selection. While this idea is somewhat attractive, a prediction is that thymic epithelial cells should be able to activate mature T cells in the absence of antigen, which does not appear to be the case.

While more work is needed in this area, experiments with APCs of the thymus seem to suggest that thymic epithelium works pretty much like other APCs in activating T cells. As with negative selection, it may be that the key lies in the developing thymocyte rather than in a special property of the APC. This, however, would not explain why different APCs seem to be involved in negative versus positive selection.

It may well be that T-cell receptors have some affinity for MHC in the absence of antigen, but that this affinity is normally too low to activate a mature T cell. The AFFINITY ARGUMENT suggests that if a T-cell receptor interacts with an MHC molecule in the thymus with high affinity, then it is negatively selected. If the affinity is lower, some signal is transduced to the T cell, and positive selection occurs. If there is no affinity, then the developing cell is simply lost. This concept depends, however, on there being at least two sites on T-cell receptors, with at least one site recognizing MHC (and not antigen). In a way, this is a variation on the dual-recognition hypothesis, posing dual sites on a single receptor.

A number of investigators have observed a phenomenon that may bear on this problem (or may not). If lymphocytes from rodents or humans are enriched and cultured, they often spontaneously proliferate. Dissection of the system demonstrated that this proliferation is due to $CD4^+$ T cells responding to class II MHC on autologous B cells, a phenomenon called AUTOLOGOUS MLR. The significance of the autologous MLR is not known, but it is possible that it represents a response induced by the weak affinity of T cells for "self"-MHC. A careful reexamination of this phenomenon might determine its relationship to positive selection.

Obviously, these ideas are difficult to address without more information. Why are different APCs apparently involved in negative versus positive selection? Why do double-positive thymocytes respond so differently when the T-cell receptor contacts the appropriate MHC plus antigen (negative selection) versus the appropriate MHC alone (maturation to single-positive thymocyte via positive selection)? It may well be that by the time you read this, cleverly designed experiments will have helped to resolve these dilemmas.

SYNTHESIS
Selection of the T-Cell Receptor Repertoire During Development

The processes described in this chapter are so complex that it is worthwhile considering the selection of the T-cell receptor repertoire one more time, attempting to put it all together. The overall scheme of thymocyte development with negative and positive selection is shown in Figure 4. We've chosen to place negative selection before positive selection for two reasons: (1) negative selection appears to act on double-positive thymocytes, but following positive selection, the thymocyte (if selected) becomes single-positive. Therefore, negative selection probably acts before positive selection. (2) Cells that are not negatively selected probably do not receive a signal to this effect, that is, they don't "know" that they've passed the negative-selection test. (They simply did not contact the appropriate MHC plus antigen that would signal negative selection.) On the other hand, positively selected cells certainly receive a signal. It would be logical (or at least convenient) if one outcome of the positive selection event was now to become resistant to negative selection. The mature single-positive cell would now be prepared to respond to the appropriate MHC plus antigen to make an immune response.

Recently, some support for this timing of negative versus positive selection has come from the transgenic mouse studies of von Boehmer and colleagues. They have found that during the development of the mouse, negative selection of thymocytes in male transgenic mice can be observed several days earlier in ontogeny than can maturation of CD8 single-positive thymocytes in female transgenics (positive selection).

These arguments, we realize, are not airtight, but they serve to create a somewhat logical picture of thymocyte maturation. The results of these selection processes are a population of T cells that fail to respond to self-antigens (at least those that could get to the thymus), are restricted to self-MHC, and bear CD4 or CD8 depending on whether they are restricted to class I or class II MHC.

There are many immune phenomena that this scheme does not explain, such as why the immune system doesn't usually respond to self-antigens that are not present in the thymus (a problem we confront in Chapter 31). Nevertheless, we've managed to get a glimpse of part of the blueprint for building an immune system that discriminates self from nonself.

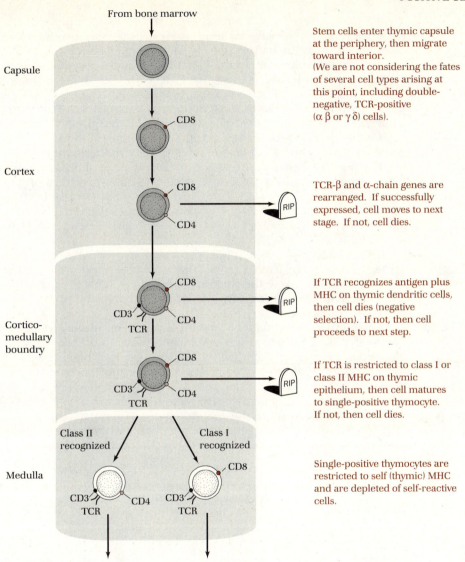

From bone marrow

Stem cells enter thymic capsule at the periphery, then migrate toward interior.
(We are not considering the fates of several cell types arising at this point, including double-negative, TCR-positive (α β or γ δ) cells).

Capsule

CD8

Cortex

CD8

TCR-β and α-chain genes are rearranged. If successfully expressed, cell moves to next stage. If not, cell dies.

CD8

RIP

CD4

CD8

If TCR recognizes antigen plus MHC on thymic dendritic cells, then cell dies (negative selection). If not, then cell proceeds to next step.

CD3

CD4

TCR

RIP

Cortico-medullary boundry

CD8

If TCR is restricted to class I or class II MHC on thymic epithelium, then cell matures to single-positive thymocyte. If not, then cell dies.

CD3

CD4

TCR

RIP

Class II recognized

Class I recognized

Medulla

CD8

Single-positive thymocytes are restricted to self (thymic) MHC and are depleted of self-reactive cells.

CD3

CD4

CD3

TCR

TCR

4   A Scheme of T-Cell Development in the Thymus. The placement of negative selection prior to positive selection in this scheme is not confirmed. The little graves are meant to represent cell death in a nondenominational way.

Summary

1.   MHC restriction in the T-cell receptor repertoire develops in bone marrow chimeras according to the MHC haplotype of the thymus. F_1

T cells that mature in a P_1 thymus respond to antigen plus P_1 APC but not P_2 APC. In $P_1 \rightarrow P_2$ chimeras, the T cells appear unresponsive, because although the mature T cells respond to antigen plus P_2 APC, the APCs in the animal are of the P_1 haplotype (since they derive from the bone marrow). This "learning" of MHC restriction is really a consequence of positive selection.

2.   Positive selection can be most dramatically observed in TCR transgenic mice. In the absence of antigen, double-positive thymocytes (CD4$^+$CD8$^+$) mature into single-positive T cells only if the MHC molecule for which the TCR is restricted is present in the thymus.

3.   Further, this restriction seems to determine the ultimate phenotype of the T cell: if the TCR is restricted to class I MHC, then the mature T cells will be CD8$^+$; if the TCR is restricted to class II MHC, then the T cells will be CD4$^+$. Therefore, positive selection is responsible for the association of CD4 vs. CD8 with class II vs. class I MHC restriction.

4.   The cell that appears to be responsible for presenting MHC molecules to developing T cells for positive selection is a resident cell of the thymus, most likely the thymic epithelial cell. This is in contrast to the bone marrow-derived thymic dendritic cell that presents antigen for negative selection.

5.   The simplest explanation for the phenomenon of positive selection is that a TCR that recognizes antigen plus a particular MHC is also capable of recognizing the MHC molecule alone. This presumably low-affinity recognition is insufficient to trigger the T cell but is sufficient to provide the necessary signals for positive selection.

6.   The combined effects of negative and positive selection during T-cell development result in the generation of a TCR repertoire capable of distinguishing self-antigens from antigens that are not normally present, and recognizing the latter in the context of self-MHC molecules.

Additional Readings

Benoist, C. and D. Mathis. 1989. Positive selection of the T cell repertoire: Where and when does it occur? *Cell* 58: 1027.

Berg, L. J., A. M. Pullen, B. Fazekas de St. Groth, D. Mathis, C. Benoist and M. M. Davis. 1989. Antigen/MHC-specific T cells are preferentially exported from the thymus in the presence of their MHC ligand. *Cell* 58: 1035.

Kisielow, P., H. S. Teh, H. Bluthman and H. von Boehmer. 1988. Positive selection of antigen-specific T cells in thymus by restricting MHC molecules. *Nature* 335: 730.

von Boehmer, H. 1990. Developmental biology of T cells in T cell-receptor transgenic mice. *Annu. Rev. Immunol.* 8: 531.

LYMPHOCYTE ACTIVATION I
From the Cell Surface to the Genes

CHAPTER

26

Overview   Up to now we have seen that antigen initiates the cellular events in the immune response by being presented to the T cell in an MHC-restricted manner by the APC. Subsets of T cells communicate with each other in the generation of cell-mediated responses, and the helper T cell communicates with the B cell in the generation of the humoral response.

One thing should already be clear about T cells: the binding of antigen to the receptor is complex. Because B cells bind antigen directly, it is tempting to treat them as mere spheres with receptors on their surfaces; but this can be a fatal oversimplification. Antigen (or antigen–MHC) initiates a cascade of intracellular events that culminate in gene activation. The cellular machinery of activation induces the cells to produce and/or respond to various growth factors, and this continues the activation process. The emerging picture reveals that little about the signal transduction from the cell membrane to the nucleus in lymphocytes may be unique to lymphocytes, and that studies in a variety of cell systems will prove to be applicable to the cells of the immune system (and vice versa). Lymphocyte activation in response to specific antigen results in proliferation and differentiation of function. Thus, clonal selection proceeds.

In this chapter, we consider the steps in lymphocyte activation up to the point at which genes become activated. In the next chapter, we continue our discussion by considering some of the products of these genes: growth factors and their receptors.

A Simplified Scheme of Lymphocyte Activation

The problem addressed in this chapter and the next is how a signal that begins at the cell membrane affects the activity of genes in the nucleus. For lymphocytes, and especially helper T cells, we

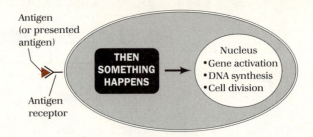

Antigen
(or presented
antigen)

THEN
SOMETHING
HAPPENS

Nucleus
• Gene activation
• DNA synthesis
• Cell division

Antigen
receptor

1   One View of Lymphocyte Activation.

will see that this is a two-tiered process. That is, a signal is generated at the membrane following recognition by the T-cell receptor, leading to the activation of growth factor and growth factor receptor genes. The products of these genes then interact on the cell membrane (on our original cell and on other cells), and this again generates a signal that leads to the activation of other genes and to cell proliferation. In this chapter, we will consider the mechanisms of the activation of lymphocytes, from antigen recognition to the gene level, and some of the first genes to be expressed. In the next chapter we will discuss the growth and differentiation factors, their receptors, and how the interaction leads to cellular differentiation and proliferation.

A simplified scheme of lymphocyte activation is shown in Figure 1, in which we see that there are a lot of gaps in our knowledge. We will attempt to give a feeling for what is known and what we *think* we know in this important process. This is shown in Figure 2, a simplified time course of events in lymphocyte activation.

Cell-Surface Events In Lymphocyte Activation

We begin where we have left off in other chapters, immediately after antigen has contacted a B cell or after antigen plus MHC (on an APC) has contacted a T cell. In a *general* sense, the events that follow are the same in all lymphocytes, regardless of whether they are helpers or effectors. The signal that originates at the cell-surface antigen receptor must be transduced into the cell by a complex and not fully understood process that culminates in gene activation. Understanding how a signal gets from the surface of a cell to where it affects gene activation is clearly a problem of general biological interest. So far, researchers have gotten only a taste of this complicated process, but many are very hungry for more. This is an area that is moving rapidly.

Receptor Cross-Linking Leads to Activation

We must first consider what binding of antigen (or antigen–MHC) to an antigen receptor actually *does*. The first hint came in 1965, when Sell and Gell showed that anti-Ig antibodies are capable of stimulating B cells in vitro. In order for this to happen, however, the antibodies have to be bivalent [intact or (Fab)₂]; Fab fragments will not work. Similar experiments were performed by Alfred Nis-

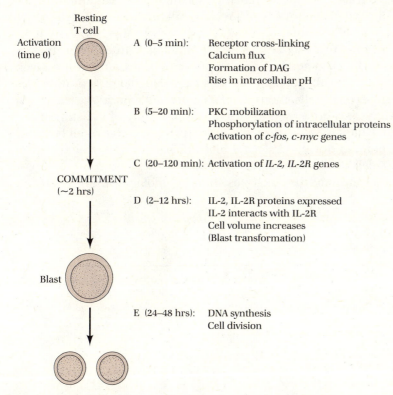

2 A Simplified Time Course of Lymphocyte Activation. Activation of a helper T cell is shown. Removal of the activation signal (e.g., antigen plus APC) prior to 2 hours stops the subsequent steps in the activation process. After 2 hours, the cell is "committed," and activation will proceed regardless of continued presence of the activation signal. By approximately 12 hours post activation, the cell has become an enlarged blast. DNA synthesis and cell division occur in 24 to 48 hours.

sonoff and colleagues (see Table 1). Experiments of this kind, performed in many different laboratories, showed the requirement for bivalent [(Fab)$_2$] versus monovalent (Fab) anti-Ig antibody. This led to the conclusion that *cross-linking* of surface Ig on B cells is an activation signal. This was also consistent with the observation that antigens with repetitive B-cell epitopes seem to be better antigens for B cells. In fact, these can often activate B cells in the absence of T cells; therefore, they are called T-INDEPENDENT ANTIGENS. There is a feeling, however, that truly T-independent antigens also provide a second signal to B cells (see below).

The activation of lymphocytes by cross-linking of antigen receptors has also been demonstrated in T cells. Jonathan Kaye and Charles Janeway found that an anticlonotype antibody (see Chapter 22) against the T-cell receptor of one of their T-cell clones was capable of directly activating the T cell. They found that an Fab fragment of this antibody not only failed to activate the cell but also blocked activation in response to intact antibody, antigen plus APCs, or allogeneic cells (normally capable of activating this clone). Presumably, then, the Fab fragment bound to the T-cell receptor and prevented its cross-linking by any of the stimuli.

In Chapter 22, we described the structure of the T-cell receptor and pointed out that the CD3 molecules are an integrated part of the T-cell receptor complex. When the T-cell receptor is cross-linked, naturally this includes the CD3 molecules. Antibodies to

Table 1   Induction of B-cell proliferation by cross-linking of surface Ig.[a]

Group	Goat anti-rabbit Ig	(Fab') goat anti-rabbit Ig	[(Fab')$_2$] rabbit anti-goat Ig	Proliferation
1	−	−	−	−
2	+	−	−	+++
3	−	+	−	+
4	−	−	+	−
5	−	+	+	+++

Source: Fanger et al., 1970. *J. Immunol.* 105: 1484.
[a]Rabbit lymphocytes are reacted with the indicated antibodies, then assessed for proliferation by uptake of ^{3}H-thymidine. The rabbit B cells proliferate if their surface Ig is bound *and* cross-linked.

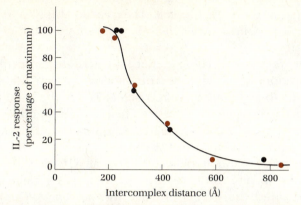

3 Immobilized MHC–Antigen Complexes Activate T-Cell Hybridomas.
Complexes of class II MHC molecules and antigenic fragments, immobilized
in a lipid planar membrane, were used to stimulate a T-cell hybridoma to
produce growth factor (IL2; see Chapter 27), which was assayed as a measure
of T-cell activation. The membranes were prepared at different concentrations
of MHC molecules (*colored* circles) or different concentrations of antigenic
peptide (*black* circles), and the distances between complexes determined by
an energy-transfer technique. [From Watts, 1988. *J. Immunol.* 141: 3708]

CD3 molecules on human, rodent, and other mammalian T cells
(and probably *any* kind of T cell, when looked at) are capable of
activating T cells, and, again, cross-linking of CD3 is important.

Tania Watts in Toronto has further examined the requirement
for receptor cross-linking on T cells in a series of elegant experiments. She found that purified class II MHC molecules placed in
a planar lipid membrane are capable of presenting antigenic peptides to T-cell hybridomas. By varying the concentrations of MHC
molecules or peptides, she determined the optimal physical distance between immobile ligands needed to activate the T cells (see
Figure 3). Thus, the evidence to date indicates that simply bringing together the cell-surface antigen receptors triggers the initial
events of lymphocyte activation.

The Two-Signal Hypothesis

The experiments discussed above showed that cross-linking of
cell-surface receptors on the surface of lymphocytes is an important step in lymphocyte activation; but is it, in fact, the whole
story? In 1972, Peter Bretscher and Melvin Cohn proposed on
theoretical grounds that two or more signals must be required for

lymphocyte activation. One signal, without the other(s), would lead to unresponsiveness of the cell. They called this the Two-SIGNAL HYPOTHESIS. Cross-linking of cell-surface receptors could be the first of these signals.

In general, most B cells are not fully activated to proliferation and Ig production by simply cross-linking the cell-surface Ig. In addition to this signal, a second signal is usually required. The second signal appears to come from helper T cells and is probably mediated by growth and/or differentiation factors. This is covered in much more detail in the next chapter.

Marc Jenkins and Ronald Schwartz at NIH developed an in vitro system to test the two-signal hypothesis for helper T cells. They compared the effects of *fixed* and *normal* APCs on T cell clones. Normal APCs plus antigenic peptides stimulated proliferation as expected. However, the fixed cells plus antigenic peptides rendered T cells *incapable* of responding to subsequent stimulation. The negative effect of the fixed cells was specific for both the class II MHC molecule and the antigenic peptide recognized by the helper T cell. That is, when the antigenic peptide was presented by fixed cells of the wrong MHC, the T cells remained able to respond to the antigen on normal APC (i.e., the inhibitory effect was not seen). Similarly, if the fixed cells bore the appropriate MHC but presented the wrong antigenic peptide, there was again no inhibitory effect. They suggested that one signal (antigen plus MHC) was given to the T cells with either the normal or the fixed APC, but that in the case of normal APC, an *additional* signal was also provided (and not provided by the fixed APC). This supported the two-signal hypothesis, in which one signal alone leads to lymphocyte unresponsiveness, and two signals lead to activation.[1]

What, then, is the nature of the second signal for T-cell activation? Jenkins and Schwartz found that if they mixed fixed APCs with normal allogeneic cells (the latter without antigen), activation rather than unresponsiveness occurred. This indicated that a cell-surface molecule other than MHC (or, at least, the polymorphic part of MHC) is also involved in activating T cells. They have called

[1] The astute reader will remember that in Chapter 20 we described important experiments in which fixed APCs presented antigenic peptides and stimulated T cells. The critical difference between those experiments and the ones described here are that in the former experiments the responding cells were T-cell hybridomas. In the experiments described here, the responding T cells were cloned T-cell lines. T-cell hybridomas thus seem to respond to one signal whereas T-cell clones require two. The latter seem to more closely mirror the actual in vivo situation. This underscores the importance of choosing the correct experimental model to study a problem and the difficulty in translating the result into the "real life" situation.

this signal the *costimulator* and have not, as yet, identified either the molecules involved or the precise nature of the signal. Below, we discuss other molecules involved in T-cell activation, but so far, none of these appear to be the costimulator molecules on the T cell or APC. We will return to these important observations in our discussion of immunologic tolerance (Chapter 31).

Other Cell-Surface Molecules are Involved in Lymphocyte Activation

In addition to the antigen receptors, a number of cell-surface molecules have been implicated in T-cell activation (and others may well be found to be involved in B-cell activation). The relationship of these molecules to the two-signal hypothesis (and to the experiments described above) is currently unknown.

CD4 and CD8

We have already discussed the association of the accessory molecules CD4 and CD8 in the context of MHC recognition by T cells, and these molecules are generally thought to play a role in T-cell activation. Antibodies to CD4 or CD8 are capable of blocking the activation of T cells bearing these molecules (discussed in Chapter 19). In addition, Janeway and colleagues have shown that anti–T-cell receptor antibodies that cause cross-linking of *both* T-cell receptor and CD4 activate T cells, whereas those antibodies that cross-link T-cell receptor but not CD4 fail to stimulate T cells. Similarly, Klaus Eichman and colleagues showed that cross-linking of either CD4 or CD8 with antibodies facilitates the ability of small amounts of anti–T-cell receptor antibodies to activate T cells. Both these studies support the idea that cross-linking of these accessory molecules *in addition to cross-linking of the T-cell receptor* plays a role in T-cell activation. As we will see below, these cell-surface molecules transduce signals into the cell, but the precise role of these signals in T-cell activation is not fully understood.

CD2 and LFA-3

Another clue to the activation signals for T cells comes from studies of molecules involved in adhesion of lymphocytes to APCs. T cells have a molecule called CD2 on their surface that interacts with its ligand, LFA-3, on APCs. The CD2 molecule, when cross-linked by anti-CD2 antibodies, is capable of directly activating T cells, perhaps via a different pathway than that involving the T-cell receptor.

Nevertheless, the interaction between CD2 on a T cell and LFA-3 on an APC has been shown by Ellis Reinherz and his colleagues to facilitate antigen recognition by T cells. In these studies they transfected mouse T-cell hybridomas with the gene encoding the human CD2 molecule. In addition, they also transfected cells with truncated genes encoding human CD2 that lacked cytoplasmic residues (and that produced a molecule incapable of directly activating T cells when cross-linked with antibodies). They found that these transfected T-cell hybridomas responded to specific antigen plus MHC on murine APC in the same way as the nontransfected cells. However, when the murine APC was transfected with human LFA-3, the (human CD2)$^+$ murine T hybridoma cells responded far better to the antigen plus MHC presented by the (human LFA-3)$^+$ APC. Thus, the human CD2 molecule on the T cell interacted with the human LFA-3 molecule on the APC to facilitate antigen presentation to the T-cell receptor. Note that this also implies that the interaction between CD2 and LFA-3 is species-specific. The researchers also found that the enhancement occurred even when the cytoplasmic region of the human CD2 was absent, suggesting that this effect is mediated by adhesion. Therefore, by increasing the adhesion between the T cell and the APC, the presentation to the T-cell receptor was improved. Other studies have suggested that the interactions between CD2 and the T-cell receptor may be more complicated than this simple picture implies.

Intracellular Events in Lymphocyte Activation

So far, we have seen that at least one signal for lymphocyte activation is receptor cross-linking. This triggers a cascade of events within the cell that results in gene induction, cell proliferation, and the other hallmarks of activation. As we'll see, precisely *how* cross-linking of the antigen receptors delivers a signal is unclear, and the first steps in this signaling are only suspected. Then we move onto more solid ground, because the "second messengers" of activation are fairly well described: ion fluxes, the phosphatidylinositol pathway, and protein kinase C. How these pathways result in gene activation is, again, only suspected, but gets us into the fascinating realm of DNA-binding proteins.

As far as we know, the events that we will now describe are the same in B cells and T cells, rodents and primates. They are characteristic (and were first described) for many receptor–ligand interactions in many different cell types. With all the strange things that lymphocytes seem to do, it is sometimes comforting to realize that they can be, after all, fairly typical cells.

We take up the story, then, just after the surface antigen receptors have been cross-linked. This, in turn, sets up a signal that, based on studies of other cell types, might then involve G proteins and/or tyrosine phosphorylation (or something completely different). We'll consider each briefly before continuing on into the cell.

G Proteins and Lymphocyte Activation

G proteins (*guanine nucleotide regulatory* proteins) act in many systems to couple cell-surface receptors to second messenger systems within the cell (Figure 4). In general, they appear as a complex of three subunits (α, β, and γ). Activation occurs when GDP, bound to the α subunit, is replaced by GTP (forming G_α-GTP). The α subunit then dissociates and directly modifies a target molecule (such as an enzyme), which, in turn, continues the intracellular signaling pathway. In the process of modifying the target, the GTP bound to the α subunit is converted to GDP, and the G_α-GDP once again reassociates with the β-γ subunits. The complex is now ready to act again. Two important targets (for our purposes) of G-protein modification are ion channels and an enzyme called phospholipase C. We will see why these are important a little later.

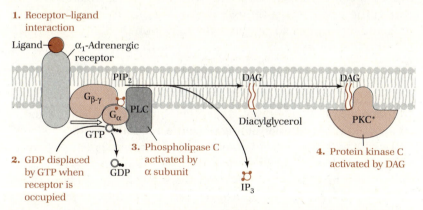

1. Receptor–ligand interaction

Ligand α_1-Adrenergic receptor

PIP$_2$ DAG   DAG

$G_{\beta\text{-}\gamma}$

G_α PLC

GTP

Diacylglycerol   PKC*

2. GDP displaced by GTP when receptor is occupied

GDP

3. Phospholipase C activated by α subunit

IP$_3$

4. Protein kinase C activated by DAG

4   G-Protein Signal Transduction Pathway. The pathway shown is for the α_1-adrenergic receptor, coupling the receptor to phospholipase C (see Figure 6). It is not known if a similar arrangement exists in lymphocytes. Upon receptor–ligand interaction, GTP replaces GDP on the α subunit, activating the G protein. This, in turn, activates the effector [in this case phospholipase C (PLC)]. The intrinsic GTPase activity of the α subunit then converts the bound GTP to GDP, and the pathway is now ready to transduce another signal.

There are a number of ways in which the role of G proteins in signal transduction pathways is studied. One is through the use of bacterial toxins, such as cholera toxin and pertussis toxin, which irreversibly block the activity of many of the G proteins. Unfortunately, however, such toxins may not affect all G proteins, and they may have other effects (such as elevation of levels of cyclic AMP). Not surprisingly, the results obtained with such toxins in lymphocyte activation have been contradictory.

More direct demonstrations of G protein involvement in lymphocyte activation have been provided for B cells by John Monroe and his colleagues. They have shown that in isolated B-cell membranes, cross-linking of the cell-surface Ig leads to the uptake of radiolabeled GTP (but not ATP) and the release of GDP. This would be expected if G proteins had been activated. Further, using a monoclonal antibody to the G_α subunit, they found that G_α becomes associated with membrane IgM following cross-linking. These studies strongly support the idea that receptor cross-linking leads to activation of G proteins, but, of course, do not prove that this association is critical for B-cell activation. Thus, G proteins are a likely, but not proven, connection between the cell-surface antigen receptors and the inside of the cell.

We've briefly considered the G proteins as a means for getting from the cell-surface receptor to the second-messenger pathways within the cell. Clearly, though, it is by no means proved that this mechanism applies to lymphocyte activation. An alternative and/ or complementary mechanism that is worth considering is that of tyrosine phosphorylation.

Tyrosine Kinases and Lymphocyte Activation

In many types of cell-surface receptors, binding of specific ligands induces conformational changes in the receptor molecules that, in turn, cause the activation of tyrosine kinases. These enzymes, which phosphorylate proteins at tyrosine residues, can be associated with receptor molecules, or, alternatively, the receptor itself can have this enzymatic activity. Once activated, the enzyme puts phosphate groups onto other proteins (and often onto itself), which can lead to activation of the target proteins and a continuation of signaling. If radioactive phosphate on ATP is present in the cell, the activated kinase will cause the radioactivity to associate with proteins. These can then be isolated and digested into single amino acids to determine if the radioactivity is on tyrosines in the protein. In this way, investigators can uncover tyrosine kinase activation during receptor signaling. More recently, antibodies have been made that directly recognize phosphorylated tyrosine, and this has greatly facilitated such studies.

Neither surface Ig nor the T-cell receptor complex (including CD3) display tyrosine kinase activity after cross-linking. However, one component of CD3 (CD3ζ), as well as CD4, CD8, and other molecules, become phosphorylated on tyrosines after T-cell activation. This has led some to speculate that tyrosine kinases might play a role in lymphocyte activation. The responsible enzyme appears to be a tyrosine kinase called p56^{lck}, which is associated with CD4 and CD8 molecules and is activated when they are cross-linked (see above for the involvement of these molecules in T-cell activation). We don't know, however, whether this phosphorylation is necessary for activation of T cells, or how p56^{lck} interacts with other intracellular signal systems. Further, no involvement of such tyrosine kinases has been shown in B-cell activation. In the next chapter we will see that some immunologically important receptors involved in growth factor effects probably do use the mechanism of tyrosine phosphorylation as a mode of signal transduction.

Tyrosine phosphorylation should not be confused with phosphorylation of serine and/or threonine, which also occurs during lymphocyte activation and is probably a function of protein kinase C (see below).

We've made this excursion into G proteins and tyrosine kinases to suggest that one or both of these mechanisms may play a role in getting a signal from the antigen receptor to the inside of the cell. It is also possible that lymphocytes use some other mechanism of signal transduction. For our purposes, though, it is only necessary to realize that mechanisms exist that allow cell-surface receptors to begin a signaling process that results in gene activation.

Now that a signal has been generated by the cross-linked receptor, intracellular second-messenger pathways become activated. In lymphocytes, these second messengers are becoming understood, and we will consider this step next.

Second Messengers and Lymphocyte Activation

When T or B cells are activated via their antigen receptors, at least two important events occur, which are likely to represent the intracellular pathways involved in signaling. These are the opening of *ion channels* in the membrane and the activation of the *phosphatidylinositide pathway*. Both these events occur within minutes of antigen receptor cross-linking.

Ion Fluxes

Calcium. Calcium enters the cell when a calcium channel opens in the cell membrane. This is called a CALCIUM FLUX. This flux can be assessed by first loading cells with a dye that fluoresces in the presence of calcium, and when the flux occurs, this fluorescence can then be accurately measured (see Figure 5). This has been observed after antigen receptor cross-linking in both B and T cells. Lymphocytes that are cultured under conditions in which calcium fluxes cannot occur fail to activate. The calcium channels on the surface of lymphocytes are different from those found on other cell types, but the precise nature of these channels is not yet known. In any case, this inward flux of calcium ions appears to be a crucial signal in lymphocyte activation as it is in many other cell types.

What does this calcium ion influx do to the cell? First, there are several intracellular enzymes that are dependent upon calcium for their function. These include protein kinase C, which is most probably an important player in lymphocyte activation (see below). In addition, calcium ions induce another protein kinase associated with CALMODULIN. It is not known, however, if calmodulin or calmodulin-dependent protein kinase plays a role in lymphocyte activation.

Most of the calcium inside a cell is stored in the endoplasmic reticulum, and the free calcium concentration within lymphocytes can also increase due to the release of this stored ion. The problem of understanding the physiological role of stored intracellular calcium is that cultured lymphocyte lines have a large amount of

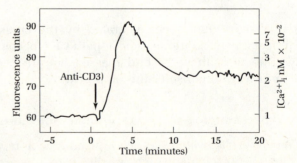

5 **Increase in Intracellular Calcium Following Receptor Cross-Linking.** Lymphocytes are pretreated with a dye that becomes fluorescent in the presence of calcium. Following cross-linking of antigen receptors (in this case, with anti-CD3), there is a rapid increase in the concentration of intracellular calcium, $[Ca^{2+}]_i$. [From Alcover et al. 1987. *Immunol. Rev.* 95: 5]

stored calcium, while resting lymphocytes may not. This can lead to differences in experimental results. Nevertheless, intracellular release of calcium occurs after activation, probably as a result of the action of products of the phosphatidylinositide pathway, discussed below.

The Na^+–H^+ Antiport.   Another ion flux that occurs during lymphocyte activation involves Na^+ and H^+ ions. Upon activation, Na^+ moves into the cell and H^+ moves out, resulting in an increase in intracellular pH. The ion channel responsible is called the Na^+–H^+ ANTIPORT, and its importance in lymphocyte activation is unclear. On the one hand, this channel is always activated when lymphocytes are stimulated. On the other hand, blocking the antiport with drugs appears to have no effect on lymphocyte proliferation. What these ion fluxes actually do in the cell is not known.

Having considered ion fluxes as one of the second messengers in lymphocyte activation, we now turn to another: the phosphatidylinositide pathway. This complex biochemical pathway has been implicated as a second-messenger system in many cell types, including lymphocytes.

The Phosphatidylinositide Pathway.   Following cross-linking of cell-surface antigen receptors, the phosphatidylinositide pathway becomes activated. This second-messenger system has been described in a number of cells, including B and T cells. It is shown schematically in Figure 6. PHOSPHOLIPASE C becomes activated to cleave PHOSPHATIDYLINOSITOL BISPHOSPHATE (PIP_2) into two active components: INOSITOL TRIPHOSPHATE (IP_3) and DIACYLGLYCERIDE (DAG). The components of this pathway are present within the membrane, and this hydrolysis occurs within minutes of lymphocyte activation. IP_3 goes on to induce the release of calcium ions from intracellular stores (which may or may not be a necessary step, given the calcium flux that also occurs and appears to be required). Probably more important is the action of DAG. This molecule causes PROTEIN KINASE C (PKC) to move from the cytoplasm to the cell membrane, where it in turn phosphorylates (on serines and threonines) several molecules, including $CD3_\gamma$, CD4, and CD8 in T cells and surface Ig in B cells. In addition, several cytoplasmic proteins become phosphorylated, though at present, the roles of these molecules are not certain.

The activation of PKC has been associated with the initial stages of lymphocyte activation by many lines of evidence. Depletion of PKC, or drugs that block its activity, prevents stimulation of lymphocyte activation through antigen receptors. Phosphorylation of surface molecules by PKC can change their activities, while phosphorylation of enzymes and other proteins in the cytoplasm can stimulate a wide range of functions. At present, we do not know which phosphorylation events are necessary for lymphocyte activation. We will discuss some events that are likely to be occurring, which in turn may be involved in gene activation, but these are currently only speculation. The intensive work that is going on in this area, however, will certainly help to put this puzzle together.

Lymphocyte Activation through Bypassing Antigen Receptors. If it is true that calcium fluxes and the phosphatidylinositide pathway are important second messengers in lymphocyte activation, then it should be possible to bypass the cell-surface antigen receptors on B cells or T cells by directly activating these messengers. In fact, this can be done, and it is probably because of such bypasses that many immunologists are confident in thinking that our notions are correct about the roles of these messengers in lymphocyte activation.[2]

In many studies, B or T cell activation has been induced by the combined actions of CALCIUM IONOPHORES and PHORBOL ESTERS. The ionophore allows calcium to flux into the cell, which, while producing some effects, is not sufficient to cause complete activation. Similarly, phorbol esters mimic DAG and activate PKC, and these also produce effects without complete activation. However, when *both* calcium ionophores and phorbol esters are added to lymphocytes, activation occurs.

This supports our current models of lymphocyte activation, but some caution is needed in interpreting these results. First, the activation produced in this way is seldom as extensive as that produced by cross-linking of the cell-surface receptors. Second, the fact that these agents activate cells does not *prove* that the same mechanisms are functioning naturally. Nevertheless, these approaches have given us some important insights into the cell biology of lymphocyte activation and tell us that we may be on the right track.

---

[2] We shouldn't, however, be *too* confident of our understanding of second messengers in lymphocyte activation. As with most concepts in immunology, even this area contains more than a little controversy, and it may well turn out that our ideas are destined to change.

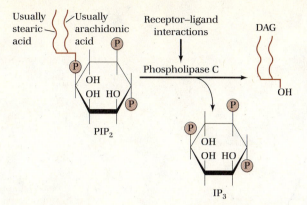

6 **Phosphatidylinositide Second-Messenger Pathway.** The cross-linking of cell-surface receptors leads to the activation of phospholipase C. This enzyme catalyzes the breakdown of phosphatidylinositol 4,5-bisphosphate (PIP_2) into 1,2-diacylglycerol (DAG) and inositol 1,4,5-trisphosphate (IP_3). DAG is involved in the translocation and activation of protein kinase C. Phospholipase C, PIP_2, and DAG function in the membrane, whereas IP_3 is released into the cytoplasm, where it can have additional effects.

SYNTHESIS
From the Membrane to the Cytoplasm

Lymphocyte activation, as we've considered it this far, is summarized in Figure 7. Following cross-linking of cell-surface molecules, including antigen receptors, a signal is generated. This signal is mediated via G proteins, tyrosine phosphorylation, or both (or via something else). The result is twofold: (1) calcium channels in the cell membrane open to allow calcium ions into the cell, and (2) phospholipase C is activated to hydrolyze PIP_2 to IP_3 and DAG. DAG then causes protein kinase C to move from the cytoplasm to the membrane, where it is activated to phosphorylate several cell-surface and cytoplasmic proteins. The entire process, from receptor cross-linking to protein phosphorylation, occurs in a matter of minutes.

We've managed, at this point, to get a signal from outside the cell to within the cytoplasm, but how does this result in gene activation? While we are sure that *something* happens next, we don't really know what the next step is. Recent advances in the process of gene activation, however, have given us some clues, and we can make some pretty fair guesses. We will consider these possibilities next.

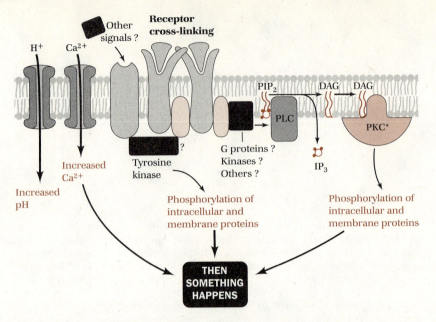

7 **Summary of Known and Hypothesized Membrane Events in Lymphocyte Activation.** Black boxes indicate processes that have not been fully elucidated in lymphocytes (or for which roles are not yet understood). Following these events, the cell activates genes involved in cell growth and differentiation, but, again, the mechanisms are not yet known.

Possible Routes from Protein Phosphorylation to Gene Activation

At this point in our scheme of lymphocyte activation, changes on the cell surface have led to changes in intracellular ion concentrations and to protein phosphorylation on the inner cell membrane and in the cytoplasm. In this section, we will suggest ways in which these events can lead to activation of specific genes. In order to do this, however, we will have to skip ahead a bit to consider the role of DNA-binding proteins in the activation of lymphocyte genes. We will then return to the problem of how these might be regulated by the intracellular signal pathways we've discussed.

Enhancers and DNA-Binding Proteins

Any eukaryotic gene that is differentially expressed in different tissues or under different circumstances is probably under the control of enhancer regions and their corresponding DNA-binding proteins. We briefly considered enhancers in our discussions of tissue-specific expression of Ig genes. You should recall that two distinct types of genetic regions, enhancers and promoters, control gene expression. Enhancers, unlike promoters, are generally neither position- nor orientation-dependent for their function.

During lymphocyte activation, some of the genes that are expressed are unique to lymphocytes and perhaps a few other cell types. Such genes have identifiable enhancer regions, and it is probably the binding of the appropriate DNA-BINDING PROTEIN to these regions that results in the transcriptional activation of the gene.

There are a number of ways in which enhancer regions for particular genes have been identified. The first step is generally an examination of the DNA "footprint" of the noncoding regions near or within a gene of interest. The basic idea is shown in Figure 8. Genomic DNA containing non-coding regions (near the gene of interest) is first exposed to extracts from the nuclei of cells in which the gene is active or inactive. For example, extracts from active versus inactive lymphocyte nuclei could be used to study the control of genes in lymphocyte activation. Proteins within the extracts with affinity for specific DNA sequences bind to the DNA. The DNA is then exposed to nucleases or chemical treatments that randomly cut the DNA at all sites not protected by bound protein. The DNA is then labeled and run on gels, often side by side with DNA labeled for sequencing. The net result is that every position corresponding to a nucleotide that is protected by a DNA-binding protein appears blank. The sequence of these protected regions is then read off the sequencing lanes.

Just because a region of DNA is specifically bound by a protein does not mean that it functions as an enhancer. To examine this possibility, a plasmid is constructed that contains the presumed enhancer, a promoter, and an indicator gene, which is usually the gene for chloramphenicol acetyl transferase (CAT). This construct is then transfected into cells, and the expression of the indicator gene is monitored (Figure 9). In the case of enhancers that may be involved in lymphocyte activation, the transfected cells are lymphoid (usually transformed lymphoid lines). Following transfection, the cells are activated (or not), and the effect of the presumed enhancer region on the expression of CAT is determined.

An example of interest is the gene for the low-affinity subunit for the interleukin-2 receptor (considered in more detail in the

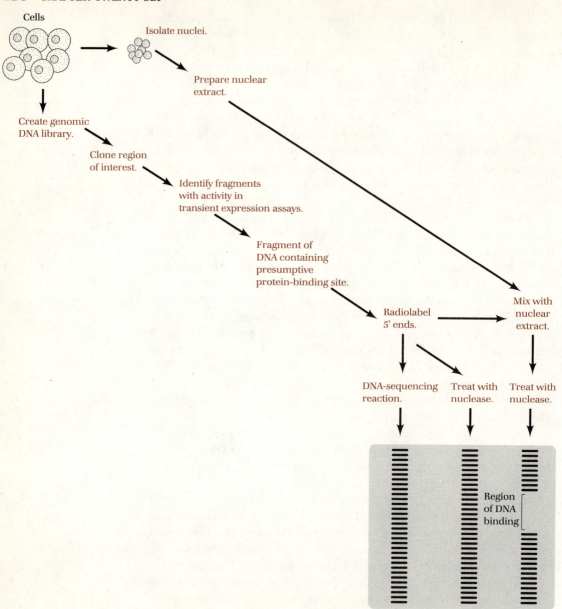

Cells

Isolate nuclei.

Prepare nuclear extract.

Create genomic DNA library.

Clone region of interest.

Identify fragments with activity in transient expression assays.

Fragment of DNA containing presumptive protein-binding site.

Radiolabel 5' ends.

Mix with nuclear extract.

DNA-sequencing reaction.

Treat with nuclease.

Treat with nuclease.

Region of DNA binding

8   DNA "Footprint" of a Protein-Binding Site. Segments of DNA that flank the gene of interest are examined for regulatory activity in a transient expression assay (see Figure 9), and active regions are identified. DNA segments are reacted with nuclear extracts (containing DNA-binding proteins) and then exposed to degradative enzymes. The portion of DNA that is bound by protein is protected from degradation, and by comparing the resulting fragments with untreated DNA and with the DNA sequence, the region of protein binding is determined.

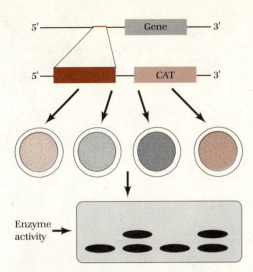

5' flanking region of a gene of interest is cloned from a genomic DNA library.

Fragments of the 5' flanking region are cloned upstream of the CAT gene (with or without promoter).

CAT constructs are transfected into different cells for transient expression.

Extracts are screened for CAT activity.

9   Transient Expression Assay. Segments of DNA that flank a gene of interest are cloned upstream from the gene for chloramphenicol acetyl transferase (CAT), with or without a promoter. The construct is then transfected into different cell types, and the expression of the indicator gene is monitored (by measuring enzyme activity). The regulatory effects of the DNA segment (e.g., promoter, enhancer, etc.) are thereby determined, as well as the tissue specificity of the effect.

next chapter). This gene is induced during the activation of T cells and is under the control of one or more enhancer regions. Each of these regions was placed into a construct containing the gene promoter for this receptor gene (together with the CAT indicator gene). When these constructs were transfected into a T-cell line and the cells were activated, enhanced expression of CAT was observed. In the absence of an enhancer region, no increased expression was observed upon activation of the transfected cell. Thus, these regions are involved in the control of the expression of this gene during T-cell activation.

Several DNA-binding proteins have been purified and characterized. In general, this is done by taking advantage of the specificity of the protein for a particular DNA sequence. The sequence of interest (identified by footprinting) is prepared and coupled to a solid matrix. Nuclear extracts containing the protein are then passed through the matrix, and subsequently, the bound protein is eluted. Heroic amounts of nuclear extract are usually required in order to purify enough protein for characterization. Another approach has been to make cDNA expression libraries from cells that produce the DNA-binding protein, and then to screen these libraries with the DNA sequences to which the protein binds. Surprisingly, this seemingly naive approach has worked in some cases, allowing a shortcut to the characterization of the protein.

One of the DNA-binding proteins that is important in expression of the interleukin-2 receptor gene mentioned above is called NFκB. This protein is also involved in the control of many other genes, including the κL chain in B cells. Different DNA-binding proteins are involved in the regulation of other genes in lymphocyte activation. The situation can get very complex, with both coordinate and independent regulation of genes by different DNA-binding proteins.

Activation of DNA-Binding Proteins in Lymphocyte Activation

In lymphocyte activation, it is very likely that many of the required DNA-binding proteins are already present (in an inactive form) in the cell before activation occurs. At present, little is known, however, about how a DNA-binding protein becomes activated to perform its functions. There are basically two ways in which inactive DNA-binding proteins in the cytoplasm have been shown to become active and move to the nucleus. (These have been shown in other systems and are not yet ascertained for lymphocyte activation.) One way is for the inactive protein to become phosphorylated. Obviously, then, the various kinases induced during lymphocyte activation have this as their goal: by phosphorylating an inactive DNA-binding protein, they cause the now-activated protein to move to the nucleus and begin activating genes. At last, the pathway from the membrane to the gene is complete!

Some DNA-binding proteins, however, are not phosphorylated. It is possible that these are present in inactive forms as a complex with an inhibitory protein. (This is the case for steroid receptors in the cytoplasm, which are inactive DNA-binding proteins until steroids bind, dissociate them from their inhibitor, and allow them to move to the nucleus.) It may be that the inhibitor is a target for phosphorylation, which causes the complex to dissociate and release the now-active DNA-binding protein. Recent evidence suggests that this may be the case for NFκB.

This is an extremely intensive area of research, and we will certainly gain a great deal of knowledge in the next few years. For the first time the control of gene activation by cell-surface events seems to be within reach.

Although we don't know the details, it may be enough for our purposes to realize that we have reached the point in our scheme at which genes are beginning to be expressed following activation. We will complete this chapter with a consideration of some of the genes expressed early in lymphocyte activation.

Early Gene Expression and Lymphocyte Activation

Within a few hours of receiving an activation signal, lymphocytes begin to express genes. Several of these genes are protooncogenes, genes that were originally identified by their ability (or the ability of slightly altered forms) to transform cells. In retrospect, it is not surprising that such genes would normally play a role in cellular activation.

The two genes that we will consider here are *c-fos* and *c-myc* (the *c* indicates that this is the cellular, rather than viral, form of the oncogene). These are expressed very early during activation, with *c-fos* mRNA usually appearing within 2 to 3 hours of culture, and *c-myc* mRNA appearing within the next few hours.

Expression of both these genes is an absolute requirement for lymphocyte activation.[3] This was shown by using a valuable molecular technique involving the control of gene function by "antisense." The basic idea behind this technique is shown in Figure 10. Cells are transfected with a construct that expresses an inverted gene sequence, yielding mRNA that is complementary to the mRNA of interest (hence, ANTISENSE RNA). When this antisense RNA is expressed in abundance, the mRNA of interest can be effectively blocked and the effects of this blocking analyzed. When this was done for both *c-fos* and *c-myc*, lymphocyte activation was prevented. Another approach is even simpler. Short stretches of antisense DNA can be easily synthesized, and when these are added to cells, the cells spontaneously take up these ANTISENSE OLIGODEOXY-NUCLEOTIDES, which then specifically block translation of the mRNA of interest. This has successfully been done for *c-myc* in T cells, where the *c-myc* antisense oligonucleotides blocked the proliferation of T cells after activation.

It is not entirely clear what roles these two protooncogenes have in lymphocyte activation. The *c-fos* gene encodes half a DNA-binding protein (the other half is encoded by another protooncogene called *c-jun*), but the role of this protein in activation has not been worked out. The *c-myc* gene produces a protein that is localized to the cell nucleus, but we know even less about what this protein does.

[3] *c-myc* and *c-fos* are activated in many cell systems, and the reader is not meant to think that they are unique to lymphocytes. Being immunologists, we are taking the parochial, lymphocyte-oriented view.

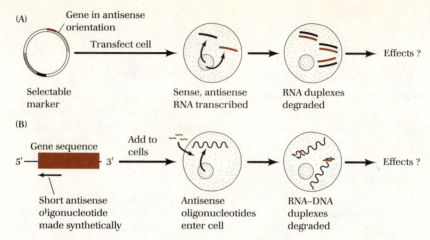

(A)

Gene in antisense orientation

Transfect cell

Selectable marker

Sense, antisense RNA transcribed

RNA duplexes degraded

Effects ?

(B)

Gene sequence

Add to cells

5'——————3'

Short antisense oligonucleotide made synthetically

Antisense oligonucleotides enter cell

RNA–DNA duplexes degraded

Effects ?

10   Control of Gene Expression by Antisense RNA or Oligodeoxy-nucleotides. (A) A gene of interest is cloned in antisense orientation into a mammalian expression vector (which also contains a selectable marker). This is then transfected into cells, which are selected for expression of the marker. Antisense RNA is expressed, and binds specifically to the appropriate mRNA in the cytoplasm, leading to degradation of the RNA–RNA duplexes. The biological effects are then assessed. (B) Small oligodeoxynucleotides corresponding to an antisense sequence (often at the translation start) of a gene of interest are synthesized. These may be chemically modified to increase their activity. The antisense oligonucleotides are added at high concentrations to cells and enter the cells in some way. These specifically bind to appropriate mRNA, forming heteroduplexes that are degraded. The biological effects are then assessed. While both approaches to the use of antisense have been successful in different systems and for different genes, other genes and systems have been resistant to control by these strategies.

Following expression of the protooncogenes, the activated lymphocyte begins to express genes for lymphokine receptors and, if it is a T cell, for lymphokines. In the next chapter we will consider the lymphokines and related factors that play roles in the immune response. We will then take up the story at the next stage: What happens when a lymphokine binds to its receptor on the lymphocyte surface?

Summary

1.   Lymphocyte activation begins when the cell-surface receptors on a B cell or T cell are cross-linked. Although this cross-linking is insufficient, on its own, to stimulate a normal cell, it is one of the primary signals.
2.   What happens next is not clear. In B cells it is likely that a signal is generated via G proteins, which in turn activate second-messenger

systems. It is equally likely that this is not what happens in most T cells; we don't know the actual transduction system in T cells.

3. Following transduction of the signal from the surface receptors, two second-messenger systems become activated: calcium ions flux into the cell and phosphatidylinositol bisphosphate breaks down to form inositol triphosphate and diacylglyceride. The latter stimulates the transduction and activation of protein kinase C. Although the second messengers have been proved to be activated in lymphocytes, alternative second messengers may exist.

4. Tyrosine kinases also become activated, and, together with protein kinase C, this leads to phosphorylation of a number of cell-surface and intracellular proteins. In ways that are not yet known, this in turn contributes to the activation of DNA-binding proteins.

5. DNA-binding proteins that bind specifically to DNA sequences are capable of controlling the transcription of genes. A number of specific DNA-binding proteins (and the DNA sequences they recognize) have been identified on genes involved in lymphocyte activation. It is very likely that such interactions represent the final step in transducing a signal from the cell-surface to the activation of specific genes.

6. Among the genes that become expressed early in lymphocyte activation are a number of protooncogenes. The products of these genes (such as those of *c-fos*) may be involved in forming DNA-binding proteins, or may have other functions not yet defined (such as those of *c-myc*). Studies have shown, however, that the expression of these genes is critical for lymphocyte activation. Other genes involved in lymphocyte activation include the genes for growth factors and their receptors.

Additional Readings

Alexander, D. R. and D. A. Cantrell. 1989. Kinases and phosphatases in T cell activation. *Immunol. Today* 10: 200.

Cambier, J. C. and J. T. Ransom. 1987. Molecular mechanisms of transmembrane signaling in B lymphocytes. *Annu. Rev. Immunol.* 5: 175.

Gelfand, E. W., G. B. Mills, R. K. Cheung, J. W. W. Lee and S. Grinstein. 1987. Transmembrane ion fluxes during activation of human T lymphocytes: Role of Ca^{++}, Na^+/H^+ exchange, and phospholipid turnover. *Immunol. Rev.* 95: 59.

Isakov, N., M. I. Mally, W. Scholz, and A. Altman. 1987. T lymphocyte activation: The role of protein kinase C and the bifurcating inositol phospholipid signal transduction pathway. *Immunol. Rev.* 95: 89.

Janeway, C. A., J. Rojo, K. Saizawa, U. Dianzani, P. Portoles, J. Tite, S. Hague, and B. Jones. 1989. The co-receptor function of CD4. *Immunol. Rev.* 109: 77.

Mustelin, T., and A. Altman. 1989. Do CD4 and CD8 control T cell activation via a specific tyrosine protein kinase? *Immunol. Today* 10:189.

LYMPHOCYTE ACTIVATION II
Growth and Differentiation Factors

Overview The principal manner by which the cells of the immune system communicate is through the elaboration of soluble factors. These growth and differentiation factors are essentially hormones made by the cells of the immune system. These factors are called lymphokines and cytokines, and they act on the other cells of the immune system to regulate their function. We have already seen some of these factors, the colony-stimulating factors, and discussed their roles in hemopoiesis. In this chapter, we will discover many more.

In the last chapter we discussed some of the events that occur within lymphocytes upon antigen recognition. Among the genes activated in this cascade of intracellular signals are those for lymphokines and their receptors. We will see that these growth and differentiation factors are essential players in the activation of lymphocytes. In this chapter we will pick up where we left off in the last: with the induction of growth and differentiation factors and their receptors.

The nature of these factors is becoming clear, and studies are now beginning to show how these molecules initiate intracellular events in the cells of the immune system. The emerging picture reveals that very little about the signal transduction from the cell membrane to the nucleus in lymphocytes may be unique, and that studies in a variety of cell systems will prove to be applicable to the cells of the immune system.

Growth and Differentiation Factors in Lymphocyte Activation

In the 1970s many laboratories carried out experiments showing that soluble factors from spleen cells could be used to augment mitogen-induced responses or to substitute for helper T cells. Each laboratory used a slightly different assay system, and each laboratory gave its factor a unique name and acronym. The array reached almost comic proportions, and it soon became clear that Nature would not be cruel enough to use this apparently endless array of factors to effect proliferation and differentiation. It was also clear that order had to be brought to the near chaotic situation. So in 1979, a group of investigators actively working in this field met at Ermatigen, Switzerland, and made a systematic comparison of all the known factors. They concluded that the only differences between most of them were the names and the manner in which they were assayed. In fact, they concluded, the bewildering array really consisted of only two factors.

A generic name that had no meaning in any known language (and would therefore have a low probability of offending anyone) was chosen to replace the names that usually described how the factor was assayed. The factors were called INTERLEUKINS because this neologism gives a vague hint of involvement in communication between the cells. The two factors were called INTERLEUKIN-1 and INTERLEUKIN-2 (IL-1 and IL-2). The prototypic factor for IL-1 was lymphocyte activating factor (LAF); that for IL-2 was T-cell growth factor (TCGF).

Since then, many more interleukins have been identified and characterized (it now appears that Nature is, perhaps, so cruel!). They receive a number only after the genes have been cloned and sequenced and at least some biological activity is known. The biochemical and biological properties of the known interleukins are given in Table 1. We have also included a list of several other factors, including the interferons and the tumor necrosis factors. You should remember that there are also colony-stimulating factors produced by cells of the immune system (see Chapter 12). It's a big list, and growing bigger all the time.

A Note on Names

Immunologists have always had a bad habit of generating a perplexing jargon, and some of the worst of it has been in the area of growth and differentiation factors. Every time something has been done about this (for example, calling all such factors *interleukins*), more problems crop up. So, the best we can do is to try to help you sort through what the various terms mean, or are supposed to mean.

- LYMPHOKINES, MONOKINES, and CYTOKINES are terms that were coined to refer to factors produced uniquely by lymphocytes,

Table 1 Some growth and differentiation factors in the immune system.

INTERLEUKINS

Factor	Chemical characteristics	Produced by	Biological actions	Other names
IL-1α,β	Mr 17Kd, pI 5.0 (α), pI 7.0 (β)	Macrophages, epithelial cells, endothelial cells, dendritic cells, Langerhans cells, B-cells, some T-cells, astrocytes, and others.	Enhances T- and B-cell activation, induces fever; induces acute-phase reactants, induces fibroblast proliferation (through PDGF), induces sleep, hemopoietic growth factor	Lymphocyte-activating factor, pyrogenic factor, hemopoietic factor-1, B-cell-activating factor.
IL-2	Mr 15.5 Kd	T cells	Promotes growth of T cells, induces p55 subunit of IL-2 receptor, NK-cell activation, B-cell growth and differentiation	T-cell growth factor, costimulator.
IL-3	Mr 30–40 Kd	T cells, epidermal cells (?)	Mast cell growth, formation of neutrophils, macrophages, megakaryocytes, and mast cells from precursors	Colony-forming unit-stimulating activity, panspecific hemopoietin, multi-CSF.
IL-4	Mr 15–16 Kd, pI 6.7 (human)	T cells, mast cells	Promotes T-cell growth, B-cell production of IgE and (with IL-5) IgA, mast-cell growth factor	B-cell growth factor, B-cell-stimulating factor-1, T-cell growth factor-2, mast-cell growth factor-2.
IL-5	Core: Mr 12.4 Kd exists as dimer, Mr 45–50 Kd	T cells	Growth and differentiation of eosinophils, B-cell proliferation and IgA production (with IL-4), thymocyte stimulation	T-cell-replacing factor, B-cell growth factor II, eosinophil differentiation factor, IgA-enhancing factor.

IL-6	Mr 19–26 Kd, pI 6.2, 6.4	Monocytes, T cells, fibroblasts, endothelial cells	B-cell differentiation and IgG production, promotes growth of hybridomas, supports growth of T-cells and thymocytes (with IL-2), induces synthesis of acute-phase proteins from hepatocytes	B-cell-stimulating factor-2, interferon-β2, hepatocyte growth factor.
IL-7	Mr 25 Kd	Bone marrow stromal cells	Stimulates pre-B and pre-T cells, enhances thymocyte proliferation (with mitogen)	Lymphopoietin-1.
IL-8	~Mr 10 Kd, pI 8 - 8.5	Monocytes, endothelial cells, fibroblasts	Neutrophil chemotaxis, T-cell chemotaxis at high doses	Monocyte-derived neutrophil chemotactic factor, neutrophil-activating factor, monocyte-derived neutrophil-activating peptide.
IL-9	Core: Mr 16 Kd, exists as dimer, ~Mr 40 Kd	Some T-cells	Stimulation of T cells and mast cells	T-cell derived p40.
IL-10	Core: Mr 17 Kd, exists as dimer, Mr 34-40 Kd	T_{H2} cells	Inhibition of antigen presentation to T_{H1} cells, stimulation of mast cells and thymocytes, induction of class II MHC	Cytokine secretion inhibitory factor.
TUMOR NECROSIS FACTORS				
TNFα	Mr 17 Kd	Macrophages, T cells, B cells	Tumor cytotoxicity, mediates endotoxic shock, induces cachexia (wasting), stimulation of fibroblasts and melanocytes, activation of macrophages and neutrophils	Cachectin.
TNFβ	Mr 17 Kd 30% homology with TNFα	T cells	Tumor cytotoxicity, B-cell activation under some conditions, many other activities shared with TNFα	Lymphotoxin.

(Continued)

447

Table 1 (*continued*)

Factor	Chemical characteristics	Produced by	Biological actions	Other names
INTERFERONS				
α-INF	At least 20 subtypes Mr 15–21 Kd	Most cells, including epithelial cells, macrophages	Anti-viral activity, enhances class I MHC expression, increases NK function	
β-INF	Mr 20–25 Kd, 16 Kd core	Fibroblasts, other cells	Anti-viral activity, enhances class I MHC expression, increases NK function	
γ-INF	Sensitive to low pH Mr 15 Kd	T cells	Activates macrophages, induces or increases class I and class II MHC on many cells, stimulates some B cells, enhances IgG_{2a} production, inhibits IgG_1 and IgE, inhibits proliferation of T_{H2} cells, anti-viral activity	Immune interferon.
TRANSFORMING GROWTH FACTOR				
TGFβ	Mr 12.5 Kd, exists as dimer, 25 Kd, activated at pH 2.	T cells, B cells	Inhibits proliferation of T cells and B cells, IgA switch factor	

monocytes (or macrophages), and other cells, respectively. Very quickly, however, it became clear that many factors were produced by many different cell types. Some investigators suggested that all factors simply be called *cytokines*, but this never caught on. Sometimes the terms are used interchangeably (*cytokines* has replaced *monokines* in many lexicons), but they are easier to say than *growth and/or differentiation factors*. Don't get too worried about what's what; in a pinch use this rule: if it came from a lymphocyte, it's a lymphokine; if it came from anything else, it's a cytokine.

- *Interleukins*, as we've seen, is a term that is meant simply to refer to factors that go between white cells. In general, this has been a popular name; however, many interleukins also act on cells that are *not* white cells (see Table 1). Also, many investigators don't like the trend toward producing a big list of numbers ("Where will it end?") and opt instead for names that are more descriptive.

- *Colony Stimulating Factors*, or *CSFs*, are growth and differentiation factors that stimulate the formation of differentiated colonies from stem cells. We saw these earlier in our discussion of hemopoiesis (Chapter 12).

- Finally, the *interferons* are a group of factors with antiviral activity. These also have effects on cells of the immune system, and we will consider one of these, γ-interferon, in more detail in this chapter.

There isn't much we can do, at present, about this complicated situation. The trouble is that growth and differentiation factors are extremely important to our current understanding of immune interactions, and there really isn't an alternative to simply memorizing the names of the most important players[1].

The Discovery of IL-2

In 1976, Doris Morgan, Francis Ruscetti, and Robert Gallo at the National Institutes of Health discovered that human T cells could be grown in continuous culture in the presence of the supernatant fluid from cultures of mitogen-stimulated cells. This discovery, as we have seen, made it possible to grow normal, nontransformed, functional T cells as clones in culture. The factor was to become known as T-cell growth factor (TCGF). At the same time, a similar finding was made in Edmonton, by Gordon Mills and Verner Paet-

---

[1] It will probably turn out that no more than ten (or so) of these are the *most* important (from the point of view of immunologists). We just don't know which ones these are.

kau, who found and characterized a "costimulator" factor that drove the proliferation of murine thymocytes. A crucial discovery was made two years later when Steven Gillis, Kendall Smith, and their colleagues at Dartmouth devised a simple, unequivocal assay for TCGF. In this assay, a TCGF-dependent cell line was grown in the presence of various concentrations of TCGF. The ability of the added TCGF to cause proliferation of these cells was then determined by quantifying the incorporation of tritiated thymidine. This situation represents one of those cases in which a standard method is needed in order for an advance to be made, because, as we have learned, many investigators had been generating "factors" and assaying them in a variety of ways. With the development of this simple, unambiguous assay, a simple and accurate means of quantifying and comparing various factors became available. The 1979 workshop mentioned earlier classified the many factors that had TCGF-like activity as a single factor, which they called interleukin 2, or IL-2.

Since then, IL-2 has been well characterized in a number of mammals, as well as other vertebrate species. It is, perhaps, the most important mediator of lymphocyte activation (or, at least, one of the most important), and its mode of action is one of the best understood. In this chapter, we will spend some time discussing the roles IL-2 plays in the immune response. The reader should be aware at the outset, however, that IL-2 is not the only important player in these processes.

Production of IL-2 by T Cells

Diverse pieces of evidence can be marshaled to show that IL-2 is a product of the T cell. First, it is elicited by T-cell mitogens such as concanavalin A (ConA) and phytohemagglutinin (PHA). Second, when a population of mouse spleen cells is treated with anti-Thy-1 and complement to eliminate T cells, it is unable to produce IL-2. Furthermore, mature T cells are the source of the material, because thymocytes, which contain only a few percent of mature functional cells, are a very poor source of IL-2. On the other hand, cortisone-resistant thymocytes, which are mature T cells, are the best source. Spleen, which contains 30% Thy-1$^+$ cells, all of which are mature and functional, is also a good source. Of the mature, functional T cells, it is the CD4$^+$ subpopulation that is responsible for most of the production, because treatment with anti-CD4 and complement reduces the ability to produce IL-2, but treatment with anti-CD8 and complement does not. This is a general finding, applicable to mammals and birds, and probably other vertebrates as well.

The Cloning of IL-2 and Other Factors

A tremendous explosion in knowledge occurred in the 1980s (and continues) with the development of methods for the cloning of genes that encode growth and differentiation factors. In general, two methods have been successfully employed in these efforts. Both require highly sensitive and rapid assays for the detection of the factor. The first involves biochemical purification of the factor to the point that some amino acid sequence information can be obtained. Based on this information, all the nucleotide sequences capable of encoding a small part of the protein are predicted and synthesized, and these oligonucleotides are then used to screen cDNA libraries (made from cells producing the factor). A second approach, shown schematically in Figure 1, uses a shortcut. cDNA from cells producing the factor is put into a eukaryotic expression vector, which has the capability of transiently expressing the cDNA when the construct is transfected into cells. This cDNA library is divided into pools, and each pool is transfected into cells, usually COS-7 (a monkey cell line). The supernatants from each transfection are tested for the presence of the factor, and a positive indicates that the gene of interest is in that pool. This pool is again divided up into smaller pools. The process is repeated until a single construct is isolated, one which contains the cDNA encoding the factor. This process sounds easier than it really is; nevertheless, a great many growth and differentiation factors have been characterized in this (or a similar) way.

With the availability of recombinant growth factors, a great deal of analysis was possible on how different factors affect different cells. In addition, purified growth factors were used to generate monoclonal antibodies capable of specifically neutralizing the activity of the growth factors. Using these tools, the roles of the different growth factors in lymphocyte activation and function began to be unraveled.

IL-2 and T-Cell Activation

When a CD4[+] T cell is activated, it often (but not always) transiently turns on the IL-2 gene via the mechanisms discussed in the last chapter (at least some of the DNA-binding proteins involved in activation of this gene have been identified, but are not yet well characterized). The production of IL-2 by the activated T cell then

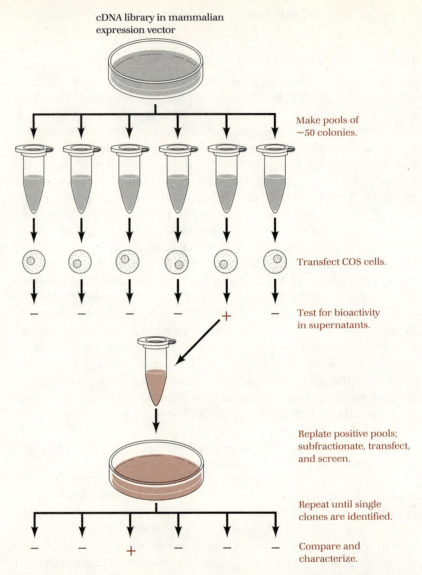

cDNA library in mammalian
expression vector

Make pools of
~50 colonies.

Transfect COS cells.

Test for bioactivity
in supernatants.

Replate positive pools;
subfractionate, transfect,
and screen.

Repeat until single
clones are identified.

Compare and
characterize.

1   An Approach to the Cloning of Genes for Growth and Differentiation Factors. cDNA is prepared from cells making a factor of interest, and a library is constructed using a vector capable of expression in mammalian cells. Small pools of the library are prepared (e.g., 50 colonies) and used to transiently transfect cells. The supernatants of the transfected cells are collected and tested for biological activity. Pools that transfer ability to make the factor are then further divided, until individual colonies are identified. The cDNA responsible for making the factor is then characterized.

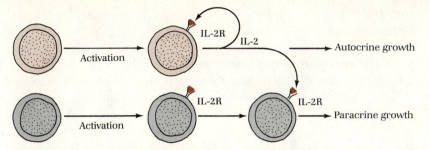

2 Autocrine versus Paracrine Growth. In the examples shown, the growth factor is IL-2, but any growth factor can stimulate these two types of growth.

plays an essential role in driving the cell to proliferate. Thus, the same cell can produce and then utilize IL-2, a process called AUTOCRINE GROWTH. On the other hand, CD8[+] T cells produce little IL-2, and require this factor from the CD4[+] T cells for maximal growth. This, then, is PARACRINE GROWTH (see Figure 2).

The importance of IL-2 in the activation of normal, resting T cells has been demonstrated in both mouse and human cells by adding anti–IL-2 antibodies, capable of neutralizing this factor, to stimulated cultures. These antibodies block the proliferation of the stimulated cells, showing that this factor is essential. With long-term T-cell clones, on the other hand, such antibodies sometimes block proliferation, and sometimes they don't. As we'll see, this is because some T cells can use a different T-cell growth factor for autocrine growth.

In order for IL-2 to contribute to the activation of a T cell, it must bind to a receptor. This receptor is expressed (in its complete form) only during the activation of the T cell. Like most things in immunology, the IL-2 receptor story is complex (and unfinished).

SYNTHESIS
Antigen-Nonspecific Mediators of
Antigen-Specific Responses

By now you know that clonal selection depends upon the specific interaction between an antigen and a lymphocyte, leading to proliferation of the lymphocyte. We have seen that T-cell receptors interact specifically with the ligand formed from MHC and antigen, and that this sets off a sequence of intracellular events leading to clonal selection.

But now we have introduced the idea that as an essential part of this process an antigen-*nonspecific* growth factor (IL-2) is released from the cell and stimulates growth in both an autocrine and a paracrine fashion. How can we reconcile this with the requirements for clonal selection?

The answer is one of unexpected elegance, and we develop it in more detail below. It is simply this: lymphocyte activation results in the surface expression of a growth factor receptor (e.g., IL-2 receptor) *that is not otherwise present on the cell*. In this way, only those cells that have come into contact with specific antigen are prepared to respond to the nonspecific signal.

In autocrine growth, the cell that has been induced to make a growth factor also begins to express a receptor for the factor. In paracrine growth, the recipient cell, upon induction, does not make a growth factor, but makes a receptor for a factor produced by another cell.

IL-2 Receptors

We have just seen that when T cells are activated by antigen (or mitogen) they produce IL-2. The IL-2, in turn, induces T cells to proliferate. It can be shown that during the course of this reaction, the IL-2 that is produced disappears from the medium (the same is true for exogenously added IL-2). Radiolabeled IL-2 can be shown to bind to the activated T cells. These facts strongly suggest that the binding of IL-2 is to a specific *receptor* (IL-2R). In fact, the kinetics of the binding of the labeled material, the saturation curves, and tissue and ligand specificities all suggest that a specific receptor is involved. The binding studies showed that IL-2 binds to the receptor with two different affinities: a high affinity ($K_d = 10^{-11}$ M) and a low affinity ($K_d = 10^{-9}$ M). Saturation studies showed that the receptors are saturated at about the same concentration of IL-2 that causes T-cell proliferation.

By chance, a monoclonal antibody against the IL-2 receptor, called ANTI-TAC or ANTI-CD25, was developed against a then-unknown molecule on activated T cells. (In addition to its usefulness as a tool, it shows the power of the monoclonal antibody technique. It is extremely difficult to produce an antibody against a single, unique antigen on the surface of a cell.) Anti-Tac blocks the binding of radiolabeled IL-2 and prevents IL-2-dependent T-cell proliferation, which strongly suggests that anti-Tac is directed against the IL-2 receptor.

When anti-Tac was used to *isolate* the receptor from the membrane (using reasoning and methods very much like those that were used to isolate the T-cell receptor; Chapter 22), it was found that this receptor molecule is a glycoprotein that consists of a single chain and has a molecular weight of 55,000. We now refer to this molecule as p55, or IL-2Rα.

It didn't take long to realize that IL-2Rα is not the whole story. The gene was cloned by Warren Leonard and Warner Greene at NIH, and almost simultaneously by Tasuku Honjo and colleagues in Kyoto. When the product of the gene was examined, they found that the binding of IL-2 to this molecule has a low affinity ($K_d = 10^{-9} M$). This was a clue that at least one more molecule was needed for high-affinity binding.

By cross-linking radiolabeled IL-2 to its receptor on activated T cells, it was possible to detect another part of the IL-2 receptor. This protein, with a molecular weight of 70 to 75 kd, is now called IL-2Rβ. The gene for this protein was cloned and characterized by Tadatsugu Taniguchi and colleagues in Osaka.

Low levels of IL-2Rβ molecules are already present on many resting T cells. This protein, by itself, binds IL-2 with an intermediate affinity ($K_d = 10^{-10} M$). Upon stimulation, the T cell activates both the gene for IL-2Rβ and that for IL-2Rα. Some of the molecules appear on the surface of the cell as a complex of both, and this complex has a high affinity for IL-2 ($K_d = 10^{-11} M$).

This high-affinity receptor has an interesting property. IL-2 binds and dissociates rapidly from IL-2Rα and only slowly from IL-2Rβ. However, with the complex, the binding of IL-2 is rapid, and its dissociation is slow. So we see that the formation of a high-affinity IL-2R occurs following activation by the expression of one of the molecules of this receptor, the IL-2Rα chain, and the association of this chain with the IL-2Rβ chain on the surface. It is this high-affinity receptor that binds physiological concentrations of IL-2.

We thought for a while that this would wrap up the IL-2 receptor story. Recently, however, additional molecules associated with the IL-2 receptor have been identified, and these are believed to also form part of the receptor. It is very likely that our picture of this important receptor will continue to change in the near future.

Signals Generated by the Interaction of
IL-2 with Its Receptor

Unlike the binding of ligands to cell-surface antigen receptors on lymphocytes, the binding of IL-2 to the IL-2 receptor complex does not generate either a calcium flux or hydrolysis of phosphatidyl-inositides (see Chapter 26). Further, blocking of protein kinase C function, or use of mutant cell lines that lack protein kinase C, demonstrated that this enzyme is not required for the growth-promoting effects of IL-2. Rather, it appears that signal transduction through this receptor depends, as in many other receptor systems, upon enzymatic properties of the receptor complex itself.

When IL-2 binds to its receptor, a tyrosine kinase activity is seen within minutes. This was shown by Gordon Mills and colleagues in Toronto, who precipitated this molecule with antibodies to phosphotyrosine after interaction of IL-2 and IL-2 receptor. The role of tyrosine phosphorylation in IL-2 receptor function is not yet understood, and at present neither the nature of the tyrosine kinase nor how it associates with the IL-2 receptor are known.

What we do know is that the outcome of the events that follow IL-2 binding to its receptor is the induction of genes and molecules necessary for entry into S phase of the cell cycle and clonal expansion of the cell. So we can now see how nonspecific initiators of growth can induce the proliferation of specific cells: the antigen induces the appearance of the receptor and the synthesis of IL-2, which reacts with the receptor. Any cell that has not been activated by antigen does not have the complete receptor, and therefore the IL-2 that is present does not affect these cells.

Growth and Differentiation Factors in Helper T-Cell Function

Profiles of Growth Factor Production by Helper T Cells

For a long time, IL-2 was believed to be *the* T-cell growth factor. In the process of studying growth and differentiation factors for B cells, however, Tasuku Honjo and his colleagues in Kyoto (among others) discovered another growth factor, which came to be called IL-4. Like IL-2, IL-4 turns out to be a T-cell growth factor that acts on its target cells via a unique receptor. Some of its properties are listed in Table 1.

Timothy Mosmann and Robert Coffman in Palo Alto examined the production of IL-2, IL-4, and other factors from cloned murine T-cell lines. They found that, in general, most helper-cell clones produced *either* IL-2 or IL-4, but not both. Further, they found that those that produce IL-2 can also produce γ-interferon, while those producing IL-4 also produce IL-5. Variations on this pattern were not found, leading them to propose that there are (at least) two types of helper cells, which they called T_{H1} and T_{H2}. A more complete listing of the growth factor profiles of these two types of helper cells is shown in Table 2.

The real importance of this finding came with the realization, by a number of investigators, that these two types of helper T cells have dramatically different *functions*. T_{H1} cells, because of the factors they produce, help in the induction of delayed-type hypersensitivity via macrophage activation, generation of CTLs, and induction of B cells to make IgG_{2a}. T_{H2} cells, on the other hand, cannot induce DTH, but rather induce B cells to make IgG_1, IgA, and IgE. Further, these cells (via their factors) appear to actually induce B cells to undergo class switching in order to produce these isotypes.

When a B cell contacts antigen, it receives part of its activation signal (as we've discussed), the remainder of which is delivered by the helper T cell (also discussed below). The isotype of antibody produced by the B cell, however, depends in part on the type of

Table 2   Profiles of growth and differentiation factors produced by murine T_{H1} vs. T_{H2} clones.[a]

Factor	T_{H1}	T_{H2}
IL-3	+ +	+
GM-CSF	+ +	+
TNF_α	+ +	+
IL-2	+ +	−
γ-INF	+ +	−
TNF_β	+ +	−
IL-4	−	+ +
IL-5	−	+ +
IL-6	−	+ +
IL-10	−	+ +

[a]Actual quantities of factors produced by individual clones may differ greatly, but the general patterns remain surprisingly constant.

helper T cell it interacts with. It then proceeds to secrete antibodies and often differentiates into a plasma cell.

The concept of T_{H1} and T_{H2} helper cells has greatly improved our understanding of what guides an immune response into a particular effector system. What, however, decides whether a T_{H1} or T_{H2} cell is involved?

Recent findings suggest that normal resting T cells are not committed to either the T_{H1} or T_{H2} pattern, but that after repeated stimulation a profile seems to be chosen. At present, the nature of this decision is unclear. This is an intensive area of research, and many questions concerning these cells are outstanding. For example, the existence of T_{H1} and T_{H2} cells in humans is controversial. In the next few years, we will certainly see some action in this important area.

In any case, the idea that growth factors from helper T cells provide the additional signals needed by antigen-induced B cells for activation seems correct. At first glance, however, this seems inconsistent with the idea that B cell activation (in cooperation with helper T cells) requires both hapten and carrier bound together. If the role of the carrier is simply to activate T cells to produce growth factors for the B cells, then why must it be linked to the hapten? We consider this question next.

The Problem of Hapten–Carrier-Linked Recognition in T–B Cooperation

Recall from Chapter 17 that the induction of an antibody response requires both the hapten and the carrier *linked together*. How does this observation fit with the picture of lymphocyte activation developing here? This question has puzzled several generations of immunologists. There has been no definitive hypothesis supported by experimental data. There are, however, reasonable models, and we will present one of them here.

Recall from Chapter 20 that B cells can present antigen to T cells. When a B cell binds a hapten (and thus its carrier) its activation pathway is induced. At the same time, the antigen and cross-linked surface Ig are internalized and processed, and peptide fragments are represented together with class II MHC on the surface. The idea is that *peptide fragments of the carrier are presented by the B cell because the carrier was linked to the hapten determinant bound by the B cell's antigen receptor*. These carrier peptides are then presented to carrier-specific T cells, which, upon activation, now release growth factors to help the B cell.

We've made two assumptions in using this model to explain the requirement for linked recognition of carrier and hapten. The first is that after antigen has entered the system (and T cells have undergone proliferation in response to the carrier presented by, say, macrophages), these T cells can then find B cells displaying the carrier. The second is that the growth factors released by the T cells operate over a very short range.

According to this hypothesis, carrier-specific helper T cells and hapten-specific B cells are able to specifically cooperate in antibody responses to the hapten because of the processes of antigen presentation by the B cell and the short range of action of growth factor from the T cell.

Helper–Effector Cooperation in Cell-Mediated Immunity

The basic principles of antigen presentation, helper-T-cell activation, and growth factor release apply not only to helper T cell–B cell interactions, but also to cell-mediated immunity (as we saw in Chapter 18). In general, the process is the same.

T_{H1}-cell clones can produce DTH when injected together with antigen into a site such as the footpad of a mouse. This response depends, at least in part, on a macrophage–T-cell interaction that is analogous to the B–T interaction considered above. The macrophage presents the specific antigen to the T cell, which in turn releases growth factors (notably γ-interferon among others) that stimulate the macrophage. In this reaction, unlike the B–T interaction, bystander activation of other resident and recruited cells appears to play an important role in the overall response.

In Chapters 17 to 19, we discussed the cellular interactions and roles of MHC in the generation of cytotoxic T cells. Upon recognition of specific antigen, these cells progress to the stage at which they express growth factor receptors and then await paracrine stimulation by helper cells. This seems to be (at least) a three-cell system, in which an APC brings the helper cell into proximity with the precytotoxic T cell.

SYNTHESIS
The Consequences of Activation

For decades immunologists tried to find the unique features of the immune system. So far, they have been able to show that the division of labor, MHC restriction, gene reorganization, and interleukin cascade all have aspects that can be considered to be unique to the immune system. But as we come to this part of the narrative, which deals with the consequences of bringing all these things together, we must leave the realm of the uniquely immunologic and enter the world of general cell biology. The events that follow receptor activation by antigen, and growth factor–receptor interaction, seem to be events common to many cell systems. Much of the research in immunology in the next decade will be cell and molecular biology that happens to use lymphocytes rather than sea urchins, transformed tissue culture cells, or the retina. The flip side of this, of course, is that facts and concepts garnered from the more traditional cell biology systems can be readily applied to the immune system. Immunologists of the future will have to be very good biologists, and may, sad to say, have to give up their identity as fearless pioneers at the frontier of an arcane field and join the ranks of the rest of the biological community.[2]

Summary

1.   T cells, macrophages, and other cells produce factors (lymphokines, monokines, and cytokines, respectively) that act on other cells in the immune system. One generic term for these factors is *interleukins*.

2.   There is a growing list of growth and differentiation factors involved in immune functions. These have a wide range of effects, either alone or in concert with others, and appear to be one of the principal ways (together with antigen presentation) that cells of the immune system communicate.

3.   Only T cells expressing high-affinity IL-2 receptors are induced to proliferate by IL-2. Activation by antigen induces the expression of low-affinity IL-2 receptors (IL-2Rα) that associate with a second, intermediate affinity chain on the cell surface (IL-2Rβ). The combination produces a high-affinity receptor for IL-2. It is likely that similar processes occur for other inducible receptors for the growth and differentiation factors of the immune system.

4.   The lymphokine IL-4 is needed for proliferation and differentiation of some B cells, while IL-2 works on others. These short-range growth factors are able to stimulate the APCs (e.g., the hapten-specific B cells that present the linked carrier).

5.   The consequences of the binding of a growth (and/or differentiation) factor to its receptor involve signal transduction from the membrane to the nucleus via second messengers. These can be distinct from the signals generated via the antigen receptor. The result, though, is the completion of lymphocyte activation, DNA synthesis, and cell

---

[2] Where many will probably become fearless pioneers of these new arcane fields.

division. Thus, in accordance with the clonal selection theory, antigen recognition by the lymphocyte is a critical requirement for clonal expansion (even if the route is somewhat roundabout).

Additional Readings

Durum, S. K. and J. J. Oppenheim. 1989. Macrophage-derived mediators: Interleukin 1, tumor necrosis factor, Interleukin 6, interferon, and related factors. In W. E. Paul, ed., *Fundamental Immunology*, 2nd ed. Raven, New York, p. 639.

Gillis, S. 1989. T cell derived lymphokines. In W. E. Paul, ed., *Fundamental Immunology*, 2nd ed. Raven, New York, p. 621.

Howard, M., and W. E. Paul. 1983. Regulation of B cell growth and differentiation by soluble factors. *Annu. Rev. Immunol.* 1:307.

Mosmann, T. R. and R. L. Coffman. 1989. T_{H1} and T_{H2} cells: Different patterns of lymphokine secretion lead to different functional properties. *Annu. Rev. Immunol.* 7: 145.

Kishimoto, T. 1985. Factors affecting B cell growth and differentiation. *Annu. Rev. Immunol.* 3: 133.

Smith, K. A. 1984. Interleukin-2. *Annu. Rev. Immunol.* 2: 283.

CYTOTOXIC EFFECTOR CELL MECHANISMS

Overview   So far, we've seen how helper cells help other cells (and themselves) through the production of growth and differentiation factors. We have also seen how B cells and antibodies perform their effector functions. But we have only hinted at the phenomena involving cell-mediated cytotoxicity, and these are the focus of this chapter.

Cytotoxicity, the killing of one cell by another, can be mediated by a number of different cell types. We have already mentioned the cytotoxic T cells, which are usually CD8$^+$ and class I MHC-restricted. The CD8$^+$ cytotoxic cells, because of their class I MHC restriction, seem to be specialized for killing cells expressing novel antigens in their cytoplasm (since this appears to be the only way that the antigen can be processed and presented with class I MHC—see Chapter 20). Other cells with cytotoxic activity will also be introduced in this chapter.

In the last few years, a great deal has been learned about *how* a cell can kill another cell, but, as we'll see, not all the mechanisms are fully understood. It seems very likely that this is an important effector function for the immune system, playing a central part in the rejection of foreign grafts, perhaps having critical roles in the resistance to some types of infectious diseases (especially viruses, but also some bacteria and protozoan parasites), and probably involved in defense against some tumors.

Types of Cytotoxic Effector Cells

We have seen that cytotoxic T cells are usually CD8$^+$, but in some cases CD4$^+$ T cells can also be cytotoxic effector cells. As we'll see, these two types of cytotoxic T cells differ, not only in their genetic restriction (class I versus class II MHC) but often in the way they mediate cytotoxicity. There are also other cells, both lymphoid and myeloid, that can be cytotoxic. The LARGE GRANULAR LYMPHOCYTES

(LGL) contain cytotoxic cells including NATURAL KILLER (NK) cells and K CELLS. The latter bear Fc receptors and are responsible for killing in the presence of specific antibody against target cells, a process called ANTIBODY-DEPENDENT CELL-MEDIATED CYTOTOXICITY (ADCC). ADCC is also a property of some myeloid cells.

Cytotoxic T Cells

As discussed in Chapters 18 and 19, CD8$^+$ cytotoxic T cells recognize internally expressed antigens that are processed and presented with class I MHC. Fairly early on, it was realized that when these cells kill a target cell, they do so without affecting other cells in the mixture. That is, if target cells are mixed with other cells that are not targets, only the targets are killed. This, it turns out, is in contrast to the action of many CD4$^+$ cytotoxic T cells. As mentioned in Chapter 19, such cytotoxic cells exist, and these are restricted to class II MHC. Unlike the CD8$^+$ cells, these cytotoxic cells often kill not only their specific targets, but also other cells that are mixed with the targets. This effect is called BYSTANDER KILLING because of its effects on "innocent bystanders" (see Table 1).

A likely explanation for this difference is that the CD8$^+$ cytotoxic T cells, upon activation, precisely deliver a lethal signal to the bound target. On the other hand, the CD4$^+$ cells, upon recognition of the antigen plus MHC, release a cytotoxic factor that kills all susceptible cells in the vicinity. As we'll see, both types of mechanisms are employed by different cytotoxic cells and may well have different functions in the body.

It should be noted that bystander killing does not imply that CD4$^+$ cytotoxic T cells are antigen-nonspecific: no bystander killing will occur in the absence of the specific antigen and APCs.

This is in contrast to another type of cytotoxic T cell that is relatively antigen-nonspecific, but displays no bystander killing. It often happens that CD8$^+$ cytotoxic T cells, especially those maintained in tissue culture, can appear to have little or no antigen specificity, but rather simply kill many different types of target cells fairly indiscriminately. These have been called *promiscuous cytotoxic cells*, and in some cases, cytotoxic T cells that start out as antigen-specific become promiscuous in culture. This will be important when we consider lymphokine-activated killer (LAK) cells, below.

Finally, one other type of cytotoxic T cell has been described: cytotoxic cells bearing the γδ T-cell receptor. Neither the general nature of the ligand for this receptor nor the biological function of these cells is known.

Table 1   Properties of conventional versus bystander T-cell killing.[a]

Anti-A effector T cell	Unlabeled "cold" target	Labeled target	Label release	Comments
Conventional	–	A	+++	Cells kill A but not B targets.
	–	B	–	
	A	A	±	"Cold" A but not B cells
	A	B	–	block killing of labeled A
	B	A	+++	targets. Presence of "cold" A does not stimulate killing of labeled B.
Bystander killer	–	A	+++	Cells kill A but not B targets.
	–	B	–	
	A	A	++	"Cold" A cells stimulate
	A	B	++	killing of labeled B targets (and fail to block killing of labeled A targets).

[a]Conventional cytotoxic T cells (CTLs), specific for cells of strain A, kill A but not B. Unlabeled A cells compete as targets and thereby block release of label from A (cold target inhibition). The presence of "cold" A cells does not trigger killing of labeled B targets. Cells capable of bystander killing, specific for cells of strain A, similarly kill A but not B. However, unlike conventional CTL killing, bystander killing is not as effectively blocked by cold targets. More strikingly, labeled B targets (bystanders) are killed if unlabeled A stimulators are present.

Natural Killer Cells

Natural killer (NK) cells are large granular lymphocytes expressing neither surface Ig nor T-cell receptor. These cells are capable of killing certain types of targets, especially certain tumor cells. But, unlike cytotoxic T cells, NK cells are not antigen-specific. This is not surprising, since they do not appear to bear unique, clonally distributed receptors and do not undergo clonal selection. Currently, the nature of the cell-surface receptors that allow these cells to identify suitable targets is unknown. They are often present in unstimulated cell populations, but their activity can be enhanced by certain growth factors, including IL-2 and γ-interferon.

The receptor on NK cells has not been identified but may show some similarity to the T-cell receptor. One of the CD3 molecules that form the nonpolymorphic part of the T-cell receptor (see Chapter 22) has been found on NK cells. This molecule (CD3ζ), however, is not associated with a T-cell receptor on NK cells, but rather with another group of molecules that might be involved in NK-cell activation.

High Doses of IL-2 Stimulate Potent Cytotoxic Cells

LYMPHOKINE ACTIVATED KILLER (LAK) cells are induced by the culture of lymphoid cells in large amounts of IL-2. Like NK cells, LAK cells are antigen-nonspecific, but LAK cells act on a broader range of targets than do NK cells. Over the last few years, LAK cells have been the basis for a controversial cancer therapy involving administration of high doses of IL-2 and/or large numbers of LAK cells to cancer patients. While animal studies and some therapeutic trials have been encouraging, there is considerable skepticism regarding the efficacy of this treatment (see Chapter 33). LAK cells appear to be derived from NK cells, cytotoxic T cells, or both. As mentioned above, cytotoxic T cells can lose their specificity in culture, and this happens more quickly in the presence of high doses of IL-2. NK cells are also stimulated by IL-2, and it may well be that both types of cytotoxic effector cell contribute to the LAK phenomenon. The receptors responsible for target cell recognition and binding by LAK cells are unknown.

Antibody-Dependent Cell-Mediated Cytotoxicity (ADCC)

Many different types of cells carry Fc receptors and are capable of participating in ADCC. These include some myeloid cells, LGLs, and a small population of T cells. In all cases, the basic idea is the same: specific antibody bound to a target cell is, in turn, bound by the Fc receptor on the effector cell. This leads to the activation of a cytolytic mechanism and destruction of the target cell.

In general, the cytotoxic effector cell of ADCC is referred to as a K CELL, but this term is usually reserved for LGL effectors that do not seem to function by any other mechanism.

Bypassing Specificity in Effector–Target Interactions

We have seen that some cytotoxic effector cells are antigen-specific while others are not (but have a restricted range of cell targets). Studies in which antigen specificity of killing by cytotoxic T cells is "bypassed" suggest that similar events occur to trigger a cytotoxic "hit" from most types of effectors.

Plant lectins such as Con A and PHA are capable of activating T cells. In addition, these substances also permit an antigen-specific cytotoxic T cell to kill any cell nonspecifically. It is likely that the target cells become coated with the lectin, which, upon binding to an effector cell, triggers the effector to deliver its lethal signal. The lectin apparently functions as an activating "glue."

These observations might help to explain how promiscuous cytotoxic T cells and LAK cells work. If these cells express high amounts of adhesion molecules, then they may more readily bind a large range of target cells (in the absence of antigen). If this binding results in effector cell activation (for any reason), then the target will be killed.

The specificity of a cytotoxic T cell can also be bypassed by coating targets with antibodies to CD3, a component of the T-cell receptor (Chapter 22). If a cytotoxic T cell contacts the target, the anti-CD3 stimulates the T cell, and the target is killed. A novel application of this idea may have therapeutic implications: "hybrid" antibodies composed of one antigen-binding site specific for a target cell (such as a tumor) and another site specific for CD3 (see Figure 1) can effectively cause any cytotoxic T cell to kill the targets. This idea has been effectively used in tumor therapy in animal models.

Mechanisms of Cell-Mediated Cytotoxicity

The mechanisms of cell-mediated cytotoxicity are not fully understood and might vary with different types of effector cells. We have already seen one mechanism used by the immune system to effect cytotoxicity: the membrane attack complex of the complement pathway (Chapter 8). As we'll see, there is reason to suspect that a similar process can be involved in cell-mediated cytoxicity. There are also reasons to suspect that this is only part of the story.

In Chapters 18 to 20, we discussed the cellular interactions involved in the activation of cytotoxic T cells, and in the previous chapters in this section (Chapters 26 and 27) we discussed the cellular events and the growth factors involved in this activation. Here, we take up the story after the cells have been activated and are ready to kill their targets. The basic mechanisms of killing, as far as we know, may be similar in the different types of cytotoxic effector cells, and we will take them together (pointing out differences where they are known). The more we learn about the mechanisms of cell-mediated cytotoxicity, it seems, the more we learn about the potential biological functions of these cells.

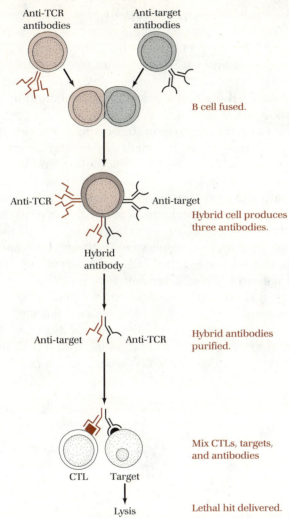

B-cell hybridomas producing:

Anti-TCR antibodies

Anti-target antibodies

B cell fused.

Anti-TCR

Anti-target

Hybrid cell produces three antibodies.

Hybrid antibody

Anti-target

Anti-TCR

Hybrid antibodies purified.

CTL

Target

Mix CTLs, targets, and antibodies

Lysis

Lethal hit delivered.

1 Cytotoxic "Bridge" Formation by Hybrid Antibodies. B-hybridoma cells producing, respectively, antibodies to the T-cell receptor and antibodies to the target cell are fused. The "hybrid hybridoma" produces the original two antibodies as well as a hybrid antibody, wherein one binding site recognizes T-cell receptor and the other recognizes the target. These hybrid antibodies are purified and are capable of bridging any cytotoxic T cell to the target cell, leading to target-cell destruction. The part of the antibody that binds the T-cell receptor presumably triggers the T cell, and the bridging to the target cell allows the lethal hit to be delivered.

The Stages of Cell-Mediated Cytotoxicity

The process of cell-mediated cytotoxicity is shown schematically in Figure 2. The first step in the cytotoxic response is adhesion of the effector cell to the target. As we know, this step is specific for MHC and processed antigen in the case of most cytotoxic T cells, but is not antigen-specific when other types of effectors are involved. In all cases, though, the result is the formation of an effector–target CONJUGATE.

Following conjugate formation, the cytoplasmic organelles of the effector cell reorganize to orient on the target cell. These include the CYTOTOXIC GRANULES, which contain a number of interesting substances (see below). In addition, the membranes of both the effector and the target become interdigitated (see Figure 3).

At this point, the cytotoxic granules in the cytoplasm of the effector cell move to the plasma membrane and release their contents. Because of the close association of the effector and target, the contents are released directly onto the target cell. The cells then disengage, and the effector cell moves off to find another target. A short time later, the original target cell dies.

Two important points should be noted. First, the effector cell *recycles*, so that one effector can kill a number of targets. Second, the interaction of the effector and target leads to a delayed death of the target. This has been called PROGRAMMING FOR LYSIS.

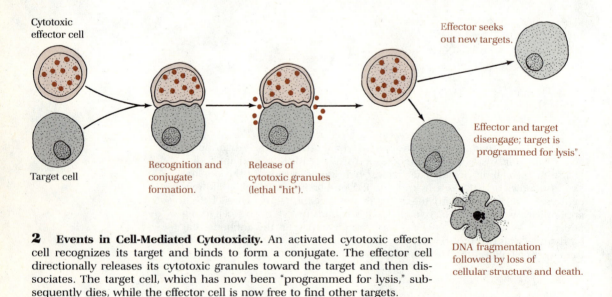

Cytotoxic
effector cell

Effector seeks
out new targets.

Recognition and
conjugate
formation.

Release of
cytotoxic granules
(lethal "hit").

Effector and target
disengage; target is
programmed for lysis".

Target cell

DNA fragmentation
followed by loss of
cellular structure and death.

2   Events in Cell-Mediated Cytotoxicity. An activated cytotoxic effector cell recognizes its target and binds to form a conjugate. The effector cell directionally releases its cytotoxic granules toward the target and then dissociates. The target cell, which has now been "programmed for lysis," subsequently dies, while the effector cell is now free to find other targets.

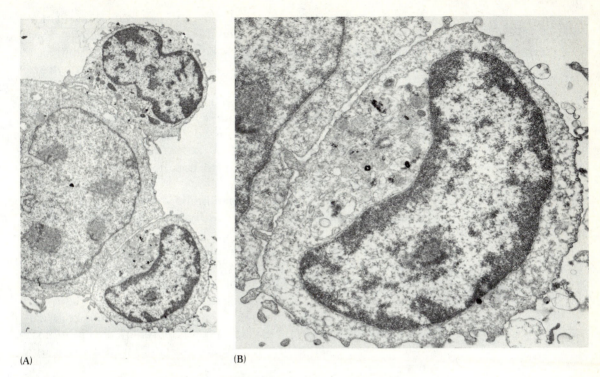

(A)

(B)

3 **Cytotoxic Effector–Target Conjugate.** Transmission electron microscopy of NK cells binding to target cells. (A) Two NK cells conjugated to a
melanoma tumor cell target seen at low magnification (×5300). (B) The NK
cell at the bottom of A seen at higher resolution (×16,000). The interdigitation
between the NK and target can be seen at the points of contact. Similar
conjugate formation and interdigitation has been observed with other cytotoxic effector cells. [From Zucker-Franklin et al., 1983. *Proc. Natl. Acad. Sci.
U.S.A.* 80: 6977; courtesy of D. Zucker-Franklin]

The precise mechanisms whereby the effector cell programs
the target for death are not fully known, but one key probably lies
within the cytotoxic granules. As discussed below, these contain
a number of substances that probably participate in the cytotoxic
effect. It should be kept in mind, however, that different cytotoxic
effector cells (or even one particular cytotoxic cell) may have *multiple* ways in which they can kill their targets. Some of these may
not involve the granules at all.

Cytotoxic Effector Cells Contain Cytoplasmic Granules

All types of cytotoxic effector cells often contain granules that can
be observed by electron microscopy. These granules are mem-

brane-bound and contain darkly staining materials. The relationship between cytotoxic function and these granules was established in correlative studies. For example, when a number of human lymphocyte clones generated in mixed lymphocyte responses (see Chapter 11) were examined, it was found that those clones with cytotoxic function (CTL, NK, or K cell) all had cytoplasmic granules. Those without cytotoxic function lacked the granules. Such correlations suggested that the granules are somehow involved in cytotoxic function.

When the granules were isolated and their contents examined, they were found to contain several interesting substances. One of these was found to produce membrane damage and was called PERFORIN or cytolysin (here we use the former term, because we now know that this molecule acts to put holes in the target-cell membranes, that is, it perforates them). Both names are still in use. In addition, several proteases are found in the granules, and these, too, may play a role in the cytotoxic function. There may also be a substance related to the tumor necrosis factors (see Chapter 27) present in the granules. Finally, a number of proteoglycans (carbohydrate-rich molecules with a protein core) are also found. We will consider each of these granule contents and the roles they may serve.

Perforin Can Produce Membrane Damage

When cytotoxic granules are isolated and their contents allowed to interact with target membranes, doughnut-shaped pores (see Figure 4) that are similar (but not identical) to those produced by activated C9 in the complement pathway (see Chapter 8) form in the targets.

One possibility was that the granules contain C9, and this idea was tested by Hans Müller-Eberhard and his colleagues. They found that a component in the cytotoxic granules is bound by anti-C9 antibodies and that this substance has the ability to damage membranes. However, it turned out that this is a protein that is different from, but related to, C9. This molecule was independently isolated by a number of different investigators, including Eckhard Podack and Pierre Henkart (who each called it something different: e.g., C9-related protein, perforin, cytolysin). The gene encoding perforin has been identified, and the predicted amino acid sequence of the protein does have a small amount of homology to C9, but it is clearly different.

It seemed likely, then, that upon recognition, the cytotoxic

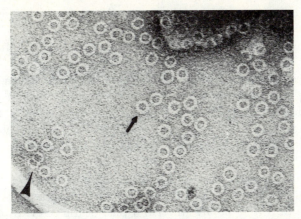

4 Perforin-Induced Pores in Target Cell Membranes. In order to visualize the holes formed by cytotoxic effector cell contact with targets, NK cells were cultured with rabbit erythrocytes in the presence of a mitogenic lectin (which bridges the effector and targets). The holes that form in the erythrocyte, which have the appearance of white rings, are identical to pores formed by purified perforin. Similar pore formation is observed with other cytotoxic effector cells. [From Podack and Dennert, 1983. *Nature* 302: 442. Courtesy of E. Podack]

effector cell releases granule perforin, which then punches holes in the target cell and causes its death. If so, then the cell would die from COLLOID OSMOTIC LYSIS, due to free flow of water and ions across the plasma membrane. This is supported, in part, by the observation that different ions flow into or out of target cells upon binding to cytotoxic effectors.

There were some problems with this idea, however. First of all, not all cytotoxic effector cells cause pore formation in their targets. Amounts of perforin vary in different cytotoxic cells, and some controversy exists as to whether some effector cells completely lack this protein. Second, the nature of the cell death induced by cytotoxic effector cells differs from that induced by the complement cascade—which argues that targets of cytotoxic cells do *not* die due to colloid osmotic lysis. We take this up next.

Cell Death by Cytotoxic Effector Cells Differs from That of Complement Lysis

Death's sting, at the cellular level, can take different forms. There are at least two different types of cell death, termed NECROSIS and APOPTOSIS (see Chapter 24). Necrosis occurs when the plasma membrane is disrupted or when the cell is metabolically poisoned. An example of necrosis is complement-mediated lysis. Apoptosis, on the other hand, begins with changes in the nucleus, leading to fragmentation of the DNA and cell death. It turns out that when cytotoxic effector cells kill their targets, the death often shows the characteristics of apoptosis. It is unlikely, therefore, that a complement-like mechanism could be the whole explanation for cell-mediated cytotoxicity.

One event that appears to be important in both apoptosis and cytotoxic killing is a flux of extracellular calcium ions into the target cell. While in some special circumstances this flux does not appear to be required for cytotoxic killing, in most cases it is. The calcium flux alone is probably insufficient to program a target cell for lysis, but it may be an important part of the pathway.

One idea, then, was that the pores produced by perforin facilitate the entry of something else into the target cell. This "something" might then trigger events leading to the death of the cell. Investigators examined the contents of the cytotoxic granules to try to find out what this something could be.

Proteases in the Cytotoxic Granules May Participate in Killing

The idea that proteases may play a role in cell-mediated cytotoxicity was based on observations that inhibitors of serine proteases are capable of inhibiting cytotoxicity. Treatment of effector cells with such inhibitors prior to the addition of target cells has no effect, but for a short time after the addition of targets, cytotoxicity is highly sensitive to inhibition. Thus, it seemed likely that some critical proteases are somehow exposed to the inhibitors as effector and target cells come into contact.

A number of observations from different laboratories have focused attention on proteases in cytotoxic effector functions. Jurg Tschopp and his colleagues have characterized seven different proteases in cytotoxic granules, which they have named *granzymes* (each one identified by a letter, A–G). Meanwhile, the laboratories of Irving Weissman, R. Christopher Bleackley, and Pierre Golstein discovered that a number of genes that are preferentially expressed in cytotoxic effector cells encode serine proteases. The relationships between the different names for the granule-associated serine proteases are given in Table 2.

Do any or all of these proteases play a role in cytotoxic effector function? Pierre Henkart and colleagues have found that a component of cytotoxic granules, different from perforin, can cause

Table 2   Synonyms for the serine proteases found in cytotoxic granules.[a]

Granzyme	Synonym(s)
Granzyme A	HF, CTLA-3
Granzyme B	CCP 1, CTLA-1
Granzyme C	CCP 2
Granzyme D	CCP 5
Granzyme E	CCP 3
Granzyme F	CCP 4
Granzyme G	CCP 6

[a]The granzymes are as described by J. Tschopp ca. 1989. Granzymes G and H, named prior to 1989, are now granzyme B; the "new" granzyme G is equivalent to CCP 6. The synonyms were described in the following laboratories: HF, I. Weissman; CCP, R. C. Bleakley; CTLA, P. Goldstein. Other synonyms also exist.

the release of DNA from isolated nuclei (that is, can cause DNA fragmentation). This activity is blocked by protease inhibitors that are also capable of blocking DNA fragmentation induced by cytotoxic T cells. They believe that the protease(s) involved in the destruction of the target-cell DNA enter the target cells via the pores produced by perforin. Their findings, however, are controversial, and we'll have to wait and see whether this idea turns out to be correct.

Tumor Necrosis Factors and Cell-Mediated Cytotoxicity

TNFα and TNFβ have been known for some time to be capable of killing certain target cells (TNFβ is also called *lymphotoxin* for this reason). Nancy Ruddle and her colleagues in New Haven demonstrated that TNF induces DNA fragmentation in target cells, suggesting that it may play an important role in at least some types of cell-mediated cytotoxicity. In fact, they showed that at least some CD4$^+$ cytotoxic T cells release TNFβ after activation, and that this is responsible for their cytotoxic activity. Further, a type of cytotoxic large granular lymphocyte has also been found to mediate its effects through production of TNF.

It is likely that cytotoxic granules in at least some types of cytotoxic effector cells contain TNF or a closely related factor. TNF may also be able to kill targets that are not normally sensitive to TNF if the factor can get inside the cell (e.g., through a perforin pore).

SYNTHESIS
Diversity among Cytotoxic Effector Mechanisms

From this discussion, we can see that there are a number of different cytotoxic cell types and cytotoxic mechanisms. There is, however, a thread of similarity between all of these. In each case, the induction of cytotoxicity begins with the binding of a cytotoxic cell to its target, and the activation of the cytotoxic effector cell. The activation may be via the T-cell receptor or another receptor on the cell surface and may be antigen-specific or nonspecific. This activation leads to the release of either long-range mediators (e.g., TNF) that can mediate bystander killing, or short-range mediators (e.g., perforin, granzymes) that program the bound target cell for lysis. Each of these different modes of activation and effector function may play a different role in immunologic defense, though as yet only a few such roles are really understood. We will consider the roles of cytotoxic effector cells further in our discussions of immunity to infectious diseases (Chapter 32), immunity to tumors (Chapter 33), and graft rejection (Chapter 37).

Cytotoxic Effector Mechanisms In Vivo

Although we do not yet fully understand the roles of granule-associated perforin and serine proteases in cytotoxicity, there is evidence that the mechanisms we've discussed are physiologically important.

When genes are identified that appear to be involved in the function of a cell type, it may be useful to examine which cells, in vivo, express these genes and under what circumstances. This can best be done by the technique of IN SITU HYBRIDIZATION. Usually, this is done as follows (see Figures 5 and 6). The cDNA for the gene of interest is cloned into a vector that allows expression of RNA. For the technique, however, we want an *antisense* RNA, which is radioactively labeled. The labeled antisense RNA is then used to treat thin sections of tissue. Cells in the tissue that expressed the gene (and thus contain normal mRNA) will now contain complexes

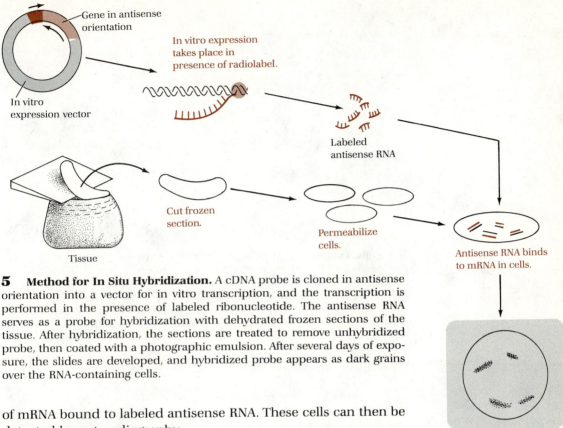

Gene in antisense
orientation

In vitro expression
takes place in
presence of radiolabel.

In vitro
expression vector

Labeled
antisense RNA

Cut frozen
section.

Permeabilize
cells.

Tissue

Antisense RNA binds
to mRNA in cells.

Stain, apply
autoradiographic
immulsion and
develop.

5   Method for In Situ Hybridization. A cDNA probe is cloned in antisense orientation into a vector for in vitro transcription, and the transcription is performed in the presence of labeled ribonucleotide. The antisense RNA serves as a probe for hybridization with dehydrated frozen sections of the tissue. After hybridization, the sections are treated to remove unhybridized probe, then coated with a photographic emulsion. After several days of exposure, the slides are developed, and hybridized probe appears as dark grains over the RNA-containing cells.

of mRNA bound to labeled antisense RNA. These cells can then be detected by autoradiography.

In this way, it was shown that T cells that infiltrate a foreign graft express the genes for perforin and the granule proteases (Figure 6). Combined with the observation that cytotoxic T cells are important in the rejection of foreign grafts, this is evidence that these genes are, in fact, expressed in vivo under the expected conditions.

Why Don't Cytotoxic Cells Kill Themselves?

Earlier in this chapter we suggested that a single cytotoxic cell kills its target and then continues on to kill others without harming itself (Figure 2). This is directly supported by studies using micro-cinematography (where we can see this happening). In all our discussions of cytotoxic mechanisms, however, we have not considered why this can happen. That is, why don't the cytotoxic cells also die in this process?

(A)

(B)

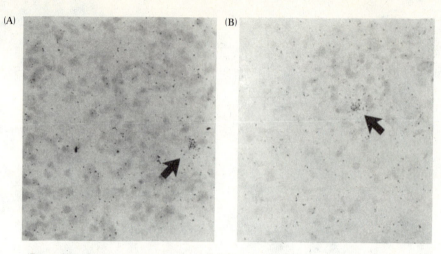

6   **Cells Infiltrating an Allogeneic Graft Express Genes for Granule Proteases.** Allogeneic grafts were removed at different days post grafting and prepared for in situ hybridization (see Figure 5) with probes for two granule-associated proteases. By day 2 post grafting (A, B) protease-expressing cells can first be seen in the graft, and these increase in number by days 6 (C, D) and 10 (E, F). G represents negative results with a control probe, and H represents negative results with skin taken from a site other than the graft. [From Mueller et al., 1988. *J. Exp. Med.* 167: 1124]

To see why this is a paradox, let's look at a model of how cytotoxic cells kill. First, a cytotoxic cell is activated via its receptor upon contact with a ligand on the surface of the target cell. This activation leads to the fusion of cytotoxic granules with the cell membrane, releasing the contents of the granules (e.g., perforin, proteases) to the outside of the cell. These substances now act across the short distance separating the effector and the target cell, to induce target-cell death. Somehow, though, the cytotoxic mediators act only on the target and not on the effector cell.

There are two general ideas regarding the directionality of the cytotoxic effect. Either the cytotoxic mediators are somehow directly placed on the target cell (and never contact the effector) or else the cytotoxic effector cells are resistant to the mediators.

The first idea is difficult to reconcile with the observation that the contents of the granules are nonspecific mediators of cytotoxicity. However, one interesting possibility, proposed by Podack, suggests that within the granules are "minivesicles" that contain the mediators. He proposes that these vesicles might have receptors on their surfaces, the same receptors that are used by the effector cell to recognize the target. When the granules fuse with

(C)

(D)

(E)

(F)

(G)

(H)

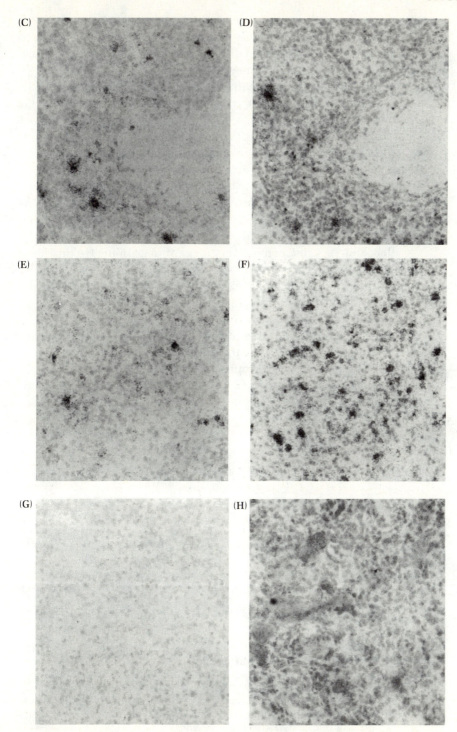

the surface membrane, the minivesicles are released, and these theoretically bind to the target cell via their receptors. This would account for the unidirectionality of the effect (as the vesicles will not bind to the surface of the effector).

The second idea, that cytotoxic effector cells are simply resistant to killing, seemed not to be correct. Some cells, such as embryonic trophoblast cells, are genuinely resistant to cytotoxic T cells (though they are susceptible to NK and LAK cells), but it has been fairly easy to show that cytotoxic cells are susceptible to being killed by other cytotoxic cells. (An example of this phenomenon is discussed in Chapter 30). Some investigators have suggested that cytotoxic cells are somewhat *less* susceptible to lysis than other targets, but this does not really explain how they can resist their own cytotoxic effects.

Bleackley has suggested a very elegant possibility. He proposes that the proteoglycans present in the granules (mentioned earlier in this chapter) coat the inner surface of granules and may be important in protecting the granule membrane from the cytotoxic mediators. Upon fusion with the surface membrane, these proteoglycans now coat the outside of the cell, protecting the membrane in the immediate vicinity of the mediators (see Figure 7). These regions of local protection would prevent the cell from killing itself, but produce, at best, only a marginal protection from other cytotoxic cells.

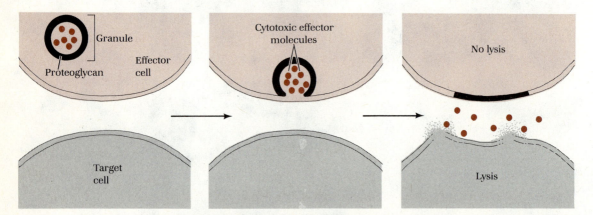

7   A Possible Mechanism for Protection of the Cytotoxic Effector Cell During Delivery of the Lethal Hit. R. Christopher Bleackley has proposed that the proteoglycans contained in the cytotoxic granules form a local protective coating during exocytosis. Thus, the cytotoxic effector is resistant to lysis only in the immediate vicinity of the released granule contents. While this clever idea accounts for many observations on effector cell protection, there is no proof of this hypothesis at present.

At present, we don't know which, if any, of these ideas are correct. As we learn more about the different cytotoxic effector cells and their mechanisms of action, we hope to resolve this paradox.

Summary

1. There are several different types of cytotoxic effector cells, including cytotoxic T cells, NK cells, K cells, and LAK cells. Although target specificity differs between these types, many of the basic mechanisms of action appear to be the same (although differences probably exist). Cytotoxic effector cells have been demonstrated to play important roles in defense against infectious diseases and tumors, and in graft rejection.

2. When a cytotoxic effector cell recognizes a target cell, a conjugate between the two forms. The cytotoxic cell introduces a lethal "hit" to the target and then disengages to seek out new targets. Some time later, the target cell dies (i.e., it has been "programmed for lysis").

3. The lethal hit that a cytotoxic effector cell delivers is probably contained in cytotoxic granules in the cytoplasm of the cell. Upon activation, the cell releases the granules, which affect the target cell.

4. One of the components of the granules is perforin, a molecule that induces pores in the target-cell membrane. These pores resemble (but differ in size from) those produced by the membrane attack complex of complement. Death induced by cytotoxic effector cells, however, differs from that induced by complement, in that only the former produces DNA fragmentation in the targets. It is likely, then, that other components of the granules also play a role in cytotoxic effector cell function.

5. The granules also contain a number of serine proteases, many of which appear to be unique to cytotoxic cells. The role of these proteases in target cell destruction is not yet known.

Additional Readings

Henkart, P.A. 1985. The mechanism of lymphocyte-mediated cytotoxicity. *Annu. Rev. Immunol.* 3: 31.

Hersey, P. and R. Bolhuis. 1987. "Nonspecific" MHC unrestricted killer cells and their receptors. *Immunol. Today* 8: 233.

Martz, E. and D. M. Howell. 1989. CTL: Virus control cells first and cytolytic cells second? DNA fragmentation, apoptosis, and the prelytic halt hypothesis. *Immunol. Today* 10: 79.

Moller, G., ed. 1988. Molecular mechanisms of T cell mediated lysis. *Immunol. Rev.* 103.

Trinchieri, G. 1989. Biology of NK cells. *Adv. Immunol.* 47: 187.

Young, J. D. E. and C. C. Liu. 1988. Multiple mechanisms of lymphocyte mediated killing. *Immunol. Today* 9: 140.

REGULATION OF THE IMMUNE RESPONSE

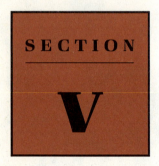

SECTION

V

It is a mystery that is hidden from me by reason that the emergency requiring the fathoming of it hath not in my life-days occurred, and so, not having no need to know this thing, I abide barren of the knowledge.

Mark Twain
A Connecticut Yankee in King Arthur's Court

Up to now we have addressed some of the problems of initiating immune responses and have seen that there is a delicate balance of cells and factors involved. It is intuitively obvious that anything as complex as this must have complex regulation. In the next three chapters we will examine what many consider to be a highly controversial area of immunology: the regulation of the response. We will discuss two distinctly different modes of regulation: the network of receptor interactions and the control of immunity by T cells. We will also discuss the ultimate problem of regulation: self–nonself discrimination. In entering this dangerous realm, the reader is urged to be both open-minded and cautious. We do not yet know the many different ways in which the immune system is regulated, or which ways are most important (or in what circumstances). We will also examine what is probably the most controversial topic in immunology: the suppressor T cell.

REGULATION BY ANTIBODY: THE NETWORK

Overview Niels Jerne has profoundly changed the thinking of immunology on two occasions. In 1955 he proposed the *natural selection theory* (see Chapter 1), which paved the way for clonal selection, which became the dominant paradigm of immunology. Then in 1973 he proposed the *network theory*, which has come to be one of the two dominant modes of thinking about the regulation of the immune response.[1] The network theory differs from other immunologic thinking because it endows the immune system with the ability to regulate itself using only itself. We will see later that this is a profound departure in biological thought and, if correct, gives biological systems a power they had not previously been thought to possess. The theory is based on the fact that antibody not only has the ability to combine with antigen (its traditional function) but also has the ability to *be* an antigen.

We learned earlier that it is possible to immunize an individual of one species with an antibody molecule from another species and make anti-idiotype antibodies. Jerne postulated that the antibody molecule can carry out these two functions (acting both as antibody and antigen) within the *same* animal, and the interplay of these two functions constitutes the makings of a regulatory system. Furthermore, amino acid sequences within the Ig molecules, by chance, share antigenic determinants with all the antigens to which the animal can respond. These sequences are called the *internal image*, and the idea of the internal image is the crucial philosophical underpinning of the theory.

---

[1] In 1985 Niels Jerne won the Nobel prize. His contributions have been so extensive that it must have been a very difficult task for the committee to decide which of them to cite in the award, so the award was simply given for "contributions."

CHAPTER

29

Epitopes, Paratopes, and Idiotopes:
The Language of the Network

Many immunologists have been put off by the vocabulary of the network, the basis of which is the idea that each member of the immune system is capable of interacting with every other member. This interaction is possible because the antigen-combining site on one antibody molecule is able to recognize an antigenic determinant on another antibody molecule. The language of the network was designed to facilitate this discussion. Accordingly, the antigen-combining site on an Ig molecule is called the PARATOPE. Suppose we immunize an animal with bovine serum albumin (BSA) and raise an anti-BSA antibody. When BSA and anti-BSA combine, the antigen combines with the paratope on the antibody. Although we have been calling this site the antigen-combining site up to now, the reader will find that with a bit of practice paratope rolls more trippingly off the tongue.

The antigenic determinant on a BSA molecule (and on other antigens as well) is called the EPITOPE, a term that has already become an integral part of immunologic vocabulary; it was introduced in Chapter 2. Thus an antigen–antibody reaction in the traditional sense is a reaction between the paratope on the Ig molecule and the epitope on the antigen molecule. In the network, the paratope on one antibody molecule can be recognized by a paratope on another antibody molecule. The first paratope thus is acting as an antigen, or epitope. The part of the combining site of the first antibody that is seen in this manner by the paratope on the second antibody molecule is called an IDIOTOPE. The sum of the unique structures (idiotopes) of an antibody molecule is called the *idiotype.*[2] Epitope, paratope and idiotope are illustrated in Figure 1.

Another way of looking at this is the following:

> We have known since Landsteiner that practically all molecules in the universe are antigens. The total of all the antigenic determinants of these antigens is the total set of epitopes. No matter how large this set is, *every* member of this set can be recognized by a paratope of the immune system of an individual (which possesses an estimated *10 million* antibodies of different specificities). [N. Jerne, personal communication]

The *vocabulary* of the network is based on the two roles of the

---

[2] Networkists often refer to idiotopes and idiotypes as *id*. To non-networkists the distinctions between the immunological and Freudian id are often blurred.

1 **The Language of the Network.** Antibody molecules contain antigen-combining sites (paratopes) and antigenic determinants (idiotopes). Antigen molecules contain determinants (epitopes) that combine with the appropriate paratope. The network thus has epitope–paratope and idiotope–paratope interactions.

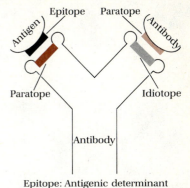

Epitope: Antigenic determinant
Paratope: Combining site
Idiotope: Antigenic determinant
             on an antibody

antigen-combining site. As seen in Part A of Figure 2, it binds antigen (as a paratope it binds to an epitope) and it offers a unique antigenic configuration (it acts as an idiotope for other antibodies). In the parlance of the network this anti-epitope antibody is called Ab1. In Part B of Figure 2 we address the *function* of the network. Because the underlying assumption of the network is that an Ig molecule has the property of both antigen and antibody, the Ab1 (produced in Part A) can act as an antibody to react via its paratope with the idiotope of a surface Ig molecule on another B cell (Figure 2B, left). Alternatively, it acts as an antigen when its idiotope is bound by the paratope of a surface Ig molecule on some other B cells (Figure 2B, right). In either case, the result is the clonal expansion of B cells bearing Ig molecules that bind or are bound by the Ab1. The antibodies induced in either way by Ab1 are collectively called Ab2.

The Internal Image

The concept central to the network theory is that each idiotope is the same as an epitope of one or several antigens. This is another way of saying that several idiotopes would cross-react with a large number of epitopes in nature. These common determinants between idiotopes in the animal and epitopes in the world outside the animal are called the INTERNAL IMAGES of antigens (Figure 3). According to the theory, the network works because all possible antigens are reflected in this cross-reactivity. This being the case, the immune system need only look into itself to see any possible

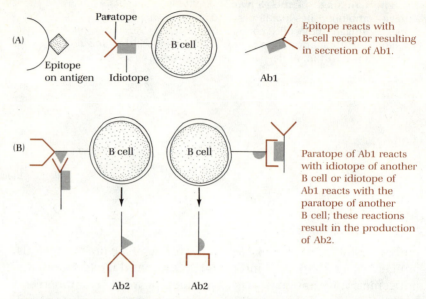

2   The Function of the Network. (A) Epitope reacts with B cell expressing a receptor with the proper paratope. This surface Ig molecule also has an idiotope. The B cell secretes antibody (Ab1) molecules with the paratope (p1) and the idiotope (i1). (B) Ab1 can react *either* with a B cell expressing an idiotope (i2) that reacts with the p1 *or* with a B cell expressing a paratope that reacts with i1. In both cases the B cells secrete antibody. Gray symbols indicate idiotopes, while brown symbols indicate paratopes. [Based on Paul and Bona, 1982. *Immunol. Today* 3: 230]

epitope within its own repertoire of idiotopes and paratopes. This is a unique idea, which if correct means that all possible reactions that the immune system can carry out with the epitopes in the world outside the animal are accounted for in the internal system of paratopes and idiotopes already present inside the animal. The mystical reader may ponder that this is akin to looking at oneself in a mirror and seeing the entire world in the reflection. Jerne in fact began a 1984 review (called "Idiotypic networks and other preconceived ideas") with a quote from Jean Cocteau: "Mirrors would be well-advised to think twice before reflecting images;" and he ends the review by saying that those who seek exterior pressures on the system "would do well to turn their vision towards the interiors of themselves, and there discover the mystery, perhaps never completely revealed, of the immune system."

SYNTHESIS
Cross-Reactivity between Paratopes and Epitopes:
The Generative Grammar of the Network

Jerne addressed the possible cross-reactivity between idiotopes and epitopes in his 1985 Nobel prize address. He likened the immune system to language and used Noam Chomsky's notion of "deep structure" of language.[3] Note in Figure 4 that a portion of the structure THE PRODUCTION OF INSULIN DEPENDS ON CELLS, is also found on the structure THE NAME OF INSULINDE WAS GIVEN TO, and on the structure A RESULT OF INSULIN DEFICIENCY. Even though they are totally unique structures (both as sentences and as epitopes and paratopes), they by chance share sequences. If these shared sequences are brought into proper position, they can interact with each other.[4]

The idea of the internal image is used in network theory to allow the immune system to regulate itself after initial confrontation with exogenous antigen. The concept is that it does it totally by its own internal viewing of itself. It can do this, the theory says, because it can see all of the outside world reflected in itself. This is heady stuff and forces us to think about biological systems in general and the immune system in particular in a unique way. We

[3] See, for example, N. Chomsky, 1971. *Problems of Knowledge and Freedom*. Vintage Books, New York.

[4] There are two published versions of the Nobel prize address. The version appearing in the *EMBO Journal* [1985. 4: 487] has this illustration. The shortened version in *Science* [1985. 229: 1057] does not.

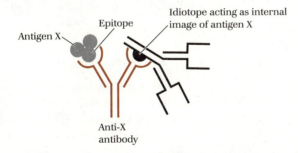

Antigen X
Epitope
Idiotope acting as internal image of antigen X
Anti-X antibody

3   **The Internal Image.** An epitope on antigen X is defined by the ability of an anti-X antibody to bind to it. If the paratope of the anti-X binds to an idiotope on a different antibody, the second antibody is said to bear an internal image of the epitope on antigen X.

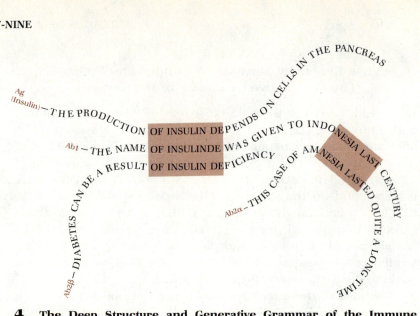

Ag (Insulin) — THE PRODUCTION OF INSULIN DEPENDS ON CELLS IN THE PANCREAS

Ab1 — THE NAME OF INSULINDE WAS GIVEN TO INDONESIA LAST CENTURY

DIABETES CAN BE A RESULT OF INSULIN DEFICIENCY

Ab2β — DIABETES CAN BE A RESULT

Ab2α — THIS CASE OF AMNESIA LASTED QUITE A LONG TIME

4 The Deep Structure and Generative Grammar of the Immune Response. An identical structure can appear on many structures in many contexts and be reacted to by the reader or by the immune system. [From Jerne, 1985. *EMBO J.* 4: 847]

can also see that it is the uniqueness of the vision that necessitates the new vocabulary.

> I see the immune system as continuously seeking a dynamic equilibrium—and by "dynamic" I mean that a vast number of immune responses are going on all the time, even in the absence of foreign antigen. The old term "immune response" suggests that the system is "at rest," waiting to "respond," whereas I think it is continuously active, interacting with self-antigens, idiotopes, factors, etc. [N. Jerne, personal communication]

Testing the Network Theory

A theory of this nature is very difficult to test experimentally, but there are several points that should be immediately testable. One that is crucial to the theory is that it should be possible to generate antibodies against the idiotype. Such antibodies are called ANTI-IDIOTYPE ANTIBODIES. The theory also predicts that it should be possible to generate antibody against one's own idiotypes—that is, AUTO–ANTI-IDIOTYPE antibodies. The theory requires that such auto–anti-idiotype antibody be regulatory. We will see below that these conditions have been satisfied. In addition to these minimal considerations, the idea of the internal image predicts that under some conditions anti-idiotype antibody should mimic antigen. We will see that this too can be shown to occur.

The Production of Auto–Anti-Idiotype Antibodies

As stated above, the first of the two criteria that have to be met for the network theory to be viable is that it must be possible to generate auto–anti-idiotype antibodies. One of the first experimental demonstrations that this can indeed be done is shown in Figure 5. Scott Rodkey in Kansas immunized rabbits with hapten–carrier conjugate; 6 months later he collected their serum and purified the anti-hapten antibodies. The purified anti-hapten antibodies were then made more immunogenic by polymerization and injected back into the *same* rabbits that had produced them. In a short time these animals began to make antibodies that reacted with their own anti-hapten antibody and with no other Ig molecules. This result shows that it is possible for an individual to make a productive antibody response against its own idiotypic determinants.

Similar results have been obtained with molecules that have the properties of lymphocyte receptors and can be found in urine after presumably being shed from the surface of lymphocytes. In

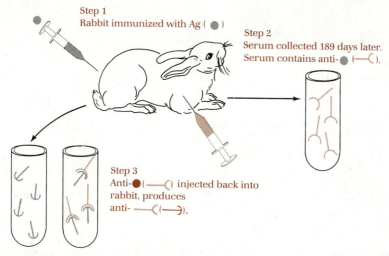

5 **Production of Auto–Anti-Idiotype Antibody.** Antigen is injected into a rabbit, which responds by producing antibody. The antibody is purified and reinjected into the same rabbit, which responds by producing anti-idiotype antibody. [After Rodkey, 1974. *J. Exp. Med.* 139: 712]

this case, the shed receptors had specificities directed against alloreactive MHC antigen. When these receptors were injected back into the animals, antibodies directed against the idiotypes of the receptors on their own lymphocytes were produced. The production of these auto–anti-idiotype antibodies caused those lymphocytes with the receptors for the alloreactive MHC to be eliminated. As a result, the animals were not able to mount responses against those MHC antigens.

The Regulatory Role of Anti-Idiotype Antibody

The second criterion the network theory must meet is that anti-idiotype antibody must be shown to be regulatory. The experiment mentioned above, in which auto–anti-receptor antibody caused the elimination of cells with that receptor and hence the elimination of the ability to react to a certain MHC, is one example of the possible regulatory role of this antibody.

Anti-idiotype antibody is also able to *suppress* the generation of the immune response (Figure 6). In this experiment spleen cells

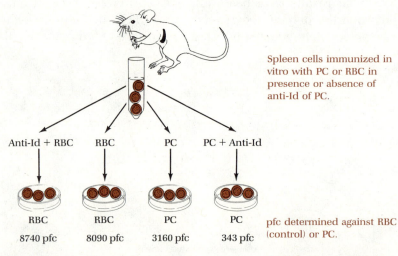

Spleen cells immunized in vitro with PC or RBC in presence or absence of anti-Id of PC.

Anti-Id + RBC   RBC   PC   PC + Anti-Id

RBC   RBC   PC   PC

8740 pfc   8090 pfc   3160 pfc   343 pfc

pfc determined against RBC (control) or PC.

Anti-Id prevents generation of anti-PC response but has no effect on anti-RBC response.

6   Anti-Idiotype Specifically Inhibits Generation of Antibody Response. Spleen cells are immunized in vitro with specific antigen (PC) or control antigen (RBC) in the presence or absence of anti-idiotype antibody to PC. Anti-idiotype antibody inhibits production of anti-PC but has no effect on anti-RBC response. [In vitro after Cosenza and Kohler, 1972. *Proc. Natl. Acad. Sci. U.S.A.* 69: 2701; in vivo after Hart et al., 1972. *J. Exp. Med.* 135: 1293] are incubated in vitro with either of two antigens, phosphorylcholine (PC) or red blood cells (RBC). An anti-idiotype antibody is added to some of the cultures. This anti-idiotype antibody was raised by purifying anti-PC and then making an antibody against the purified antibody. In the cultures that contain anti-idiotype antibody and PC, there is a 90% reduction in cells producing anti-PC. In contrast, the cultures that received the RBC and anti-idiotype make responses comparable to those without anti-idiotype. Remember that in this experiment the anti-idiotype is against the anti-PC antibody, so the RBC immunization is not affected. This experiment shows that an anti-idiotype antibody can *down-regulate* the immune response.

The experiment in Figure 6 shows that anti-idiotypic antibody can suppress the immune response, but it is also possible to *enhance* the immune response with anti-idiotype antibody. For example, if an anti-idiotype antibody is produced against an antibody to group A *Streptococcus* in a guinea pig, it is found that when mice are treated with the IgG1 fraction of this antibody they are primed for a secondary response to the *Streptococcus* even though they have not received a primary injection. There are at least two possible explanations. One is that the paratopes of the anti-idiotype antibodies (Ab2) reacted with idiotopes on the surface of antigen-specific B cells, cross-linking them and activating the cells. The second explanation could be that the idiotopes on the Ab2 reacted with the paratopes on antigen-specific B cells, effectively being seen as antigen (i.e., internal images). The first explanation assumes that the majority of B cells bearing the recognized idiotopes are specific for the antigen.[5] In any case, the end result is that the anti-idiotype antibody acts to enhance the immune response.

Here we have two examples of anti-idiotype antibody behaving in a *regulatory* role, a condition that is essential for validation of the network theory.

The Ability of Anti-Idiotype to Mimic Antigen

Another prediction of the network theory is that anti-idiotype antibodies should under some conditions mimic antigen. This prediction is based on an essential tenet of the theory, namely, that the internal images within the immune system reflect the epitopes outside the system. If this is true, then one should be

---

[5] Networkists think of antibodies other than Ab1 as bearing idiotopes that are reactive with those on Ab1. Such antibodies are called the nonspecific set and play important roles in complex network models that we will not go into here.

able to use the idiotopes of antibodies to raise antibodies whose paratopes will bind to an epitope of choice.[6] This use of the internal image has been demonstrated with several antigens, with hormone receptors providing some of the more dramatic examples.

The chain of reasoning for these experiments, which are diagramed in Figure 7, goes as follows: Hormones bind to receptors. Antihormone antibody binds to the hormone. And antibody against the antihormone binds to the antihormone. Because both receptor and antihormone antibody bind to the hormone and because the antihormone additionally can bind to the anti-antihormone, it follows that the anti-antihormone could bind to the receptor. This is a long way of saying that the anti-idiotope could bind to the receptor. If this chain of reasoning is correct, we should be able to raise an antibody against a receptor without ever using the receptor as antigen. The ligand and the internal images should let us end up with antireceptor antibody. This was first done by Sege and Peterson with insulin in 1978.

An illustrative experiment is seen in Figure 8. In these studies,

[6] The reader should be able to follow this sentence, which is written entirely in networkese. If you can't, do not pass go; return to start and try again.

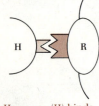

Hormone (H) binds receptor (R).

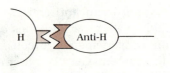

Hormone binds antihormone antibody.

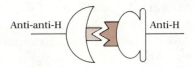

Antihormone antibody binds anti-antihormone antibody.

Therefore, anti-Id of antihormone should bind to receptor of hormone.

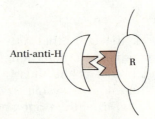

7 **Generation of Anti-receptor Antibodies.** Because both receptor and anti-hormone antibody bind to the hormone, and anti-hormone binds to anti–anti-hormone, then anti–anti-hormone should bind to receptor.

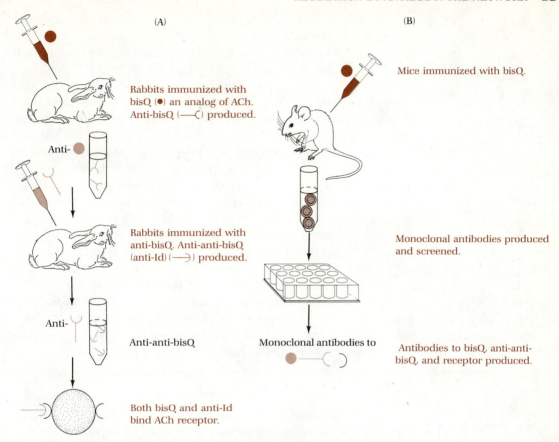

(A)

Rabbits immunized with
bisQ (●) an analog of ACh.
Anti-bisQ (——Ç) produced.

Anti-●

Rabbits immunized with
anti-bisQ. Anti-anti-bisQ
(anti-Id) (——⊋) produced.

Anti-Y

Anti-anti-bisQ

Both bisQ and anti-Id
bind ACh receptor.

(B)

Mice immunized with bisQ.

Monoclonal antibodies produced
and screened.

Monoclonal antibodies to

Antibodies to bisQ, anti-anti-
bisQ, and receptor produced.

8 Anti-receptor Antibodies Can Be Produced Using the Network. Two experiments to show that antireceptor antibodies can be produced using the network. (A) Rabbits are immunized with bisQ and produce anti-bisQ. The purified anti-bisQ is reinjected, and rabbits produce anti–anti-bisQ, which reacts with the ACh receptor. [After Wasserman et al., 1982. *Proc. Natl. Acad. Sci. U.S.A.* 79: 4810] (B) Mice are immunized with bisQ, and monoclonal antibodies are generated. These antibodies can be shown to react to bisQ, anti-bisQ, and the receptor. [After Cleveland et al., 1983. *Nature* 305: 56]

Bernard Erlanger and his co-workers in New York developed an antibody against the acetylcholine (ACh) receptor using the principles of the network. As seen in Figure 8A, rabbits were immunized with a molecule called bisQ, a highly active agonist (an agonist is a substance that reacts with the receptor to cause a response) of the ACh receptor (AChR). The resulting anti-bisQ antibody had all the properties of an anti-ACh antibody, that is, it could react with ACh to prevent its binding to the receptor. The anti-bisQ was purified and used to immunize another set of rabbits to produce anti-idiotype antibodies. The resulting anti-idiotype antibody (i.e., the anti-antibody) had the characteristics of an anti-receptor antibody. It could bind to the receptor and prevent binding of ACh—the result we would predict from Figure 7.

Erlanger and his co-workers also showed that animals produce auto–anti-AChR antibody (Figure 8B). First they immunized mice with bisQ and then produced monoclonal antibodies, using the cells in the spleens of these animals. They reasoned here that if the network theory is correct, the injection of antigen elicits antigen-specific antibody, and subsequently the animals generate regulatory anti-idiotype antibody. But there should also be antibody against the physiological hormone receptor, because just as an anti-idiotype antibody can mimic antigen by binding to an antigen receptor, so can it mimic a hormone by binding to the hormone receptor. When the clones were screened, it was found that indeed antibodies of all three specificities were produced, namely, anti-bisQ, anti-idiotype, and anti-ACh receptor antibodies.

Experiments like these show that all the elements of the network are in place and operative during the course of an immune response. The question, of course, remains about their physiological role in the immune response.

Summary

1.   The network theory of immune regulation introduces a new concept and a new vocabulary to the immune response.

2.   The vocabulary of the network uses the term *paratope* to define an antigen-binding site on an antibody molecule; the term *idiotope* defines the structures on Ig molecules that are seen as antigenic determinants by other antibody molecules; and *epitopes* are antigenic determinants on other molecules of the universe of antigens.

3.   The concept of the network introduces the idea that the idiotopes on an antibody molecule are shared by many antigens and cross-react with a large number of epitopes. Thus a paratope can react with an epitope on a large number of antigens. This results in the whole universe of antigens being reflected in the interacting elements of the immune system. These are *internal images* of the antigens.

4.   The immune system is seen as regulating itself through a network of interactions initiated by antigen. For example, an epitope on the antigen reacts with a paratope on a B-cell receptor and causes antibody formation. This first antibody is called Ab1. Ab1 has a paratope (p1), which binds the epitope, and Ab1 is itself antigenic because it bears an idiotope, i1. Another B cell has a receptor with specificity for i1 and is therefore stimulated to produce antibody. This second

antibody is Ab2, which has a paratope and idiotope, p2 and i2. The p2 binds i1 on Ab1, and the i2 induces a B cell with a paratope for i2 to make Ab3. Ab3 has p3 which binds i2. In this way the immune system responds once to an external stimulus and from then on carries out a network of internal responses to regulate itself.

5. Regulatory auto–anti-idiotype molecules can be found in animals undergoing an immune response.

6. The network theory predicts that anti-idiotype antibody to an anti-hormone antibody should have the internal image of the hormone receptor. Anti–anti-hormone can be shown to function as anti-receptor antibody.

Additional Readings

Golub, E. S. 1980. Idiotypes and networks. An introduction. *Cell* 22: 641.

Green, M. I. and A. Nisonoff, eds. 1984. *The Biology of Idiotypes.* Plenum, New York.

Jerne, N. K. 1960. Immunological speculations. *Annu. Rev. Microbiol.* 14: 341.

Jerne, N. K. 1973. The immune system. *Sci. Am.* 229: 52.

Jerne, N. K. 1974. Toward a network theory of the immune system. *Annals Immunol.* 125C: 373.

Jerne, N. K. 1984. Idiotype networks and other preconceived ideas. *Immunol. Rev.* 79: 5.

Jerne, N. K. 1985. The generative grammar of the immune system. *EMBO J.* 4: 847.

Meyer, D. I. 1990. Receptor anti-idiotypes. Mimics—or gimmicks? *Nature* 347: 424.

Zanetti, M. and D. H. Katz. 1985. Self-recognition, autoimmunity, and internal images. *Curr. Topics Microbiol. Immunol.* 119: 111.

REGULATION BY T CELLS

Overview   While antibodies and the network may be important in the regulation of the immune response, most studies suggest that T cells also play a major role. We've already considered how T cells help immune responses through the release of lymphokines. In addition, T cells can suppress the immune response by a number of mechanisms. The contrast between regulation by the network and by T cells is an important one at both the biological and philosophical levels. Regulation of the immune response by T cells is brought about in a manner compatible with clonal selection. That is, lymphocytes display receptors for the universe of antigens with which the immune system can react, and one function of T cells is to suppress the immune response. In this view antigen is seen as playing its normal role of selecting cells with the appropriate receptors. These cells then exert a regulatory influence.

T cells that suppress immune responses may not belong to a unique T-cell subset with a specialized function, but may instead represent regulatory activities of helper and cytotoxic T cells. In this chapter we will describe the discovery that T cells can suppress immune responses and follow this field into its controversial areas. We will discuss the complex interactions which have been associated with regulatory T cells and examine some of the new directions which the field is taking. By considering both sides of the controversies, we hope to give a feeling for the dynamics of immunologic research. In some ways, the suppressor cell story is a microcosm of the sociological aspects of immunology.

Suppression of Immune Responses by T Cells

By the mid-1960s it was clear to most cellular immunologists that the T cell is crucial in the immune response, because it is able to be both an effector cell in cell-mediated responses and a helper cell in both humoral and cell-mediated responses. At that time

Richard K. Gershon at Yale concluded that the T cell could also be a *regulatory* cell that could suppress the immune response. It is important, 25 years after the fact, for the reader to recognize what a creative leap this idea was. It was met with almost universal skepticism.

Along with the uniqueness of the idea, the complexity of the experiment may have been another reason why the idea of the suppressor T cell was not readily accepted. Figure 1 is a figure from the original 1970 Gershon and Kondo paper describing the experiments. The large number of groups and apparent vastness of the experiment worked as a real impediment to immunologists at the time. Groups of adult mice were thymectomized, lethally irradiated, and reconstituted with syngeneic bone marrow. Some of them were injected with thymus cells and others were not. Some groups then received repeated doses of high concentrations of antigen. The idea here was to induce a state of immunologic tolerance (discussed in detail in Chapter 31). After several weeks of this treatment, half the mice received an injection of thymus cells as a source of helper cells and were challenged with an immunizing dose of antigen. The antibody responses were then quantified, and it was found that the groups that had received thymus cells at the time of bone marrow reconstitution did *not* produce anti-RBC antibody.

This result fulfilled Gershon's prediction—that under certain conditions, antigen seen by thymus-derived cells can induce not only helper and effector cells but also cells able to suppress the immune response. The groups of mice that received the antigen *before* they were reconstituted with thymus (i.e., in the absence of a thymus) made good antibody responses, but the groups that received the antigen while they had thymus cells did not. Thus the presence of a thymus during part of the response prevented the animals from making antibody. The cells responsible for this suppression were found to be T cells (see below) and were termed SUPPRESSOR T CELLS.

T cells capable of suppressing immune responses have since been described in a wide range of systems. One problem that arose in this regard was that these effects were all attributed to "suppressor T cells," implying that there was only one mechanism (and cell type) that could produce such effects. We now know that there are a number of ways in which T cells (as well as other cells) can inhibit immune responses. Before embarking on a discussion of the suppressor T-cell controversies, therefore, we will first consider how more "conventional" T cells can suppress immune responses.

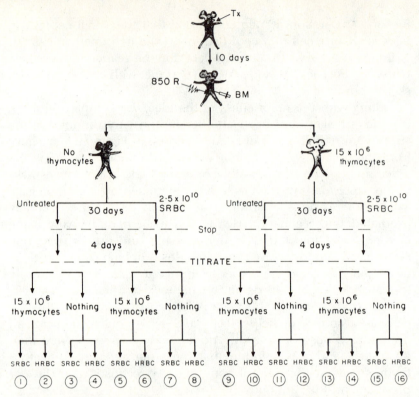

1   Suppressor T Cells and "Infectious Tolerance." The complex "plan of experiments" from Gershon's original paper on suppressor T-cells. Animals were thymectomized, and some were reconstituted with thymocytes (as a source of T cells). Repeated injections with sheep red blood cells (SRBCs) as antigen followed; then animals were injected with thymocytes (as a source of help) and rechallenged with SRBCs or horse red cells (HRBCs). Animals that received thymocytes and were repeatedly injected with SRBCs failed to respond to SRBCs (but responded to HRBCs) even after additional thymocytes were injected. Lack of response, i.e., tolerance, was dominant. [From Gershon and Kondo. 1970. *Immunology* 18: 723]

Helper T Cells Can Suppress Immune Responses

In Chapter 27 we discussed the evidence for two types of CD4$^+$ helper T cells. Type 1 helper cells (T$_{H1}$) produce IL-2 and γ-interferon upon activation, while type 2 helper T cells (T$_{H2}$) produce IL-4 and IL-5. It is now known that γ-interferon, released from T$_{H1}$ cells, inhibits the proliferation and function of T$_{H2}$ cells (while having no effect on T$_{H1}$ cells). T$_{H2}$ cells also produce a lymphokine capable of suppressing T$_{H1}$ cells.[1]

[1] This lymphokine, believe it or not, is IL-10. It is so new that it just barely made the list in Chapter 27.

These observations have very important ramifications for our understanding of immune regulation. For example, we know that T_{H2} cells and the lymphokines they produce are required for the generation of IgE antibody, which is a critical component of one type of allergy (see Chapter 34). In mice, induction of an IgE response can be inhibited by the administration of γ-interferon. This, of course, has clinical implications for the control of allergy. In addition, immunization protocols that decrease allergic responses have been in use for a number of years, although their mechanisms of action have been unclear. It is possible that these protocols work by preferentially inducing T_{H1} cells, which in turn suppress T_{H2} cell function.

These findings have also been important in understanding immune responses to parasitic infections. The *Leishmania* parasite (see Chapter 32) can produce either lethal or transient infections, depending on the mouse strain infected. T cells from infected, susceptible strains can suppress effective immune responses in resistant strains. These inhibitory T cells have now been shown to be $CD4^+$ T_{H2} cells, which inhibit the beneficial immune response elicited by T_{H1} cells. Treatment of susceptible strains with either γ-interferon or anti–IL-4 antibodies, both of which block T_{H2} induction, renders the susceptible animals resistant to infection.

Cytotoxic T Cells Can Suppress Immune Responses

Another way in which T cells can suppress immune responses is through the action of cytotoxic T cells. Conceptually, this could occur if the cytotoxic cells killed other T cells (or B cells) bearing specific idiotypic determinants related to antigen recognition. In this sense, this sort of suppression would be a variant of the network. Another way in which cytotoxic cells could suppress immune responses would be by killing the active APCs, thus removing the stimulus before an immune response could be generated. There is evidence supporting the idea that these processes *can*, at least, occur. We are not sure, however, that they normally do.

Hans Binz and Hans Wigzell did a series of experiments to test whether cytotoxic T cells can be generated that have an apparent specificity for idiotypic structures on other T cells, and what effects such T cells have on the generation of specific immune responses. The general plan of their experiments is shown in Figures 2 and 3. T cells were activated in an allogeneic MLR, and the activated T cells were separated from the nonactivated cells. The activated T-cell blasts were then used to immunize syngeneic mice. After

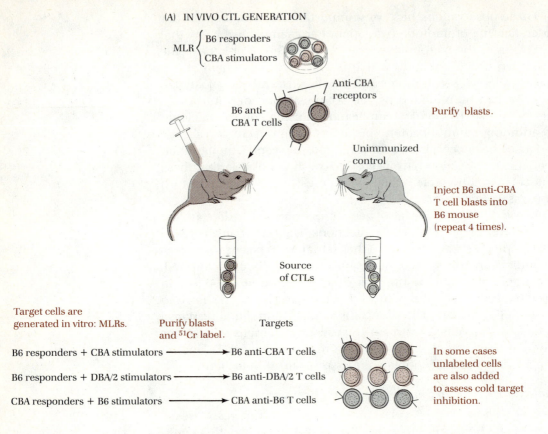

(A) IN VIVO CTL GENERATION

MLR { B6 responders / CBA stimulators

Anti-CBA receptors

B6 anti-CBA T cells

Purify blasts.

Unimmunized control

Inject B6 anti-CBA T cell blasts into B6 mouse (repeat 4 times).

Source of CTLs

Target cells are generated in vitro: MLRs.

Purify blasts and ^{51}Cr label.

Targets

B6 responders + CBA stimulators → B6 anti-CBA T cells

B6 responders + DBA/2 stimulators → B6 anti-DBA/2 T cells

CBA responders + B6 stimulators → CBA anti-B6 T cells

In some cases unlabeled cells are also added to assess cold target inhibition.

(B)

CTL from	"Cold" targets	Percent killing of ^{51}Cr-labeled blast cell targets		
		B6 anti-CBA	B6 anti-DBA/2	CBA anti-B6
B6	—	−0.11	0.55	−0.39
B6 immunized 4 times with B6 anti-CBA blasts	—	72.52	1.47	−0.17
	B6 anti-CBA	18.73	Not done	Not done
	B6 anti-DBA/2	60.08	Not done	Not done

several immunizations, cells from the immunized mice were tested for their ability to kill T-cell blasts (Figure 2). They found that T cells from the immunized animals were capable of killing syngeneic T-cell blasts generated against the original stimulator but not against a different stimulator. Thus, they attained one of their goals: they had generated CTLs capable of killing syngeneic T cells bearing unique idiotype determinants related to T-cell specificity.

◄**2** **Cytotoxic T Lymphocytes (CTLs) That Recognize Specific Antigen Receptors on Syngeneic Cells Can Be Generated In Vivo.** (A) Plan of the experiment. An MLR with B6 responder cells and CBA stimulator cells is generated, and the blasting T cells (see Chapter 26) are purified. These cells are B6 anti-CBA T cells (since they responded in the MLR). The B6 anti-CBA T cells are then used to immunize B6 mice several times. Unimmunized mice serve as controls. Spleen cells from these mice are then tested for the presence of CTLs using target cells generated in MLRs. The target cells are purified B6 blast cells after responding to CBA or DBA/2 stimulator cells, or CBA blast cells after responding to B6 stimulators. The blast cells are labeled with ^{51}Cr and cultured with the CTLs. In some cases, unlabeled blast cells are added to test for cold target inhibition of the cytotoxicity (see Chapter 28). (B) Results. Cells from B6 mice immunized with B6 anti-CBA T cells contain CTLs capable of killing B6 anti-CBA blasts, but not B6 anti-DBA/2 blasts or CBA anti-B6 blasts. The killing of labelled B6 anti-CBA blasts was inhibited by unlabelled B6 anti-CBA blasts, but not by unlabelled B6 anti-DBA/2 blasts. These results show that CTLs can be generated that specifically kill syngeneic T cells bearing unique antigen receptors. The ability of such CTLs to specifically suppress immune responses is examined in the experiment shown in Figure 3. [After Binz and Wigzell, 1978. *J. Exp. Med.* 147: 63]

(Remember that these experiments were performed before the T-cell receptor had been identified.) The question now became, Could these idiotype-specific CTLs suppress immune responses?

Figure 3 shows the experiment designed to answer this question. Binz and Wigzell injected the T cells from the blast-immunized animals into normal recipients, and found that the injected cells contained a Thy-1$^+$, CD8$^+$ T cell capable of reducing the recipients' ability to generate mixed lymphocyte responses to the original stimulator cells. This suppression was specific, i.e., MLRs generated against a different stimulator were normal. They interpreted their results as follows. Since the T cells used for immunization are specific for an antigen, they bear unique idiotypic structures on their T-cell receptors. CTLs generated in the immunized animals recognize these unique structures and thereby kill any syngeneic T cells specific for the original antigen. If this is a general phenomenon, it represents one mechanism for the down-regulation of specific immune responses by T cells.

Patrick Flood and his colleagues then extended these results into a model of T-cell-mediated tumor rejection. Using a fibrosarcoma that is actively rejected by normal, syngeneic animals, they generated T-cell blasts specific for the tumor and used these T cells to immunize animals. They then showed that these animals had a reduced ability to resist the tumor, in that most of the immunized animals developed tumors when injected with the

(A) Test suppressor activity of in vivo-generated CTL.

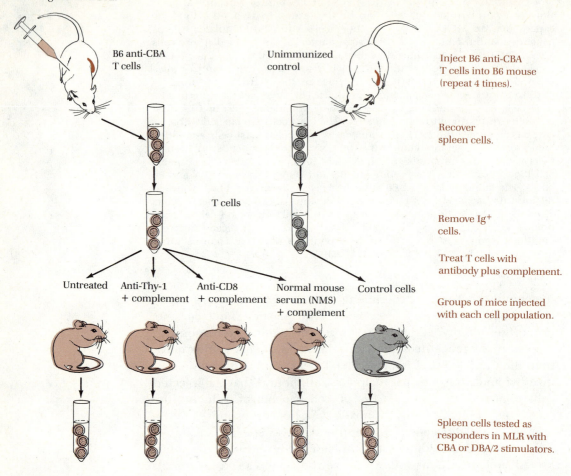

B6 anti-CBA T cells

Unimmunized control

Inject B6 anti-CBA T cells into B6 mouse (repeat 4 times).

Recover spleen cells.

T cells

Remove Ig$^+$ cells.

Treat T cells with antibody plus complement.

Untreated | Anti-Thy-1 + complement | Anti-CD8 + complement | Normal mouse serum (NMS) + complement | Control cells

Groups of mice injected with each cell population.

Spleen cells tested as responders in MLR with CBA or DBA/2 stimulators.

(B) Results

MLR from B6 mice, 1 month after adoptive transfer of treated cells from blast-immunized animals

Cells transferred from	Treatment of transferred cells	[^{3}H]Tdr incorporation in cpm	
		CBA stimulators	DBA/2 stimulators
B6	Anti-Ig column	201,905	210,428
B6 immunized 4 times with B6 anti-CBA blasts	Anti-Ig column	40,691	198,934
	Anti-Thy-1 + complement	131,439	178,316
	NMS + complement	52,075	191,399
	Anti-CD8 + complement	111,830	193,148

◄ **3** **CTLs That Recognize Specific Antigen Receptors on Syngeneic Cells Can Act As Suppressor Cells.** (A) Plan of the experiment. Spleen cells from the mice used in the experiment in Figure 2 were depleted of B cells by passage over an anti-Ig column. The enriched T cells from the blast-immunized mice were further treated with normal mouse serum, anti-Thy-1, or anti-CD8, plus complement. These fractionated T cells or T cells from control mice were then injected into normal B6 recipients. One month later, spleen cells from these recipient mice were tested for their ability to respond in an MLR to CBA or DBA/2 stimulator cells. (B) The result, expressed as [^{3}H]TdR incorporation (cpm) of the MLR, show that animals that received CD8$^+$, Thy-1$^+$ cells from blast-immunized mice showed a decreased ability to respond to CBA stimulators (underlined groups). Recall from Figure 2 that the blast cells used to immunize mice were B6 anti-CBA, and that CTLs from the immunized mice could specifically kill these blast cells. Taken together, the data from Figure 2 and this figure suggest that CTLs were generated that were capable of killing syngeneic T cells specific for CBA stimulators, and when transferred into syngeneic animals, these CTLs eliminated T cells with anti-CBA specificity but not those with anti-DBA/2 specificity. [After Binz and Wigzell, 1978. *J. Exp. Med.* 147:63]

fibrosarcoma. None of the animals that were immunized with nonresponsive T cells (the nonresponding T cells from the same cultures) developed tumors. Like Binz and Wigzell, they then demonstrated that these immunized animals generated cytotoxic T cells capable of killing T-cell blasts responding to the original fibrosarcoma but not T-cell blasts generated against a similar (but antigenically different) fibrosarcoma.

These studies suggested that cytotoxic T cells could suppress immune responses by recognizing and killing T cells that bear a specific idiotype (presumably on the T-cell receptor). More recent studies open the possibility that cytotoxic T cells may also have the capacity to control immune responses by killing active APCs. Michael Bevan's laboratory has shown that a peptide fragment of a protein antigen (ovalbumin) can associate with class I MHC on the surface of cells to act as a target for ovalbumin-specific cytotoxic T cells, without a requirement for cytoplasmic processing of the antigen (see Chapter 20). They then showed that if this peptide is injected into mice, ovalbumin-specific cytotoxic T cells are generated. We can imagine that if such peptides can be generated naturally, then CD8$^+$ cytotoxic T cells could then be activated and would, perhaps, kill cells attempting to present the protein to the immune system. Although this has not been demonstrated, we should consider this (or some variation on this theme) as a possible way for T cells to suppress immune responses.

Other mechanisms are related to the regulation of immune

responses by the release of lymphokines from activated T cells. Some CD8$^+$ cells are known to produce γ-interferon upon activation, which could lead to the suppression of some types of immune responses (see above). Similarly, some CD4$^+$ cells, upon recognition of antigen plus class II MHC, release the lymphokine TNFβ (lymphotoxin, see Chapter 27), which is cytotoxic for some types of cells and might inhibit some immune responses. Other lymphokines, perhaps undiscovered, might similarly inhibit immune responses in related ways.

We've gone to some lengths to describe how T cells might be able to suppress immune responses without resorting to completely novel mechanisms in order to set the stage for the "suppressor T-cell controversy." This is because, as we'll see, there are suggestions that at least some T cells control immune responses by a completely different route that appears to violate much of what we know about how T cells work. The question for you to decide, as a reader, is whether this completely different process might provide new insights into how T cells regulate immunity. Part of the problem is that the study of immune regulation is difficult, and not all the information is yet available.

Antigen-Specific Suppressor T Cells and Factors

If suppressor cells are to be of regulatory significance during an immune response, they must be antigen-specific; and there are countless examples of such antigen specificity. An early example comes from the experiments of Tomio Tada and his co-workers in Tokyo (Figure 4). Mice were primed with carrier, and their spleen or thymus cells were transferred to unirradiated recipients, which were then challenged with hapten and carrier. The response of the recipients to the hapten was suppressed under these conditions. Treating the cells from the primed donor with anti-Thy-1 and complement before transfer abolished their ability to induce suppression of the unirradiated recipients. Treating the donors with a carrier different from the one used in the hapten–carrier conjugate at challenge gave no suppression. These experiments indicate that there is antigen-specific suppression carried out by T cells. More recently, Lee Herzenberg at Stanford coined the term EPITOPE-SPECIFIC SUPPRESSION to describe this phenomenon, which she showed to be readily reproducible.

A similar early discovery was made by Baruj Benacerraf and his co-workers, using GAT-nonresponder mice. Mice of the DBA/1 strain are low responders to the polymer glutamate, alanine, tyro-

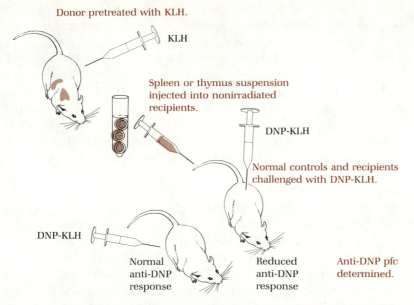

Donor pretreated with KLH.

KLH

Spleen or thymus suspension injected into nonirradiated recipients.

DNP-KLH

Normal controls and recipients challenged with DNP-KLH.

DNP-KLH

Normal anti-DNP response

Reduced anti-DNP response

Anti-DNP pfc determined.

4   Generation of Antigen-Specific Suppressor T Cells. Mice are primed with the carrier (KLH), and the spleen or thymus cells are injected into unirradiated hosts. After challenge with hapten bound to the carrier (DNP-KLH), the recipients make a reduced anti-DNP response. This phenomenon is now known as *epitope-specific suppression*. Note that this experiment does not demonstrate that "suppressor T cells" are a unique subset. [After Tada et al., 1974. *J. Exp. Med.* 140: 239]

sine (GAT). Gershon had predicted earlier that nonresponder mice might have suppressor cells activated more readily than responder strains. Treating nonresponder strains with GAT and then adding their cells to cultures with cells from responder strain animals was found to render the responder cells nonresponsive. Thus the nonresponder strains made cells able to suppress the cells from the responder strain. Treatment of the nonresponder cells with anti–Thy-1 and complement abolished their ability to suppress, showing that there are suppressor T cells that are responsible for the lack of response.

Thus, suppressor cells are Thy-1$^+$ and therefore appear to be T cells. The immediate question that came to mind was: What is the CD profile of the cells? The answer to this question originally looked simple, but as often happens, the problem was more complicated than originally conceived. There seemed to be very complex cell interactions involved in the generation of suppressor cells, and each of the interacting cells had a different phenotype. It could be shown, at first, that the cell carrying out the suppression (i.e., the suppressor effector cell) is $CD8^+$ in mice, rats, and humans. Later, a $CD4^+$ cell was described that appears to induce these $CD8^+$ cells, and this was called the suppressor inducer cell. Another marker that became available for murine suppressor T cells was "I-J." We will discuss this very problematic marker in more detail below, but for now we'll treat it like any other marker.

We have seen that T cells, in contrast to B cells, can bind antigen only in the context of self-MHC molecules. Suppressor T cells, however, may be an exception to this statement. The experiment diagrammed in Figure 5 shows evidence for this. Antigen-specific suppressor cells are induced in mice, and then the B cells are removed from the spleen-cell population by either passing the cells over a column or incubating them on a petri dish coated with rabbit anti–mouse Ig (RAMIG). The B cells, which are Ig^+, adhere to the surface; the Ig^- cells, which are T cells, are removed. The T-cell population is then passed over a column (or incubated on a plate) coated with the specific antigen used to induce the suppressor cells. A small proportion of the cells adhere to this surface. These cells are gently removed from the surface and compared with the T cells that did not adhere to the antigen-coated surface. As seen in the figure, both populations are $Thy-1^+$. The adherent cells are also strongly $CD8^+$, whereas the non-antigen-binding cells are strongly $CD5^+$. The antigen-binding population is able to carry out suppression when incubated with normal cells and antigen. Anti–I-J antibodies plus complement removed the suppressive activity detectable in these cells (see below for a discussion of the problems associated with this marker).

These experiments suggested that the effector cell in suppression differs from other T cells in its ability to bind antigen directly. It must be recalled, however, that these cells do not bind antigen by means of a surface Ig, because neither the antigen-binding nor the nonbinding populations adhered to the anti-Ig-coated surfaces. This result implies that the antigen-specific receptor on the suppressor T cell is somehow different from that on helper and cytotoxic T cells. This is considered in much more detail below, because it, like I-J, is part of the suppressor T-cell controversy.

Antigen-Specific T-Suppressor Factors

One of the first demonstrations of the antigen-specific suppressor factor involved the IgE response to the hapten dinitrophenol (DNP). Tada and his co-workers found that when they sublethally irradi-

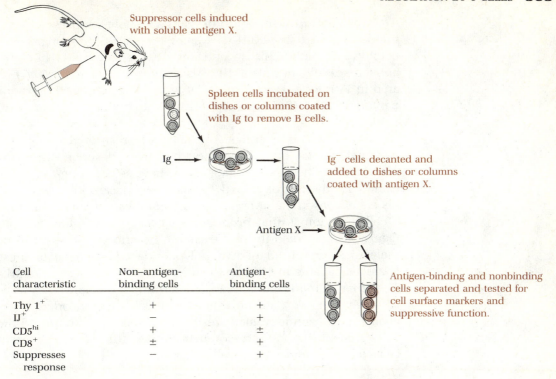

Suppressor cells induced with soluble antigen X.

Spleen cells incubated on dishes or columns coated with Ig to remove B cells.

Ig ⟶

Ig⁻ cells decanted and added to dishes or columns coated with antigen X.

Antigen X ⟶

Antigen-binding and nonbinding cells separated and tested for cell surface markers and suppressive function.

Cell characteristic	Non–antigen-binding cells	Antigen-binding cells
Thy 1$^+$	+	+
IJ$^+$	−	+
CD5^{hi}	+	±
CD8$^+$	±	+
Suppresses response	−	+

5 **Some Characteristics of Suppressor T Cells.** Suppressor cells are induced by injection of soluble antigen, and the spleen cells are depleted of B cells. The T cells are then separated by their ability to adhere to antigen-coated surfaces, and the populations are compared for surface markers and function (suppression). Surface markers were determined by cytotoxicity with complement. The suppressive cells were antigen-binding, Thy-1$^+$, CD5^{lo}, CD8$^+$. The suppressive activity was also removed by treatment with anti–I-J plus complement (not shown). [After Okumura et al., 1977. *J. Exp. Med.* 146: 1234; and Taniguchi and Miller, 1977. *J. Exp. Med.* 146: 1450]

ated rats and immunized them with DNP conjugated to *Ascaris* (DNP-Asc) plus pertussis vaccine, a good anti-DNP response, which was mostly IgE, occurred. To determine whether a cell-free supernatant fraction could induce suppression, Tada and co-workers sonicated thymocytes and spleen cells from these immunized animals and subjected the lysate to ultracentrifugation. They obtained an extract that was able to suppress an ongoing anti-DNP IgE response when injected into rats. The factor was antigen-specific (extracts from normal cells did not work, nor did extracts from cells immunized to other antigens).

Tada's group went on to develop a soluble suppressor factor in the mouse using KLH, a system that all immunologists felt comfortable with. This second suppressor factor was not only antigen-specific, but also MHC-restricted. If the factor was generated in F_1 mice that were H-2$^{k/d}$, it would suppress each parental haplotype (i.e., H-2^k and H-2^d), but not strains of other MHC haplotypes.

By the late 1970s, antigen-specific, MHC-restricted soluble factors that carried out suppression had been described by many laboratories. The next advance (as we have seen happen so often) came with the use of cloned T cells. First, Masaru Taniguchi and his colleagues, then several other laboratories, established cloned T-cell hybridomas that produced such factors (see, for example, Figure 6). The majority of the factors described appeared to be molecules composed of two polypeptide chains. One of these chains is capable of binding to antigen attached to a solid matrix. The other, in many cases, bears a determinant recognized by anti–I-J antibodies. To date no genes responsible for encoding these chains have been identified, despite some efforts. Like I-J and the T-cell receptor of suppressor hybridomas, this is an important basis for the suppressor T-cell controversy.

The Suppressor T-Cell Controversy

We have gone into some detail about the study of suppressor T cells, and you might consider this excessive considering that there seem to be a lot of problems regarding their properties. However, this area of study played a major role in the development of immunology in the 1970s and early 1980s, when the skepticism came to a head. Let's consider the problems in more detail, so that you can decide on your own what should be done about them.

The controversy surrounding suppressor T cells can be broken down into two general categories or questions: (1) Do suppressor T cells represent a distinct functional subpopulation of T lymphocytes, as do helper and cytotoxic T cells? (2) Do any T cells regulate immune responses via mechanisms requiring the proposal of new processes in the immune system (e.g., antigen-specific factors)? Some people have combined these into one big question, asking, "Do suppressor T cells exist?"

Lee Herzenberg has put the controversy into context by relating her thoughts when one of her students asked her whether

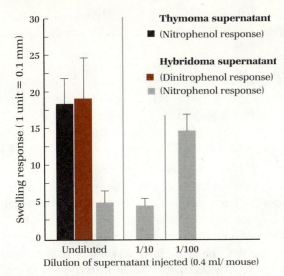

6 **Action of an Antigen-Specific T Suppressor Factor In Vivo.** Groups of animals were immunized with either nitrophenol or dinitrophenol. On the day before antigen reexposure, mice were given an injection of supernatant from a nitrophenol-specific T-suppressor hybridoma, or from the parent thymoma (the tumor line used to make the hybridoma). Cell-mediated immunity was assessed by ear swelling in response to the antigen. The nitrophenol (but not dinitrophenol) response was suppressed by injection with the hybridoma supernatant. This suppressive effect decreased (i.e., responses increased) with dilution of the hybridoma supernatant. In related experiments, animals were immunized with both antigens; the factor again only suppressed responses to nitrophenol. Similar T-hybridoma-derived suppressor factors have been described for dinitrophenol (and other antigens). [Data from Minami et al., 1981. *J. Exp. Med.* 154: 1390]

"she still believed in suppressor T cells." At first she considered retorting that "believe" shouldn't apply to a large body of experimental data, but rather that we should be concerned with the interpretation of that data. Then, as she says, she reconsidered the question in these terms: The controversy surrounding suppressor T cells is a microcosm of the transition, between the 1970s and the 1980s, between cellular and molecular experimentation in immunology. Cellular immunology gave a strong "yes" to suppressor T cells, while molecular immunology failed to find any evidence to account for either the cells or their function. So the questioner really was asking, "Do you have more faith in the experimental evidence of cellular immunology (as practiced in the 1970s and early 1980s) or in the lack of evidence from molecular immunology?" It is an important and valid question.

Let's consider the controversy from the point of view, first, of the skeptic. This can be summarized in what we call the five "no's" of suppression.

The Five "No's" of Suppressor T Cells

The case against either question 1 or 2 regarding suppressor T cells (see above) is embodied in five general statements. As we'll see below, these statements may be more or less valid, so don't take them at face value (yet). These are

- "No" Number 1: There are *no* cell-surface markers that uniquely identify suppressor T cells as a functional population.
- "No" Number 2: There are *no* (or few) cloned, long-term T-cell lines with suppressive activity.
- "No" Number 3: T-cell hybridomas that produce antigen-specific suppressor factors have *no* (or variable) T-cell receptor gene rearrangements. (This is discussed in much more detail below.)
- "No" Number 4: "I-J," a marker that has been associated with murine suppressor T cells and antigen-specific factors, maps into the I region (class II MHC), but *no* corresponding gene is present. (This is discussed in more detail below.)
- "No" Number 5: Antigen-specific T-cell factors have been characterized as proteins, but *no* genes encoding these factors have been identified.

In general, all these arguments, especially if taken together, make a pretty strong case against suppressor T cells as unique and/or antigen-specific factor-producing cells. The arguments that have carried the most weight are those of No's numbers 3, 4, and 5 (partly because they argue effectively for both sides of the controversy).

Now let's take the position of the suppressor T-cell advocate. This will give a feeling for why any controversy at all exists in the face of such damning charges.

The Arguments for Suppressor T Cells and Factors

The main argument in support of suppressor T cells and factors is that they have been described (and continue to be described) by many different laboratories around the world. And while the phenomenon of suppressor T-cell factors has been observed by many, the field is at an impasse until something new is found. Ideally, this would be the identification of genes encoding such factors (No number 5, above). In a way, this is the critical point:

if such genes are unambiguously identified, the controversy is resolved; on the other hand, failing to find such genes only continues the controversy without resolution, until eventually the advocates decide to give up (which will only resolve the issue in practice). Nevertheless, the failure thus far to identify these genes has tended to put the issue out of the minds of many immunologists (and given the number of things to attend to in immunology, this is not unreasonable).

The same arguments hold, in a way, for No's number 1 and number 2. Finding specific surface markers and/or developing methods to readily clone suppressor T cells will help in the research but won't really resolve the controversy.

Right now, the key to the story seems to lie in the T-cell receptor (No number 3) and, perhaps, in the I-J puzzle (No number 4). To see why, we will have to go into these stories in a bit more detail.

The T-Cell Receptor in Suppressor T-Cell Hybridomas

Shortly after the cloning of the first TCR gene, genomic DNAs from a number of different T cells, including cloned T helper and cytotoxic cells and suppressor T-cell hybridomas, were examined for rearrangement of this gene. When these were digested with endonucleases and probed with a β-chain cDNA (see Figure 7), it was found that all helper and cytotoxic T cells contained rearranged DNA (seen as new restriction fragments not found in the germ line; see Chapter 23). In contrast, suppressor T cells appeared not to rearrange this gene, indicating that these cells do not use the β chain of the T-cell receptor.

This finding was quickly confirmed by Mitchell Kronenberg and Leroy Hood. Further, they found that in several of the suppressor T-cell hybridomas, the entire chromosome housing the β-chain gene from the original T cell was lost, leaving only those of the thymoma fusion partner (this can happen in hybridoma cells, which start with double the normal number of chromosomes, then spontaneously shed some).

This finding was fine with both the skeptics and the advocates (at least for a while). Some of the latter asserted that, after all, suppressor T cells and their factors can bind directly to antigen (unlike other T cells) and that therefore they use a different T-cell receptor. Many favored the γδ T-cell receptor as a candidate, but quickly found that expression of the γ-chain gene does not correlate with suppressor cells. In fact, part of the problem with the

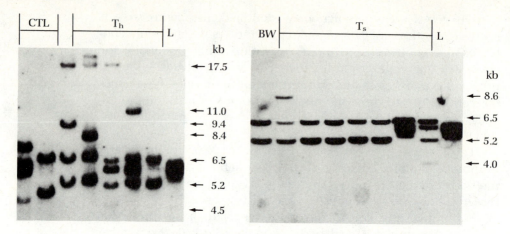

7 **TCRβ Genes in Suppressor T-Cell Hybridomas.** Southern blots of DNA from (A) cytotoxic (CTL) and helper (T$_h$) T-cell clones, and (B) suppressor T-cell (T$_s$) hybridomas. Note that in most of the cases, there is no rearrangement of the β chain in the suppressor cells. [From Hedrick et al., 1985. *Proc. Natl. Acad. Science U.S.A.* 82: 531]

reasoning around this time was that few seemed to notice (or be concerned) that T-cell receptor genes are *sometimes* rearranged and expressed in these suppressor T-cell hybridomas. People were hot to find new genes in these cells.

It wasn't until some time later that anyone questioned the original experiments. David Weiner and Mark Greene reasoned that perhaps the failure to *consistently* find T-cell receptor gene expression in suppressor T-cell hybridomas was a methodological problem, rather than a bona fide reflection of the nature of these cells. After all, helper T-cell hybridomas, if left too long in culture, often lose chromosomes bearing T-cell receptor genes. Unlike suppressor T-cell hybridomas, though, helper T-cell hybridomas are regularly recloned and kept in culture for relatively short periods of time. Therefore, Weiner and Greene selected an apparently T-cell-receptor-negative suppressor T-cell hybridoma and separated a very small population of T-cell-receptor-positive cells from the rest. They did this on the basis of cell-surface expression of the CD3 marker. They found that these CD3[+] cells were the only ones in the cloned population that were capable of producing their antigen-specific factor. Further, they showed that the CD3 molecules were associated with a conventional T-cell receptor. Thus, although the cells were cloned, it appeared that in culture they were losing chromosomes bearing T-cell receptor genes (and losing function) over time.

This result was quickly verified by Vijay Kuchroo, Martin Dorf, and their colleagues, using several other suppressor T-cell hybridomas. Further, they showed that removing T-cell receptor from the surface of these cells resulted in a loss of antigen-binding activity. This lab and others showed that the T-cell receptor genes in these suppressor T-cell hybridomas are rearranged, suggesting that this is a "conventional" T-cell receptor.

Now, several other investigators have found cell-surface T-cell receptors (and mRNA) associated with suppressor T-cell hybridomas. The next step was to examine the antigen-specific factors. Robert Fairchild and John Moorhead found that antigen-specific factors produced from suppressor T-cell hybridomas could be bound by antibodies to the T-cell receptor. They also showed that an anti-TCR C_α antibody was capable of binding suppressor factors from either hybridomas or "bulk" suppressor T-cells, and that this antibody was binding to the antigen-specific chain of the factor.

Recently, there has been renewed interest in the subject of suppressor T cells and antigen-specific factors as a result of this work. It's too early to say that any resolution of the suppressor T-cell controversy is at hand, but at least there is some action in the field. One idea that's being considered is that suppressor T cells may bear a T-cell receptor that has an affinity for antigen (perhaps in the absence of MHC), and that somehow, in soluble form, this receptor gives antigen specificity to the suppressor factor.

Despite these encouraging findings, and even if the T-cell receptor story becomes clear, there remains a major dilemma for the suppressor T-cell advocates to solve. This is the conundrum of I-J.

The I-J Enigma

The finding that T suppressor effector cells are $CD8^+$ distinguished them from T helper cells but did not allow them to be distinguished from T cytotoxic cells, which are also $CD8^+$. This is important, because one possible explanation for the phenomenon of suppression is that suppressor T cells are cytotoxic cells that are killing the helper T cells or the effector cells (see above). However, a cell-surface marker that seemed to be unique for the suppressor T cell was discovered in 1976. It was found that an antiserum raised by immunizing the congenic strain B10.A(3R) with cells from B10.A(5R) (or vice versa) gave an antiserum that seemed to react exclusively with T suppressor cells. Mapping studies showed that the gene was located in the I region (class II) of the MHC. This locus was called *I-J* and was found to map between I-E_α and I-E_β

(the genes for the two chains of I-E). Both suppressor cells and the soluble suppressor product were shown in some cases to react with I-J antiserum. Monoclonal antibodies to I-J haplotypes were generated, and studies seemed to be shaping up. But then events took a sudden change.

When the genes of the I region were isolated, cloned, and sequenced, there was not enough DNA between $I-E_\alpha$ and $I-E_\beta$ to account for the I-J molecule. Further, the genetic crossovers in both B10.A(3R) and B10.A(5R) were found to be located within the same region, the intron between $I-E_{\beta1}$ and $I-E_{\beta2}$. No obvious DNA sequence differences between these strains could be found. There was no I-J gene in the I region. Thus, the I-J enigma: How can a cell-surface marker map to a part of a chromosome where there is no gene?

The answer remains unclear, but there may be some clues. More recent studies by Tada and his colleagues have shown that I-J, unlike MHC molecules, appears to differentiate adaptively. Most of these studies focused on the $I-J^k$ marker (identified by monoclonal antibodies in $H-2^k$ mice). They found that $I-J^k$ can be expressed by T cells in non-$H-2^k$ animals immunized with antigen on $H-2^k$ cells. They suggested that $I-J^k$ is actually a receptor for I-E molecules. Flood and colleagues took this a step further. They showed that $H-2^b$ mice, made transgenic for the E_α^k gene (and thus expressing E_α^k, E_β^b) could produce suppressor factors bound by anti-$I-J^k$ antibodies.

I-J has only been described in the mouse, and the problems associated with it have been severe. While there are glimmerings of progress on these problems, it is a possibility that the I-J enigma will simply not be solved. Like many aspects of the suppressor T-cell controversy, the fact that the phenomenon was reproducible in different laboratories was no guarantee that it would be quickly understood.

SYNTHESIS
How to View the Suppressor T-Cell Controversy

This chapter is necessarily different from all the other chapters in the book, because the subject of suppressor T cells is different from all other subjects in modern immunology. Thinking about suppressor T cells dominated much of the immunology of the 1970s, and just 10 years later it became (almost) a forbidden topic. If nothing else, this is a valuable lesson in how science works. We think, however, that there is more value in this discussion than just as a history lesson.

Somewhere along the line, the study of suppressor T cells and antigen-specific factors went wrong. Some investigators, including a few of those who were mentioned here, are attempting to set it right. At least we will find a basis for some of the phenomena, and we will then have to decide how important they are.

It is not uncommon for a popular finding to be due to a trivial artifact, a situation that can undermine volumes of theoretical speculation. What would be strange, however, would be for a set of findings, repeated extensively in many systems in many laboratories, to be either illusory or artifactual. What we've tried to do in this chapter is to lay out the story as fairly as we could and to leave it to the reader to decide where, and whether, the work should proceed.

The resolution of the suppressor T-cell controversy could either resign this chapter to a footnote in immunologic history or dramatically alter the way we view the immune response. The latter would be no small thing, and therefore these few pages may not be a waste of good ink.

Summary

1. T cells can regulate immunity by a number of mechanisms, including interactions between helper T-cell subsets and the action of cytotoxic T cells against syngeneic, antigen-specific cells. Often, T cells that inhibit immunity are referred to as "suppressor T cells," but this does not mean that they represent a unique T-cell subset.

2. One important way in which T cells regulate immune responses is via the lymphokines they produce. T_{H1} cells produce lymphokines that inhibit the function of T_{H2} cells, and vice versa. Because the lymphokines produced by these different helper cells have distinct functions, the effects of such cross regulation can be dramatic.

3. One controversial mechanism of suppressor T-cell function is the production of antigen-specific regulatory factors by T cells. While these factors have been demonstrated in many systems, little is known of their molecular or chemical nature.

4. The suppressor-cell controversy asks two questions: (1) Is there a unique population of T cells with suppressor function? and (2) Is there a unique mechanism (e.g., antigen-specific factors) of suppression? Many immunologists would answer no to both questions, but interesting observations that contrast with this view have been made. The relative paucity of molecular information on suppressor cells and factors raises a third question: Should suppressor cells be studied?

Additional Readings

Gejewski, T. F., S. R. Schell, G. Nau and F. W. Fitch. 1989. Regulation of T cell activation: Differences among T cell subsets. *Immunol. Rev.* 111: 79.

Hodes, R. J. 1989. T cell mediated regulation: Help and suppression. In Paul, W. E., ed. *Fundamental Immunology*, 2nd ed. Raven, New York, p. 587.

Ishikura, H., V. Kuchroo, S. Abromson-Leeman and M. E. Dorf. 1988. Comparisons between helper and suppressor T-cell induction. *Immunol. Rev.* 106: 93.

IMMUNE TOLERANCE

Overview Because immunology grew out of the study of infectious diseases, the imagery of its language still carries allusions to battle against invading hordes of hostile microbes and the protection of the sanctity of body. Paul Ehrlich was one of the first to write about (and demonstrate) the fact that in the process of protecting itself from external invaders, the body must take care not to react against itself. He called this bio-taboo against self-reactivity *horror autotoxicus*. The field of immunologic tolerance is the rethinking of this idea.

The condition in which an animal "tolerates" an antigen by not making a response to it is called *immunologic tolerance*. In Chapter 24, we saw that at least part of this process involves negative selection of self-specific T cells during maturation in the thymus. This, however, is only a part of the story. In this chapter we will examine the experimental approaches to the question of self–nonself discrimination. We will see that tolerance can be induced to a wide range of antigens in both the newborn and the adult and that both B and T cells can be rendered tolerant. Tolerance may act at the level of lymphoid development (central tolerance) or may render mature lymphocytes specifically unresponsive (peripheral tolerance). Furthermore, we will see that there are at least two mechanisms of tolerance: one involving loss of cells during maturation, and one involving loss of cellular activity without removal of the cells (clonal anergy). The latter can apparently occur with or without the activation of regulatory T cells.

CHAPTER

31

Self and Nonself

The central question in immunology has always been: How can the immune system discriminate between "foreign" and "self"? Until immunologists were in a position to understand the fundamental processes by which responses to foreign antigens are carried out, there was little hope of understanding how responses to self were prevented. This is not to say that immunologists were not always aware of the question; rather, it shows the need to be able to frame a question that is amenable to the formulation of a testable hypothesis. At the turn of the century Paul Ehrlich stated the problem in Latin (which makes even the most banal concept sound imposing) by calling the process of not making autoresponses HORROR AUTOTOXICUS. He had observed that although an individual will make antibody responses to nearly any injected substance, including tissues from other individuals of the same species, it will not respond to injected samples of its own tissues. Of course, he was not in a position to predict a mechanism.

The Concept of Self-Learning

The question of how the immune system prevents (or is prevented from) autoreactions was not seriously dealt with until 1949, when F. M. Burnet and F. Fenner published a monograph called *The Production of Antibodies*. Burnet and Fenner were heavily influenced by the work of Ray Owen at the California Institute of Technology, a geneticist who was at that time interested in blood groups of cattle. He noted that the apparent incidence of *monozygotic twins* in cattle as indicated by his blood tests was much greater than farmers and breeders knew to actually be the case. Owen then drew upon F. R. Lillie's 1916 observation that *dizygotic twin* fetuses in cattle very often exchange blood because the placentas are so close together. When Owen treated the red cells of cattle that expressed both X and Y blood groups with anti-X antibody and complement, he found that some of the cells were not lysed. The unlysed cells could be shown to be expressing the Y blood group. He concluded that the apparent monozygotic twins were really chimeras, that is, they were dizygotic twins that had shared the precursors of the blood cells of the other in utero. Because of this sharing, as adults each twin produced the red cells of the other and did not make immune responses to the other's red cell antigens. They were, in fact, treating the red cells (and precursors) of the other twin as if they were their own. Somehow the early contact with antigen rendered the animal able to tolerate the antigen without responding to it.

Burnet and Fenner put this very important observation into a theoretical framework by postulating that "self" is distinguished from "nonself" during embryonic development. They postulated a process called SELF-MARKING in which at some point in development the individual marks its own tissue in some unspecified manner. After this marking occurs, any antigen that enters the system will lack the self-marker and thus be identified as foreign. In the twin cattle, the precursors of the red cells had been shared and thus were marked. To test the hypothesis experimentally, Burnet and Fenner injected fertilized eggs with influenza virus and then determined whether the chickens that developed from these eggs had the ability to make anti-influenza antibody. Unfortunately, although all the animals made antibody responses, it was because of the experimental system chosen. Later, in other systems, it was shown that introduction of antigen into the newborn does in fact result in IMMUNOLOGIC TOLERANCE.

We now know that "marking" of self-tissue is not the mechanism of tolerance. Instead, it is a *learning* of self by the immune system. Part of this education is during development and is due to selection events such as negative selection (Chapter 24), as well as other mechanisms, as we'll see. For now, however, we will simply consider the concept that the immune system learns what self is.

Induction of Tolerance in the Newborn

Experimentally Induced Neonatal Tolerance

Because Burnet and Fenner had cast the phenomenon of self-tolerance in terms of Owen's discovery that dizygotic twin cattle are blood-cell chimeras, in 1951 Peter Medawar and his co-workers in England showed that a large proportion of these cattle could accept skin grafts from the other twin. Medawar and his group then went one step further. They intentionally established chimeras in laboratory animals to determine whether these could now accept allogeneic skin grafts. In these experiments, Rupert Billingham, Leslie Brent, and Medawar injected lymphoid cells from C57BL/6 mice into *newborn* mice of the A strain (Figure 1). When these animal reached maturity (about 6–8 weeks), they were grafted with skin from mice of the same strain (A), or from two different strains (C57BL/6 or CBA). The A-strain mice that had not been injected at birth rejected the skin from both CBA and C57BL/6. In contrast, those A-strain mice that had been injected with the C57BL/6 cells rejected the CBA skin but *did not* reject the C57BL/6 skin (Figure 2). This meant that contact with foreign tissue at a very early stage of life (the experiments were also conducted by injecting mice in utero) allowed them to *tolerate* the specific foreign skin as if it were self. The results were consistent with the

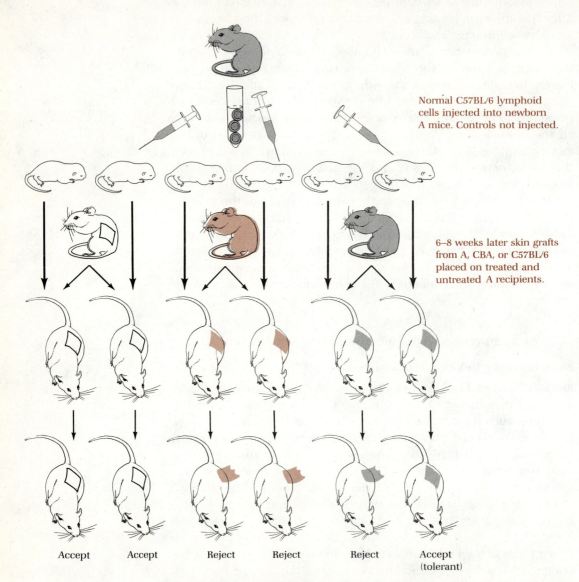

Normal C57BL/6 lymphoid cells injected into newborn A mice. Controls not injected.

6–8 weeks later skin grafts from A, CBA, or C57BL/6 placed on treated and untreated A recipients.

Accept Accept Reject Reject Reject Accept (tolerant)

1 Induction of Tolerance in the Newborn. Lymph node cells from C57BL/6 mice are injected into newborn A mice. When these mice reach 6–8 weeks of age, they, along with normal A mice, are grafted with skin from either A, CBA, or C57BL/6 mice. The A and CBA skins serve as controls (the A skin should be accepted and the CBA skin rejected). The C57BL/6 skin is rejected by untreated mice; but those mice receiving the neonatal injection of C57BL/6 tissue are rendered tolerant, and they accept the grafts. [After Billingham, Brent, and Medawar, 1956. *Phil. Tran. R. Soc. London* B 239: 257]

Burnet–Fenner hypothesis and opened the way for the experimental testing of the mechanism of self–nonself discrimination.

At about the same time, but for quite different reasons, Milan Hasek in Prague was carrying out experiments that proved to be a test of the idea in chickens. Hasek had manipulated chick embryos (he made a deliberate synchorial parabiosis between chick embryos in the shell) so that they were exchanging blood. After hatching, the parabionts were separated and found to be incapable of making antibodies to each other's red cells or of rejecting grafts of the other's skin.

The "experiment of nature" that Owen had been astute enough to explain could now be repeated in the laboratory, and the stage was now set for inducing *immunologic tolerance*—the ability to tolerate the presence of an antigen without making a response to it—in the newborn, so that self–nonself discrimination could be studied experimentally. In 1960 Burnet and Medawar shared the Nobel prize for their work. In his lecture Burnet stated that "when Medawar and his colleagues showed that immunological tolerance could be produced experimentally the new immunology was born."[1]

[1] In humans, the "tolerogenic window" appears to occur well before birth, making clinical application of the phenomenon tricky. Prior to this, it was seriously suggested that newborns be grafted with hemopoietic tissue from other primates, rendering them tolerant. Should they someday require an organ graft, the chimp or baboon would be the donor. Human tolerance induction became a moot point before the ethics of such a practice became a consideration.

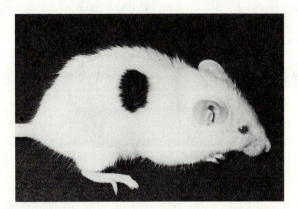

2   Tolerant Mouse with Allogeneic Skin Graft. An A-strain mouse injected neonatally with lymph node cells from a C57BL/10 mouse. As an adult it received a skin graft from C57BL/10, which grew luxuriantly. [Photo courtesy of P. B. Medawar]

The Triplett Experiment

The thinking up to this point led to the idea that the developing immune system "learns" about self by being in the presence of self-antigens. Another way of saying this is that an antigen is "foreign" unless it and the immune system make physical contact before the functional differentiation of the immune system. This idea was tested by E. L. Triplett in 1961 in an elegant experiment. Triplett reasoned that if a self-component could be removed from the animal before the immune system developed, its unique antigens would not be "learned"; and if it were returned to the animal at a later time, it should be recognized as foreign. The frog is a perfect experimental tool for this experiment because all stages of development occur where the researcher can get at them. Triplett began by removing the pituitary glands from embryonic frogs. As they develop, these hypophysectomized animals are colorless, but they turn dark almost immediately after they receive a pituitary graft. If the graft is accepted, the animals remain dark; but if it is rejected, they revert to the colorless state. This provides a good method for assaying the response, if any, to the replaced pituitary.

Triplett grew the pituitary that he had removed from an individual frog as an implant in the dermis of a feeding tadpole. When the original hypophysectomized (and now colorless) animal grew to the proper stage, *its own* pituitary was reimplanted. The frog very quickly became dark; but after about 40 days most of such animals became colorless again—they had rejected their own pituitary glands. In other words, they treated their own tissue, which had been temporarily removed, as if it were foreign.

The possibility that the antigens on the frog's pituitary had changed during the time it resided in the intermediate host was tested by performing a partial hypophysectomy, that is, leaving a piece of the pituitary in the animal and growing part of it in a tadpole. If the antigens had changed while growing in the tadpole, then the new piece would be recognized as foreign and rejected when reimplanted. Such pieces were not rejected, indicating that they had not acquired new antigens. This experiment very clearly shows that tolerance to an antigen requires that the antigen be present and come into contact with the immune system at a crucial stage of development. This idea has been a basic assumption in all studies of immune tolerance.

More recently, Nicholas Cohen and his colleagues in Rochester have performed experiments that cast doubt on the validity of the

Triplett experiment. As sometimes happens in science, however, the experiment had already affected the field to guide it into fruitful areas of research. We now know that whether or not the original experiment turns out to be correct in detail, its general conclusions have held up.

Negative Selection and Neonatal Tolerance

In Chapter 24, we introduced the concept of negative selection during T-cell development in the thymus. Clearly, this is one important way in which "self" is learned. If a developing T cell (at the appropriate stage of development) recognizes its specific antigen, it dies. If not (and if it is positively selected) it matures, ready to make immune responses.

Recall that the presence of Mls in a mouse leads to the deletion of T cells bearing Mls-reactive T-cell receptors. Using a protocol for the induction of neonatal tolerance, H. Robson MacDonald and his colleagues in Lausanne have shown that similar negative selection can be induced in Mls$^-$ mice by the injection of Mls$^+$ cells. Thus, neonatal tolerance induction can lead to negative selection. Presumably, the tolerizing cells make their way to the thymus and present their "self"-antigens to developing T cells.

Similar results have now been obtained with soluble superantigens (see Chapter 24). Staphylococcal enterotoxins stimulate T-cell populations bearing particular TCR-V$_\beta$'s (much as Mls antigens do). Injection of such antigens into neonatal mice causes negative selection of these T cells and tolerance to the superantigen.

With the use of TCR transgenic mice, it will soon be apparent whether neonatal induction of tolerance to protein antigens (which are not superantigens) is also associated with negative selection. As we'll see below, however, negative selection is not the whole story, and other forms of tolerance exist in which T cells are not deleted.

Induction of Tolerance in the Adult

Central versus Peripheral Tolerance

When we consider the induction of tolerance in a fetal or neonatal individual, it may be reasonable to suppose that the effects can be ascribed to tolerization of developing cells rather than to cells that have already attained antigenic reactivity. Since maturation of lymphocytes probably continues throughout life, such tolerance processes occur continuously. Tolerance that exerts its effects on developing lymphocytes is referred to as CENTRAL TOLERANCE. Negative selection of developing T cells is one example (others are given below).

Tolerance, however, can also be induced when antigen-reactive cells have already matured. Such tolerance may proceed through independent mechanisms and has therefore been given a different name: PERIPHERAL TOLERANCE.

As we'll see, the mechanisms of central and peripheral tolerance may be the same or different for B cells and T cells. In addition, both may function at the same time.

Immunologic Paralysis

Introduction of antigen into the newborn, an action that results in tolerance, was quite naturally thought to be a means of studying the way the immune system develops "natural" tolerance to self. This seemed reminiscent to some people of a phenomenon known since the mid-1940s and called IMMUNOLOGIC PARALYSIS. At that time Fenton had shown that the injection of a low dose (0.025 mg) of pneumococcal polysaccharide protects mice from a lethal infection of *Pneumococcus* organisms by eliciting antipolysaccharide antibody. However, when immunization was carried out with a high dose (100 mg), little or no antibody was produced. It was not known whether the high dose of antigen prevented the mice from responding to the antigen, or whether they were making a response but the high concentration of slowly catabolized antigen in the body was absorbing the antibody as it was produced. When the phenomenon was later reexamined, it was found that there was indeed a state of tolerance: the mice were not producing antipneumococcal antibody. This result indicates that tolerance can be induced not only to tissues in embryonic development, but also to foreign antigens in the adult.

Induction of Adult Tolerance

We now know that tolerance in the adult can be induced in several ways. Some of these are listed here.

Form of the Antigen. A protein antigen such as bovine γ-globulin (BGG) can be ultracentrifuged to remove the aggregates. Injection of the *aggregate-free* antigen into adult mice results in a state of specific tolerance (Figure 3). Similarly, injection of hapten conjugated to a nonimmunogenic carrier results in tolerance to the

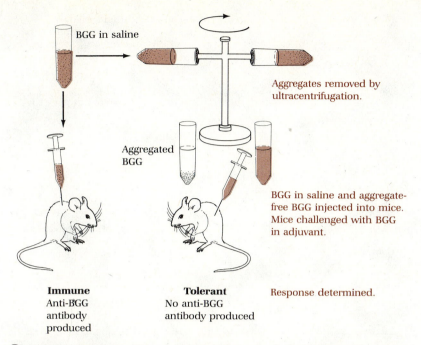

BGG in saline

Aggregates removed by ultracentrifugation.

Aggregated BGG

BGG in saline and aggregate-free BGG injected into mice. Mice challenged with BGG in adjuvant.

Immune
Anti-BGG antibody produced

Tolerant
No anti-BGG antibody produced

Response determined.

3 **Effect of Antigen Form on Response.** The form of the antigen determines whether the response will be immunity or tolerance. BGG in saline is ultracentrifuged to remove aggregates. Injection of aggregate-free BGG induces tolerance (the mice do not make anti-BGG when challenged with BGG in adjuvant). Pretreatment with unfractionated BGG does not result in tolerance. This figure does not show that injection of the aggregates also results in anti-BGG antibody production. [After Dresser, 1962. *Immunology* 5: 161]

hapten. For example, DNP conjugated to aggregate-free antigen results in tolerance to the hapten and to the carrier.

When the injected hapten is conjugated to a *self*-component, such as serum, tolerance to the hapten also is induced (Figure 4). Mice are injected either with autologous serum or a DNP–autologous serum conjugate. After a suitable interval they are challenged with DNP-KLH, and the number of anti-DNP antibody-forming cells in the spleen is determined. It is obvious from the figure that treatment with hapten conjugated to autologous serum renders the animals tolerant to challenge with the hapten conjugated to the immunogen.

Another tolerogenic form of antigen also involves conjugation with self-components. When antigens are coupled to syngeneic APCs and injected intravenously, tolerance results. This can also be demonstrated for minor histocompatibility antigens (such as

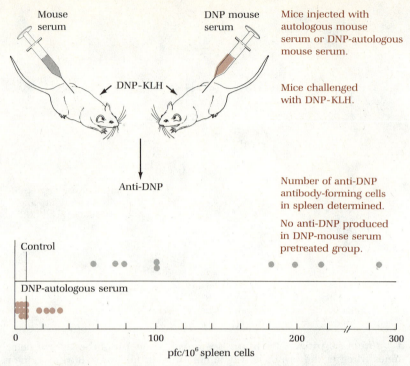

Mouse serum

DNP mouse serum

Mice injected with autologous mouse serum or DNP-autologous mouse serum.

DNP-KLH

Mice challenged with DNP-KLH.

Anti-DNP

Number of anti-DNP antibody-forming cells in spleen determined.

No anti-DNP produced in DNP-mouse serum pretreated group.

Control

DNP-autologous serum

0   100   200   300

pfc/10^6 spleen cells

4   Tolerance to a Hapten. Immunization with DNP conjugated to autologous serum results in tolerance to DNP. Groups of mice are pretreated with either untreated autologous serum or DNP-autologous serum. After challenge with DNP-KLH, the DNP-serum treated group fails to produce anti-DNP antibody; that is, they are tolerant to DNP. [After Borel, 1971. *Nature New Biol.* 230: 180]

Mls) on MHC-matched cells. In this method, the injected cells and the host must share MHC alleles if tolerance is to be produced. We will discuss some possible reasons for this below (although you should have already guessed that it is likely to have something to do with the T-cell receptor).

Antigen Concentration.   Treating animals with extremes of antigen concentration also induces tolerance. Earlier we noted that a very high dose of pneumococcal polysaccharide results in immune paralysis. A very dramatic example of the effect of low dose as well as high dose can be seen in the now classic 1964 experiment by Mitchison (Figure 5). Groups of mice were injected with various doses of soluble bovine serum albumin (BSA) three times a week for up to 16 weeks. In this way the effect of dose and time could

be determined. The animals were then challenged with an immunogenic form of BSA and the anti-BSA antibody titers determined.
When the data were plotted, it was found that high doses of
antigen induced tolerance (as expected). Also as expected, slightly
lower doses did not induce tolerance. But the surprise was that
very low doses were tolerogenic. This phenomenon is called LOW-
ZONE TOLERANCE and has been observed with several antigens. Similarly, very high doses of antigen have the capability of inducing
HIGH-ZONE TOLERANCE.

Route of Antigen Administration. Tolerance induction can also

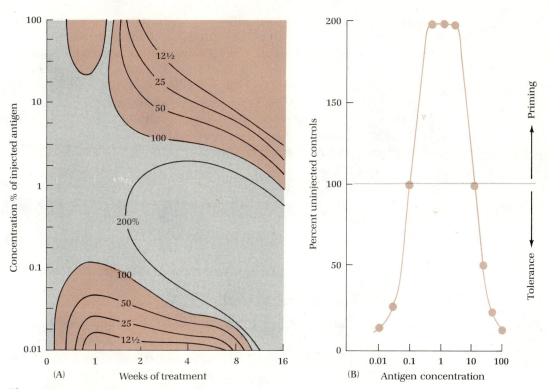

5 **High-Zone and Low-Zone Tolerance.** (A) "Contour map" showing that
repeated injection with a midrange dose of antigen for 2 or more weeks
results in enhanced immunity (*gray*), whereas treatment with either a high
or a low dose results in tolerance (*brown*). Numbers (and their contour lines)
represent percentage of a normal primary response (i.e., greater than 100%
represents priming for a secondary response, less than 100% represents
degrees of tolerance). (B) Conventional graph shows a subset of the data. [After
Mitchison. 1964. *Proc. R. Soc. London* B 161: 275]

depend on the anatomic site at which the antigen enters the body. Two such sites that have received some attention are the gut and the anterior chamber of the eye. Obviously, it would be disadvantageous to constantly generate immune responses to all the different foods we eat, leading to the idea of ORAL TOLERANCE. Similarly, immune responses in the anterior chamber of the eye would obstruct vision, rendering the eye useless; this gives us the idea of ANTERIOR CHAMBER–ASSOCIATED IMMUNE DEVIATION (ACAID). Thus, we have viewed the tolerance-inducing properties of these sites as logical, even if they are not well understood.[2]

Antibody-Induced Tolerance. Tolerance can also be induced by administering antibody. This has been observed in experimental systems both in vivo and in vitro. For example, various amounts of anti–polymerized flagellin (anti-POL) antibody were added to cultures of normal spleen cells. The cultures were then immunized to either POL or sheep red blood cells (SRBCs) as a specificity control. It was found that the presence of anti-POL antibody in the cultures inhibits the POL response by the cultures but has no effect on the SRBC response; that is, a state of specific tolerance to POL has been induced by pretreatment with anti-POL.

The preceding examples make it abundantly clear that tolerance can be induced to a wide range of antigens in either embryonic, neonatal, or adult animals. As we now prepare to examine the mechanism(s) of tolerance, the reader must ask whether or not all or any of these forms of tolerance are indeed the experimental counterparts of "natural tolerance."

Mechanisms of Immune Tolerance

Induction of Tolerance in T Cells

So far we have established that tolerance can be induced in both newborns and adults to a variety of antigens in a variety of ways. To understand the mechanism (or, almost certainly, the mechanisms) of tolerance induction, it is important to know whether

---

[2] There are several ideas about why the presence of antigen at these sites induces tolerance. One possible reason for the phenomenon of oral tolerance, suggested by Ann Fergusson, is that the gut "filters" the antigen, removing aggregates and allowing aggregate-free antigen into the system. She and her colleagues have provided evidence in favor of this idea, though work from other laboratories suggests that the situation may be considerably more complicated. The anterior chamber of the eye is somewhat more mysterious: Tom Ferguson (no relation) has shown that ACAID does not occur in the dark. This is an observation which is so utterly puzzling that it *must* be important.

tolerance can be established in both B and T cells. The first approach to this question was carried out by Jacques Chiller and his colleagues in La Jolla (Figure 6). The plan of the experiment was to repopulate irradiated recipients with combinations of normal and tolerant bone marrow and thymus cells to determine which population is tolerant. Tolerance was induced by injecting deaggregated human gamma globulin (HGG) into adult mice. After a suitable interval, bone marrow and thymus cell suspensions were made and used in combination with normal bone marrow and thymus cells to repopulate irradiated recipients. In this manner groups of recipients were repopulated with tolerant thymus and normal bone marrow, normal thymus and tolerant marrow, tolerant thymus and tolerant marrow, and normal thymus and normal marrow. All the groups were then challenged with antigen in the immunogenic form, and the ability of the recipients to make an anti-HGG response was tested.

As shown in Figure 6A, groups receiving *either* tolerant bone marrow cells or tolerant thymus cells were tolerant, showing that both populations can be rendered tolerant. The experiment was carried out in such a manner that the kinetics of induction could also be investigated. Figure 6B shows that T-cell tolerance is acquired quickly and lasts a very long time. In contrast, B-cell tolerance appears later and wanes quickly. This was interpreted to mean that T-cell tolerance is easier to induce and lasts longer than B-cell tolerance.

Using cloned T helper cells, it has been shown, first by Jonathan Lamb and colleagues in London, then by William Weigle and others in La Jolla, that tolerance can be induced in T cells in vitro. The more recent experiments of Jenkins and Schwartz at NIH (mentioned in Chapter 26) confirmed and extended these findings. In these experiments (Table 1), a cloned murine T-cell line that responds to a peptide fragment of pigeon cytochrome *c* was incubated with fixed APC plus the antigenic peptide. After an interval, the cells were washed and antigen plus fresh APC were added to one group. Interleukin-2 was added to another group to show that the cells still had the ability to respond to signals. It can be seen that preincubation with fixed APC did not affect the ability of the cells to respond to IL-2. In contrast, preincubation with fixed APCs plus antigen did prevent the cells from subsequently responding to antigen. Appropriate specificity controls showed that the loss of ability to respond only occurred with preincubation with the correct antigen and MHC. More recent experiments have shown

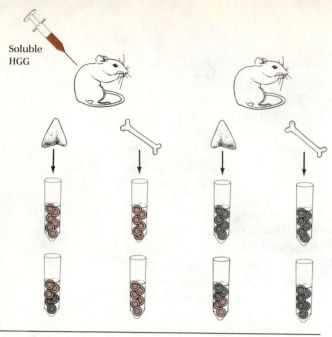

Soluble
HGG

Thymus and bone marrow cells prepared from normal and tolerant mice.

Cells mixed in combinations and injected into irradiated recipients.

Thymus	Tolerant	Tolerant	Normal	Normal
Bone marrow	Normal	Tolerant	Tolerant	Normal

Recipients challenged with immunogenic HGG.

(A) Tolerant   Tolerant   Tolerant   Immune

Anti-HGG responses determined.

6   Tolerance in B and T Cells. (A) Tolerance is induced with deaggregated HGG (dHGG). Bone marrow and thymus cells from the tolerant mice are injected into irradiated recipients along with normal thymus or bone marrow. After challenge with antigen, the mice receiving either tolerant thymus or tolerant bone marrow cells are tolerant. (B) Kinetics of tolerance induction in thymus and bone marrow cells. Thymus cells are tolerant early and remain tolerant. Bone marrow cells become tolerant later and lose tolerance faster. [After Chiller et al., 1971. *Science* 171: 813]

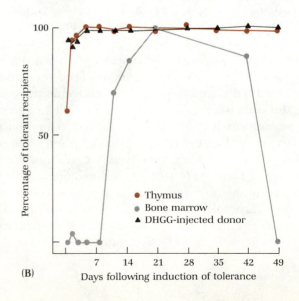

Percentage of tolerant recipients

- ● Thymus
- ● Bone marrow
- ▲ DHGG-injected donor

(B)   7   14   21   28   35   42   49

Days following induction of tolerance

**Table 1   T-cell unresponsiveness induced in a
T-cell clone in vitro.**[a]

Preincubation conditions		Restimulation response to	
Fixed APC	Antigen	APC-Ag	IL-2
Syngeneic	−	++++	+++
Syngeneic	+	+	+++
Allogeneic	−	++++	+++
Allogeneic	+	++++	+++

Source: Data from Jenkins et al., 1987. *Immunol. Rev.* 95: 113.

[a] A T-cell clone was incubated overnight with fixed syngeneic
or allogeneic APC, ± the antigenic peptide. Cells were then
washed and recultured either with antigen plus APC or with
IL-2. Proliferation of the cells was determined after 3 days.

that this unresponsiveness can also be produced using antibodies
to the T-cell receptor (in the absence of APC). Such experiments
show that T cells can in fact be rendered tolerant and that this
state of anergy is the result of a signal through the T-cell receptor.

Interestingly, the induction of tolerance in T-cell clones in vitro
is not blocked by the addition of IL-2 (even though the cells proliferate to this lymphokine). The anergic state appears to make the
cells incapable of producing growth factor in response to antigen.
The cells do, however, increase their expression of IL-2 receptors,
suggesting that if the same phenomenon goes on in vivo, then
tolerance might be overcome (at least temporarily) in the presence
of added IL-2. Experiments by Peter Medawar and colleagues,[3] and
more recently, by Nossal and colleagues (in MHC transgenic mice,
discussed later) suggest that this might indeed be the case. More
work will be needed, however, to ascertain the relationship between states of tolerance in vitro and in vivo.

Induction of Tolerance in B Cells

Eleanore Metcalf and Norman Klinman, in a very elegant series of
experiments (Figure 7), showed that B cells at *early* stages of differentiation can be rendered tolerant. Using a spleen microfocus-
forming assay, they found that B cells from immature animals
were rendered tolerant by confrontation with antigen. More re-

---

[3] These were among the last experiments that Sir Peter published, showing that injecting
IL-2 causes "tolerated" allogeneic skin grafts to be rejected.

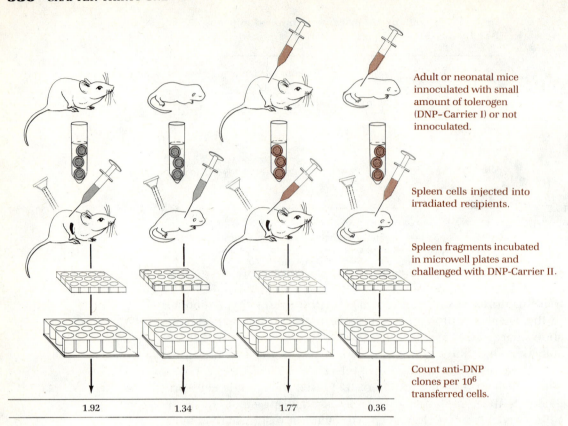

Adult or neonatal mice innoculated with small amount of tolerogen (DNP–Carrier I) or not innoculated.

Spleen cells injected into irradiated recipients.

Spleen fragments incubated in microwell plates and challenged with DNP-Carrier II.

Count anti-DNP clones per 10^6 transferred cells.

1.92   1.34   1.77   0.36

7   Tolerance Induction in Neonatal B Cells. Adult and newborn mice are pretreated with DNP carrier I to induce tolerance to DNP, and the spleen cells of these tolerant mice or untreated controls are injected into irradiated recipients. Spleen fragments from the recipients are then cultured in vitro with DNP carrier II to induce anti-DNP antibody. Nontreated spleens give foci of antibody formation, but spleen cells from pretreated newborns do not. [After Metcalf and Klinman, 1976. *J. Exp. Med.* 143: 1327]

cently, others have shown that similar results are obtained with surface Ig-negative pre-B cells isolated by flow cytometry.

Mature B cells can also be rendered tolerant by direct contact with antigen. In these studies—done by many groups but especially by Gus Nossal in Melbourne—it appears that somehow the antigen-specific receptors (i.e., the sIgM) must be affected so that receptor reorganization cannot be accomplished. (The importance of receptor cross-linking was discussed in Chapter 26.) In this form of tolerance induction, the receptors become unable to transduce the signal to the cell. For this reason the mechanism is called RECEPTOR BLOCKADE.

Little doubt remains that both B cells and T cells can be rendered tolerant; what remains to be learned is the mechanism of this tolerance.

SYNTHESIS
Clonal Deletion, Clonal Abortion, Clonal Anergy, or Tolerant Cells?

In the original version of the clonal selection theory, Burnet explained the phenomenon of immunologic tolerance by postulating the *deletion* of clones. He predicted that lymphocytes that came into contact with antigen early in their differentiation would be killed, that is, the clones would be deleted rather than induced to proliferate, as adult lymphocytes are. Nossal and his colleagues have carried out a very large series of experiments over the years addressing this crucial question. The experiments of Metcalf and Klinman have shown that young B cells are rendered tolerant by contact with antigen, and the experiments by Nossal's group have shown that receptor blockade could occur. Nossal has concluded that the sensitivity to loss of function by young B cells after contact with antigen is seen just after the emergence of surface IgM and before the cells express IgD. He postulated that tolerance is the result of an interruption of the differentiation of the cell, an interruption preventing clones of mature B cells of that specificity from developing. He called this phenomenon CLONAL ABORTION, to indicate that the differentiation process has been aborted before the full functional expression of the clone can be achieved.

If tolerance is due to the elimination of antigen-specific clones, then antigen-binding B cells for the specific antigen should be absent from tolerant animals. When Nossal tested this point, he found, however, that essentially normal levels of these cells were present (Figure 8). This result led him to conclude that tolerance is not due to *physical* elimination of B cells but rather to a "recognition and storage of negative signals" that prevents the cells from making responses to the antigen even though they have the receptors. Because the cells are present but not functional, he called this phenomenon CLONAL ANERGY.

If the idea of clonal anergy is correct, then the next experiments in tolerance studies must be an identification of the nature

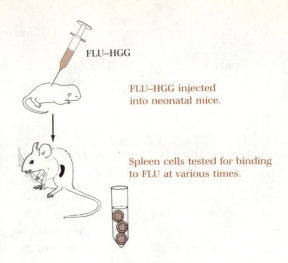

FLU–HGG

FLU–HGG injected into neonatal mice.

Spleen cells tested for binding to FLU at various times.

Weeks after injection	Antigen-binding cells per 10^6 cells	
	Control	FLU–HGG
1	119	67
2	146	117
4	147	118
6	161	150

8   Tolerant Mice Have B Cells that Bind Antigen. Neonatal mice were rendered tolerant to the hapten fluorescein (FLU) by treatment with FLU-HGG. The number of FLU-binding cells is determined 1, 2, 4, or 6 weeks later. [After Nossal and Pike, 1980. *Proc. Natl. Acad. Sci. U.S.A.* 77: 1602]

of the anergy. Why do the cells that are capable of binding antigen not respond to it, and what is the nature of the "negative signals"?

Clonal Anergy to a "Self"-Antigen in Ig-Transgenic Mice

Transgenic technology has provided dramatic support for the idea that clonal anergy functions to render self-reactive B cells tolerant. Chris Goodenow and colleagues in Melbourne "constructed" two types of transgenic mice (see Figure 9A). One set were made transgenic for the hen-egg lysozyme (HEL) gene, thus making this protein a "self"-antigen in these mice. Not surprisingly, these animals were incapable of making an antibody response to HEL.

The second type of transgenic mice was generated using Ig H- and L-chain genes from an HEL-specific B-cell hybridoma. Further, the H-chain transgene contained both the μ and the δ C-region genes. All the B cells in these transgenic mice expressed cell surface IgM and IgD that bound HEL, and spontaneously produced anti-HEL antibody.

These researchers then mated the two types of transgenic mice to determine the effects of bearing HEL as a "self"-antigen on the development of the HEL-specific B cells. They found that these animals had numbers of HEL-binding B cells that were equivalent to those in Ig-transgenic animals without the HEL transgene. The difference, however, was that the B cells in these double-transgenic animals had IgD on their surfaces but lacked IgM (Figure 9B). Furthermore, the B cells from these animals were incapable of making an anti-HEL response, even in the presence of normal helper T cells.

This experiment demonstrates that clonal anergy in B cells can be a mechanism of self-tolerance, in a model that attempts to be as physiological as possible. It does not, however, tell us how this anergy comes about, nor the relative roles of IgM versus IgD expression, since the observed effects may be a function of the transgenic setting rather than a real reflection of the normal process. Nevertheless, these animals will certainly be valuable for the analysis of the cellular biology of B-cell anergy and have provided strong support for the existence and importance of this phenomenon.

In combination with the above studies, these results tell us that, for B cells, clonal anergy appears to be an important mechanism of central tolerance. We do not yet know if this is also an important mechanism of peripheral tolerance in B cells.

T-Cell Anergy

In Chapter 24, we described how T-cell receptor–transgenic mice have been used to study the process of negative selection of self-reactive T cells during thymic maturation. What happens, though, when such T cells mature in an animal lacking the self-antigen, which is then tolerized to the antigen?

Since T cells bearing a particular TCR V_β make responses to Mls antigens, several groups examined the effects of induction of peripheral tolerance to Mls. Following tolerance induction in the adult animals, there is no loss of these T cells, and yet the cells fail to respond to Mls. Hans-Georg Ramensee and colleagues in Tübingen showed that these T cells from tolerized animals were unable to produce IL-2 upon activation but did express IL-2Rα (see Chapter 27). Thus, the tolerant cells express TCRs that recognize the antigen (Mls), but the activation of these cells is defective. In other words, the T cells are anergic.

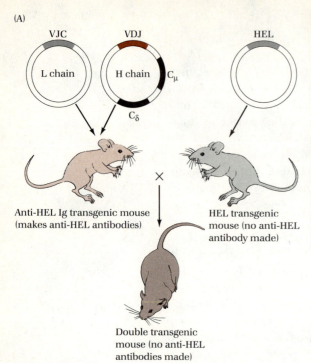

(A)

VJC

L chain

VDJ

H chain C_μ

C_δ

HEL

Anti-HEL Ig transgenic mouse
(makes anti-HEL antibodies)

×

HEL transgenic
mouse (no anti-HEL
antibody made)

Double transgenic
mouse (no anti-HEL
antibodies made)

9   Tolerance in Transgenic Mice Expressing a Foreign Antigen and the Igs that Bind It.
(A) Light- and heavy-chain genes for an antibody that binds to hen-egg lysozyme (HEL) were cloned into a vector for transgenic expression. The H-chain gene carries C regions for both μ and δ, allowing expression of either isotype (by RNA splicing). Transgenic mice carrying these transgenes (Ig-transgenic) were bred with transgenic mice carrying the gene for HEL to produce double-transgenic mice. The double-transgenic mice do not produce antibody in response to HEL. (B) FACS analysis of B cells from transgenic mice. Cells were stained with antibodies to the Ig transgenes (IgD[a] and IgM[a]) or with fluorescent-labeled HEL (lysozyme). The double-transgenic mice have IgM[−], IgD[+], HEL-binding B cells. [From Goodnow et al., 1988. *Nature* 324:676]

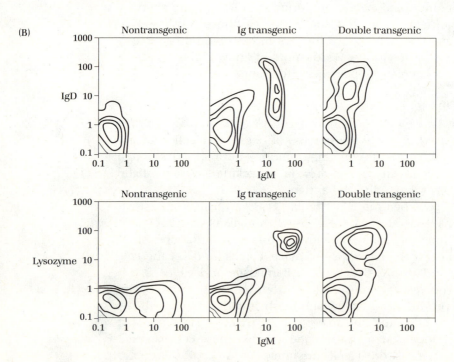

(B)

Nontransgenic   Ig transgenic   Double transgenic

IgD

1000
100
10
1
0.1

0.1 1 10 100   1 10 100   1 10 100

IgM

Nontransgenic   Ig transgenic   Double transgenic

Lysozyme

1000
100
10
1
0.1

0.1 1 10 100   1 10 100   1 10 100

IgM

In a different set of studies, animals were made transgenic for allogeneic MHC genes (class I or II) that were driven by the insulin promoter. This resulted in the allogeneic MHC molecules being expressed only in the β-islet cells of the pancreas (the cells that produce insulin). Peripheral T cells from these animals were unable to respond to the allogeneic MHC, even though the pancreatic MHC was not expressed in the thymus. Manipulation of these cells with growth factors (such as IL-2) demonstrated that cells with the potential to respond to the transgenic MHC were present, albeit nonresponsive. Thus, in addition to negative selection, it appears that T cells can be rendered anergic by an as-yet-unknown mechanism.

In T cells, then, central tolerance appears to be mediated primarily by negative selection, while peripheral tolerance appears to proceed primarily by clonal anergy.

SYNTHESIS
Return of the Two-Signal Hypothesis

Such findings bring us back to the experiments of Ronald Schwartz and colleagues that we discussed in Chapter 26. Recall that they had observed that presentation of antigen on fixed APC led to the inactivation of T-cell clones. This was reminiscent of the *two-signal hypothesis* of Bretscher and Cohn, which suggested that if only one of two signals is given to a lymphocyte, tolerance rather than activation ensues.

The signal that, in the absence of a second signal, appears to lead to anergy is that of the antigen–MHC complex. The second signal, which has been called the *costimulator*, is uncharacterized but appears to be constitutively present on dendritic cells but absent from macrophages until they are stimulated. This second signal overrides the tolerance-inducing signal given by signal 1 and allows activation to occur. Once anergy has been induced, however, signal 2 is ineffective. It is proposed, then, that treatments that lead to peripheral tolerance do so by providing signal 1 in the absence of signal 2.

These ideas seem to fit the in vivo data and provide a way to study T-cell anergy in vitro. Clearly, an understanding of the cellular mechanisms underlying clonal anergy of T cells will have important consequences for the understanding of immune tolerance.

"Active" Tolerance and the Breakdown of Tolerance

The Veto Concept

Another possible cellular mechanism for the functional elimination of clones has been proposed by Richard Miller in Toronto. He has introduced the notion of the VETO CELL. As we know, lymph node populations that contain precytotoxic cells (pCTLs) give rise to cytotoxic T cells (CTLs) when incubated with stimulator cells. But Miller has shown that when spleen cells from the appropriate strain of athymic nude mice (*nu/nu*) are included in the initial incubation, the pCTLs do not develop into CTLs (Table 2). His experiment employed cells from three mouse strains: BALB/c, B10, and RNC, which differ in MHC and background genes. The BALB/c responder lymph nodes develop CTLs to either B10 or RNC stimulator cells, even in the presence of BALB/c nude spleen cells. But when the BALB/c lymph node cells are incubated with RNC nude spleen cells, they do not develop CTLs to the RNC cells even though they develop normal levels of CTLs to B10. Thus the inability to respond is specific.

Miller has suggested that a cell in the *nu/nu* spleen can "veto" a developing clone so that tolerance can be established. According to this model (Figure 10), whenever a pCTL for self is generated, it comes into contact with the veto cell, which eliminates it.

Suppressor Cells in Tolerance

When the idea that suppressor cells could be a major mode of regulation of the immune response was introduced, many groups began to look for the presence of suppressor cells in the tolerant state. There is evidence that they exist in tolerance induced in both adults and newborns to a wide variety of antigens ranging

Table 2 Veto cells in the *nu/nu* spleen.

Responder	Stimulator	Target	Killing
BALB/c lymph node	RNC	RNC	Yes
	B10	B10	Yes
BALB/c lymph node + BALB/c *nu/nu* spleen	RNC	RNC	Yes
	B10	B10	Yes
BALB/c lymph node + RNC *nu/nu* spleen	RNC	RNC	No
	B10	B10	Yes

Source: Data from Miller, 1980. *Nature* 287: 544.

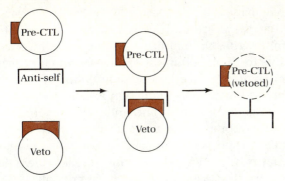

10 **The Veto Concept.** Veto cells deliver a cytotoxic "hit" to any cell that recognizes MHC (or MHC plus antigen) on the veto cell. Thus, cells that react against the veto cell (i.e., have receptors that are anti-self) are removed. "Vetoing" of pre-CTLs (shown in the figure) has been demonstrated, but the mechanism could theoretically function against any cell.

from serum proteins to allogeneic tissues. (The first experiment showing suppressor cells utilized tolerized animals as a source.) Bear in mind, however, that the existence of such cells as a discrete population is very controversial (see Chapter 30). Suppressor cells have been described that inhibit reponses to self antigens and can, in some cases, be a means of maintaining nonresponsiveness to self. Even though it was often stated that this is the true role of the suppressor cell, the evidence for such a statement is still far from conclusive. It is usually not possible to demonstrate such suppressor cells unless the tolerant animal is challenged just prior to removing the cells, and even then they often fail to appear. It is possible that suppressor cells represent a "backup" system to prevent autoimmunity, especially in cases in which the antigenic challenge bears both self and foreign epitopes. If helper T cells recognize the foreign epitopes, suppressor cells (recognizing the self-epitopes) might prevent the helper T cells from inducing immune responses to the self-epitopes. While this has been shown in several systems, it is by no means proved that suppressor cells normally perform this function. Even if it were, we have no good idea how they perform this function (in terms of precise mechanisms). Given the status of the suppressor-cell controversy (see Chapter 30) it may be some time before we know the answer.

Naturally Occurring Self-Reactivity

We have just developed arguments and evidence to justify the logical idea that the body must not react against itself. However, there are some cases in which there appears to be naturally occurring autoreactivity without disease. There is a fairly large literature showing that there are both T and B cells that react to normal tissue components. Normal humans and mice, for example, have cells reactive to thyroglobulin, and many normal individuals have titers of anti–autologous erythrocyte antibody in their serum. But what is more convincing is that when cells are activated polyclonally with mitogens, both cells and antibodies against a wide range of self-antigens appear. The finding of naturally occurring autoreactivity has important implications for our understanding of diseases that result when self-tolerance breaks down (i.e., autoimmune diseases, discussed in Chapters 35 and 36)

Experimentally Induced Self-Reactivity and the Breaking of Tolerance: The Weigle Phenomenon

There are several ways to experimentally induce immune responses against self-antigens, and many of these are discussed in the chapters on autoimmunity. Here we discuss the ramifications of this induction for our understanding of tolerance.

During the 1960s, William Weigle in La Jolla observed that experimentally induced tolerance could be "broken" if closely related antigens were injected into the tolerant individual. For example, he tolerized animals to BSA by intravenous injection of the deaggregated protein. These animals failed to respond to BSA, but did respond to methylated-BSA (mBSA). After injection of mBSA, the animals once again responded to BSA as well. The tolerance was broken. The first part (that tolerant animals respond to the related antigen) is fairly easy to understand–cells are responding to the new determinant (to which they are not tolerant). Why, however, this disrupts the tolerance to the original antigen is far less clear.

Nevertheless, this phenomenon can be shown for some forms of self-tolerance as well. For example, if mice are injected with rabbit thyroglobulin, they generate a response not only to the foreign antigen, but to their own thyroglobulin as well. This can result in an autoimmune state.

In order for these phenomena to occur, there must be T cells that can recognize the antigens, even if they are normally unresponsive (i.e., the tolerance must be due to anergy and/or suppression rather than negative selection). The presence of T cells capable of reacting to self-antigens has been demonstrated most dramatically for autologous insulin. Judith Kapp and her colleagues generated T-cell clones from mice immunized with pork insulin and showed that, depending on the mouse strain, many of these T cells reacted equally well to mouse insulin. Their evidence suggested that active suppression was normally responsible for preventing the expansion of these cells.

Such observations appear to go against many of the things we have discussed in this chapter. Rather than be upset with this, the student should be relieved that there are still some things to be discovered regarding the vitally important area of tolerance in the immune system.

SYNTHESIS
What Maintains Self-Tolerance?

We have now seen that there are several mechanisms for the maintenance of a tolerant state to a specific antigen. Which ones are actually important for the maintenance of self-tolerance? The simple answer is "all of them," but there is no more evidence in support of this answer than there is for any one mechanism.

In order to address this question, we should look to a different question: What is the failure in self-tolerance that leads to autoimmunity? As we'll see in Chapters 35 and 36, we just don't know the answer to this question yet. Nevertheless, we might be able to get a few clues by examining some anomalies in the process of self-tolerance.

Cyclosporin A is a potently immunosuppressive drug that is used to inhibit graft rejection in transplant recipients (discussed in Chapter 37). Curiously, cyclosporin A also interferes with the negative-selection process, allowing potentially self-reactive T cells to leave the thymus and enter the periphery. In some cases, this can lead to an autoimmune condition. Negative selection, then, is apparently responsible for self-tolerance.

Cyclosporin A-induced autoimmunity, however, only occurs if there are no mature T cells present in the system at the time of cyclosporin A treatment (that is, the treatment must begin just following birth in mice, or just after lethal irradiation and bone marrow transplant). Mature T cells can prevent the induction of this autoimmune state, by an as-yet-unidentified process.

Another puzzle is the observation that in neonatal animals expressing Mls, T cells with Mls-reactive V regions appear to avoid negative selection and can be found in the peripheral lymphoid organs. One possible explanation for this might be that at this early time, the Mls antigens are not yet expressed. But if this is so, why don't these potentially Mls-reactive T cells respond later on? Several investigators in the early 1970s showed that T cells present in the neonatal spleen are capable of proliferating to syngeneic, adult cells (whether this was due to Mls was not investigated). We know, however, that these animals remain healthy, and therefore these T cells remain unresponsive (and become, at best, an extremely minor population). Therefore, some mechanism of peripheral tolerance seems to be active in maintaining self-tolerance.

The study of tolerance, including self-tolerance, is not complete, even though we have learned so much in the last few years. Puzzles and paradoxes exist, and some of these might provide the clues we need to better understand the central problem of self–nonself discrimination.

Summary

1. The question of how the immune system discriminates between self and nonself is the most fundamental question in immunology. The condition in which the immune system eliminates or prevents responses to a specific antigen is called immune tolerance. One mechanism of tolerance is negative selection, but there are others.

2. In newborn and adult animals tolerance can be induced to a wide variety of antigens. In the adult, the form and concentration of the antigen are crucial factors in determining whether there will be a response or tolerance.

3. Tolerance can be induced in both B cells and T cells. In general, tolerance in T cells is longer-lasting.

4. Tolerance that acts upon developing lymphocytes (e.g., negative selection) is called central tolerance. Peripheral tolerance, which acts on mature cells to prevent responses, also exists (and appears not to involve negative selection).

5. The mechanisms of tolerance induction vary and are not completely understood. Two alternative mechanisms are deletion of clones and inability of clones to respond. Deletion could be physical (negative selection) or functional (deletion by receptor blockade or by aborted differentiation of a clone, as in developing B cells). The inability of clones to respond to antigen could also be due to negative signals in the tolerant cell (clonal anergy). Although clonal anergy has been demonstrated, the cellular mechanisms are not known.

6. Immune regulation by T cells may play a role in maintenance of some forms of tolerance, and veto cells (which kill any cells that recognize them) may be important in others. Most likely, these will be found to have roles in different forms of peripheral tolerance, although more work is needed to address the mechanisms of different types of immune tolerance.

Additional Readings

Miller, J. F. A. P., G. Morahan and J. Allison. 1989 Immunological tolerance: New approaches using transgenic mice. *Immunol. Today* 10: 53.

Mueller, D. L., M. K. Jenkins and R. H. Schwartz. 1989. Clonal expansion versus functional clonal inactivation: A costimulatory signalling pathway determines the outcome of T cell antigen receptor occupancy. *Annu. Rev. Immunol.* 7: 445.

IMMUNITY AND IMMUNOPATHOLOGY

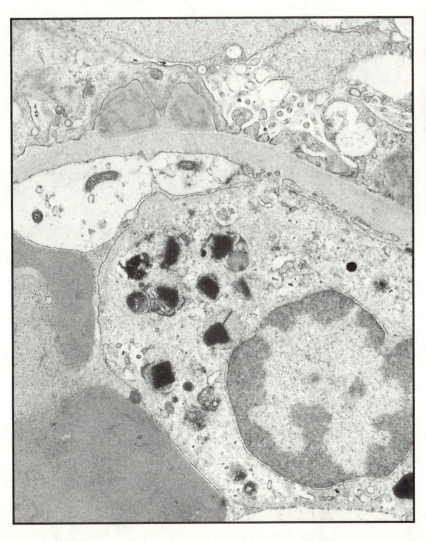

PART

3

IMMUNITY AND IMMUNOPATHOLOGY

The practical application of what I have said is very close to the problem which I am investigating. It is a tangled skein, you understand, and I am looking for a loose end.

Arthur Conan Doyle, *The Case Book of Sherlock Holmes*

The purpose of these chapters on immunity and immunopathology is to attempt to put some of the consequences—both good and bad—of the actions of the immune system into a context in which they will be explained by all that has gone before. These chapters are not a catalog of clinical woes but will let the reader see how the knowledge we have gained about the immune response can be applied to the human condition. Perhaps the reader will also see that despite all our understanding of immunology, we have not made overwhelming progress into many of these important problems. These problems put our ideas to the test; sometimes they make us humble, and sometimes they provide us with new approaches to learning more about the basic biology of the system.

THE RESPONSE TO EXTERNAL INVADERS
Immunity to Parasites

CHAPTER

32

Overview In Chapter 1 we introduced the idea that the primary subject of the book, the specific immune response, is part of the complex means used by the body to achieve the state of immunity: the ability to resist disease. The specific immune response first appeared with the evolution of the chordates. This means that 99.999% of the rest of the animals in the world (give or take a few), many of which arose long before the chordates, have been doing quite well without it. Their world is as full of potential pathogens as is the world of the animals in the phylum Chordata, so the majority of animals are able to survive with other defense mechanisms. In this chapter we will see that the basic means of achieving immunity is through nonspecific defense mechanisms. These nonspecific mechanisms are also used by the chordates, which have added the specific immune response. The specific response has been integrated into many of the nonspecific mechanisms, thereby making them more efficient.

We will see that the combination of specific and nonspecific immune responses works to protect the organism from external invaders (bacteria, viruses, protozoans, worms) and may have evolved in such a manner as to play a role in the defense against internal invaders such as tumors. Whether the disease is due to external or internal invasion, the invader survives at the expense of the host and is therefore called a parasite. The study of immunity can therefore be a study of the host–parasite relationship. The outcomes of host–parasite relationships depend on factors that allow one or the other to win the battle. The host first uses its nonspecific factors, which begin with an attempt to prevent the potential parasites from invading. If this fails and the external invader enters the host, the inflammatory response marshals phagocytic cells to the site. These cells ingest and kill the invading organisms. The specific immune response is used to augment various aspects of nonspecific immunity. As we'll see, however, this Machiavellian view of host attack assumes a relatively helpless parasite, which is often not the case. Parasites employ evasive strategies to elude the immune response, such that we can often only hope for a peaceful settlement with no clear-cut winners.

The Response to External Invaders: Host–Parasite Relationships

At the outset we defined immunity as the ability to resist infection and remain free from disease. The specific adaptive immune response that we have been studying in this text is one part of the armamentarium the body uses to achieve this end. Even the use of the term *armamentarium* shows that this process has been visualized as a battle between two opposing forces, one good and one very bad. Because history is always written by the winners, we will be looking at how the good guys do it.[1]

All animals live in a world filled with potentially hostile and harmful species. Perhaps as a result of their neurological development, humans have elevated the natural acts of predation and defense, which the rest of the biological world uses for survival, to the high arts of murder, warfare, and apartheid. But even in the absence of these fine arts, the average member of the higher biological phyla is constantly prey to parasites and predators. We study these in the life cycles of animals and in the interdependence of various species. Public television alone has filled our hours with images of mating moose and predatory panthers in an attempt to personalize nature (or perhaps more correctly, Nature). But if one species is dependent upon another for its survival, the only way the first species can maintain itself is to develop a relationship that is beneficial to itself without eliminating the second species. When two species are mutually beneficial and dependent, their relationship is called COMMENSALISM. But if one species survives at the expense of the other, the relationship is called PARASITISM. Infectious diseases are examples of parasitism. Because the infectious agent benefits at the expense of the organism it has infected, it is the PARASITE. The organism that is parasitized is called the HOST. The "perfect parasite" has evolved a relationship with its host that may be very harmful to the host but still allows enough

[1] Of course, parasites are alive and well, but if we are not winning the battle, we are still the only ones who can write.

members of the host species to survive to ensure the continued existence of the parasite. The outcome of the infection is determined at several levels by the relationship that is established between the host and the parasite—that is, the host–parasite relationship.[2]

Factors Affecting the Host–Parasite Relationship

PHYSIOLOGICAL INCOMPATIBILITY between the two potential interactants is one factor that can affect the potential host–parasite relationship. For example, if a bacterium survives at an optimal temperature of 56°C (a thermophilic bacterium) and the body temperature of the host is 37°C, the host has a NATURAL RESISTANCE to the parasite. Similarly, if the optimal temperature of the invading organism is 37°C but the host is a frog whose body temperature is 26°C, the invader will not grow.

The intact host also has a series of ANATOMICAL BARRIERS that can prevent or deter the infectious agent. The skin is an animal's first line of defense. If the skin remains intact, an invading organism (which requires the temperature, moisture, and nutrients that are inside the body) will be prevented from reaching a compatible environment and will die. Breaks in the skin, therefore, are breaks in the host's defense system because they allow the potential parasite access to a favorable growth environment. A "parasite's-eye view" of a vertebrate host is shown in Figure 1.

All animals have bacteria that live in and on them, either as perfect parasites or as commensals. These microorganisms constitute the NATURAL FLORA of the host. Mammals, for example, rely on the bacteria of the gut to produce vitamin K, which they are incapable of producing themselves. (The gut is really outside the body, being a lumen around which the body is formed.) In many cases, these organisms of the natural flora act to prevent the growth of invading organisms. But the balance is a very delicate one; and given a change from "normal" conditions, members of the natural flora can become harmful. For example, normal human skin has populations of the bacterium *Staphylococcus aureus*. These organisms cause no harm when they are on the skin, but if the skin is broken and the staphylococci are given access to the inner milieu, they can cause pustules or even severe systemic

---

[2] The term *parasite* is also used to identify a class of invading organisms, such as trypanosomes and schistosomes, but we will use the term in its general meaning. We use the more specific terms *protozoans* and *helminths* to refer to these particular parasites.

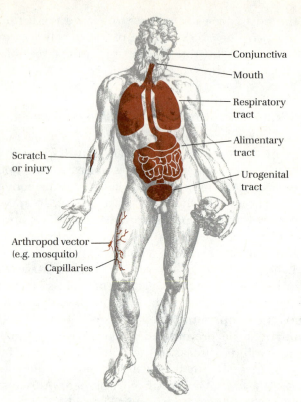

Conjunctiva

Mouth

Respiratory
tract

Alimentary
tract

Urogenital
tract

Scratch
or injury

Arthropod vector
(e.g. mosquito)

Capillaries

1   Parasite's Eye View of a Classic Host. From a parasite's point of view, the vertebrate host is a series of anatomical barriers that have to be breached in order to enter or leave the body.

infections. The common bacterium of the gut, *Escherichia coli*, is a necessary part of our natural flora, but if it leaves the gut and enters the body as a result of trauma to the gut wall, the result can be severe peritonitis.

HOST SECRETIONS can also be a factor in preventing the invading organisms from gaining a foothold. For example, secretions such as saliva, tears, and nasal secretions contain the enzyme LYSOZYME, which cleaves a sugar linkage that is very common in the cell walls of bacteria. The invading organism that lands on a surface bathed by lysozyme-rich secretions is liable to be killed before it can do much harm. Organisms that are ingested and reach the stomach are subjected to extremely low pH, and if they are susceptible to low pH (as many bacteria are), they are killed. Another extremely important secretion is MUCUS, which plays important roles in forming a barrier and in the clearance of invaders.

Rapid Responses to Infection: Fever, Acute-Phase Proteins, and Tumor Necrosis Factor

Most people think of fever as an undesirable consequence of an infection, but some evidence suggests that low-grade fever is a host defense reaction. Many pathogens are temperature-sensitive, and a slight increase in the core temperature of the host can drive the infection into the cooler, distal regions, or even destroy it. Such small increases in body temperature also dramatically enhance many specific and nonspecific immune mechanisms, adding to the benefits imparted by the fever. Of course, high fevers are dangerous and must be treated.

Elevated temperature has been thought throughout the years to be one of the body's defenses. In fact, during the last century it was noticed that syphilis was often cured if the patient contracted malaria. Reasoning that it was the bouts of fever in malaria that cured the syphilis, clinicians attempted to induce fever by inducing "artificial malaria" with mercury. (This led to the adage "one night with Venus and a lifetime with Mercury.") It is in the realm of the possible that fever may have evolved as another, albeit very dangerous, way of increasing nonspecific immunity. A substance that causes fever is called a PYROGEN.

Many gram-negative bacteria, when lysed, liberate some of their wall components, called ENDOTOXINS, which can then activate the alternative pathway of complement (Chapter 8) and lead to further lysis. Most bacterial endotoxins are pyrogens, acting directly upon the thermoregulating center in the hypothalamus.

Other, endogenous pyrogens include IL-1, IL-6, and the interferons (see below). These may be produced in response to endotoxin, or as a consequence of the specific or nonspecific immune responses to infection. Another consequence of producing such mediators (especially IL-6) is the induction and release of large amounts of ACUTE-PHASE PROTEINS from the liver. Concentrations of these proteins can increase 100-fold within a day of infection. One example is a serum protein called C-REACTIVE PROTEIN, (so called because it binds to the C protein of pneumococci). C-reactive protein binds to the surfaces of a variety of bacteria and fungi and functions to activate complement and increase phagocytosis.

Bacterial endotoxins rapidly induce another response in myeloid cells—the release of tumor necrosis factor (TNF). This cytokine has a very wide range of effects, many of which are probably beneficial to the host at normal concentrations. Unfortunately, however, an endotoxin-stimulated cell can devote itself to producing large amounts of TNF, such that 1% of all the protein the cell produces is this molecule. At higher concentrations, the effects of TNF become pathologic, resulting in a potentially lethal condition called ENDOTOXIC SHOCK, which can occur when the bacterial infection is severe. TNF is believed to be the major mediator of endotoxic shock.

Interferon

The responses of the host that occur after infection with viruses and lead to a state of immunity are similar to those we have been describing, with the exception of the production of INTERFERON. In 1957 Isaacs and Lindenmann discovered that, once freed of virus, the supernatant fluid obtained from cultures of cells that had been infected with virus protected other cells from infection. They called the substance that had the ability to interfere with virus infection interferon.

Interferon has been the subject of innumerable review articles and investigations by not a few biotech companies. There is reasonable agreement about its role in viral immunity, but because there are several types of interferon, each made by a different cell type, the other roles we can assign to it are controversial. α-interferon (INF-α) is produced by leukocytes; β-interferon (INF-β) is produced by fibroblasts; and γ-interferon (INF-γ) is produced by stimulated T cells (see Chapter 27).

It must be remembered that interferon is produced by the host cells infected with the virus. This reaction is a form of biological altruism, because the production of interferon will not save the infected cell. The interferon is exported and used by other cells. When these cells become infected with the virus, the interferon causes the cells to produce molecules that prevent the replication of the infecting virus. The events occurring in these cells that react with interferon are only partly understood. Reaction of interferon with an interferon receptor causes what is called the INTERFERON-INDUCED ANTIVIRAL STATE. A sequence of events results, among other things, in the inhibition of viral protein synthesis through degradation of viral mRNA. The first event is the induction by interferon of a molecule called 2,5-A POLYMERASE. If a cell that has interacted with interferon (and is now producing 2,5-A polymerase) becomes infected with virus, the virus activates the polymerase to produce an unusual 2,5-OLIGOADENOSINE (2,5-A). The presence of 2,5-A in turn activates a preexisting, inactive molecule called RIBONUCLEASE L. It is ribonuclease L that degrades single-stranded RNA.

In this manner the cycle of virus reproduction is interfered with and the infection is either stopped or the process slowed down enough to enable the specific immune response to eliminate the infecting virus. Interferon-mediated events are nonspecific, because interferon induced by one virus can cause in other cells the appearance of the interferon-induced antiviral state that will protect them from infection by other viruses, namely, the activation of ribonuclease L, which has no specificity for either host or viral mRNA. In theory, *any* transcription events required by the host cell will be inhibited.

The activation of the 2,5-A-polymerase–endoribonuclease system is not the only mechanism of interferon action. Interferons also induce the synthesis of other proteins, such as a double-stranded-RNA-dependent protein kinase. In addition, interferons often induce genes involved in specific immune responses (such as MHC genes). The overall picture is quite complex, as one might expect for an important antiviral defense mechanism.

The Inflammatory Response

It is likely that under ordinary circumstances the first lines of defense discussed above are all that most members of the species need in order to carry on their day-to-day activities of preying upon and being preyed upon. Another, very powerful, nonspecific defense, called the inflammatory response, has evolved for those instances when these first-line defenses are not enough.

The Cardinal Signs of Inflammation

The INFLAMMATORY RESPONSE is the vascular lymphatic and local tissue reaction elicited in higher animals by the presence of micoorganisms or nonviable irritants. This complex response, aspects of which are seen throughout the animal kingdom, has evolved as the most effective defense mechanism in the animal world.

The various aspects of the inflammatory response can be seen by the response to a simple thing like a sliver of wood in the finger. The piece of wood becomes inserted under the skin, and after a few hours the area becomes red. After a while one notices that there is swelling and pain, and, if the area is large enough, one notices that it is perceptibly warmer than the surrounding tissue. These are the conditions that have been known since the time of the ancients as INFLAMMATION.[3]

The Greek physician Celcus (ca. 30 B.C. to A.D. 38) described the "four cardinal signs of inflammation," a term that is still used. These four signs are REDNESS (*rubor*), SWELLING (*tumor*), HEAT (*calor*), and PAIN (*dolor*). The first person to write extensively on inflammation was the great Galen (A.D. 130–200), who added a fifth sign, LOSS OF FUNCTION. The first of the more modern physicians to write on inflammation was John Hunter (1728–1793).

The redness and heat are caused by an increase in blood flow to the area of trauma and by constriction of the blood vessels that carry blood away from the area. The constriction occurs immediately after the trauma. Capillary permeability increases; consequently both fluids and blood cells leave the capillaries and cause swelling and pain (a result of increased pressure). From our point of view, however, the most important thing to occur is the exit of phagocytic cells from the capillaries to the extracellular spaces. The most common cell types accumulating at the site of infection are phagocytic leukocytes, primarily GRANULOCYTES (including NEUTROPHILS, EOSINOPHILS, and BASOPHILS).

Granulocytes in Inflammation

The granulocytes are one of the body's most efficient scavenger systems. They are cells that have the ability to engulf particles by the process of phagocytosis and in some cases to destroy them. Thus the inflammatory response acts as a means of bringing scavenger cells to the site of a breach in the first line of defense.

During the inflammatory response, the capillary endothelial surfaces become sticky, thus causing granulocytes to attach to the capillary walls. The granulocytes then leave the capillaries by migrating between the cells of the capillary walls. Many microorganisms elaborate CHEMOTACTIC FACTORS toward which the cells migrate after leaving the capillaries. One group of important chemotactic factors is the FORMAMYL PEPTIDES that are found in many microbes and have been used extensively to study chemotaxis.[4] The complement component C5a, which can be generated by

---

[3] Pus, which is a consequence of inflammatory responses, was described in Egyptian papyri of the second millennium B.C. as being related to the demons of disease. The school of Hippocrates noted the reddening of the skin and called it *erysipelas* (literally, "redness of the skin"). They called the swelling *oidema*, which we now call edema.

[4] These peptides are produced only by prokaryotic organisms and have the amino acid sequences f-Met-Phe and f-Met-Leu-Phe.

either the classical or the alternative pathway, is also a powerful chemotactic agent. In addition, the complement components C3a and C5a are both ANAPHYLOTOXINS—substances that cause the release of histamine from mast cells, thus causing further increase of vascular permeability.

There are some cases in which the inflammatory response itself can cause the symptoms of the disease. For example, in tuberculosis, the invading organisms (*Mycobacterium tuberculosis*) enter the lung tissue and induce an inflammatory response. The defensive cells that arrive, first granulocytes and then monocytes, ingest the tubercle bacilli, but the parasite in this case has evolved a defense mechanism of its own. *Mycobacterium tuberculosis* has a cell wall that prevents it from being destroyed after it is phagocytized; in fact, it grows inside the monocytes and eventually kills them. Thus there is a chronic inflammatory response going on in the lung, with more monocytes being attracted to the site. Eventually the mass of inflammatory cells causes so much damage to the lung tissue that the symptoms of tuberculosis become manifest: shortness of breath, tiredness, loss of weight, and the classic symptoms of the cough and bloody sputum. In most cases of parasitic invasion, however, the inflammatory response is an efficient and beneficial response.

Phagocytosis

The granulocytes and macrophages that are attracted to the site of infection and inflammation PHAGOCYTIZE the microbes. The notion of phagocytosis as a general defense mechanism was championed by Elie Metchnikoff (1845–1916). This marvelously eccentric man had for complicated reasons resigned his professorship at Messina in 1882 and was relaxing on the shores of the Mediterranean when the whole business of immunity became clear to him.

> I was resting from the shock of the events which provoked my resignation from the University and indulging enthusiastically in researches in the splendid setting of the Straits of Messina.
>
> One day the family had gone to a circus to see some extraordinary performing apes. I remained alone at my microscope, observing the life in the mobile cells of the transparent starfish larva, when a new thought suddenly flashed across my brain. It struck me that similar cells might serve in the defense of the organism against intruders. Feeling that there was in this something of surpassing interest, I felt so excited that I began striding up and down the room and even went to the seashore in order to collect my thoughts.

I said to myself that, if my supposition was true, a splinter introduced into the body of a starfish larva, devoid of blood vessels or of a nervous system, should soon be surrounded by mobile cells as is to be observed in a man who runs a splinter into his finger. This was no sooner said than done.

There was a small garden to our dwelling, in which we had a few days previously organized a "Christmas tree" for the children on a little tangerine tree; I fetched from it a few rose thorns and introduced them at once under the skin of some beautiful starfish larvae as transparent as water.

I was too excited to sleep that night in the expectation of the result of my experiment, and very early the next morning I ascertained that it had fully succeeded.

That experiment formed the basis of the phagocyte theory, to the development of which I devoted the next twenty-five years of my life. [Metchnikoff, quoted in Humphrey and White, *Immunology for Medical Students*, 3rd ed., p. 14]

Metchnikoff, clearly no shrinking violet, soon became embroiled in a controversy over the relative roles of the phagocytic cells and the humoral factors (i.e., antibody) in immunity. We now know that both are important and that the antibody (from the specific immune response) enhances some aspects of the phagocytic process (from the nonspecific response).

The mechanism of phagocytosis is very well studied, but we will go into only enough detail to see how the process is used in immunity. After microbes contact the surface of a phagocytic cell, the cell membrane folds around the particles, bringing them into the interior of the cell. The microbes are now in a vacuole called a PHAGOSOME, whose membrane is formed by the cell membrane of the phagocytic cell. Another characteristic feature of phagocytic cells is the presence of large, prominent GRANULES. The different types of granules distinguish the different types of granulocytes (the names of the cells—*neutrophil*, *eosinophil*, and *basophil*— derive from the types of dye that color the characteristic granules).

Some of these granules are in fact LYSOSOMES, which are essentially bags of proteolytic and other degradative enzymes. DEGRANULATION occurs when the phagosome and several lysosomes fuse, causing the lysosomes to dump the contents of their granules into the phagosome (forming a PHAGOLYSOSOME). The lysosomal contents, along with PEROXIDE and SUPEROXIDES (which are products of the metabolic process during phagocytosis) then aid in the killing of the microbes that have been ingested. This degranulation is different from that of mast cells (mentioned in Chapter 7 and discussed in Chapter 34), and the two should not be confused.

The reader will no doubt have seen the similarity between the process of phagocytosis and that of antigen processing (Chapter 20). The former can lead to the latter if the phagocytic cell is an APC (e.g., it bears class II MHC). Not all phagocytic cells can present antigen, however, and not all APCs are phagocytic. Nevertheless, the cells with both characteristics, such as many macrophages, form an important link between the nonspecific and the specific immune defense mechanisms (see below).

Holes, Burns, and Toxins

Peter Lachman has summarized nonspecific immunologic effector mechanisms into the categories of holes, burns, and toxins.[5] Not only is this a useful way to remember them, but it also illustrates the relatively few ways that a large number of effector cells and molecules work.

Holes is meant to represent the formation of lytic pores produced by such mechanisms as the membrane attack complex of the complement cascade (Chapter 8) or perforin from cytotoxic effector cells (Chapter 28). As we've seen, these holes might kill by letting water and ions flow freely across the membrane (colloid osmotic lysis) or by allowing other molecules to migrate in (e.g., cytotoxic effector molecules).

Burns is meant to represent the action of free oxygen radicals that destroy cells by rapid oxidation (burning). Free oxygen radicals are produced by a number of different cells (e.g., macrophages, neutrophils, eosinophils) by several different biochemical pathways. For example, peroxides and superoxides in lysosomes (see above) kill by "burning."

Toxins include cytokines (interferons, TNF), lysozymes, and other molecules with direct or indirect actions on parasites.

Together, the holes, burns, and toxins produced by the non-specific effector mechanisms of the immune system play major roles in the control of infection. They are so effective that we might tend to think that the specific components of the immune system are of relatively minor importance. This view, in fact, is held by a fair number of researchers studying immunity to infectious disease (and is not necessarily wrong).

Two things, however, should be kept in mind. First, individuals who are deficient in the specific immune system (B and T cells) have a greatly increased chance (over normal individuals) of con-

---

[5] Lachman actually used *plugs* in place of *holes*. Either term would do, but *plugs* suggested to us something being stopped up rather than leaking.

tracting a lethal infection. Second, specific immunity to infectious disease is a very well documented phenomenon; in fact, it is the historical basis for the field of immunology (Chapter 1). Therefore, specific immune responses *are* extremely important in protection from infectious disease. We now consider why this is.

SYNTHESIS
The Interplay between Nonspecific and Specific Immunity

The events of the inflammatory response, which we have just described, are independent of the specific immune system and are common (with some variations) throughout much of the animal world. Because they have served so many species so well for so long, there can be little argument that inflammation and phago-cytosis are efficient in evolutionary terms. But as we move further along in evolution, there is greater emphasis on the survival of the individual, and the efficiency of the nonspecific factors has been augmented in the vertebrates by interaction with the specific immune system.[6]

The realization that the nonspecific and specific immune systems work together in immunity came about only after a rather acrimonious battle between the proponents of the "humoral" school, who argued that antibody and complement could account for all immunity, and those of the "cellular" school, who argued that phagocytosis alone is sufficient. It was Almoth Wright in England who eventually brought the two ideas together by showing that the two could work together. Wright coined the term OPSONIN (from the Greek *opsono*, "I prepare food for") for the activity of antibodies that enhance the phagocytic process. As John Humphrey points out in the introduction to his classic textbook (Humphrey and White, *Immunology for Students of Medicine*, 1963), Wright was an enthusiast so well known that he appears, thinly disguised, as Sir Colenso Ridgeon in G. B. Shaw's *The Doctor's Dilemma*:

> Drugs can only repress symptoms: they cannot eradicate disease. The true remedy for all diseases is Nature's remedy. Nature

---

[6] This is a transparent bit of hand waving, because we don't really know why the specific immune system is restricted to, and so important for, the vertebrates. The fact of the matter is, when our immune system fails in severe immunodeficiency diseases (Chapter 38 and 39) lethal infection can rapidly overwhelm us. It's just not the same with invertebrates (which, though susceptible to infectious disease, seem to do moderately well). It's an interesting puzzle to think about.

and Science are at one, Sir Patrick, believe me; though you were taught differently. Nature has provided in the white corpuscles as you call them—in the phagocytes as we call them—a natural means of devouring and destroying all disease germs. There is at bottom only one genuinely scientific treatment of all diseases, and that is to stimulate the phagocytes. Stimulate the phago-cytes. Drugs are a delusion. Find the germ of the disease; prepare from it a suitable antitoxin; inject it three times a day quarter of an hour before meals; and what is the result? The phagocytes are stimulated; they devour the disease; and the patient recovers—unless, of course, he's too far gone. That, I take it, is the essence of Ridgeon's discovery.

Opsonization is discussed in some detail below. For most of the rest of this chapter, we will examine how the specific immune system functions to augment the nonspecific components of the immune system, via many of the processes with which you should already be familiar. We will then take a look at why these important defense mechanisms don't always work, or not as well as we'd like. (If they did, we wouldn't really need this chapter, would we?)

The Specific Immune Response and Infectious Disease

We now enter the arena of host defense, which, as far as we know, is a hallmark of only the vertebrate immune system. We'll begin with the antibodies. There are several things that antibodies do: they can neutralize a biologically active molecule, induce the com-plement pathway, stimulate phagocytosis, or participate in anti-body-dependent cell-mediated cytotoxicity (ADCC).

Neutralization by Antibody

Antibodies bind to their antigens, and this binding can have impor-tant consequences for host defense. If the antibodies bind to a site that is critical for biological function of a molecule, the effects of the molecule can be NEUTRALIZED. In this way, specific antibodies can block the binding of a virus or a protozoan to cell-surface receptors (see Plate 7-1). Similarly, bacterial (and other) toxins can be bound and neutralized by appropriate antibodies.[7] This action

---

[7] This is the basis for the first successful treatment for diphtheria. Horses were immu-nized with the bacterial toxin, and serum from the horses was injected into patients. The antibody neutralized the toxin and helped to control the disease. Repeated expo-sure to the horse serum caused a different problem, however: serum sickness, caused by an adverse immune reaction to the foreign (horse) proteins (see Chapter 34).

of antibody is clearly independent of any other specific or non-specific effector mechanism. However, regardless of whether a bound antibody neutralizes its target, the resulting antigen–antibody complex may now interact with other defense mechanisms, resulting in destruction and/or clearance of the antigen. One such interaction is the process of opsonization, considered next.

Opsonization

Phagocytic cells can ingest a wide range of particles, from bacteria to polystyrene beads; but the efficiency of phagocytosis is enhanced severalfold if the particle that is to be phagocytized has reacted with antibody. The coating of the particle with specific antibody that enhances phagocytosis is called OPSONIZATION. Assume that the sliver of wood that broke the skin in the earlier example of phagocytosis had some bacteria on it. In such a simple circumstance the nonspecific system is almost always able to clear up the local infection caused by the organisms on the wood or pushed from the skin into the tissue. If, however, there are too many microbes, or if they have enough of a counterdefense and are not cleared, their presence induces the formation of a specific antibody. As the antibody is produced, its concentration in the serum increases, and at some point enough antibody is present at the site of inflammation to react with the microbes. The microbes are now opsonized, and the rate at which they are ingested by the phagocytic cells increases dramatically.

Phagocytic cells have receptors on their surfaces for the Fc portions of Ig molecules (Fc RECEPTORS). The antibody reacts with the microbe through its Fab portion, a reaction producing an Ag-Ab complex. This reaction leaves the Fc portions of the antibody exposed. When these Fc portions react with the Fc receptor on the surface of the phagocyte, there is greatly enhanced membrane movement, which is needed to start the process of ingestion and the formation of the phagosome (Figure 2). It should be emphasized that Fc receptors react only with the Fc portion of Ig that is part of the Ag-Ab complex or has been aggregated in some physical manner. If this were not the case, the receptors would constantly be occupied with the Fc of serum Ig.

Another important opsonin is the complement breakdown product C3b. Regardless of whether C3b is produced as a consequence of the classical or alternative pathways (Chapter 8), the presence of C3b on a particle increases its ability to be phagocytized. The receptor for C3b on phagocytes is a close relative of the

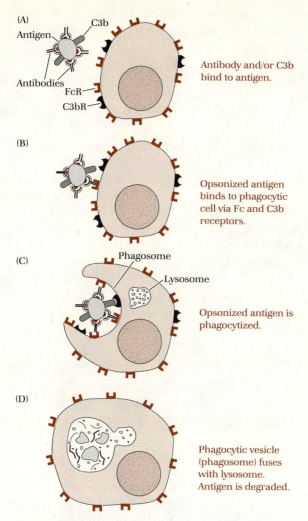

(A)

Antigen — C3b

Antibodies

FcR

C3bR

Antibody and/or C3b bind to antigen.

(B)

Opsonized antigen binds to phagocytic cell via Fc and C3b receptors.

(C)

Phagosome

Lysosome

Opsonized antigen is phagocytized.

(D)

Phagocytic vesicle (phagosome) fuses with lysosome. Antigen is degraded.

2   Opsonization. (A, B) Opsonized antigen (reacted with antibody and complement) reacts at the cell surface with Fc and C3b receptors. (C) The particle is brought inside the cell by invagination of the cell membrane, thereby forming a phagosome. (D) The phagosome fuses with a lysosome.

LFA molecules involved in cell–cell adhesion (mentioned in Chapter 26).

Antibody-Mediated Cytotoxicity

The binding of antibody to an infectious organism (or an infected cell) can result in cytotoxicity via several mechanisms. The activation of the classical complement pathway by antibody (Chapter 8) results in the destruction of many kinds of bacteria and some protozoans.

Another antibody effector mechanism is ADCC (Chapter 28). Certain cells bearing Fc receptors bind to IgG antibody and release a lethal "hit" when the antibody binds its antigen. ADCC is effective against *Schistosoma* and *Trichinella* helminths (Figure 3) and other parasites.

There is another important antibody effector mechanism that we have not yet discussed. This mechanism involves IgE antibodies and appears to be important for the control of some helminth (worm) infections, such as *Ascaris* and *Nippostrongylus*.[8] In some way, the helminth induces T cells to release IL-4, which, in turn, induces B cells to produce IgE (against helminth antigens). The IgE antibodies bind to mast cells, and upon antigen contact, the mast cells release substances with several activities. These activities include making the endothelia "leaky" (allowing cells and fluid to

---

[8] Such responses are important in the defense against nematodes (roundworms) and may be less effective (or not occur) against the platyhelminths (flatworms).

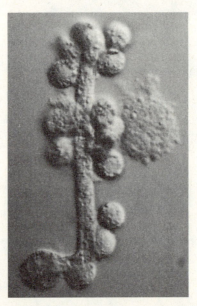

3   ADCC Against Helminths. A newborn larva of *Trichinella spiralis* is under attack by ADCC. In *T. spiralis* infections, the effector cells (shown here) are eosinophils, which bear Fc receptors. Specific antibodies arm the cell, which releases a lethal hit upon interacting with the parasite. [Courtesy of T. Lee, University of Calgary]

penetrate) and recruitment of eosinophils. The eosinophils also bind IgE and use this to bind and assault the helminth with destructive enzymes. Meanwhile, other substances produced by the mast cells cause contractions of the smooth muscles and secretion of mucus, both of which enhance expulsion of the parasite.

Overall, this a very powerful defense reaction. Unfortunately, this defense reaction may also manifest in response to innocuous substances in the environment, resulting in common allergies. These immediate-type hypersensitive responses are discussed in more detail in Chapter 34.

Cytotoxic T Cells

Cytotoxic T cells, at first glance, appear to be an example of a specific immune effector mechanism that does not exploit the nonspecific components of the immune system. On the other hand, the cytotoxic effector mechanisms, discussed in Chapter 28, are used by other (nonspecific) cell types; cytotoxic T cells appear merely to couple the activation of these mechanisms to the T-cell receptor. This coupling provides the cytotoxic T lymphocyte with a unique role in the spectrum of host defenses.

$CD8^+$ cytotoxic T cells bear T-cell receptors that recognize antigenic peptides complexed with class I MHC molecules (if you don't remember why, see Chapter 25). Since antigens are only processed with class I MHC if they are present in the cell cytoplasm (Chapter 20), the cytotoxic T cells are therefore specialized to recognize infected cells. All viruses and many bacteria and protozoans infect cells, and their antigens are presented with class I MHC on the cell surface. Such infected cells can be recognized by cytotoxic T cells, which lyse the cells and induce destruction of the parasite (and cellular) DNA (Chapter 28). Thus, not only is the infected cell destroyed, but so are the parasites, preventing their escape from the damaged cell.

T Cell–Macrophage Interactions

Macrophages are one of the most important "bridges" between nonspecific and specific immune mechanisms. In addition to the phenomenon of opsonization, macrophages interact with the specific immune system by virtue of two of the things they do well: (1) phagocytosis and digestion and (2) antigen presentation to T cells. It often happens that macrophages ingest bacterial or protozoan parasites that are then incompletely (or not at all) destroyed within the cell. This may be due to evasion by the parasite (discussed in the next section) or simply because of excessive numbers of the parasites. Due to the antigen-presenting capacity of some macrophages, however, antigen-specific T cells can be recruited to participate in the response.

Intracellular antigens, presented with class I MHC, or antigens present within the phagosomes, presented with class II MHC, can stimulate T cells ($CD8^+$ and $CD4^+$, respectively) to release lymphokines. (Of course, presentation with class I MHC can also stimulate $CD8^+$ cytotoxic cells, as discussed above.) The lymphokines INF-γ and GM-CSF, released by $CD8^+$ T cells and some $CD4^+$ T cells (T_{H1}, see Chapter 27), have the ability to stimulate macrophages, including the stimulation of intracellular destructive mechanisms. The activated macrophages kill their intracellular parasites (Figure 4). Such responses may play important roles in the immunologic control of some bacterial (e.g., *Listeria*) and protozoan (e.g., malaria, South American trypanosome, and *Leishmania*) infections. INF-γ, in addition to activating macrophage destructive mechanisms (hence its nickname, MAF, or macrophage-activating factor) also stimulates increased expression of class II MHC molecules on the macrophages. These, in turn, have an increased ability to stimulate T cells, resulting in a positive-feedback loop (positive from the point of view of the host, that is).

In addition to the activation of intracellular destructive mechanisms, T cells can also induce macrophages to kill extracellularly and efficiently. Stephanie James and Carol Nacy have dissected the interactions that lead to intracellular versus extracellular killing by macrophages and concluded that these are independent macrophage effector functions, probably under the control of different lymphokines (though some lymphokines, such as INF-γ, will activate both). This form of killing may be important for defense not only against large, extracellular parasites, but also against parasites that infect cells other than macrophages.

T cell–macrophage interactions don't necessarily stop there. MIGRATION INHIBITORY FACTOR (MIF) is yet another lymphokine produced by T cells that results in the recruitment of more macrophages. Other growth and differentiation factors then induce collagen synthesis and fibroblast proliferation that effectively walls off the infected region. These effects are characteristic of a condition called DELAYED-TYPE HYPERSENSITIVITY (or type IV hypersensitivity), discussed in more detail in Chapter 34. Such responses play important roles in the control of some viral, bacterial (e.g., tuber-

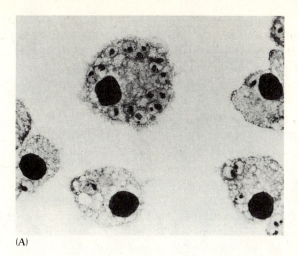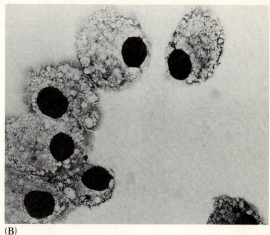

(A)   (B)

4 **γ-Interferon Induction of Macrophage Killing of Intracellular Parasites.** (A) The macrophages have ingested *Leishmania* parasites, which survive in the cell. (B) The macrophages have killed their intracellular parasites shortly after exposure to γ-interferon. [Courtesy of M. Belosovic, University of Alberta]

culosis, leprosy), and protozoan (e.g., *Leishmania*) infections. Chronic responses of this type, resulting in granuloma formation (see Chapter 34) are made against trichinella cysts and the eggs of schistosomes and are responsible for the pathological effects of these helminths.

Parasite Strategies for the Evasion of the Immune Response

If the immune system were 100% efficient, we wouldn't have infectious disease. Not surprisingly, however, parasites have evolved an array of mechanisms for avoiding the immune response. In addition to telling us why we get sick, an overview of these mechanisms also gives us some insights into which aspects of the immune response play predominant roles in eradication of parasites (i.e., if the parasite has evolved ways to evade a particular immune mechanism, then that mechanism is likely to have been a key factor in preventing the parasite's survival, at least at some point in evolution).

Some of the evasion mechanisms are fairly obvious; these relate to size and location. Obviously a very big organism is more difficult to kill than a smaller organism. Some helminth (worm) and arthropod (e.g., tick) parasites fall into this category (tapeworms can grow to over a meter in length). Where in the body a parasite lives is also obviously relevant to its susceptibility to immune assault. Areas with limited access by some of the effector mechanisms of the immune system (e.g., eye, gut, brain) are favored sites for many of the most serious disease-causing parasites.

Parasites evade immunity in a number of ways. They can vary the antigens that they express, shed them in response to immune attack, or simply bury them beneath a layer of host molecules. Parasites can be resistant to immune effector mechanisms by producing substances that inactivate the immune molecules. Alternatively, parasites can produce substances that suppress immune responses. Eukaryotic parasites can undergo dramatic structural changes associated with different stages in the life cycle.

Considering all of the ways that parasites evade immunity can lead the reader to question how we *ever* gain immunity to an infectious disease. Such a view is in stark contrast to our suggestions that the immune system is so competent and uses so many effector mechanisms that few parasites slip through the defenses. Almost certainly, the real situation is that immune effector mechanisms and parasite evasion strategies combine to *limit* the severity of infectious disease. In the absence of antibiotics or other interventions, many people died from infectious disease, but obviously enough survived that we are here today.

Antigen Shedding, Cloaking, and Variation

From the point of view of a parasite, the vertebrate immune response is an extremely potent selective pressure for evolutionary change. Not surprisingly, then, antigenic molecules in parasites are targets for selection and therefore often display variations that may improve the parasite's ability to evade immunity. Three "strategies" for antigen-related evasion are SHEDDING, CLOAKING, and VARIATION.

Antigenic shedding depends on the way in which major antigens are anchored in the parasite's membrane. When antibodies bind to a surface antigen, the antigen is released from the parasite, thus avoiding antibody effector mechanisms. The parasite overproduces these antigens, which then serve as a sort of "smoke screen," preventing effective immunity. One consequence of shedding large quantities of antigen is that antigen–antibody complexes form in the host, which may precipitate in host tissues, with immunopathologic effects. This is referred to as IMMUNE COMPLEX DISEASE, or type III hypersensitivity (discussed in Chapter 34), and can cause skin rashes, kidney failure, arthritis, and other problems.

Another strategy involves antigenic cloaking. The parasite coats itself in a thick layer of host proteins, such that antibodies and effector cells might become "blinded" to the presence of the parasite. While such cloaking has been observed, it has not been formally proved that cloaking is an effective evasion of immunity.

Antigenic variation is, perhaps, the most important (or at least most studied) of the evasion strategies, in part because such variation makes vaccine development especially tricky. There are two basic ways in which antigenic variation can occur: antigenic DRIFT and antigenic SHIFT. Drift is relatively simple. Point mutations in genes that encode parasite antigens can alter the epitopes on the antigen, such that immunologic memory to the original antigen is not triggered by the mutant. Accumulation of such point mutations in a parasite population can result in multiple infections in the same host, because immunity to one variant will not necessarily ensure immunity to others. Antigenic drift has been found in most parasites (including viruses, bacteria, and protozoa), but its importance varies among individual species.

Antigenic shift is a bit different, in that the new antigen that appears is often very different from the previous one. In influenza viruses, antigenic shift is the cause of new epidemics, because following a relatively rare shift, the virus behaves as a brand new disease (at least as far as immune systems are concerned). This type of antigenic shift in viruses is often due to reassortment of antigen genes between two different viruses. Tremendous variability in the parasite can result from a combination of antigenic drift and shift (Figure 5).

One of the best studied cases of antigenic shift is in the African trypanosome, a protozoan parasite. Unlike most other parasites, the trypanosome can alter its major antigen during the course of infection, thus completely evading the immune system (see Figure 6). This VARIABLE SURFACE GLYCOPROTEIN, or VSG, is encoded by more than a hundred (possibly a thousand) different genes in the parasite (Figure 7). Some of these genes lie at the telomeric end of the chromosome, and in a way that is not understood, their promoters activate one at a time to produce antigenically distinct VSGs during the course of an infection. But to make matters worse, other VSG genes can move into these sites to yield more varieties. Yet more variation occurs when different VSG genes recombine to produce

5 **Antigenic Variation in Influenza.** The relationships among influenza viruses, based on the NH_2-terminal amino acid sequences of the HA1 antigen. Branch points represent percentage amino acid sequence difference. Since antibodies to HA1 can neutralize the virus infection, the extensive variation in this antigen allows the parasite to effectively evade immunity (i.e., responses to one subtype are unlikely to affect another). [From Air et al., 1987. In Cruse and Lewis, eds., *Antigenic Variation: Molecular and Genetic Mechanisms of Relapsing Disease*, p. 28]

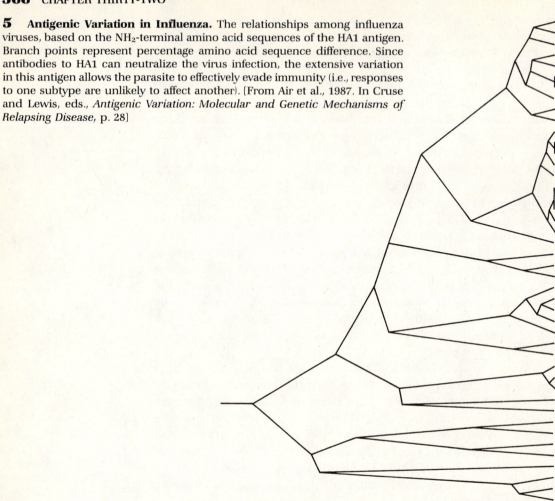

Amino acid sequence difference (percent)

new forms. Though the molecular mechanisms are very different, it seems as though this parasite uses the same strategy to produce antigens that the immune system uses to produce antibodies. In this case, the immune system has been beaten at its own game.[9]

[9] It is useful to point out that in these parasites, a variety of clonal selection is also going on. The immune response to the infection (say, against antigenic form A) effectively eliminates those parasites that express the antigen. Any parasite that has undergone antigenic variation, though, escapes (is selected) and expands until another immune response can act on this new population (to select new variants).

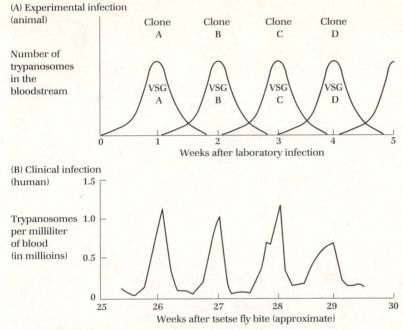

(A) Experimental infection (animal)

Clone A   Clone B   Clone C   Clone D

Number of trypanosomes in the bloodstream

VSG A   VSG B   VSG C   VSG D

0   1   2   3   4   5

Weeks after laboratory infection

(B) Clinical infection (human)

Trypanosomes per milliliter of blood (in millioins)

1.5

1.0

0.5

0

25   26   27   28   29   30

Weeks after tsetse fly bite (approximate)

6   Antigenic Variation in African Trypanosomes. (A) Controlled infection produced in a laboratory animal by injection of an African trypanosome expressing variable surface glycoprotein A (VSG-A). The immune response eliminates nearly all the parasites except rare individuals that have shifted to expression of VSG-B (which is not cross-reactive with VSG-A). Individual parasites from each peak can be isolated and the genes encoding the particular VSG identified (see Figure 7). (B) African trypanosome infection in a human host. [From Ross and Thompson, 1910. *Proc. R. Soc. London* B 82: 411]

Destruction or Suppression of Immune Effector Mechanisms

In addition to the above evasion strategies, parasites can directly alter immune responses by a wide range of mechanisms. For example, some parasites produce enzymes that destroy antibodies or complement components, or prevent phagocytosis. Alternatively, parasites that enter cells can avoid intracellular destruction by a number of mechanisms. The following examples involve protozoan parasites, but similar mechanisms may exist for bacteria as well.

Avoiding intracellular destruction requires that the parasites escape the action of lysosomal enzymes (see Figure 2). *Toxoplasma* does this by preventing the fusion of the phagosome with the lysosome. The South American trypanosome, *T. cruzi*, escapes from the phagosome into the cytoplasm before the phagolysosome

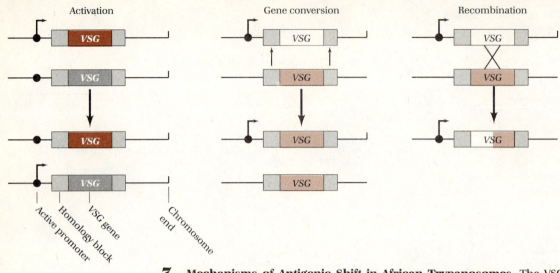

Activation | Gene conversion | Recombination

Active promoter / Homology block / VSG gene / Chromosome end

7 Mechanisms of Antigenic Shift in African Trypanosomes. The VSG undergoes antigenic shift by several different mechanisms during trypanosome infection. VSG genes located near the telomeres have promoters that differentially activate to express different genes (*activation*). Other genes located in other chromosomal regions can replace active genes via *gene conversion*, which depends on blocks of homology that flank the VSG genes. A third, rare mechanism involves *recombination* between genes to yield unique VSG genes. [Adapted from Pays, 1989. *Trends Genet.* 5: 389]

can form. Two other parasites, *Leishmania mexicana* and *Trypanosoma dionisii* have developed ways to survive the attack by lysosomal enzymes. The former produces enzyme inhibitors, and the latter manages to be resistant to the oxygen free radicals (burning). These few examples show that many evasion strategies are effective for avoiding an immune effector mechanism.

For an immunologist, one of the most interesting ways that a parasite can avoid immunity is by suppressing or subverting the immune response. Studies on viruses, bacteria, fungi, protozoans, and helminths have identified situations in which infection leads to a marked reduction in immunity. This might affect the response to the parasite itself, or even open the door to secondary infections.

Recently, studies on *Leishmania* infections in mice have demonstrated one way in which such subversion of the immune system can occur (Figure 8). To understand these studies, it is important to recall that T cells that make one set of lymphokines can regulate the subset that makes a different set (T_{H1} vs. T_{H2} cells, see Chapter 30). Frederick Heinzel and Richard Locksley in San Francisco examined the expression of lymphokines from T cells

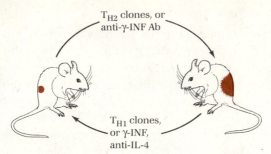

T_{H2} clones, or
anti-γ-INF Ab

T_{H1} clones,
or γ-INF,
anti-IL-4

Infection in resistant animals
manifests as a small
lesion that regresses.

Infection in susceptible animals
manifests as a progressive
lesion often resulting in death.

RESPONSE:
Predominantly T_{H1},
which protects against
parasite and inhibits T_{H2}.

RESPONSE:
Predominantly T_{H2},
which does not protect against
parasite and inhibits T_{H1}.

8   T Cell-Derived Growth Factor Profiles Determine Resistance versus Susceptibility in *Leishmania* Infections. Mice are genetically susceptible or resistant to infection with *Leishmania*. Those that display resistance tend to generate T_{H1}-type responses, while those that are susceptible generate responses suggesting T_{H2} activation. Susceptibility or resistance can be altered, however, by the administration of antibodies to relevant lymphokines, or by injection of cloned, *Leishmania*-specific T cells of one or the other type. Why the host–parasite interaction favors one or the other helper cell type (or lymphokine profile) is not known.

in susceptible and resistant mice with parasite infections. They found that expression of γ-interferon correlates with resistance to the parasite, while susceptible animals express IL-4. Meanwhile, Phil Scott and Alan Sher at NIH showed that animals that are susceptible to infection can be rendered resistant by injection of anti–IL-4 antibodies. Conversely, Michael Belosevic and Carol Nacy showed that anti–γ-interferon antibodies convert resistance to susceptibility. F.-Y. (Eddy) Liew at Wellcome Labs in England further showed that T-cell clones that produce resistance produce γ-interferon (i.e., are T_{H1}-like) while those that inhibit effective immunity produce IL-4 (i.e., are T_{H2}-like). Altogether, this work suggests that one way for a parasite to alter the immune response in its favor is to (somehow) shift the balance of T_{H1} and T_{H2} cells (and/or the pattern of lymphokines that is induced from T cells). The reader should recall, however, that the existence of such helper cell subsets in humans is still controversial (Chapter 30), and therefore their importance in human disease should be treated with caution.

Life Cycles and Immunity

The eukaryotic parasite is often a complex organism, going through a number of changes associated with its life cycle in the host. Each type of parasite goes through different characteristic stages, and, in general, each of these has a different name in different parasites. For simplicity, however, we'll generalize for the purposes of our discussion (Figure 9). Parasites enter the body in the form of an INFECTIVE STAGE, which rapidly changes to a form we'll call the GROWTH STAGE. This is most often the form that causes disease. At some point, some of the growth-stage parasites undergo a further change to a TRANSMISSION STAGE, which is the form that leaves the body. This is also the sexual stage of most parasites. Often, the parasite must then enter a different species of host organism (usually an invertebrate) in order to generate more infective-stage parasites. These hosts are considered the PRIMARY HOSTS and act as VECTORS to spread the parasite to the SECONDARY HOSTS, such as us. In Figure 10, actual life cycles are shown for three protozoan parasites and one helminth parasite.

Each stage of the life cycle of a parasite is usually endowed with a set of STAGE-SPECIFIC ANTIGENS. An immune response directed

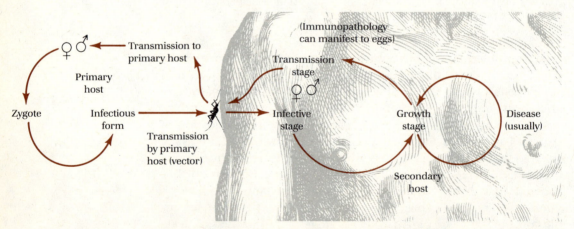

9 Generalized (and Simplified) Life Cycle of a Protozoan or Helminth Parasite. Many variations on this basic theme exist (for example, many parasites are asexual). The primary host, usually an invertebrate, acts as a vector to transmit the parasite to secondary hosts (such as humans). Immune intervention may be directed at any stage of the parasite's life cycle to which the secondary host is exposed, but often the response to one stage is ineffective against another. Actual, though simplified, life cycles of several parasites are shown in Figure 10.

at one stage of the parasite's life cycle may therefore not affect the same parasite at another stage. In this way, the parasite can effectively evade many types of responses. Much research into vaccines for such parasites is concerned with directing immunity to a particular stage and studying the effects of such immunity on infectivity, growth, and transmission of the parasite.

The Immune Response as Disease

In some cases, the disease that is associated with an infection is not a direct result of the action of the parasite itself, but rather of the immune response to the parasite. We have already mentioned examples of this when we discussed granuloma formation and immune complex disease. It is not always easy to know, however, whether preventing the immunopathologic consequences of an infection is always for the best. For example, the skin rash that accompanies measles infection is not a direct effect of the virus but a consequence of the immune response. However, some individuals don't display this rash, but in such cases there is a high risk of neurological damage as a consequence of the infection.

In the case of the helminth *Schistosoma* parasite, the disease that develops is the consequence of granuloma formation against the eggs of the worm. As the granulomas enlarge, small blood vessels become blocked (especially in the liver), resulting in disease. Not everyone responds to the parasite in this way, and the disease, though debilitating, is not especially dangerous otherwise.

One of the least understood immunopathologic consequences of parasite infection may be autoimmune disease. Either because of parasite mimicry of host antigens or by some other mechanism, individuals with a genetic predisposition for autoimmunity may have the disease "triggered" by a viral or bacterial infection. Thus, the complexities of the host–parasite interrelationship have consequences outside the realm of infectious disease. The field of immunology arose as an offshoot of the study of infection and continues to benefit from such research.

Summary

1.   Immunity, the ability to resist and remain free from disease, is achieved by a variety of specific and nonspecific means. A parasite is an organism that functions at the expense of another, and the host–parasite relationship is determined by a delicate balance of factors.
2.   The host may have natural immunity because of physiological

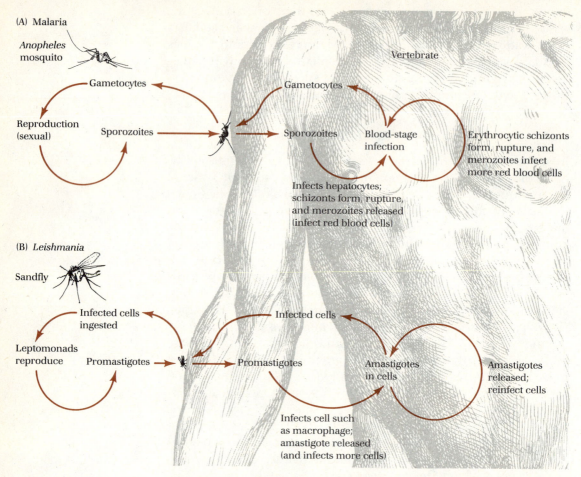

(A) Malaria

Anopheles
mosquito

Gametocytes

Reproduction
(sexual)

Sporozoites

Vertebrate

Gametocytes

Sporozoites

Blood-stage
infection

Erythrocytic schizonts
form, rupture, and
merozoites infect
more red blood cells

Infects hepatocytes;
schizonts form, rupture,
and merozoites released
(infect red blood cells)

(B) Leishmania

Sandfly

Infected cells
ingested

Leptomonads
reproduce

Promastigotes

Infected cells

Promastigotes

Amastigotes
in cells

Amastigotes
released;
reinfect cells

Infects cell such
as macrophage;
amastigote released
(and infects more cells)

10   **Simplified Life Cycles of Some Protozoan and Helminth Parasites.**
Simplified life cycles, based on the general scheme in Figure 9, are shown for
several protozoan parasites (A, B, and C) and a helminth parasite (D). Different
names (e.g., merozoite, promastigote, etc.) describe the form of a particular
parasite at a particular stage.

incompatibility with the potential parasite. Natural physical barriers
such as the skin and mucosa also prevent potential pathogens from
invading the host. In addition, host secretions may repel or destroy
invaders.
3.   When an invader penetrates these first lines of defense, the host
uses the inflammatory response as a potent nonspecific defense. The
inflammatory response ultimately leads to the accumulation of phagocytic cells at the site of infection. Phagocytes ingest and kill the
invading organisms. Interferon is produced by virus-infected cells and
may be of importance in viral immunity.

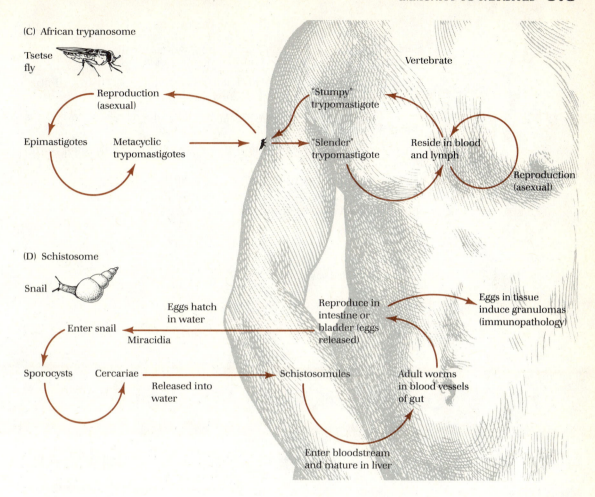

(C) African trypanosome

Tsetse fly

Reproduction (asexual)

Epimastigotes → Metacyclic trypomastigotes

Vertebrate

"Stumpy" trypomastigote

"Slender" trypomastigote

Reside in blood and lymph

Reproduction (asexual)

(D) Schistosome

Snail

Enter snail

Eggs hatch in water

Miracidia

Sporocysts → Cercariae

Released into water

Schistosomules

Reproduce in intestine or bladder (eggs released)

Eggs in tissue induce granulomas (immunopathology)

Adult worms in blood vessels of gut

Enter bloodstream and mature in liver

4. There is an interplay of the nonspecific immune system and the specific reactions to antigens on the parasites. Such interactions include antibody activation of the complement pathway, opsonization, and T cell–macrophage interactions.

5. Parasites have evolved a number of effective strategies for evading immune responses. These include antigen shedding, antigenic variation, resistance to immune effector mechanisms, and suppression (or alteration) of immune responses. In addition, some parasites have complex life cycles that may also allow them to escape effective immunity.

6. In some cases, it is the immune response, rather than the invading organism, that produces the pathologic condition associated with a disease. It is often not completely clear whether or not we would be worse off without these pathologic immune responses.

Additional Readings

Bach, M. K. 1982. Mediators of anaphylaxis and inflammation. *Annu. Rev. Microbiol.* 36: 371.

Cerami, A. and B. Beutler. 1988. The role of cachectin/TNF in endotoxic shock and cachexia. *Immunol. Today* 9: 28.

Mims, C. A. 1987. *The Pathogenesis of Infectious Disease*, 3rd ed. Academic Press, New York.

Playfair, J. H. L., ed. 1989. Immunity to infection. *Curr. Opinion Immunol.* 1: 425.

Scott, P., E. Pearce, A. W. Cheever, R. L. Coffman and A. Sher. 1989. Role of cytokines and CD4[+] T cell subsets in the regulation of parasite immunity and disease. *Immunol. Rev.* 112: 161.

THE RESPONSE TO INTERNAL INVADERS:
Immunity to Tumors

Overview Up to now we have been discussing the response of the organism to *external* invaders and have developed the idea that because the specific immune response did not appear in evolution until the chordates, the vast majority of the animal kingdom defends itself against external invaders with nonspecific immunity. This raises the question of why the chordates should have needed the specific immune system. Lewis Thomas addressed this question in 1959 and concluded that the reason probably was not for defense against external invaders. Rather, he reasoned, as organisms grow more and more complex and live longer, the chance for neoplastic growth of cells increases. Thomas introduced the idea that the specific, adaptive immune response may have evolved in response to the need to protect the body from *internal* invaders, specifically neoplasia. Burnet expanded upon this theory, and, as the immune surveillance theory, it became the dominant paradigm in tumor immunology.

In its most simple form, immune surveillance argues that there are tumor-specific antigens associated with neoplastic cells and that the immune system acts as a surveillance system to identify and destroy any cells that begin to express these new antigens, and thus, to prevent tumor growth before it really begins. As we'll see, the immune surveillance theory makes a number of predictions, some of which have not stood the test of time. This has led, not surprisingly, to a modified form of the theory, which suggests that specific and nonspecific host defense mechanisms protect us from some types of cancer, and that, possibly, these mechanisms might be manipulated to fight others. This optimistic view is still controversial, but it has provided us with some new approaches to immunotherapy.

Immune Surveillance

The original immune surveillance theory, as stated by Burnet, was simply put:

> The thesis is that when aberrant cells with proliferative potential arise in the body they will carry new antigenic determinants on their cell surfaces. When a significant amount of new antigen has developed, a thymus-dependent immunological response will be initiated and eventually eliminates the aberrant cells in essentially the same way as an [allograft] is destroyed. [Burnet 1970, *Prog. Exp. Tumor Res.* 13: 1]

Several predictions that come from this theory seemed to be directly testable. First, the theory suggests that tumor cells should bear antigens that can be recognized as foreign by the immune system. These might be either unique molecules or else a normal molecule to which the immune system is not tolerant (e.g., a molecule normally expressed in very low amounts or only during early ontogeny). Second, the mechanisms of tumor rejection, according to the theory, should be related to those of graft rejection. These mechanisms, discussed in Chapter 37, include the action of cytotoxic T effector cells and the macrophage–T-cell interactions discussed in the previous chapter. Finally, if, as the theory tacitly predicts, immunity evolved as a mechanism of tumor prevention, then immunodeficient states should result in an increased frequency of cancer.

The theory, however, was not as simple to test as people hoped. Each of these predictions was supported or rejected by different experiments and observations. Part of the problem is that cancer is not a single disease, and what might be true for one type of cancer is often not true for another. Another problem came from the use of transplantable tumor cell lines in experimental animals; results of these experiments could not always be extended to spontaneously arising tumors.

In this chapter, we will use the immune surveillance theory and its predictions as a sort of outline of the development of this field and attempt to formulate a modified, if optimistic, theory.

Tumor-Specific Antigens

We saw much earlier in this book that the discovery of the MHC was intimately associated with the experimental models of tumors. It had been noted at the beginning of this century that when animals were inoculated with tumors they often rejected them, and they rejected a second injection of the same tumor even more rapidly. The logical explanation for this was that the host was responding to something unique on the tumor, perhaps a tumor-specific antigen, and mounting an immune response to the tumor. But, as we saw in Chapter 15, with the development of inbred strains of mice, the rejection could be shown to be due not to responses to tumor-specific antigens but to normal antigens encoded in the MHC. Even so, the idea that the immune system is involved in the defense against tumors is an attractive one. But if the immune system really does play a role, the basic requirement is that there be TUMOR-SPECIFIC ANTIGENS, that is, antigens that are present on tumors but are not found on normal cells and tissues. It would be to these antigens unique to the tumor that the immune response would react.

The Demonstration of Tumor-Specific Immunity

In the 1950s, the results of some experiments strongly indicated the existence of tumor-specific antigens. The basic design of these classic experiments (Figure 1) is to remove a tumor from an animal and then rechallenge the animal with the same tumor. If there are tumor-specific antigens, the animal should have made an immune response to them while the tumor was growing. When the tumor is *reintroduced*, the immune response should cause it to be rejected. In the experiments by Foley, for example, tumors were induced in C3H mice with methylcholanthrene (MCA; see below) and then caused to regress by looping some surgical thread around the base of the tumor and "strangling" it by drawing the knot tight. Deprived of its vascular supply, the tumor "dried up" in a few days and disappeared. When the mice were later challenged by implanting the same tumor, it was found that they were able to reject it. Untreated controls all died of the tumor. However, when the same experiment was attempted with spontaneous mammary tumors, it was found that these tumors grew. Thus the response to spontaneous tumors differed from the response to induced tumors. We will return to this fact later.

This basic experiment was repeated and then modified by Richmond Prehn and colleagues, who used surgical excision (as well as the strangulation) and obtained the same result as Foley. In addition they added another control: they injected groups of mice with normal tissue and showed that the tumors grew in these mice at the same rate as in the uninjected controls. This

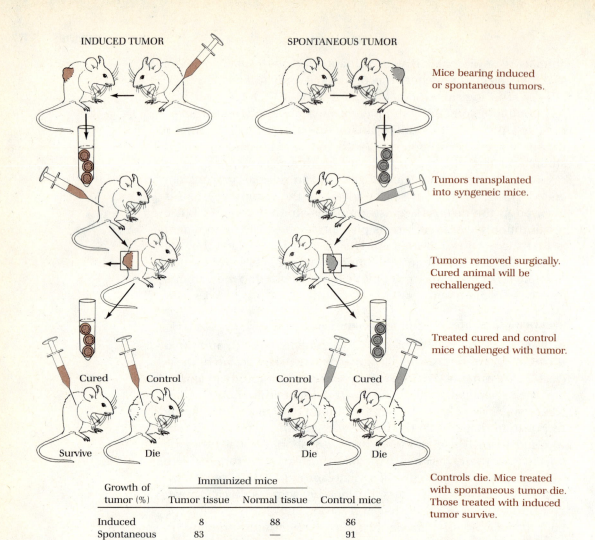

INDUCED TUMOR   SPONTANEOUS TUMOR

Mice bearing induced
or spontaneous tumors.

Tumors transplanted
into syngeneic mice.

Tumors removed surgically.
Cured animal will be
rechallenged.

Treated cured and control
mice challenged with tumor.

Cured   Control   Control   Cured

Survive   Die   Die   Die

Controls die. Mice treated
with spontaneous tumor die.
Those treated with induced
tumor survive.

Growth of tumor (%)	Immunized mice		Control mice
	Tumor tissue	Normal tissue	
Induced	8	88	86
Spontaneous	83	—	91

1   Immunity to Induced and Spontaneous Tumors. An induced or spontaneous tumor is removed from the animal and "stored" in a syngeneic mouse. Later the tumor is removed from the host mouse and reimplanted into the mouse in which it originated. Normal mice are inoculated with tumor at the same time as controls. The controls die, showing that the tumor is still active. Reintroducing the induced tumor into the original animal does not lead to death, but reintroduction of the spontaneous tumor into the original animal shows that there is no protection. [After Foley, 1953. *Cancer Res.* 13: 835; Prehn and Main, 1957. *J. Natl. Cancer Inst.* 18: 769; and Klein et al., 1960. *Cancer Res.* 20: 1561]

showed that there must have been something on the tumor that was different from its counterpart on normal tissue. Finally, George Klein and his co-workers in Sweden carried out similar experiments in which the tumor was induced and then surgically removed. These mice were able to reject the tumor when it was later reimplanted.

Figure 1 shows that for the induced tumors there was clear-cut TUMOR IMMUNITY, which was not seen with the spontaneous tumors. Thus the crucial experiments had been done, and the stage was now set for developing the idea that the immune system plays a role in the host response to tumors.

Types of Tumor Antigens

The tumor antigens that led to tumor rejection in the above experimental systems are often referred to as TUMOR-SPECIFIC TRANSPLANTATION ANTIGENS. They may be unique to a particular tumor, unique to a class of tumors, or present on many different tumors (as well as normal tissues). For example, some tumors that are induced experimentally with the carcinogen MCA stimulate immunity in the autochthonous host (i.e., the one with the tumor). This immunity may extend to other tumors, induced by other chemical or physical carcinogens or transplanted from some spontaneously arising tumors. The responsible antigens are considered tumor-specific if they are absent from normal syngeneic tissue.

The frequency of such tumor antigens detected in this way is probably an underestimate, because many tumor antigens do not normally induce rejection of the tumor. These antigens may be detected by either monoclonal antibodies or cloned T cells, which, in the case of human tumor antigens, may have considerable value for diagnosis and therapy (see later in this chapter). Studies of tumor antigens reveal they are of many different types. These include (but are not limited to) viral antigens (especially in animal tumors, but also in some human malignancies), embryonic and fetal antigens, and carbohydrate antigens.

The reason that at least some tumors express antigens not normally found on the tissue of origin is not entirely known. Several causes have been suggested. For example, tumor cells may amplify the production of proteins normally found at very low levels in the tissue (too low to induce self-tolerance), such that the protein becomes immunogenic. Alternatively, the transformed status of the cell might result in the expression of genes that are normally silent in the untransformed cell, resulting in the production of unexpected proteins. A third possibility is that the rapidly growing cells may produce mutant proteins. Examples exist for each of these possibilities.

One type of tumor-specific antigen is known to be almost absolutely unique to the tumor: the Ig or T-cell receptor on the surface of a transformed lymphoid cell. Since it is generated by the diversity mechanisms we have discussed, it represents a practically unique molecule in the body. Unfortunately, these molecules do not appear to be potent transplantation antigens, and the generation of specific agents against them (such as anti-idiotype or clonotype antibodies) is a relatively slow process if we wish to exploit them for immune therapy.

Viruses, Oncogenes, and Tumor Antigens

Many of the tumor antigens that have been identified in mice have turned out to be encoded by DNA or RNA tumor viruses. Mice harbor (and are susceptible to) large numbers of these viruses, which often become activated upon exposure to cancer-causing agents. Such viruses cause cancer by the expression of viral ONCO-GENES, genes that are very closely related to genes found in the host genome (protooncogenes, or cellular oncogenes). The cellular oncogenes encode a number of different types of proteins important for cell growth, including growth factors, growth factor receptors, and regulatory DNA-binding proteins. By mimicking the cellular genes, the viral oncogenes can produce a state of deregulated growth in the cell. The tumor antigens, then, may be products of the virus, or of deregulated cellular genes.

The excitement surrounding the discovery of the role of viruses in cancer was subdued with the realization that most human tumors are not associated with viruses. There are some exceptions, however. Epstein-Barr virus, which causes mononucleosis, can also induce a B-cell lymphoma, Burkitt's lymphoma, and an epithelial malignancy, called nasopharyngeal carcinoma. Human T-cell leukemia viruses (HTLV-I and II) can also induce cancer. Although other examples will probably be found, human tumors, for the most part, do not seem to be induced by viruses.

All tumors, however, do seem to be linked to the activation of an oncogene (any one of many). The products of cellular oncogenes, even if they reach the cell surface, are not necessarily unique antigens, but their deregulation could lead to the expression of apparently novel proteins (by the above mechanisms).

Embryonic and Fetal Antigens

The idea that cancer cells may express normally silent genes led to the notion that the most therapeutically effective tumor antigens should be those normally expressed only in early development. These have been called ONCOFETAL ANTIGENS. Indeed, tumor antigens that cross-react with normal embryonic tissue were described as early as 1932. The best studied example of such an antigen is the CARCINOEMBRYONIC ANTIGEN (CEA), expressed on human colonic cancers and also on fetal tissue. More recently, however, CEA has also been found to be expressed at low levels on normal adult tissues. Thus, CEA may be an example of increased expression of a "quiet" rather than a silent gene. Many apparent oncofetal antigens probably fall into this category.

The distinction may be important. First of all, the concept of oncofetal antigens suggested that tumors represent a state of dedifferentiation of a cell, returning it to a state of rapid growth resembling that of embryonic development. If we could understand how embryonic cells are regulated during development, we could then control the growth of tumor cells. If, however, tumors are a different sort of entity (which they most likely are), then this approach to tumor control loses some credibility. (This is not to say that this isn't still a nice idea.) Another reason that the distinction is especially important relates to some of the strategies of tumor therapy, discussed later in this chapter. Such strategies depend upon the tumor antigen's being absolutely unique in the body; otherwise, the therapeutic agent (such as an antibody coupled to an extremely potent toxin) will destroy the normal tissue displaying low levels of the antigen.

Carbohydrate Tumor Antigens

Cell-surface carbohydrates are important cellular interaction molecules in many systems, and they appear to play several roles in the physiology of cancer. From the point of view of tumor immunity, cell-surface carbohydrates may have a special relevance. For example, CEA is heavily glycosylated, consisting of approximately 50% carbohydrate. The antigenicity of this molecule is influenced by the carbohydrate structures. The role of carbohydrate antigens in tumor immunity, however, extends beyond the role of carbohydrate on glycoproteins, as we'll see.

In Chapter 2, we discussed the nature of antigens, including the ability of carbohydrates to be recognized by antibodies. For most of the book, however, our discussion of antigens has been practically limited to proteins. There are two reasons for this: first, most of immunology has focused on protein antigens, and second, T cells simply don't appear to respond to carbohydrate antigens (at least, such responses have been very difficult to study). Nevertheless, carbohydrate antigens on tumor cells hold considerable promise as unique, tumor-specific antigens. This is because of the nature of carbohydrates. Unlike protein antigens, carbohydrates are not directly encoded in the genes. Instead, carbohydrates are produced as a result of the interactions of many enzymes, working in concert. If a cell contains a unique ensemble of such enzymes (even though each enzyme is a normal protein, represented in different cells in the body), the resulting carbohydrate can be a unique molecule. A large number of carbohydrate antigens on tumor cells have been identified, and many of these appear to be tumor-specific. In several cases, these antigens even appear to be specific for a particular type of tumor, which increases the potential for the development of agents (e.g., specific antibodies) for use in diagnosis and therapy.

There are two major types of carbohydrate tumor antigens. MUCINS are mostly carbohydrate (75–80%) and often appear in altered form on tumor cells. Antibodies against specific mucins are currently being used to detect certain types of cancers (sometimes well before the tumor is apparent by other criteria). In addition, some altered mucins have potent immunosuppressive effects and/or block immune effector action against the cell. GLYCOLIPIDS come in two varieties: sialic acid–containing and blood group–like. Many of the attempts to generate a "cancer vaccine" have focused on this class of antigen.

One of the best studied carbohydrate antigens is the TF ANTIGEN. Thompson-Friedenreich, while studying human red blood cells, noticed that after the cells were stored for a while they appeared to agglutinate spontaneously. The effect turned out to be an experimental artifact (but an interesting one): contaminating bacteria produced neuraminidase, which removed neuraminic acid residues from cell-surface carbohydrates. Antibodies present in the human serum then reacted with the exposed (*cryptic*) antigen. It turns out that antibodies to the exposed carbohydrate antigen, or closely related antigens, often react with a variety of tumors. Curiously, individuals with a genetic defect that results in the presence of such antigens on red cells (in noncryptic form) have a high risk of developing cancer. One might be tempted to believe that this is because such individuals are tolerant to the exposed antigen and fail to make effective responses to the arising tumors. However, since carbohydrates are important in the regulation of activity of many cell types, it is alternatively possible that defects leading to altered structures could increase tumor risk for other reasons.

Mechanisms of Tumor Rejection

The mechanisms of tumor rejection mostly parallel those of protection against infectious disease. Both nonspecific and specific effector mechanisms can be involved, depending upon the tumor and the experimental (or clinical) situation. Nevertheless, certain generalizations can be made.

For the most part, antibody responses to tumors seem to be poorly correlated with a demonstrable resistance of the host to the tumor. In general, complement-mediated lysis of tumor cells is difficult to demonstrate and is unlikely to be of much benefit in vivo. Alternatively, ADCC (see Chapter 28) can be demonstrated to act on tumor cells in vitro and may impart some benefit in vivo.

ADCC = ab dependent cell-mediated cytotoxicity

Two types of specific immune response have been shown to be effective in preventing tumor growth in experimental systems. These are the CD8$^+$ cytotoxic T cell and the T cell–macrophage responses discussed in the last chapter. Protein tumor antigens, since they are produced within the cell, can be processed and presented with class I MHC (Chapter 20) and thereby serve as targets for the cytotoxic T cells. Alternatively, released tumor antigens can be processed and presented with class II MHC to induce CD4$^+$ T cells, which, in turn, activate macrophage effector mechanisms. Such activated macrophages kill tumor cells in vitro and can be observed, together with T cells, in some rejecting tumors in vivo.

The importance of each type of effector mechanism in protection against cancer may depend on the type of tumor. One side-prediction of the immunosurveillance theory is that any cancer that arises has been effectively selected so as *not* to induce specific immunity. If so, then our analysis of antitumor effector mechanisms is skewed by the systems under study. Two lines of evidence converge on this point. In many cases, tumors are immunosuppressive, and thus the relevant effector mechanisms don't come into play. On the other hand, immunodeficient individuals may not have an increased incidence of cancer, suggesting that the whole idea of immunosurveillance may well be wrong. We consider both these lines of evidence later on. Before doing so, however, another type of effector mechanism believed to be important in protection against cancer should be considered. This is the natural killer cell.

Natural and Lymphokine-Activated Killer Cells

If the evidence for the two basic requirements of the immune surveillance theory (unique tumor antigens and impaired immune function) is open to question, is there *any* evidence that the immune system plays a role in defense against tumors? In the course of looking for specific cytotoxic T cells that lyse chromium-labeled tumor target cells, it was noticed that normal individuals have high levels of cells cytotoxic for some tumor targets. These were called natural killer cells, or NK cells (Chapter 28), because they exist, apparently, in the absence of immunization with the antigens on the tumor cells.

The NK cells are a subpopulation of lymphocytes, which are identified morphologically as large granular lymphocytes (LGLs). As discussed in Chapter 28, NK cells lack diverse antigen receptors (such as surface Ig or TCRs) but presumably bear a receptor that allows them to recognize target cells. These cells also bear Fc receptors (but not complement receptors). This fact allows NK cells to carry out ADCC in addition to the lysis of targets in the absence of antibody. Interferon enhances NK-cell activity.

NK cells are able to lyse a fairly wide range of cells, both tumor and normal. They do this with no known MHC restriction, and, as mentioned, in the absence of prior contact with antigen. Little is known about the nature of the structures on the surface of the target cells with which the NK cells react. The possible role of NK cells in tumor immunity is a much-discussed question. We do not know the range of specificities possessed by these cells, so we cannot even begin to predict the range of structures on newly emergent tumor cells that would be recognized.

If lymphocytes are cultured in very large amounts of IL-2, an effector cell type related to NK cells is generated. These are the LAK (lymphokine-activated killer) cells (also discussed in Chapter 28). Although similar to NK cells, LAK cells kill a broader range of tumor cells. Cells appearing to have this activity have been found among the cells that infiltrate human tumors. LAK cells were believed to hold tremendous promise for tumor therapy, and although the initial results of clinical trials were problematic, new approaches to their use may still prove valuable (discussed later in this chapter).

Immune Regulation and Cancer

Since the 1960s, it has been clear that tumors regulate antitumor immunity in interesting ways, many of which we still don't really understand. For example, an animal bearing an experimental tumor that grows progressively (i.e., is not controlled by an anti-tumor response) may nevertheless be able to reject small numbers of cells from the same tumor injected into another site. This phenomenon of CONCOMITANT IMMUNITY suggested that immune responses to tumors might be generated in a tumor-bearing individual but might sometimes not be able to function in the environment of an established tumor.[1]

This phenomenon may be related to dose effects of tumor cell administration, which are reminiscent of the low- and high-zone tolerance effects discussed in Chapter 31. With many immunogenic tumor lines, injection of a number of tumor cells into an animal produces a tumor that grows for a time and then regresses as antitumor immunity acts against it. In several cases, however, injection of a very small or a very large number of cells results in the tumor growing progressively, that is, the animal has not produced effective antitumor immunity. These phenomena are referred to, respectively, as TUMOR SNEAK-THROUGH (since the small number of tumor cells appears to "sneak" past the immunity) and TUMOR BURDEN (since the burden of a large tumor challenge appears to overwhelm immune defenses).

More recently, the ability of some tumors to control immune responses has become better understood. For example, a potently immunosuppressive neuroblastoma cell line was found to produce transforming growth factor β, (TGFβ) which was shown to suppress T-cell and NK-cell function. It is not yet known, however, whether the production of TGFβ contributes to the ability of such tumors to evade immunity. One experiment, though, suggests that it does. A fibrosarcoma line that normally induces CTLs in vivo and is actively rejected by the immune system was transfected with a TGFβ gene. The resulting lines then failed to induce CTLs either in vivo or in vitro. Further, the transfected cell line (but not control lines) grew progressively in transiently immunosuppressed hosts. This requirement for transient immunosuppression, however, suggests that TGFβ production alone does not allow the cells to completely evade immunity. Other immunosuppressive substances from other types of tumors have also been identified, but again, their role in evasion of immunity has not been established. This is clearly an important question from both theoretical and practical points of view.

[1] It was this phenomenon that led Richard Gershon to propose the existence of suppressor cells. Rather than pursue his studies on concomitant immunity, he designed the experiment discussed in Chapter 30 and devoted the rest of his career to the study of regulatory T cells.

A large number of studies have implicated suppressor T cells in the evasion of immunity and progressive growth of tumors, and although, in some cases, manipulation of the immune system to remove the suppressive function has had dramatic effects, the status of the suppressor-cell controversy (see Chapter 30) has necessarily held these studies up to criticism. Nevertheless, more careful investigation of the mechanisms of immune regulation by T cells in some of these systems is bound to yield some important information.

One of the best studied systems for understanding T-cell regulation in evasion of antitumor immunity is that of skin cancer induced by ultraviolet (UV) light, one of the most common forms of cancer known. Margaret Kripke, Steve Ullrich, and their colleagues in Houston found that tumors induced by UV light in mice could be transplanted to other UV-irradiated animals, but not to normal animals. This UV-induced unresponsiveness to the tumors is associated with T cells that suppress antitumor immunity when injected into otherwise normal mice. This suppression appears to be specific for UV-induced tumors, since tumors induced by other means are rejected normally. This phenomenon of UV-induced suppressor T cells has been studied by a number of investigators, but as with other suppressor-T-cell phenomena, the mechanisms of the observed immunoregulation remain elusive (see Chapter 30).

Immune Deficiency and Cancer

The fact that under some conditions tumor-specific antigens can be demonstrated is a strong point in favor of the immunosurveillance theory. But the theory raises the question of why we develop cancer. The answer, according to immune surveillance in its purest form, is that the tumor either overpowers the immune system or develops when the immune system is not functioning well. The prediction would be that one would see more cancer in older individuals, because as the animal ages, its immune function, like other bodily functions, operates at lower efficiency. This is well known to be the case. One might also expect to see more tumors early in life, when the system is just beginning to function. Childhood leukemias are a well-known disease of the young. How then does the theory handle the tumor overpowering the immune system? The prediction is that tumors are either immunosuppressive or arise when the animal is in a state of impaired immune function.

The literature abounds with examples of tumor-bearing experimental animals and humans having depressed immune function.

These cases led to a general acceptance of the immune surveillance theory. But in 1975 Osias Stutman in New York did an extensive analysis of the literature and concluded that "there are almost as many exceptions as there are positive associations between immune deficiencies and increased risk for tumor development" [Stutman 1975, *Adv. Cancer Res.* 22: 261].

Furthermore, since the theory postulated that the T-cell response would eliminate the tumors as they developed, the prediction would be that the athymic nude mouse should have a very high incidence of tumors. In fact, these animals are essentially free of spontaneous tumors. Originally it was argued that nude mice do not live long enough to develop tumors, but when these mice are maintained under germ-free conditions so that their life span is increased, they develop tumors at roughly the same rate as do *nu/+* heterozygous littermates of the same age.

This observation was confounded, however, when investigators examined NK-cell activity in nude mice. Not only do nude mice have NK cells (which may have a role in tumor surveillance), but the numbers and/or activity of these cells is significantly enhanced over that of normal animals. It is possible, therefore, that surveillance by NK cells (or similar mechanisms) suffices in these animals. On the other hand, normally rejected tumors (even human tumors) grow very successfully when injected into nude mice. This could be taken as evidence that T cells in normal animals are, in fact, active in surveillance, or that the NK cells in nude mice are not.

It should also be remembered that in the original experiments protective responses to tumor-specific antigens were demonstrated only on induced tumors and not on spontaneous tumors. This finding raises the possibility that the responses that were observed and the protection that the responses afforded are laboratory artifacts. Induced tumors or spontaneous tumors that have been passaged for many generations may simply be different from spontaneously arising tumors.

On the other hand, studies on the relationships between immunodeficiency or pharmacologic immunosuppression and cancer continue, and not all the facts are in. Individuals with immunodeficiency diseases definitely show an increased incidence of some cancers, especially cancers of the immune system, but this may be more related to the genetic basis of their immunodeficiency than to a breakdown in immune surveillance. Immune surveillance almost certainly operates in cancers induced by viruses, such as Epstein-Barr virus (see above), in which cancer appears to be a consequence of both the action of the virus and a failure of the immune system to respond to it. Since most cancers in humans do not appear to be induced by viruses, however, the issue of whether immune surveillance operates in most cancers is still unresolved.

SYNTHESIS
Modified Immunosurveillance Theories

The lack of support for Burnet's original immune surveillance theory has required that the theory be modified (some would say "scrapped"). Several modified versions of the theory have emerged, and a brief discussion of these modifications may help the reader to put the issues into perspective.

George Klein has suggested that while immune surveillance exists in principle, it can act only on highly immunogenic tumors. Tumors that do not induce rapid, effective responses might change to avoid effective immunity. Since tumors, in general, are rapidly dividing cells, the same principles of clonal selection that we know for the immune system and for external invaders (see Chapter 32, footnote 8) can apply. That is, the immune system will destroy the immunogenic tumor cells, effectively selecting for less immunogenic variants. These variants may have lost their expression of tumor antigens or MHC molecules, or may have gained an ability to suppress immune function by some mechanism. Such selection can be demonstrated using highly immunogenic tumor lines that become progressively less immunogenic (and more lethal) as they are passed through immunocompetent animals.

If this is indeed the case, however, there may still be prospects for cancer immunotherapy, but if so, what form should it take? The reader has probably concluded by now that at the present time it is very difficult to assign relative weights to the importance of nonspecific and specific aspects of immunity in resistance to invaders (either external or internal). Richmond Prehn, whose work was so instrumental in the initial formation of the immune surveillance theory, has argued as follows:

> The evidence overall seems to suggest that immunological surveillance of nascent tumors, as originally conceived, may not exist in most tumor systems. On the other hand, there is a late acting and inefficient immunological defense mechanism. Hopefully, this mechanism may be subject to augmentation for purposes of immunotherapy. [R. Prehn, in F. H. Bach and R. A. Good, eds., *Clinical Immunobiology*, vol. 2, p. 191]

The issue, therefore, changes from whether the immune system normally surveys the body and eliminates transformed cells to whether the immune system (or an engineered component of it) *can* survey the body to eliminate cancer cells. It is a subtle distinction, but it has major ramifications, especially for the development of immunotherapy (and biotechnology companies). Therefore, we have nicknamed this modified theory "The technoimmune surveillance theory." It is based on the idea that components of the tumor–immune system interaction, such as antibodies, T cells, lymphokines, tumor antigens, or tumor cells themselves, can be modified and used to combat cancer. The rest of this chapter is devoted to this idea.

Immune Diagnosis and Immunotherapy of Cancer

There are many different approaches to the diagnosis and therapy of cancer. Since this is a textbook of immunology, however, we will concern ourselves only with those approaches that have an immunologic basis. We warn the reader, however, that many of the nonimmunologic approaches to therapy have a much better "track record" than those we will discuss. The future of immune diagnosis and therapy of cancer will probably depend upon combinations of immunologic with nonimmunologic strategies.

Antibodies in Tumor Diagnosis and Therapy

In our discussions of tumor antigens, we suggested that some efforts to identify tumor-specific antigens by using monoclonal antibodies have met with some success. One of the major benefits of identifying such an antibody will be its use in tumor diagnosis. In general, if a tumor can be located before it is large, then the prognosis following surgery and/or chemotherapy is greatly enhanced. Two approaches to diagnosing tumors employ tumor-specific antibodies.

One such approach relies on the hope that tumor-specific antigens, produced by a tumor, may appear in detectable levels in serum before the tumor reaches a dangerous size. Conventional antibody detection systems, such as RIA and ELISA (see Chapter 11) are used for screening, and in many preliminary studies this appears to have some diagnostic value in identifying some types of cancers. Clearly, the specificity of the antibodies, the reliability of the assay, and the frequency with which such cancers produce the tumor-specific antigen detected by the assay all will contribute to the value of this diagnostic approach.

A second approach to diagnosis is tumor IMAGING using antibodies coupled to a radioactive label (or other visualizable marker). If the antibodies are relatively specific (i.e., do not normally bind to the tissues in which tumors bearing the antigen may appear) then this approach may have tremendous value in identifying and localizing tumors. Such tumor imaging is under intensive study in many centers around the world and has already proved valuable for a number of types of cancer.

A potentially promising area that is receiving much attention is the use of IMMUNOTOXINS. Immunotoxins are antibody molecules to which a toxin or drug has been covalently conjugated. The rationale is that if one has a monoclonal antibody directed against a tumor antigen, it can serve as a vehicle to deliver the toxin to the tumor cells and kill them. Ricin (a plant toxin) and diphtheria toxin are two very commonly used agents. The toxins consist of a toxic polypeptide (called the A chain) that is disulfide-bonded to a cell surface-binding polypeptide (called the B chain). The most potent immunotoxins are composed of the A chain of the toxin linked to the antibody molecule. Several immunotoxins are undergoing clinical trial. Clearly, this approach requires that the antibody be extremely specific for the tumor; otherwise normal cells bearing the antigen will also be destroyed. Nevertheless, many ingenious strategies to get around this problem are being tested, and we will almost certainly be seeing this type of cancer therapy used clinically in the coming years.

Another interesting approach to the use of antibodies in tumor therapy takes advantage of the ability of antibodies to form a bridge between cytotoxic effector cells and tumor-cell targets (see Chapter 28). Hybrid antibodies, with one binding site for a tumor antigen and another for CD3, can cause any cytotoxic T cell (i.e., not specific for tumor cells) to kill tumor cells. Such antibodies, or other variations, may have some promise for therapy.

The use of antibodies for tumor diagnosis and therapy, while valuable, doesn't really have the "feel" of an *immune* therapy (at least to us), except in the sense of passive immunity. The treated patient would presumably be no more resistant to reappearance of the cancer than would someone treated by chemotherapy. Hopes for immune therapies that involve active immunity on the part of the patient have led to other approaches, all of which have had (at best) limited success. We now consider these strategies.

Adjuvant Therapy

Based upon the assumption that the immune system can play an important role in the destruction and elimination of tumors, much effort has been put into attempts to enhance the ability of the immune system to carry out these ends. A great deal of the effort has gone into attempts to nonspecifically increase the activity of the system. The most commonly used approach uses the idea of ADJUVANTS—nonspecific amplifiers of immune function. The organism used in some countries to vaccinate against tuberculosis is called BCG (bacillus Calmette-Guérin). For reasons poorly understood, this bacterium enhances phagocytosis, antibody formation, and cell-mediated responses. It was hoped that by treating patients with this organism, both the nonspecific and antigen-specific mechanisms would be increased. Unfortunately, there has been only limited success with this method.

Tumor Vaccines

The possibility that specific tumor antigens may be associated with certain types of spontaneously arising tumors in humans has stimulated a search for potential tumor vaccines. These might be used to treat patients who either have a tumor or are at high risk after removal of a tumor. Though these studies have gone on for many years, the quest for vaccines has been confounded by difficulties in preparing antigenic tumor extracts. For example, in a number of studies, the apparent immune response to the tumor vaccine was actually to a xenogeneic enzyme used to produce the extract. It has also been necessary to identify safe but effective adjuvants for the immunization protocol.

In recent years, efforts with some types of tumors, especially the highly malignant melanomas, have produced some promising results. For example, Malcolm Mitchell and his colleagues in Los Angeles have produced a melanoma vaccine by mechanical disruption of melanoma cell lines. Patients injected with the extract generate DTH responses to the vaccine, circulating cytotoxic T cells to melanoma cells, and, in some cases, partial or complete regression of the tumor. Other laboratories have reported equally encouraging results.

Though controversial, efforts to generate a tumor vaccine are of obvious importance and may be the best hope we have of immunotherapy in some types of cancer. This may be an example of an area of study in which researchers have lost some of their initial enthusiasm because of relatively slow progress, but which may nevertheless return to the limelight (as will those scientists who stuck with it). While we probably shouldn't get our hopes too high, we probably also shouldn't exclude the possibility that vaccines for some types of cancer may someday exist.

IL-2 and LAK-cell Therapy

In Chapter 28, we mentioned the phenomenon of LAK cells, lymphoid cells that have potent cytotoxicity and are generated under the influence of high doses of IL-2. Steven Rosenberg and his colleagues at the NCI in Bethesda observed that administration of IL-2 and/or in vitro-generated LAK cells into tumor-bearing animals had dramatic antitumor effects in a number of tumor models. An example, using a nonimmunogenic sarcoma line that produces liver metastases, is shown in Table 1. Administration of a high dose of recombinant IL-2 greatly reduced the number of liver metastases observed 3 days after injection of tumor cells, and this effect was even more striking with administration of LAK cells and IL-2. Similar results were obtained using cell lines that produce lung metastases. Many investigators, using other tumor lines and variations on this therapeutic strategy, have shown that such therapies are genuinely effective—at least in animals.

Initial enthusiasm for attempting such therapies in cancer patients has waned somewhat because of the extremely toxic effects of administration of IL-2 in humans (this seems to be due to nonimmunologic effects of IL-2 at high doses in vivo). Although LAK and/or IL-2 therapy has had limited success in some forms of kidney cancer and melanoma, the procedures are extremely expensive, time-consuming, and dangerous. Many investigators feel that the potential benefits of such therapy are too small to justify the harm done to patients. Nevertheless, there are several reported cases of complete remission with this therapy, and in about 20% of cases there is some benefit. It is possible that new strategies will provide a safer, more effective therapy.

SYNTHESIS
Cancer and Immunology

Immune therapy for cancer is not the only reason to study tumor immunology, nor is it the only way to fight cancer. While

Table 1   In vivo effect of LAK cells ± IL-2 on tumor metastasis in mice.[a]

Cells injected	Number of metastases	
	−IL-2	+IL-2
PULMONARY TUMORS		
None	228	152
Cultured spleen	183	156
Fresh spleen	214	191
LAK cells	200	20
HEPATIC TUMORS		
None	246	53
Cultured spleen	250	50
Fresh spleen	245	60
LAK cells	193	1

Source: Data from Rosenberg and Lotze, 1986. *Annu. Rev. Immunol.* 4: 681.

[a] Groups of mice were injected with tumor cells on day 0. On days 3 and 6, animals received injections of fresh splenocytes, splenocytes cultured without IL-2, or splenocytes cultured with IL-2 (LAK cells). Some groups also received IL-2 injections every 8 hours between days 3 and 10. Lungs or livers of the mice were then examined for metastases (small tumor foci). Note that the best protection (color) was afforded by treatment with both LAK cells and IL-2. However, the benefits of this therapy are offset by the toxic effects of the treatment.

some types of immune diagnosis and therapy of cancer hold promise, we should keep in mind that the study of tumor immunology has also taught us a great deal about the immune system and can be justified on this basis alone. The discovery of the MHC, the nature of antibodies (as myeloma proteins), the study of cytotoxic effector cells, the generation of monoclonal antibodies, and the molecular bases of antigen recognition and lymphocyte activation (to name a few) all owe a debt to the study of cancer. If we someday find new ways to treat cancer as a result of such studies, all the better.

Summary

1.   The immune system may play a role in the response to tumors. The immune surveillance theory states that neoplastic cells that express tumor-specific antigens will be recognized by the immune system and removed. Cancer would develop only when the immune system failed or when a tumor had evaded immunity.

2.   Effective tumor immunity has been demonstrated in a number of animal models, especially those involving experimentally induced tumors. Specific and nonspecific effector mechanisms that play a role in tumor immunity include the actions of activated macrophages, cytotoxic T cells, NK cells, and lymphokine-activated killer cells.

3.   One mechanism by which tumors appear to evade immunity is by a form of clonal selection, in which less immunogenic variants of the tumor are selected by the immune system, resulting in a tumor that is not rejected. Another evasion strategy is the suppression of effective immune responses by the tumor (or by the conditions under which the tumor is induced), although in most cases either the mechanism of the suppression or its role in tumor growth (or both) is unknown.

4.   Many of the predictions of the immune surveillance theory have failed to be confirmed (or are very controversial), and evidence has accumulated that suggests that immune surveillance against tumors does not occur (or only in certain circumstances). This, however, does not exclude the possibility that the tumor or components of the immune system can be engineered in such a way that immune therapy can be developed.

5.   Approaches to immune diagnosis and therapy in cancer, with more or less success, include tumor imaging with monoclonal antibodies, immunotoxins (composed of a tumor-specific antibody conjugated to a toxin or drug), adjuvant therapy and/or development of tumor "vaccines," and therapy with IL-2 plus LAK cells.

Additional Readings

Doherty, P. C., B. B. Knowles and P. J. Wettstein. 1984. Immunological surveillance of tumors in the context of major histocompatibility complex restriction of T cell function. *Adv. Cancer Res.* 42: 1.

Hakamori, S. 1984. Tumor-associated carbohydrate antigens. *Annu. Rev. Immunol.* 2: 103.

Kripke, M. L. 1984. Immunologic unresponsiveness induced by ultraviolet radiation. *Immunol. Rev.* 80: 87.

Olsnes, S., K. Sandvig, O. W. Petersen and B. van Deurs. 1989. Immunotoxins—entry into cells and mechanisms of action. *Immunol. Today* 10: 291.

Ortaldo, J. R. and R. B. Herberman. 1984. Heterogeneity of natural killer cells. *Annu. Rev. Immunol.* 2: 359.

Rosenberg, S. A. 1988. Immunotherapy of cancer using IL-2: Current status and future prospects. *Immunol. Today* 9: 58.

Schreiber, H. 1989. Tumor immunology. In W. E. Paul, ed., *Fundamental Immunology*, 2nd ed. Raven Press, New York, p. 923.

Vitetta, E. S. and J. W. Uhr. 1984. The potential use of immunotoxins in transplantation, cancer therapy, and immunoregulation. *Transplantation* 37: 535.

HYPERSENSITIVITY

Overview   Up to now we have been focusing on the mechanism of the immune response and the protective effect of the response. In this chapter we will see that the normal functioning of the immune system can have harmful effects. We will examine a series of reactions known as hypersensitivity or allergy. The discovery of hypersensitivity came at the time when the protective effects of antibody were discovered, and so the two have grown up together. A conceptual advance in the study of hypersensitivity was the classification of the various forms of disease into four groups, based on the immune mechanism that causes the symptoms. Three of these types of hypersensitivity are mediated by antibody. Type I hypersensitivity is brought about by the fixation of IgE to mast cells and the subsequent reaction of that bound IgE with the allergen, causing degranulation of the mast cells. Type II hypersensitivity occurs when antibody binds to the surface of cells, leading to cell lysis by the activation of the classical complement pathway or by the action of ADCC. Antigen–antibody complexes that precipitate in tissues and the subsequent antibody effector mechanisms that are induced are the basis of type III hypersensitivity. A fourth type of reaction (type IV hypersensitivity) is caused by the interaction of T cells with macrophages, fibroblasts, and other cells.

Immunity and Hypersensitivity

Origins of the Idea That an Immune Response Can Be Harmful

The immune response has undoubtedly evolved into its complicated and diverse state because it has survival value to the species. However, like all good things, there are aspects of the immune response that can be harmful to the individual. The original discovery of the immunologic nature of the harmful effect of antibody was made in the early 1900s by the French physician Paul Richet. His description of the discovery is of interest not only because it shows how the "prepared mind" works, but also because it gives us a glimpse of science in the Grand Style of a lost era.

> During a cruise on the yacht of Prince Albert of Monaco, the Prince advised me to study *Physalia*[1] poison, together with our friends Georges Richard and Paul Portier. We found that it is easily dissolved in glycerol and that by injecting this glycerol solution, the symptoms of *Physalia* poisoning are reproduced.
>
> When I came back to France and had no more *Physalia* to study, I hit upon the idea of making a comparative study of the tentacles of *Actinia* which can be obtained in large quantities, for *Actinia* abound on all the rocky shores of Europe.
>
> Now *Actinia* tentacles, treated with glycerol, give off their poison into the glycerol and the extract is toxic. I therefore set about finding how toxic it was, with Portier. This was quite difficult to do, as it is a slowly acting poison and three or four days must elapse before it can be known if the dose be fatal or not. I was using a solution of one kilo of glycerol to one kilo of tentacles. The lethal dose was of the order of 0.1 liquid per kilo live weight of subject.
>
> But certain dogs survived, either because the dose was not strong enough or for some other reason. At the end of two, three or four weeks, as they seemed normal, I made use of them for a new experiment.
>
> An unexpected phenomenon arose, which we thought extraordinary. A dog when injected previously even with the smallest dose of 0.005 liquid per kilo, immediately showed serious symptoms: vomiting, blood diarrhoea, syncope, unconsciousness, asphyxia and death. [Charles Richet, 1913. Nobel lecture. In *Nobel Lectures in Physiology and Medicine, 1901–1921*, p. 475.]

Richet termed this phenomenon ANAPHYLAXIS. In his Nobel lecture he tells why he coined the term:

> First I feel I must explain and indeed justify the use of the word itself, for it may seem somewhat barbarous at first glance. This neologism I invented twelve years ago on the assumption, which I think is still valid, that a new idea calls for a new word in the name of scientific precision of language.
>
> *Phylaxis*, a word seldom used, stands in the Greek for protection. *Anaphylaxis* will thus stand for the opposite. Anaphylaxis, from its Greek etymological source, therefore means that state of an organism in which it is rendered hypersensitive, instead of being protected. [p. 471]

---

[1] The Portuguese man-of-war.

Richet soon established that this "hypersensitivity" is transferable by serum and that the active material(s) are the same as antibodies. This fact is important in the historical context because the first Nobel prize, given in 1901, was to Emil von Behring for his work on the serum therapy of diphtheria, that is, on the *protective* effect of antibody. Indeed, the period was full of the excitement and hope that the combined efforts of two new sciences, bacteriology and immunology, would end the scourge of infectious diseases through immunization and serum therapy. Richet was astute enough to recognize that even though antibody could be protective, it also could be destructive.

We will see in this chapter that "anaphylaxis" has come to be used for only one type of harmful immunologic reaction and that the term *hypersensitivity* (which Richet used in the quotation above) has become the generic technical term for harmful immune reactions.

The Need for Sensitization

There are many manifestations of hypersensitivity, none of them pleasant and all having in common the fact that they are initiated by an immune reaction to an antigen and occur in or on a host who has become SENSITIZED (i.e., has previously made an immune response to that antigen). Thus hypersensitivity in all its many and varied forms is the result of *restimulation* with the offending antigen. The distinction is made between *sensitizing* and *immunizing*, because not all secondary responses are hypersensitivity reactions. In common parlance, the latter are called ALLERGIC REACTIONS and those antigens involved in hypersensitive or allergic responses are called ALLERGENS.

Because hypersensitivity reactions occur to a wide variety of allergens and at any number of areas and organs of the body, they come in what at first appears to be a bewildering variety. For years this catalog of dread was the realm of the allergist, who treated the particular symptoms as well as the times allowed. However, as more was learned about the mechanisms of the immune response, both in experimental animals and in humans, it became clear that there were some unifying principles. In the 1950s Gell and Coombs devised a classification system based upon the *nature of the immunologic reactions* rather than on the symptoms.

The Gell and Coombs Classification of Hypersensitivity

The GELL AND COOMBS CLASSIFICATION divides hypersensitivity reactions into four groups based upon features that they have in common. The characteristics of the groups are presented below and diagrammed in Figure 1.

- Type I: Type I reactions are those caused by the fixation of IgE to mast cells with the subsequent release of pharmacologically active substances that produce the symptoms. These responses are also called IMMEDIATE-TYPE HYPERSENSITIVITY, because the response can appear within seconds of challenge. Examples of type I diseases are anaphylaxis, atopy, and urticaria ("hives"). Most common allergies (e.g., hay fever, dust allergy) are due to this type of response.

- Type II: Type II reactions are caused by the action of antibodies—usually IgG and IgM—on target cells and the activation of complement or other antibody effector mechanisms, leading to inhibition of function and/or destruction of the cells. Examples of type II diseases are erythroblastosis fetalis and transfusion reactions. Many antibody-mediated autoimmune diseases—such as autoimmune hemolytic anemia (in which the antibodies bind to red blood cells) and myasthenia gravis

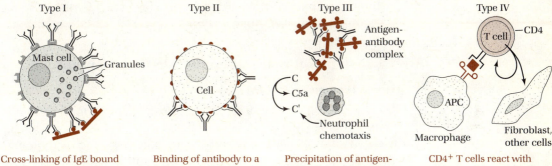

Type I

Mast cell — Granules

Cross-linking of IgE bound to mast cell causes release of active compounds from granules.

Type II

Cell

Binding of antibody to a cell triggers complement and other antibody effector mechanisms.

Type III

Antigen-antibody complex

C
C5a
C'
Neutrophil chemotaxis

Precipitation of antigen-antibody complexes triggers complement and other effector mechanisms (including recruitment of granulocytes).

Type IV

T cell — CD4

APC

Macrophage

Fibroblast, other cells

CD4+ T cells react with antigen + MHC and release lymphokines, which in turn stimulate proliferation of T cells, macrophages, fibroblasts, and other cells.

1   The Classification of Hypersensitivity Reactions. Type I reactions: Allergen reacts with IgE bound on mast cells (but produced by B cells), causing degranulation of the mast cell and release of granule contents. The mast cell mediators produce the symptoms. Type II reactions: Antibody binds to an antigen on the surface of cells. Antibody effector mechanisms then cause the symptoms (e.g., destruction of the cells). Type III reactions: Antigen–antibody complexes deposit in tissues, activating antibody effector mechanisms (including granulocyte chemotaxis and inflammation as a result of activation of the complement cascade). Type IV reactions: T cells respond to presented antigen and activate other cells (e.g., macrophages, fibroblasts), causing the symptoms.

(in which the antibodies bind to acetylcholine receptors on muscle cells)—are mediated by type II reactions.

In some cases the binding of antibodies to a cell-surface receptor stimulates a function in the cell. One example is Graves' disease (see Chapter 35) in which antibodies stimulate cells of the thyroid.

- Type III: Type III reactions are those in which antigen–antibody complexes form and precipitate, causing damage by activation of antibody effector mechanisms in a vital organ. An example of this type of reaction is immune complex glomerulonephritis, which can be induced by antibodies binding to high concentrations of antigens. These antigens may be from an infectious disease or a tumor, or may be abundant self-antigens (such as DNA released from cells destroyed in type II reactions). Because of the latter, type II and type III hypersensitivity can coexist in some autoimmune diseases.

- Type IV: Type IV reactions are cell-mediated reactions, induced by interactions of T cells with other cells, such as macrophages and fibroblasts. These are called DELAYED-TYPE HYPERSENSITIVITY (DTH) reactions, because they generally require about a day (or longer) to manifest. Allergic contact dermatitis is the principal example of diseases of this type.

Type I Reactions: Immediate Hypersensitivity

Atopic Diseases

Allergic rhinitis, or hay fever, is the most common form of immediate hypersensitivity or ATOPIC DISEASE. Although the responsible allergen often differs between individuals (e.g., ragweed pollen, grass pollen, dust[2]), the symptoms are similar. While a large proportion of the population suffers from hay fever, the nonallergic individual often has trouble realizing the extent of the misery that hay fever and similar syndromes inflict on the sufferer:

> I am suffering from my old complaint, the hay-fever (as it is called). My fear is, perishing by deliquescence; I melt away in a basal and lachrymal profluvia. My remedies are warm pidiluvium, cathartics, topical application of a watery solution of opium to eyes, ears and the interior of the nostrils. The membrane is so irritable, that light, dust, contradiction, an absurd remark . . . sets me sneezing; and if I begin sneezing at twelve, I

[2] The allergen in dust is really the feces of the house dust mite, *Dermatophagoides pteronyssinus*.

don't leave off till two o'clock, and am heard distinctly in Taunton, when the wind sets that way—a distance of six miles. [Sidney Smith to Dr. Holland, 1835]

Less frequent forms of atopic disease are bronchial asthma and atopic dermatitis. A rarer form is gastrointestinal food allergy.

Atopy

It was known for a long time that these clinical manifestations are due to antibody that somehow causes the mast cells to release histamine and other vasoactive amines. The released agents cause the contraction of smooth muscle and the other symptoms described by poor Sidney Smith. The antibody was known to have the ability to fix to the skin and (for convoluted historical reasons that we will not go into, dealing with the reagin of the old syphilis tests) was called *reaginic* antibody. What made reaginic antibody so special was not known until Kimishige and Teruko Ishizaka showed that the property of fixing to tissue, specifically to mast cells and basophils to cause their degranulation, is unique to the IgE class of Igs. The route they took to this discovery was discussed, along with the properties of IgE, in Chapter 7. 6. (p. 100)

Mast Cell Degranulation

Mast cells are found in connective and subcutaneous tissues, particularly around venules and near mucosal surfaces (Figure 2). They harbor a large number of granules (Figure 3) that contain an array of pharmacologically active mediators. The strategic location of mast cells and their ability to effect rapid physiological changes by releasing these mediators underscores the importance of these "sentinel" cells, not only in allergy, but in many other processes. In atopic disease, the discharge of the granules (degranulation) is triggered when an allergen reacts with specific IgE, bound to the surface of the mast cell.

In an especially elegant series of experiments the Ishizakas showed that IgE binds to the mast cell via the C_H3 and C_H4 domains of the Fc and that the reaction of the mast cell-bound (or fixed) IgE after reaction with allergen causes the receptors to aggregate. Somehow this receptor reorientation results in mast cell degranulation. This classic experiment is shown in Figure 4. (The nature of the receptor is discussed below.) When IgE is allowed to react with mast cells (Figure 4A), there is binding; but this binding alone does not result in degranulation of the mast cells. Degranulation requires both binding of the IgE to the cell and binding of

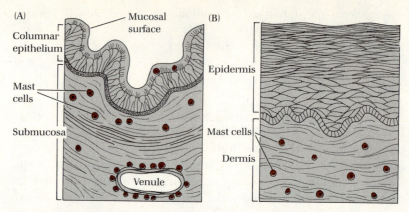

(A) Columnar epithelium / Mucosal surface / Mast cells / Submucosa / Venule

(B) Epidermis / Mast cells / Dermis

2   Mast Cell Distribution. (A) In the bronchial tissue, mast cells are found near the mucosal surfaces and in the submucosa, as well as around venules. (B) Skin mast cells are in the dermis. It can be seen that these "sentinel cells" are near interfaces with the external environment or between venous and arterial circulations. [From Austen, 1983. In Dixon and Fisher, eds., *The Biology of Immunologic Disease*, p. 224; with permission]

allergen to the Fab portion of the IgE (Figure 4B). Thus, if the IgE is not specific for the allergen, there will be no degranulation.

Why should the reaction of allergen at the antigen-combining site of molecules whose Fc portion is attached to the cell have this effect? It was known that the membrane of the cell is a fluid mosaic

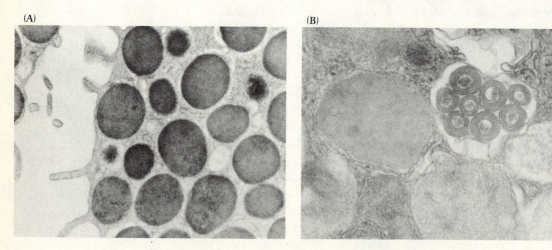

(A)   (B)

3   Internal Structure of Mast Cells. Granules within a single rat peritoneal mast cell (A; ×50,000) and within a single human mast cell (B; ×174,000). These granules contain active agents responsible for many of the symptoms of type I hypersensitivity. [From Austen, 1983. In Dixon and Fisher, eds., *The Biology of Immunologic Disease*, p. 224; with permission]

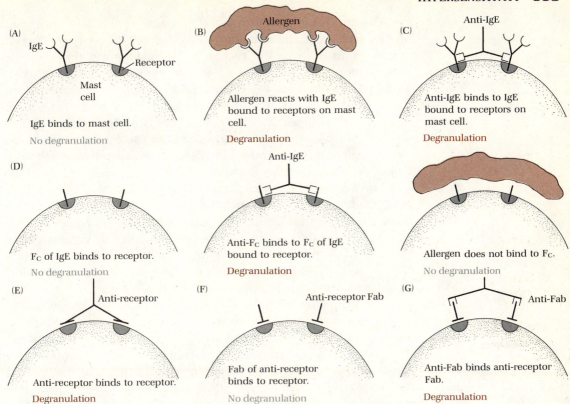

(A) IgE — Receptor — Mast cell
IgE binds to mast cell.
No degranulation

(B) Allergen
Allergen reacts with IgE bound to receptors on mast cell.
Degranulation

(C) Anti-IgE
Anti-IgE binds to IgE bound to receptors on mast cell.
Degranulation

(D) Fc of IgE binds to receptor.
No degranulation

Anti-IgE
Anti-Fc binds to Fc of IgE bound to receptor.
Degranulation

Allergen does not bind to Fc.
No degranulation

(E) Anti-receptor
Anti-receptor binds to receptor.
Degranulation

(F) Anti-receptor Fab
Fab of anti-receptor binds to receptor.
No degranulation

(G) Anti-Fab
Anti-Fab binds anti-receptor Fab.
Degranulation

4 IgE-Induced Mast Cell Degranulation. Experimental conditions that do or do not lead to mast cell degranulation are shown. As a general rule, any manipulation that causes FcRε cross-linking results in mast cell degranulation. [Based on the experiments of Ishizaka and Ishizaka, 1975. *Prog. Allergy* 19: 60]

with floating islands of proteins, many of which are receptors, and that antibody to the "islands" could move them in the plane of the membrane (patching and capping), and thus it was postulated that degranulation is the result of movement and reorientation of some molecule in the mast cell membrane. The membrane molecule involved must be a receptor for the IgE Fc. To test this idea, IgE was allowed to react with mast cells in the absence of allergen (as in Figure 4A); but instead of allergen, anti-IgE antibody was added. If the degranulation is due to the reorientation of the receptors, then the anti-IgE should have the same effect as allergen, that is, moving the receptors. This is exactly the result obtained (Figure 4C). The anti-IgE reacted with the receptor-bound IgE and caused degranulation.

This finding suggested that the crucial event is the binding of the Fc portion to the mast cells and that the function of allergen is merely to reorient the receptors. To further test this idea, Fc fragments of IgE (with no Fab, and therefore no antigen-binding sites) were allowed to react with the mast cells (Figure 4D). Once the Fc fragments had bound to the receptors, anti-IgE was added. Remember, the class-specific determinants on Ig H chains are in the Fc portion, so the anti-IgE bound to the Fc fragments. This also resulted in degranulation. In contrast, when allergen was added to the bound Fc, there was no degranulation.

The argument was made even more convincing (Figure 4E, 4F, and 4G) by showing that an antibody to the Fc receptor on the mast cells caused degranulation. However, an Fab fragment of the anti-receptor antibody (which is monovalent and cannot cause cross-linking), even though it bound to the cell, did not induce degranulation. When an anti-Fab was added to the surface-bound Fab, there was cross-linking and degranulation.

The conclusion from these experiments is that reorientation of the receptor for IgE on mast cells leads to the production of a signal for the granules to fuse with the membrane and release their contents. Under natural conditions, the reorientation is induced by the reaction of allergen with the IgE that is attached to the mast cells. An allergic individual therefore is one who has responded to the allergen by producing anti-allergen antibodies of the IgE class. The IgE is bound to that person's mast cells via the Fc receptors on the mast cells. This is like turning the mast cell into an armed bomb waiting for the firing pin to be detonated. Contact with the allergen is the triggering device.

Why does degranulation cause the symptoms? As seen in Table 1, the granules of the mast cells are an armory of pharmacologically active materials. The opening of this Pandora's box causes alteration in capillary permeability, smooth muscle contraction, and so on, depending upon the surface that is affected (skin, lung, etc.)

The biochemical events that occur after receptor binding have been studied extensively and present a very complicated picture. The main events involve the activation of the adenylate cyclase system, which converts ATP to cAMP. However, several interconnected systems are known to be involved, so that phospholipid metabolism, protein phosphorylation, prostaglandin production, and intracellular pH all come into play.[3] The complex picture is

---

[3] The triggering of mast cell degranulation by cross-linking of surface receptors (in this case Fc receptors) should be familiar from Chapter 26. The subsequent second-messenger effects in mast cells, though differing from those of lymphocytes, are not unique.

Table 1   Mast-cell mediators of hypersensitivity.[a]

Active agent	Activity
GRANULE CONTENTS	
Histamine	Increases vascular permeability; elevates level of cAMP
Heparin	Anticoagulation
Serotonin	Increases vascular permeability
Chymase	Proteolysis
Hyaluronidase	Increases vascular permeability
Eosinophil chemotactic factor	Attracts eosinophils
Neutrophil chemotactic factor	Attracts neutrophils
SYNTHESIZED AFTER ACTIVATION	
Slow reacting substance of anaphylaxis (SRS-A)	Increases vascular permeability; causes contraction of bronchial muscles
Prostaglandins	Contraction of bronchial muscles; vascular dilation
Platelet aggregating factor	Aggregates and activates platelets
Growth factors	Stimulation of mast cells, eosinophils, T cells, and B cells

[a] Following mast cell degranulation, the contents of the granules are released and mediate the functions shown. These are responsible for the "immediate" effects, occurring within minutes of contact with antigen. Following activation, the mast cell synthesizes and releases additional mediators, responsible for later effects. SRS-A is a mixture of leukotrienes (LTC_4 and LTD_4) produced from arachidonic acid via the lipoxygenase pathway. Prostaglandins are produced from arachidonic acid via the cyclooxygenase pathway. Growth factors include IL-4 and IL-5, usually thought of as T cell-derived lymphokines.

diagrammed in Figure 5. The intracellular level of cAMP is affected by β-adrenergic compounds such as epinephrine. The mast cell, in fact, has receptors for both α- and β-adrenergic compounds, so they can be used in therapeutic strategies.

The IgE Receptor and Its Regulation

From all of the above, it is clear that the crucial event initiating the process leading to degranulation is the binding of IgE to the mast cell. The IgE receptor ($Fc_\epsilon R$ I) on the mast cell has been studied extensively. The availability of both human and rat mast cell tumors has made these studies possible. The receptor is a six-

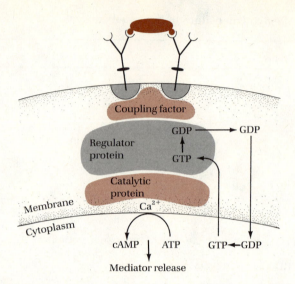

5 **Mast Cell Degranulation.** The intracellular consequences of receptor reorientation in mast cell degranulation. The reorientation causes the catalytic subunit to activate a G protein (see Chapter 26) and the formation of cAMP, resulting in mediator release. [Based on Winslow and Austin, 1982. *Fed. Proc.* 41: 22]

subunit molecule. Two α chains (α_1 and α_2), each with a molecular weight of 55,000, are associated with two β chains (β_1 and β_2) (molecular weight 33,000) and two disulfide-linked γ chains (molecular weight 9000). The γ chains and one β chain are not exposed on the cell surface and may be important for signal transduction. The α chains are the sites of IgE C-region binding, which occurs with high affinity. In addition to mast cells, basophils also possess these high-affinity IgE receptors.

There are also lower affinity IgE receptors (Fc$_\epsilon$R II), found on other cells such as eosinophils. The role of eosinophils in IgE responses was discussed in Chapter 32. This receptor also appears to be present on some B cells, T cells, and macrophages (especially alveolar macrophages). While the structure of this receptor has not been described, molecular analysis of the gene encoding the low-affinity receptor predicts a molecular weight of 36,000 with extracellular, membrane, and cytoplasmic regions. Interestingly, Fc$_\epsilon$R II shares antigenic determinants with a B-cell marker, CD23, which in soluble form may represent an IgE-binding factor. The function of neither CD23 nor soluble IgE-binding factor from B cells is well understood.

Causes of Type I Hypersensitivity

Since it became clear that an IgE response to an allergen results in allergy, a central question in allergy research has been: Why is it that some individuals respond in this manner and others do not? There is clearly a *genetic* component, because atopic diseases such as hay fever can be familial traits. For example, although 38% of atopic individuals have no parental history of atopy, there is a 75% chance that if both parents are atopic, the child will suffer the same fate. If only one parent is atopic, there is a 50% chance of the child's also being atopic. Even though no single HLA haplotype has been associated with atopy, within a family the atopic individuals tend to have the same haplotype.

It is known that certain adjuvants promote the production of IgE in experimental animals, converting what would be an IgG response into an IgE response. The most effective promoters are the helminth (nematode) parasites *Nippostrongylus brasiliensis* and *Ascaris suum* (see Chapter 32). Conjugating haptens to these agents or injecting ordinary antigens along with them results in a preferential IgE response. But even though this technique allows one to study the response in experimental systems, it does not answer the question about the natural response.

One avenue of approach that is being pursued is the notion that a balance between IgE-inducing and IgE-suppressing factors occurs in all individuals. In allergic individuals there is an "allergic breakthrough" because the suppressive factors have become less potent than the enhancing factors. This model is illustrated in Figure 6.

The nature of some of these enhancing and suppressing factors is known. IL-4 (a product of T_{H2} cells; see Chapter 27) induces IgE production and also stimulates mast cell growth. γ-Interferon (from T_{H1} cells) inhibits IgE production, as well as inhibiting the expansion of T_{H2} cells. Based on such observations, many investigators believe that the balance of these two helper-cell types (and/or the profile of lymphokines produced) influences the appearance of allergy.

Other factors that affect the IgE response may also function to control allergy. Ishizaka and colleagues, for example, have described an IgE B-CELL GENERATING FACTOR, which induces an increased number of IgE-bearing B cells, and IgE-POTENTIATING FACTOR. Both of these are made by T cells. These enhancing factors are balanced by IgE-SUPPRESSIVE FACTOR. These factors appear to be

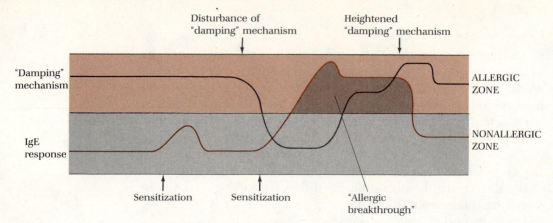

Disturbance of "damping" mechanism

Heightened "damping" mechanism

"Damping" mechanism

ALLERGIC ZONE

IgE response

NONALLERGIC ZONE

Sensitization

Sensitization

"Allergic breakthrough"

6   Allergic Breakthrough. When the magnitude of the IgE response is below a threshold (gray region), there are no allergic symptoms. When it crosses the line, allergic symptoms occur. In normal (that is, nonatopic) individuals, the response remains in the lower section because of a "damping" mechanism that prevents the conversion of the response to IgE (a net balance of suppressive factors and enhancing factors). A disturbance of the damping mechanism causes the IgE response to cross the line and produce an "allergic breakthrough." When the "damping" mechanism corrects itself, IgE production falls below the line. [Redrawn from Katz et al., 1979. *J. Immunol.* **122**: 2191; with permission]

distinct from known lymphokines and apparently differ only in their glycosylation (which is controlled by glycosylation factors, also produced by T cells). If the nature of these factors becomes clear, they may be of great usefulness in the control of allergic responses.

Strategies for the Control of Type I Hypersensitivity

The first step in attempting to control a type I hypersensitive response is to identify that such a response is occurring. The methods of quantifying IgE are seen in Box 1. Once the response has been identified, several strategies can then be employed in attempting to control such a response. New strategies are currently being explored, based on what we know of the causes of allergy (discussed above).

The mast cell has receptors for adrenergic compounds, and these alter the intracellular levels of molecules involved in degranulation; therefore, one strategy for control of the symptoms is to decrease the rate of degranulation. Epinephrine, for example, has been used for over 40 years for this purpose. If the release of the active molecules cannot be prevented, symptoms can be treated with drugs that block the action of the molecules, for example, antihistamines.

One strategy that has had a long history and some success is the attempt to DESENSITIZE the atopic individual. Sufferers of allergy have known that they can get "shots" for their diseases. The "shots" are not some wonder drug; rather, they contain small amounts of purified allergen. The strategy is to inject as pure a form of the allergen as possible in small doses and attempt to convert the immune response from one producing IgE to one producing predominantly IgG. In this way it is hoped that the IgG will compete for the allergen before it can react with any mast cell-fixed IgE. With the description of enhancing and suppressing factors, the rationale has changed; according to the current model the purified allergens may induce the production of suppressive factors.

Type II Reactions: Cytolytic Reactions

Type II allergic reactions are those brought about by antibody reacting with antigen on the surface of a cell. These reactions can cause the activation of the complement cascade or ADCC and ultimately the lysis of the cell. The specific manifestation of the reaction depends upon the cell type on whose surface the reaction is occurring. The result of the reaction is often the destruction of the cell and hence the loss of the function the cell carries out, with all the attendant difficulties that follow.

ERYTHROBLASTOSIS FETALIS is a type II reaction that can now be controlled through immunologic means. When an Rh^- mother delivers an Rh^+ fetus, she may become sensitized to the baby's Rh^+ erythrocytes during delivery. In such cases she will produce anti-Rh antibodies, which may cross the placenta and destroy the fetal erythrocytes of her next child if it too has Rh^+ red blood cells. This fetal hemolysis results in the overproduction of immature erythrocytes, or ERYTHROBLASTS (hence the name of the disease). This disorder can result in a variety of difficulties, including an aborted fetus or damage to the child's central nervous system because of the release of bilirubin and other factors. An Rh^- mother is prevented from becoming sensitized by receiving an injection of anti-Rh antibodies at the time she delivers her first Rh^+ child. This form of immunoregulation has proved remarkably successful.

Probably the best studied type II hypersensitive response is

Determining IgE Levels

Radioimmunosorbent test (RIST) for presence of IgE

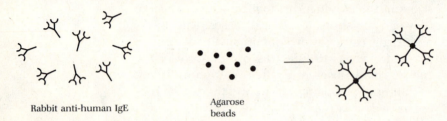

Rabbit anti-human IgE   Agarose beads

1. Rabbit anti-human IgE is conjugated to agarose beads.

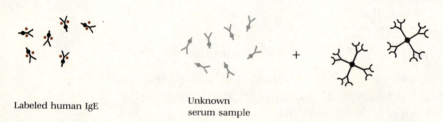

Labeled human IgE   Unknown serum sample

2. Radiolabeled human IgE and unknown serum sample are added to the anti-human IgE–agarose complex.

(a)   (b)

3. (a) The IgE present in the unknown serum competes with the labeled IgE for sites on anti-IgE.

(b) No IgE is present in the unknown serum, so all the labeled IgE is bound.

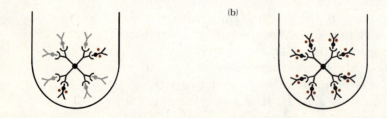

(a)   (b)

4. Centrifuge and count label in pellet. A low count (a) indicates competition for sites and therefore presence of IgE in the unknown serum. A high count (b) indicates a low level of competition and therefore a low level of IgE in the unknown.

BOX
1

Radioallergosorbent test (RAST) for presence of specific IgE

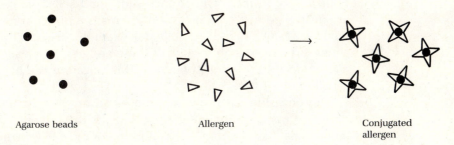

Agarose beads   Allergen   Conjugated allergen

1. Allergen is conjugated to agarose beads.

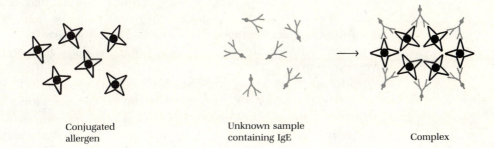

Conjugated allergen   Unknown sample containing IgE   Complex

2. Unknown serum and conjugated allergen are mixed. If specific antibody to the allergen is present, it will form a complex with the conjugated allergen.

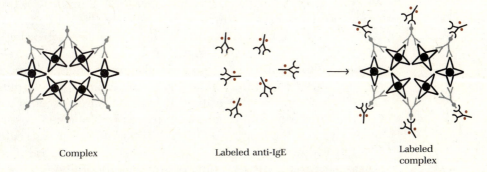

Complex   Labeled anti-IgE   Labeled complex

3. Allergen–antibody complex is mixed with labeled anti-IgE. The complex is centrifuged and the amount of radioactivity is measured. The labeled antibody binds only to antigen-specific IgE.

the transfusion reaction, which occurs when a recipient of a transfusion receives blood from a donor who differs in blood type, especially ABO antigens (discussed in Chapter 2). Because many environmental antigens (such as pollen) cross-react with ABO antigens, many of us have antibodies to other blood types without having ever received a transfusion. If these antibodies have an opportunity to react with transfused blood cells, the donor cells are destroyed in a type II response. This is a problem not only for blood transfusion; kidney cells, for example, also bear ABO antigens, and a mismatch for one of these antigens can lead to hyperacute rejection of a transplanted kidney, again by a type II hypersensitive response.

On occasion, an individual makes an antibody response to a drug that results in hemolysis because the drug interacts with red blood cells. This response and subsequent red cell destruction can result in HEMOLYTIC ANEMIA. Another form of drug-related type II reaction is an "innocent bystander" phenomenon. Some drugs such as quinine and quinidine induce antibody responses that result in drug–antibody complexes that become adsorbed onto circulating platelets. When complement reacts with the complex, lysis of the platelets ensues and produces THROMBOCYTOPENIA.

Another autoimmune disease that produces damage by type II hypersensitivity is GOODPASTURE'S SYNDROME, in which antibodies are produced to the basement membrane of the glomeruli of the kidney. This disease is different from immune complex glomerulonephritis, discussed below.

Type II hypersensitivity reactions occur by the antibody effector mechanisms discussed in Chapters 7 and 8. Cells are destroyed by the activation of the classical complement pathway, or by myeloid cells bearing Fc receptors for the antibody (ADCC). If the antibody is bound to a tissue, the release of complement breakdown products can produce further effects. C3a and C5a cause smooth muscle contraction and release of granules from basophils, all of which increase vascular permeability (which leads to swelling as plasma leaks out of the blood vessels). In addition, C5a recruits and activates neutrophils to the region, increasing the destruction.

A less common form of type II hypersensitivity occurs when an antibody binds to a receptor on the surface of a cell in such a way that the cell becomes activated. An example of disease caused by such a stimulatory mechanism is Graves' disease. This and other diseases caused by the binding of antireceptor antibodies are discussed in more detail in Chapter 35.

Type III Reactions: Antigen–Antibody Complex Diseases

In type III hypersensitivity diseases, the deposition of antigen–antibody complexes results in tissue damage. The prototype reaction is the ARTHUS REACTION. In the experimental form of this reaction, antigen is introduced into the skin of an immunized animal. After a few hours an inflammatory reaction is discernible at the site, followed in 12 hours by induration. The reaction can develop to such a point that the area becomes necrotic. Histologic examination of the site shows that the area has been infiltrated by a large number of neutrophils.

The mechanism of the Arthus reaction is very similar to that of type II hypersensitivity: the deposition of antigen into the skin of the immune animal causes antigen–antibody complexes to form at the site of injection. These complexes fix complement, and the split products of complement act as potent chemotactic factors for neutrophils. The Ag-Ab complexes are then ingested by the neutrophils that have been attracted to the scene. The ingestion of the immune complex causes them to degranulate, and the contents of the neutrophil granules cause tissue damage. The increase in vascular permeability that accompanies the activation of the complement cascade (discussed above) leads to edema (swelling). In humans, several conditions are known to be due to the Arthus reaction. Hay fever conjunctivitis, usually a type I reaction, has a severe form that is caused by the Arthus reaction. Hypersensitive pneumonitis is also caused by this reaction.

In normal antibody responses, antigen–antibody complexes (also called IMMUNE COMPLEXES) are cleared by the action of complement and the reticuloendothelial system. Type III hypersensitivity can occur, however, when these clearance mechanisms are defective (such as in some complement deficiencies) or when the quantities of antigen (and antibody) are very high. When the concentration of immune complexes becomes too high, they precipitate from the body fluids, and the sites in which they precipitate are those in which type III diseases occur. These include the skin, the ciliary body of the eye, and the glomeruli of the kidney, all sites in which proteins become concentrated. Precipitation of immune complexes can also occur by turbulence, such as in the arteries or the joints. Deposition of immune complexes in the joints, for example, is responsible for some types of arthritis, when the complexes induce type III hypersensitivity.

SERUM SICKNESS is a classical form of type III allergic disease. This was discovered when serum therapy for diphtheria was commonly used. The antitoxin was produced in a horse and administered to humans. If individuals received multiple injections of the passive antibody, they often became sensitized and produced antibodies to components in the horse serum. The result was a severe form of arthritis and glomerulonephritis caused by deposition of the antigen–antibody complexes.

IMMUNE COMPLEX GLOMERULONEPHRITIS is a very well studied allergic disease. In this case complexes deposit on the glomerular basement membrane, resulting in kidney damage by type III hypersensitivity. There is another, very similar disease in which autoantibodies to the basement membrane bind and produce damage: Goodpasture's syndrome, mentioned above. The two diseases can be distinguished from one another by the pattern of antibody on the basement membrane, which can be visualized by staining with anti-Ig antibodies. In the immune complex disease, the staining shows a "lumpy-bumpy" pattern, produced by the precipitated antigen–antibody complexes. In Goodpasture's syndrome, the antibody is evenly deposited on the basement membrane (because, in this type II disease, the antibody is *directed* against the membrane). The distinction between these two kidney diseases is one of the best examples of the differences between type II (Goodpasture's: antibodies *against* the tissue) and type III (immune complex glomerulonephritis: antibodies deposited *on* the tissue).

Type IV Reactions: Delayed-Type Hypersensitivity

The final type of hypersensitivity reactions are those called the DELAYED-TYPE HYPERSENSITIVITY or DTH reactions. These reactions are mediated not by antibody but by T lymphocytes. Historically the first delayed hypersensitivity reaction was seen by Robert Koch when he injected a small amount of fluid from tubercle bacilli cultures and found that an area of induration developed after 48 hours. This test is now used as a clinical screening procedure to determine whether an individual has come in contact with *Mycobacterium tuberculosis* (the tuberculin test). It has also been modified for use with another mycobacterium, *M. leprae*. The most common form of DTH disease is CONTACT DERMATITIS (or contact hypersensitivity) such as that caused by poison ivy and allergies to clothing. These reactions begin at about 24 hours and reach a maximum at 48 or even 96 hours. This response is in sharp contrast to that of the immediate-type reaction, which can occur within minutes.

Contact hypersensitivity reactions are initiated by T cells, which react with antigen that either has been deposited on the skin or has become covalently attached to skin cells. In the latter case, haptens such as dinitrobenzene, when painted onto the skin, can cause severe reactions. The reaction of the T cells with the antigen results in their activation and the release of lymphokines, some of which are probably chemotactic for monocytes and macrophages. It is the accumulation of these cells that results in tissue damage. It will be recalled from Chapter 18 that in the mouse the effector T cell for DTH expresses CD4, and that the effector cells that carry out DTH and those that carry out cytotoxicity are different.

Classes of Type IV Hypersensitivity

All type IV hypersensitivity responses depend upon T cells, but four classes of response can occur, depending upon the nature of the antigen, the location of the response, and the other cells involved (see Table 2). None of these responses depend upon the presence of antibody. One class of type IV response, contact hypersensitivity, has already been mentioned above, and is characterized by (1) localization to the epidermis and (2) involvement of macrophages as the primary effector cell. $CD8^+$ T cells can also act as effectors in this response, especially when haptens or other agents that can directly modify class I MHC molecules serve as the antigen. In the contact hypersensitivity response, the Langerhans cells of the skin (which express class II MHC molecules) are believed to be the APCs, stimulating $CD4^+$ T cells.

Another class of DTH response is very similar to contact hypersensitivity in that macrophages are the primary effector cells. This class of response is often referred to as TUBERCULIN-TYPE, because the response to tuberculin is a prototypical example. Unlike contact hypersensitive responses, tuberculin-type responses are not restricted to a particular anatomic location. Dendritic cells, macrophages, or other APCs are responsible for stimulating $CD4^+$ T cells, which, in turn, recruit and stimulate macrophages. Studies using antigen-specific T-cell clones have demonstrated that the growth and differentiation factors that characterize T_{H1} cells (see Chapter 27), that is, IL-2 and γ-interferon, are important in this response. We do not yet know whether the same type of helper cells mediate the other classes of type IV hypersensitivity.

Table 2   Characteristics of classes of type IV hypersensitivity.

Class	Time of onset	Duration	Effector cells
Contact	24 hours	48–72 hours	Macrophages
Tuberculin-type	24 hours	72–96 hours	Macrophages
Granuloma	7–14 days	Weeks	Macrophages, fibroblasts
CBH[a]	12–24 hours	24 hours	Basophils, granulocytes

[a] Cutaneous basophilic hypersensitivity (CBH) is also known as Jones–Mote reaction.

In our discussion of T cell–macrophage interactions in immunity to infectious diseases (Chapter 32) we considered DTH as an important defense mechanism. The tuberculin-type reaction is one way that this defense mechanism can appear. If the antigen persists, however, another class of type IV hypersensitivity can manifest: the GRANULOMATOUS RESPONSE. In this reaction, recruited macrophages and fibroblasts proliferate and produce collagen, effectively walling off the antigen. In addition, multi-nucleated GIANT CELLS appear, which probably represent fusions of several macrophages under the influence of GM-CSF. In Chapter 32, we discussed situations in which this form of response may be beneficial as well as cases in which this is the source of the pathologic lesions of a particular disease.

The fourth class of DTH differs from the others in that the primary effector cell in the response is the basophil. Like contact hypersensitivity, it can occur in the epidermis, but it persists for only a relatively short period of time (approximately 24 hours). This class, called CUTANEOUS BASOPHILIC HYPERSENSITIVITY (CBH) or JONES-MOTE RESPONSE, can be produced experimentally by immunization with antigen in the absence of adjuvant. It is seen in guinea pigs and humans, but not in mice. Probably because of the latter, the precise mechanisms and roles for this response are not well understood.

Summary

1.   Hypersensitivity reactions are reactions in which antibody or T cells react with antigen on surfaces of cells or in tissues, causing the release of pharmacologically active substances that damage the cells.

2. Type I reactions are those mediated by IgE. IgE fixes to mast cells via an Fc receptor for IgE on the mast cell. When the fixed IgE reacts with allergen, a complex series of reactions occurs, culminating in the degranulation of the mast cells. The granules contain active substances that cause the symptoms of allergy. This response is also referred to as immediate-type hypersensitivity, because the response can occur in seconds.

3. Type II reactions occur when antibodies bind to antigens on the surface of cells. The resulting antigen–antibody complex leads to the destruction (or, in some cases, stimulation) of the cell. Destruction proceeds via activation of complement or ADCC.

4. Type III reactions are those in which antigen–antibody complexes precipitate and cause damage by activating complement or ADCC in the organ in which they are deposited. The difference between this type and type II reactions is the nature of the antigen: in type II, the cell-surface antigen is bound by antibody, leading to the response. In type III, the antigen is normally in solution; when bound by antibody the complex precipitates. Type III responses, such as the Arthus reaction, often take several hours to appear after antigenic challenge.

5. Type IV reactions are induced by antigen-specific T cells, which are $CD4^+$ and therefore different from $CD8^+$ cytotoxic T cells. The effector cells in these responses are generally myeloid cells, although other cells may be involved. These reactions are called delayed-type hypersensitivity because they require at least 12 to 24 hours after antigen exposure to appear (depending on the class of response). There are four classes of type IV response, distinguished by their anatomical location and the effector cells involved.

Additional Readings

Bloy, C., Blanchard, D., Lambin, P., Goossens, D., Rouger, P., Salmon, C., Masoureclin, S. P. and Cartron, J.-P. 1988. Characterization of the D, c, E, and G antigens of the Rh blood group system with human monoclonal antibodies. *Mol. Immunol.* 25: 925.

DeWeck, A. 1983. Regulation of IgE responses. In J. Ring and G. Burg, eds. *New Trends in Allergy*. Springer-Verlag, Berlin.

Druet, P. and Glotz, D. 1984. Experimental autoimmune nephropathies: Induction and regulation. *Adv. Nephrol.* 13: 115.

Ishizaka, K. and T. Ishizaka. 1989. Allergy. In W. E. Paul, ed. *Fundamental Immunology*, 2nd ed. Raven Press, New York, p. 867.

Metzger, H., Alcaraz, G., Hoffman, R., Kinet, J. P., Pribluda, V. and Quarto, R. 1986. The receptor with high affinity for immunoglobulin E. *Annu. Rev. Immunol.* 4: 419.

Rose, N. R. and H. Friedman. 1980. *Manual of Clinical Immunology*, 2nd ed. American Society for Microbiology, Washington D. C.

Theofilopoulos, A. N. and Dixon, F. J. 1979. The biology and detection of immune complexes. *Adv. Immunol.* 28: 89.

AUTOIMMUNITY I
Autoantibodies

CHAPTER

35

Overview The central challenge for the immune system is to respond to foreign antigen while not making harmful reactions to self-components. In previous chapters we have explored the mechanisms of central and peripheral tolerance that help to explain this remarkable immunologic feature. We know, for example, that there is nothing special about antigens that are "self," except the fact that they are present throughout the development of lymphocytes. They are processed and presented like foreign antigens and, without the mechanisms of tolerance, should be capable of inducing immune responses. Nevertheless, the idea that self–nonself discrimination is a central property of the immune system was so firmly entrenched in immunologic theory that it took many years to realize that sometimes the process fails. One of the most confounding problems of modern immunology is the fact that a large number of diseases are autoimmune, that is, they are caused by the reaction of the immune system to self-antigens. It is intuitively obvious that a breakdown in the mechanisms that prevent self-reactivity can have dire consequences; the resulting diseases include rheumatoid arthritis, diabetes mellitus, systemic lupus erythematosus, and many other diseases. In this chapter we will examine some of these autoimmune diseases that come from destructive self-reactions.

The Response to Self

In most cases, the defects that lead to destructive anti-self responses are not known. The destruction can be a general one, affecting many tissues, or may be restricted to only one cell type. It may be mediated either by antibodies (discussed in this chapter) or by T cells (discussed in the following chapter). Animal models of many of the human autoimmune diseases have been studied for many years and have provided a great deal of information about autoimmune responses. We will explore the theories that have been proposed to account for these responses and consider some of the recent clues as to how they can happen, and perhaps be controlled. In no other area are our concepts of the functioning of the immune system more forcefully challenged than in the study of such diseases. We don't promise any clear answers to the mysteries of autoimmunity, but we hope that by discussing the problem we will show that there is still some important work to do in the field of immunology. Autoimmunity exists, and this fact has to be explained if we are to understand the immune system thoroughly.

Horror Autotoxicus Revisited: The Delayed Discovery of Autoimmunity

Ehrlich termed the inability of the immune system to react to self *horror autotoxicus*. He performed experiments between 1900 and 1910 in which he deliberately attempted to immunize animals against their own tissues and failed to do so. This confirmed, in his mind, the obvious correctness of his idea of *horror autotoxicus*, and he stated that a response to self tissues, such as autologous red blood cells, "would be difficult for anyone to believe and would be an occurrence which clinical observation has not yet verified."

Ehrlich's beliefs led to the general notion that autoimmunization is impossible, an idea that probably contributed to the delay in recognizing the existence of autoreactivity and autoimmune disease. As early as 1903, the first documented description of an autoimmune disease, a form of hemolytic anemia, was published by Donath and Landsteiner but was not pursued. Later, in 1933, Rivers, Sprunt, and Berry induced a nervous system disorder, encephalomyelitis, by injecting foreign nervous tissue into monkeys. Since, however, no antibodies were found that reacted with autologous nervous tissue, it was agreed that this could not be an immune-mediated phenomenon. (Landsteiner and Chase did not publish their work on the cellular transfer of delayed-type hypersensitivity until 1942, and we now know that autoimmune encephalomyelitis is mediated by T cells. This is discussed in more detail in the next chapter.)

In 1946, Boorman, Dodd, and Loutit employed a test designed a year earlier by Coomb to detect nonagglutinating antibodies against red blood cells and showed that there are anti-red cell antibodies in some types of anemia. This defined the disease autoimmune hemolytic anemia and might have established the existence of autoimmune disease, but did not sway the scientific community. Autoimmunity, it was still believed, could not happen.

Arguably, the landmark experiment that established the existence of autoimmunity was performed in the 1950s by Ernest Witebsky and Noel Rose in Buffalo. They showed that the immunization of rabbits with rabbit thyroglobulin gives rise to anti-thyroglobulin antibodies and, more importantly, inflammation of the thyroid (thyroiditis).[1] Ivan Roitt and his colleagues in London quickly followed up on this finding with their observations showing the presence of such anti-thyroglobulin antibodies in human thyroiditis. Shortly thereafter, animals that are predisposed to develop autoimmune disorders were discovered, and the notion that autoimmunity was impossible was banished forever.

Burnet and the Forbidden Clone

It was around this time that Jerne, Talmadge, and Burnet introduced the ideas that developed into the paradigm of clonal selection. One of the most attractive aspects of clonal selection was that it could be used to explain self-tolerance and autoimmunity. As discussed in Chapter 31, Burnet proposed that self-reactive clones are deleted during their development, and we saw in Chapters 24 and 31 how this is true for developing T cells (and essentially true for B cells, in that they are inactivated). Based on this theory of tolerance, Burnet reasoned that autoimmunity is due to the evasion of clonal deletion by a few autoreactive cells. These cells would then appear as FORBIDDEN CLONES, able to respond to self and induce autoimmune disease.

Armed with the knowledge that autoimmunity is a real phenomenon of clinical (as well as theoretical) importance, and with a theory in place to explain it, many immunologists and physicians now embarked on studies to identify the types and causes of autoimmune disease. Not surprisingly, AUTOANTIBODIES (antibodies that react to self-antigens) were studied extensively before T cells were discovered, but more recently the role of AUTOREACTIVE T CELLS in some types of autoimmunity has been recognized and heavily investigated (see Chapter 36). Before launching into a discussion of the different types of autoimmune diseases and their possible

---

[1] The suffix *-itis* generally refers to an inflammation. Arthritis is an inflammation of a joint, testitis is inflammation of the testes, uveitis is inflammation of the uvea of the eye, encephalomyelitis is inflammation of the brain and spinal cord, etc. It is useful to learn a few of these words in order to follow the literature in autoimmunity, not to mention impressing your friends.

mechanisms, however, we'll consider a little about what is known about autoantibodies. One of the things that will become apparent, even at this point, is that the basic idea of the forbidden clone is at least partially wrong.

Autoantibodies and Autoantigens

General Properties of Autoantibodies

With the recognition that autoantibodies exist, the question became very much like the question General Custer asked at Little Big Horn when he first saw all the Indians: How did they get there and are they really dangerous? Because of the traditional orientation of immunology toward infectious diseases, there was a tendency to think in terms of a single cause—probably an infectious organism—as the etiological agent of those diseases in which it could be shown that there was reaction to self. Because we knew how to deal with them, it was not only logical but comforting to think that a bacterial or viral agent had produced the damage to the tissue resulting in disease, and that the antibody to self-components (autoantibody) was a secondary event. But slowly the awareness that the antibodies might be the cause of the symptoms grew; even if the initial insult was from external sources, the pathogenesis was immunologic. A vast spectrum of autoantibodies have since been described and characterized, and general properties of these antibodies and the autoantigens they recognize have emerged.

Some examples of a number of diseases involving autoantibodies and the autoantigens they recognize are given in Table 1. Autoantibodies can be directed against antigens found in all cells, such as DNA, ribonucleoproteins, mitochondrial components, or the cytoskeleton. Alternatively, an autoantibody can be specific for an antigen that is found in only one or a few types of cells, such as thyroglobulin, heart myosin, acetylcholine receptor, or clotting factor VIII. The latter types of autoantibodies are each associated with (and cause) different diseases. Regardless of whether the antibody is to a ubiquitous or a tissue-restricted antigen, however, one remarkable thing is clear: *autoantibodies are not self-specific.* That is, an autoantibody to an autoantigen in an individual with an autoimmune disease will bind to the same antigen in a healthy individual. Further, such antibodies are characteristically directed to phylogenetically conserved regions of the antigen such that they will bind to similar antigens from unrelated species.

Table 1   **Antigens in autoimmune diseases.**

Disease	Antigen type[a]					
	A	B	C	D	E	F
Systemic lupus erythematosus	+		+		+	
Sjögren's syndrome	+				+	
Scleroderma	+					
Polymyositis	+		+			
Chronic active hepatitis	+				+	
Mixed connective tissue disease	+					
Insulin-dependent diabetes	+	+				+
Primary biliary cirrhosis	+					
Pernicious anemia	+					+
Autoimmune thyroiditis	+	+				+
Idiopathic Addison's disease	+					
Vitiligo	+					
Gluten-sensitive enteropathy	+					
Graves' disease	+	+				
Myasthenia gravis		+				
Autoimmune hemolytic anemia			+			
Autoimmune neutropenia			+			
Idiopathic thrombocytopenia purpura			+			
Rheumatoid arthritis			+		+	
Cirrhosis			+			
Multiple sclerosis			+			
Pemphigus vulgaris			+	+		
Autoimmune infertility			+			
Goodpasture's disease				+		
Bullous pemphigoid				+		
Discoid lupus				+		
Dense deposit disease					+	

Source: Modified from Smith and Steinberg, 1982. *Annu. Rev. Immunol.* 1: 175.

[a] A, intracellular; B, receptors; C, cell membrane components; D, extracellular; E, plasma proteins; F, hormones.

Another important property of autoantibodies is that they do not only appear in autoimmune disease. NATURAL AUTOANTIBODIES are often found at low concentrations in the sera of normal individuals, and hybridomas or virally transformed B-cell lines from normal humans and animals have been found that produce such antibodies. There is the possibility, therefore, that some types of autoimmunity are triggered not by self-antigen, but rather by a polyclonal activation of all B cells, including those that produce autoantibodies.

Some, but not all, of the cells that make natural autoantibodies belong to a subset of B cells that bear the CD5 marker (previously, we have discussed this marker only in the context of T-cell subsets, but some B cells bear it as well). This subset, so far described in rodents and humans, is unusual because it is a self-replenishing population. Injection of CD5$^+$ B cells into an irradiated mouse will provide a continuing source of these cells, whereas CD5$^-$ B cells will only survive transiently in such a situation. It has therefore been suggested that a deregulation of these cells could result in some types of autoimmunity.

Another very interesting property of autoantibodies is that they can be encoded by the germ-line V regions. Although more information is needed, at least some autoantibodies that have been analyzed do not show evidence of somatic mutation. This is important because one way that B cells can seem to avoid tolerance is to express a surface Ig that is not initially anti-self (and therefore no B-cell anergy occurs in the cell's development) but that becomes anti-self following somatic mutation. The possibility of such somatically mutated antibodies becoming anti-self was shown by Matthew Scharff and colleagues in New York, who found that a single point mutation in an anti-phosphorylcholine antibody gene altered the specificity so that the antibody now reacted with DNA. Nevertheless, it is now clear that at least some autoantibodies do not arise in this way and instead are directly encoded by the germ-line genes. This puzzling state of affairs forces us to reconsider what we know about B-cell tolerance.

B-Cell Tolerance and Autoantibodies

In Chapter 31, we discussed a little of what is known about B-cell tolerance. Two points may be particularly important here. First of all, recall that experimental B-cell tolerance wanes more rapidly than does T-cell tolerance. Secondly, unlike central T-cell tolerance (negative selection; see Chapter 24), tolerized B cells do not die but instead only become unresponsive. While we don't know why these differences between B and T cells exist, these differences are probably important for solving the puzzle of autoantibodies.

As mentioned above, one explanation for the appearance of autoantibodies in the face of self-tolerance could be based on somatic mutation in the Ig V regions after the cells have passed the stage at which they can be tolerized. This could well be *an* explanation, but it does not take into account those autoantibodies that don't show evidence of somatic mutation (i.e., their V regions match those of the germ line). We are left with two other, not mutually exclusive, possibilities. Either some B cells avoid tolerance induction to self-antigens, or else there is a way that even tolerant B cells can be stimulated. The first possibility is likely to occur in cases where the antigen is not available to the B cell at the time of development. These include autoantigens that are inside cells as well as those that are restricted to organs in inaccessible anatomical locations. We will consider such autoantigens and their importance later on in this chapter. The second possibility is an interesting one, but so far the conditions for the activation of anergic B cells have not been found.

In any case, it is clear that not all autoantibodies cause disease, and therefore, the problem of autoreactive B cells may not be a major one for the immune system. If those B cells bearing autoantibodies are not induced, then not enough autoantibody will be produced to cause any problems. Bear in mind that an autoantibody need not destroy its target to cause problems. Type III hypersensitivity (due to deposit of antigen–antibody complexes) is common in many types of autoimmune diseases. It is often the level of autoantibody that influences the disease state, as well as the specificity and isotype (and therefore function) of the antibody. How autoantibodies may be induced (and cause problems) is considered in more detail below.

There is a completely different idea about autoantibodies (especially natural autoantibodies) that comes from the minds of those who work with the network (and are used to contrary positions). They argue that natural autoantibodies are a necessity for immune homeostasis and self–nonself discrimination. Such antibodies, at low concentration, and their induced anti-idiotypes, form an immunologic self-portrait that regulates itself. Without such a picture of self the immune system would have nothing with which to compare antigen to determine if it is not self. Like many ideas that are based on the network, this one is internally consistent but very difficult to test rigorously.

How Are Autoantibody Responses Induced?

So far, we have come to grips with the fact that many B cells in the body are capable of producing autoantibodies. Sometimes, these antibodies are harmful (see below). If we can determine why a particular antibody is produced so as to lead to disease, we will have gained some understanding of the autoimmune process.

One of the best understood mechanisms for induction of auto-antibodies depends on the presence of antigens in which some epitopes are similar or identical to self and others are not. If such an antigen were to enter the system, T cells that recognize the foreign epitopes would expand and stimulate B cells that recognize other determinants. Those B cells bearing receptors that bind to the "pseudo-self" epitopes would be induced to make autoantibodies (see Figure 1).

Two types of antigens of clinical importance have these characteristics. Some drugs, when injected into the body, tightly associate with self-molecules or cells. If these complexes are at a high enough concentration, T cells that recognize the drug can stimulate B cells to make antibodies to the self-components. (Antibodies may also be made to the drug, and these may have effects resembling autoimmunity, since the drug is closely bound to self, but such responses are not, formally speaking, autoimmune).

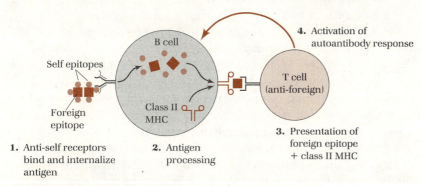

1 **Induction of Autoantibody Secretion by Antigens That Bear Both Foreign and "Self" Epitopes.** If an antigen bears B-cell epitopes that closely resemble self epitopes *and* T-cell epitopes that are foreign, then the antigen can induce the production of autoantibodies. Autoreactive B cells bind via sIg to the epitopes resembling self on the antigen, internalize the antigen, and process it. The foreign, T-cell epitopes processed from the antigen are presented by class II MHC molecules on the B cell, thus activating helper T cells, which, in turn, stimulate the B cell to secrete its antibody. Since this antibody reacts to both the "mimic" and self antigens, the result is an autoantibody response.

A second class of antigens with this property occurs in parasites that display ANTIGENIC MIMICRY. That is, parts of the antigen so closely resemble self-molecules that an antibody to the antigen acts as an autoantibody. Rather than protecting the parasite from immune attack, however, the result can be autoimmunity. One of the best examples of this occurs in RHEUMATIC FEVER initiated following infection with group A streptococci. These organisms have an antigen that cross-reacts with heart myosin. In some patients, often children, the sequela of a "strep throat" is heart disease ("rheumatic heart"), as well as kidney disease and arthritis due to immune complexes. Although we can envision why this type of response to the bacteria can cause this autoimmune disease, it is not at all clear why it affects only some individuals infected with the bacteria.

Given that some parasites mimic self-antigens, the immune system may be designed in such a way that it has the option, so to speak, of maintaining a mild anti-self response in order to more efficiently rid itself of a parasite. If so, then it would not be surprising if such responses were tightly regulated by the network, T cells, or other mechanisms. Destructive autoimmune responses that occur without the presence of an obvious parasitic threat might then involve defects in such regulation. While much work has suggested that immunoregulatory defects often accompany autoimmune states, our knowledge of immune regulation is still too limited to gain much insight into autoimmunity.

Some autoimmune conditions might not be induced in normal ways at all, but instead might be a consequence of polyclonal B-cell activation, as discussed above. Indeed, injection of animals with B-cell mitogens, such as lipopolysaccharide, can lead to a transient production of autoantibody. Such responses are rapidly damped by regulatory mechanisms but attest to the validity of the idea. A genetic defect in B-cell function that allows B cells to overreact to stimuli could lead to autoimmunity as a consequence of elevating the overall level of natural antibody, including autoantibody. Such hyperreactivity in B cells is seen in some autoimmune-prone mouse strains (such as NZB, see below).

Autoantibodies and Autoimmune Disease

Organ-Specific and Non–Organ-Specific Autoimmune Diseases

At this point it will be useful to examine several autoimmune diseases and the roles played by autoantibodies. In the next chapter we will discuss autoimmune diseases in which T cell-mediated immunity plays the major role.

Autoimmune diseases can affect a single tissue or be widespread throughout the systems of the body. Table 1 lists some autoimmune diseases and characterizes them in terms of the distribution of the autoantigens. Some diseases occur at a specific site; for example, in Graves' disease there is an antibody against the receptor for thyroid-stimulating hormone (see below). The primary site of the disease is the thyroid gland, and the symptoms of the disease are all attributable to the actions of these antibodies. In contrast, some diseases, such as systemic lupus erythematosus, are non–organ-specific, and in these disorders there are antibodies to a large range of tissues that affect many systems. But for these diseases it is difficult to know whether an antibody is the initiating event of the pathologic condition or a by-product of tissue damage.

Organ-Specific Autoimmune Diseases Involving Antibodies

Antireceptor Diseases

There are several diseases in which the pathologic condition is known to be caused by antireceptor antibodies. The point we want to make in this section is that the reaction of the antibody with the receptor can have very different results. Some of these results are illustrated in Figure 2.

MYASTHENIA GRAVIS (MG) is a neuromuscular disorder of humans that is characterized by weakness and rapid fatigue of skeletal muscles. The clinical features of the disease were first noted in 1672 and were thoroughly described by 1900, when it was noted that there was great similarity between the symptoms of MG and curare poisoning. In the 1930s it was noted that patients treated with anticholinesterase drugs showed great improvement. Because cholinesterase is known to be involved in nerve impulses at the neuromuscular junction, it was concluded that the disease is due to some malfunction at that site. In the 1960s, using microelectrode techniques, it was found that the amplitude of miniature endplate potentials (MEPPs: the amount of depolarization at the presynaptic nerve terminal) was reduced by 80% at the neuromuscular junction in MG patients. This finding suggested that there is a *presynaptic* defect in the disease. One possibility was that there is a reduced number of acetylcholine (ACh) molecules as a result of some unknown defect in the motor nerve terminals.

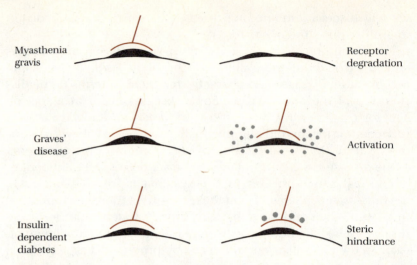

2 **Mechanisms of Anti-Receptor Autoimmune Diseases.** Auto-anti-receptor antibody reacting with a receptor can result in disease by several mechanisms. (A) Myasthenia gravis: Anti-acetylcholine receptor (AChR) antibody causes degradation of the receptor; as a result acetylcholine fails to stimulate the cell. (B) Graves' disease: Anti-thyroid stimulating hormone receptor (TSHR) antibody binds to the receptor and activates the cell. This reaction causes an unregulated production of thyroid hormones. (C) Insulin-resistant diabetes: Anti-insulin receptor antibody blocks the receptor and thus prevents insulin from acting.

In the 1970s it became possible to study the ACETYLCHOLINE RECEPTOR (AChR). Because α-bungarotoxin (α-BuTx) binds specifically and irreversibly to the AChR of skeletal muscle, it can be radiolabeled and used to quantify the number of AChRs. When this was done, it was found that the neuromuscular junctions in MG patients bind only 11 to 30% of normal amounts of ligand. Furthermore, treatment of experimental animals with α-cobra toxin, a procedure that reduces the number of AChRs, causes the characteristics of human MG in these animals. These findings indicated that the defect in MG is not presynaptic but *postsynaptic*, and that the events involved are not those preceding the release of ACh but those that follow.

The *autoimmune* nature of MG was inferred from the finding that in MG patients there is a high incidence of thymus abnormality (an association with other autoimmune diseases), reduced levels of complement, and the presence of anti-skeletal muscle antibody. These facts led to a search for antibody reactive with the AChR; and in the 1970s several groups independently identified such anti-AChR antibodies in MG patients.

The fact that MG patients have anti-AChR antibody in their serum and the fact that there are fewer available receptors in the disease might lead to the conclusion that the effect of the antibody is merely a steric blocking of the receptor site. This is not the case. Daniel Drachman and his colleagues at Johns Hopkins have shown that the anti-AChR antibody acts in this disease by causing an *accelerated degradation* of AChR (Figure 3). The anti-AChR antibody, either as the intact IgG or as (Fab)$_2$, when bound to the receptor causes degradation of the receptor (Figure 3A and B). In contrast, Fab can bind to the receptor but cannot cause degradation (Figure 3C). Treating the bound Fab with anti-Ig does cause degradation. The similarity between these experiments and those of the Ishizakas on the degranulation of mast cells by IgE will not be lost on the reader, and the interpretations are similar. When reaction of antibody with the receptor produces cross-linking of receptors, degradation occurs. In an analogous manner, when the ACh receptors are cross-linked by treatment with α-BuTx, degradation also occurs (Figure 3E). So we see that anti-AChR antibody can cause degradation of receptors and that the symptoms of the disease result from the loss of AChRs.

GRAVES' DISEASE is another autoimmune disease in which anti-receptor antibodies play a role in the pathogenesis. Patients with Graves' disease suffer from overproduction of the thyroid hormones thyroxine and triiodothyronine. In normal individuals the pituitary secretes thyroid-stimulating hormone (TSH), which binds to TSH receptors on thyroid cells. This binding activates the adenylate cyclase system and causes the thyroid cells to produce thyroxine and triiodothyronine. As with most hormone systems, there is a very delicate feedback control of the amount of TSH produced and consequently of the amount of thyroid hormone released. Patients with Graves' disease produce *antibodies to the TSH receptor*. The binding of these antireceptor antibodies, however, has an effect very different from that produced by the binding of anti-AChR antibodies to the ACh receptor. In this case, the binding of antibody to the receptor has the same effect as the binding of TSH—the production of thyroid hormone. In other words, the antibody acts like the ligand and triggers the cell to produce the hormone. Of course, the antireceptor antibodies are not under the same hormonal feedback control, so the thyroid keeps producing, and then overproducing, hormones. The symptoms of this disease are due to the antibody-stimulated overproduction of thyroid hormone.

In some cases of INSULIN-RESISTANT DIABETES there are anti-insulin

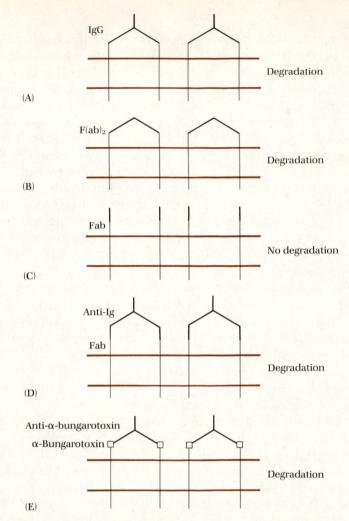

IgG

Degradation

(A)

F(ab)₂

Degradation

(B)

Fab

No degradation

(C)

Anti-Ig

Fab

Degradation

(D)

Anti-α-bungarotoxin

α-Bungarotoxin

Degradation

(E)

3 Degradation of the Acetylcholine Receptor by Antibody. (A, B) Either intact antibody or Fab₂ causes degradation of the acetylcholine receptor (AChR). (C, D) Monovalent Fab does not cause degradation, but the addition of anti-Fab does. (E) Bungarotoxin does not cause degradation, but the addition of anti-bungarotoxin does. These findings imply that cross-linking of receptors is crucial for their degradation. [After Drachman, 1978. *N. Engl. J. Med.* 298: 120]

receptor antibodies that react with the insulin receptor and partially block it. This competition prevents the insulin molecule from reacting with the receptor, resulting in the symptoms of the disease. This is a rare form of diabetes that should not be confused with diabetes mellitus, an autoimmune disease caused by T cells (discussed in the following chapter).

Antireceptor antibodies need not react with cell surfaces to cause disease. An example is seen in PERNICIOUS ANEMIA. In the small intestine, dietary vitamin B_{12} is normally bound by *intrinsic factor*, a soluble receptor that participates in the transport of the vitamin across the mucosa. In pernicious anemia, autoantibodies to intrinsic factor block the binding to the vitamin, and as a result the vitamin cannot be absorbed. This leads to a vitamin deficiency that in turn leads to anemia.

Thus these autoimmune diseases are caused by antireceptor antibodies, but in each case the antibody has a very different mechanism of pathogenesis. Autoantibodies that are not directed against receptors can cause disease as well, and we now consider some cases of such diseases.

Hemolytic Anemias

There are many reasons for the development of anemia in an individual, only some of which are due to autoimmunity (see pernicious anemia, above). Even in cases of autoimmune hemolytic anemia, it is important to determine if the disorder is one of the sequelae of another disease (even another autoimmune disease such as lupus erythematosus; see below) or is due to an autoimmune response to the patient's erythrocytes.

The autoimmune hemolytic anemias are divided into WARM ANTIBODY TYPE and COLD ANTIBODY TYPE, and are distinguished on the basis of laboratory tests. In the warm type, which is the more common, the patients have antibody on their red cells. This condition can often be diagnosed by the addition of anti-Ig, which causes agglutination of the red cells in vitro. This assay is called the COOMBS TEST. The symptoms associated with warm autoantibody hemolytic anemia are anemia; fever, jaundice, and splenomegaly associated with hemolysis; and congestive heart failure. Very commonly these signs are associated with other autoimmune disorders or leukemia. When the disease is not associated with another disease, it often follows viral infection.

Cold agglutinin disease is associated with very high titers of agglutinating IgM antibodies, which react optimally in the cold. The specificity of this IgM is usually to the I or Ii red cell antigen. Clinically, hemolysis occurs in the patients when they become cold, and the treatment consists of keeping the patients warm and waiting for a spontaneous resolution.

Note that autoimmune hemolytic anemia is an excellent example of type II hypersensitivity (see Chapter 34). When the anti-red cell antibodies bind, the classical complement pathway is activated, resulting in lysis of the cell. If the autoantibodies reach high concentrations, however, immune complexes may precipitate in the joints and kidneys, resulting in type III hypersensitivity. Such effects are not uncommon and can be a major contributor to disease.

There is a whole class of autoimmune hemolytic anemias that are known to be *drug-induced*. A wide range of drugs, from insulin to sulfonamides to chlorinated hydrocarbons, are implicated. In these cases the pathologic condition may be caused by the drug's binding to red cells that are, in turn, bound by antidrug antibody, allowing them to be lysed by complement. This is not an autoantibody response but has the appearance of autoimmunity. As we mentioned above, however, such interactions with drugs can result in true autoimmunity (see Figure 1). The drug may become bound to the red cell and act as a carrier to stimulate anti-red cell antibody responses.

Autoimmune Thyroiditis

Another organ-specific disease associated with antibody is autoimmune thyroiditis, or HASHIMOTO'S DISEASE. But unlike the antireceptor diseases discussed above, it is not clear whether the antibody is the cause or the effect of the disease. The thyroid in Hashimoto's disease is filled with inflammatory cells; and antibodies to thyroglobulin, cytoplasmic antigens, and cell-surface antigens of the thyroid can be found in the serum. The role, if any, of these antibodies, however, is not known.

The OBESE CHICKEN is an experimental model of autoimmune thyroiditis that resembles the human disease in many ways. In this model, the severity of the disease is greatly reduced by neonatal bursectomy (removal of the bursa). In Chapter 16 we noted that this treatment greatly reduces the number of B cells in the bird, and this suggests that B cells (and probably the antithyroglobulin antibody) play important roles in the pathogenesis of the disease. On the other hand, neonatal thymectomy accelerates the disease, suggesting that T cells may play a role in limiting the autoimmunity. Recent advances in the characterization of the immune system of the chicken may help to refocus attention on this autoimmune model and unravel some of its secrets.

Goodpasture's Syndrome

We noted in Chapter 34 and in this chapter that one outcome of circulating immune complexes is type III hypersensitivity in the kidney, resulting in glomerulonephritis and kidney damage. There is a disease that shows a similar effect, but without the circulating complexes. GOODPASTURE'S SYNDROME is a form of type II hypersensitivity caused by autoantibodies to the glomerular capillary basement membrane. The role of these antibodies in causing the disease was conclusively demonstrated by eluting the autoantibodies from the kidney of a patient who had died from the disease. These antibodies were then injected into a monkey and caused the same glomerulonephritis that had killed the patient. While there is little doubt that the autoantibodies cause the disease, there is also very little information about how these autoantibodies are induced.

There are many other organ-specific autoimmune diseases that are caused, at least in part, by autoantibodies. There is also a class of non–organ-specific autoimmune diseases that are associated with autoantibodies, but in which the antibody response is directed to a broad array of autoantigens.

Non–Organ-Specific Autoimmune Diseases Associated with Antibody

Systemic Lupus Erythematosus

SYSTEMIC LUPUS ERYTHEMATOSUS (SLE) is an autoimmune disease that is widespread and non–organ-specific. It is characterized by fever, skin rashes, polyarthritis, effusions in the pleural, pericardial and peritoneal cavities, and central nervous signs. SLE patients have reduced complement levels and high levels of immune complexes in their serum and glomeruli. In fact, the life-threatening lesion is often a progressive IMMUNE COMPLEX-MEDIATED GLOMERULONEPHRITIS. Deposits of autoantibody and complement can be found in the glomeruli as immune complex deposits that may be focal, membranous, or diffuse. SLE is a type III hypersensitivity disease (as opposed to Goodpasture's syndrome, which is a type II hypersensitivity disease).

Antibodies to intracellular components, cell-surface membrane components from various cell types, serum components, and nucleic acids are seen in SLE patients. Because of the great variety of antibodies and the spectrum of symptoms, SLE is another autoimmune phenomenon in which it has proved difficult to tell which of the antibodies are the cause of the disease and which are the result of tissue damage.

Animal Models of SLE

The availability of several animal models for SLE has been useful in the attempt to analyze the importance of the immune abnormalities and autoantibodies seen in human SLE. However, even with these models it is still not clear which are the most important factors in this multifactor disease.

In New Zealand, M. and F. Bielschowsky observed that New Zealand black (NZB) mice die with widespread and diverse symptoms of hemolytic anemia, glomerulonephritis, and vasculitis, all very reminiscent of human SLE. Another mouse, New Zealand white (NZW), does not develop autoimmune disease; but the F_1 mice [(NZB $\times$ NZW)F_1] develop severe disease. Backcrosses and extensive genetic studies have shown that the disease is not inherited as a single dominant trait. From these genetic studies it has become clear that some of the factors that contribute to the disease are susceptibility factors. For example, NZW mice contribute at least two genes to the susceptibility to disease of the (NZB $\times$ NZW)F_1, and NZB contributes one. At least one of these three genes is in the MHC, and one is linked to the MHC. The nature of the genes or their influence is not known. The NZB model of SLE has been studied very extensively; but as in the human disease, it has been difficult to analyze either for cause and effect relationships or for the relative importance of the pathologic changes.

Edwin Murphy and John Roths at the Jackson Laboratory in Bar Harbor developed two other strains of mice, called MRL/l and BXSB, that develop an SLE-like disease. MRL/l mice carry an allele, *lpr*, that is associated with a spectacular enlargement of the lymph nodes (LYMPHADENOPATHY) to hundreds of times their normal size. The cells that reside in these abnormal nodes are themselves abnormal: they are T cells bearing the $\alpha\beta$ TCR but lacking CD4 or CD8 and show defects in activation. What role these cells have in the development of lupus-like disease is unknown. BXSB mice are also unusual in that the disease associated with this strain is seen only in males. In contrast, most autoimmune diseases show a higher incidence in females.

While the immunologic defects that lead to autoimmunity in these mice are not known, the effects are associated with the bone marrow. When (NZB $\times$ NZW)F_1 bone marrow is transferred into irradiated recipients of other strains, the recipients develop the disease. Similarly, transplantation of bone marrow from a male into a female BXSB mouse results in disease, whereas female bone marrow transplanted into male recipients does not. In MRL mice, transplantation of bone marrow from the nonautoimmune strain MRL/n into irradiated MRL/l recipients does not lead to disease.

The role of the thymus microenvironment in these autoimmune strains differs. In MRL/l mice, neonatal thymectomy prevents the disease. Thymus abnormalities do not seem to be involved, however, since transplantation of a normal MRL/n thymus into such thymectomized mice restores the occurrence of disease. Thus, T-cell maturation is a requirement for the disease in MRL/l mice, but the abnormal T cells that arise do not appear to be a consequence of defects in the thymic epithelia. In contrast, neonatal thymectomy of $(NZB \times NZW)F_1$ mice or male BXSB mice does not prevent disease and in some cases accelerates it. Thus, if anything, the role of T cells in the disease in these strains seems to be a protective one.

All the strains that develop lupus-like disease have several other features in common. In all of them it is very *difficult to induce immunologic tolerance* to serum protein (human IgG) in adult life. This defect, at least in NZB and $(NZB \times NZW)F_1$ mice, seems to be due to an abnormality in pre-T cells. In all the strains there is also an *increased Ig production*, although the class varies in different strains. All strains have *lymphoid abnormalities* such as lymphoid hyperplasia and increases in T-cell or B-cell numbers. As in the human disease, *glomerulonephritis* is a prominent feature of the experimental disease in all the strains.

As previously stated, it is not clear which antibodies are the initiators of the pathologic condition in SLE and which the result of the initial tissue damage. Moreover, the disease is clearly the result of several factors. The autoantibody that is responsible for the immune complexes could be the result of nonspecific activation of B cells. The inability to induce tolerance in these strains could indicate that the mechanism for maintenance of self-tolerance is impaired. Thymus disorders and T-cell defects could result in a loss of regulatory T-cell function, which might allow the polyclonal activation of T and B cells. Many or all of these could be correct, but we do not know the reason for the initiation of the events that bring them all together.

The autoimmune diseases we have considered so far are thought to be predominantly associated with the production of autoantibodies. In the next chapter, we will examine those autoimmune diseases that appear to be caused by autoreactive T cells. In either type, however, the fundamental question remains: What has gone wrong with the mechanisms of tolerance so that such autoreactivity can occur? As we've seen (and will see in the next chapter), some answers to this question have been suggested, but we still have a lot more to learn.

Summary

1.   In those cases in which tolerance fails, and there are reactions against self-tissue or self-components, the result is autoimmunity. Autoimmune diseases can be brought about by antibody or by T-cell-mediated mechanisms. Such mechanisms are best understood in animal models of autoimmune disease in which genetic predispositions to autoimmunity exist. In many models, autoimmunity is induced by administration of an autoantigen.

2.   Autoantibodies specific for self-proteins (autoantigens) are responsible for causing a number of different diseases. This is especially true for autoantibodies that react against red blood cells or important cell-surface receptors. Autoantibodies can be encoded by germ-line V-region genes or can arise by somatic mutation.

3.   Not all autoantibodies cause disease. Natural autoantibodies have been identified in sera or can be generated using B cells from normal individuals. Autoantibodies that do not directly cause disease can, however, produce type III hypersensitivity.

4.   There are autoimmune diseases in which the reactions are organ-specific or tissue-specific and those in which the specificity is not obvious, either because of many sites of reaction or because of secondary effects.

5.   Autoantibodies to self-antigen in an autoimmune individual generally react to the same antigen in other individuals or even other species. This is because the epitopes recognized by most autoantibodies appear to be evolutionarily conserved.

6.   Foreign antigens that bear B-cell epitopes that cross-react with autoantigens can cause autoimmunity when T cells recognize foreign epitopes on the antigen. The T cells then trigger autoreactive B cells.

Additional Readings

Schwartz, R. S., ed. 1990. Autoimmunity. *Curr. Opinion Immunol.* 2: 565.

Schwartz, R. S. and S. K. Datta. 1989. Autoimmunity and autoimmune diseases. In W. E. Paul, ed. *Fundamental Immunology*, 2nd ed. Raven, New York, p. 819.

Theofilopoulos, A. N. and F. J. Dixon. 1985. Murine models of systemic lupus erythematosus. *Adv. Immunol* 37: 269.

AUTOIMMUNITY II
Autoreactive T Cells

Overview In the last chapter we saw that the generation of anti-bodies against autoantigens is not an unusual event, even though it violates the principles of self–nonself discrimination by the immune system and can often have dire consequences. While some autoimmune diseases are caused by (or at least associated with) such autoantibodies, others appear to be mediated by auto-reactive T cells. In this chapter we will discuss some of the latter type of autoimmune diseases.

The existence of autoreactive T cells in some autoimmune diseases might be due to defects in the mechanisms of central and/or peripheral tolerance. If we can come to understand these defects, we will not only have a chance to prevent autoimmunity but will also have a deeper knowledge of the processes of tolerance. In this chapter, we will consider how autoreactive T cells might arise and how, through our grasp of T-cell activation and function, they might someday be controlled.

Autoimmune Diseases Involving Autoreactive T Cells

We pick up this chapter where the last one left off—a considera-tion of several autoimmune diseases in humans and in animal models. Here, however, we will begin with those diseases that appear to be mediated through autoreactive T cells and the cell-mediated responses they induce.

Multiple Sclerosis

Multiple sclerosis (MS) was described as a clinical entity in 1868 by Charcot. Clinically it is a highly variable disease, which usually begins between the second and fifth decades of life. The common signs are sensory and visual motor dysfunction. In the *chronic form* the patient has periods of remission. But with each remission there is greater neurological dysfunction. A *benign form* exists and is characterized by mild exacerbations followed by a complete recovery.

The pathologic lesions of MS are confined to the nervous system. Macroscopic lesions of 1 to 4 cm called PLAQUES are scattered throughout the white matter. The term *multiple sclerosis* was initially used to describe the wide distribution of the lesions in the white matter. Microscopically the disease is characterized by a *breakdown of the myelin sheath*. The demyelinated lesions have a perivenous distribution and contain macrophages and lymphocytes. There is loss of myelin basic protein (see next section) in the area of the lesions.

The etiology of MS is unknown. Both chronic infectious agents and autoimmunity have been invoked, and in fact both might be important. MS patients have been shown to have immune complexes; but these are considered to be secondary, because levels are low compared with those seen in SLE. Similar levels are seen in the demyelinating diseases amyotrophic lateral sclerosis (Lou Gehrig disease) and subacute sclerosing panencephalitis. On the other hand, MS patients show an altered ratio of $CD4^+$ to $CD8^+$ cells,[1] and T cells are found within the regions of demyelination. These facts have led to the general conclusion that MS is a T-cell-mediated autoimmune disease. The similarity between the human disease and the model animal disease, experimental autoimmune encephalomyelitis, has strengthened this belief.

Animal Models of MS

Injection of experimental animals with CNS tissue emulsified in complete Freund's adjuvant (an oil–water emulsion containing mycobacteria) results in characteristic lesions of the central nervous system, producing a neurological disease called EXPERIMENTAL ALLERGIC ENCEPHALOMYELITIS (EAE). As stated above, this experimental disease mimics MS in so many ways that it is considered the best experimental model of the human disease. The fact that the symptoms can be transferred to normal animals by T cells and T-cell clones, but not by serum, from a diseased animal has strengthened the conclusion that the disease is a cell-mediated one.

---

[1]Changes in the CD4/CD8 ratio among peripheral blood T cells is seen in many disease situations, but the reasons for these changes are seldom clear. In the late 1970s, such alterations were overinterpreted as a change in the balance of helper versus suppressor cells. This sort of overinterpretation led to wild assertions to the effect that autoimmunity is caused by a loss of suppressor cell control over autoreactive helper cells. While this *could* be true (in some sense) we should try to exercise a little more caution in interpreting peripheral blood lymphocyte marker profiles.

One antigen in brain that is involved in the disease has been studied extensively. When the basic protein component of myelin, called MYELIN BASIC PROTEIN, is injected into animals in adjuvant, all the symptoms are produced. Analysis of the basic protein has shown that there are ENCEPHALITOGENIC PEPTIDES, but a peptide that is encephalitogenic in one species may not be in another. Encephalitogenic peptides not only may initiate the disease but also may regulate it, because circulating basic peptide has been shown to reduce the activity of the effector T cells in the disease. It is particularly interesting that some T cells found within the cerebral spinal fluid of MS patients have been found to respond to myelin basic protein.

In mice, the induction of EAE is very strain-dependent, that is, in some mouse strains the disease can easily be induced but not in others. Scott Zamvil and Larry Steinman at Stanford found that in one mouse strain, PL/J, the vast majority of the T cells that respond to myelin basic protein use a particular T-cell receptor ($V_{\alpha 2}$ or 4, $V_{\beta 8.2}$). More recently, the T-cell receptors that are used to recognize myelin basic protein in another strain, SJL, have been identified by Lee Hood and colleagues at the California Institute of Technology. These observations are reminiscent of Burnet's idea of the forbidden clone: one or a few autoreactive T cells escaping from tolerance and causing disease. However, it seems that it is always the *same* few clones, from one animal to another. There is also evidence that similar restrictions in T-cell receptor usage occur in MS and possibly other human autoimmune diseases.

The restricted usage of one or a few T-cell receptors to recognize autoantigens in the autoimmune process has important implications for the therapy of autoimmune disease. We will consider these implications in the last section of this chapter.

Rheumatoid Arthritis

One of the most common diseases is the autoimmune disease RHEUMATOID ARTHRITIS, commonly known as rheumatism. It is a disease associated with (but not restricted to) advanced age, and a large percentage of the population experiences some form of rheumatic discomfort at some time in their lives. The disease is characterized by a chronic inflammation of the joints, which is associated with autoantibodies against the Fc portion of the patient's IgG. These antibodies are called RHEUMATOID FACTOR (RF), and are either IgM or IgG. They form immune complexes with IgG molecules, which for many years were thought to be the cause of the disease. While RF may contribute to the pathology of rheumatoid arthritis, the role of autoreactive T cells has been more recently considered. The joints of rheumatoid arthritis patients contain large numbers of T cells, and it is thought to be very likely that these T cells actually cause the disease via a DTH reaction. The question is: What antigens do these T cells recognize? There are at least two candidates, both of which are interesting.

There are several forms of collagen, but one form, type II collagen, is restricted in distribution primarily to cartilage. Autoreactive T cells to this form of collagen might help to explain the symptoms of rheumatoid arthritis. David Trentham and colleagues have shown that approximately 75% of patients with rheumatoid arthritis generate cellular immune responses to type II collagen (as well as type III). The idea that a cell-mediated response to collagen might account for autoimmune arthritis is also supported by some animal models of the disease (see below).

Another candidate antigen was identified in animal models of rheumatoid arthritis. This antigen is one of the STRESS PROTEINS (also called *heat shock proteins*, or hsps). The antigen is found in mycobacteria as a 65-kd protein, identified as hsp 60 (hsp 70 is also a potential candidate). T cells from the joints of arthritis patients respond not only to bacterial hsp 60 and 70, but, perhaps more importantly, also to *human* hsp 70 (which shares at least 50% homology with the bacterial protein). Stress proteins are of particular interest, because they are expressed preferentially in cells that have been stressed (hence the name) by such things as viral or bacterial infection. Such proteins might not normally be presented to the immune system to induce tolerance. As we'll see below, responses to these stress proteins are capable of causing rheumatoid arthritis in some animals. It is also interesting that some T cells bearing the $\gamma\delta$ T-cell receptor recognize mycobacterial stress proteins, although whether this cell population plays any role in autoimmune disease is not known.

Animal Models of Rheumatoid Arthritis

It is not a coincidence that the two best-studied animal models of rheumatoid arthritis employ the two candidate antigens mentioned above. This is because the animal models suggested that these antigens might be involved and led to their being tested in patients.

In some strains of mice, rats, and squirrel monkeys, injection of type II collagen (with small amounts of adjuvant) leads to the development of COLLAGEN AUTOIMMUNE ARTHRITIS. T cells invade the joints (even at sites distant to the injection) and cause inflammation and damage. Some (but not all) T-cell lines that react to type II collagen are capable of transferring the disease to normal animals, strongly implicating such T cells in the disease. Anticollagen antibodies are also generated, and these may contribute to the disease as well.

The ability of collagen to induce autoimmune arthritis is linked to the MHC haplotype of the responding animal. This fits in well with the role of T cells in the disease. Like those found in EAE (see above), the T cells that react in collagen autoimmune arthritis show a very restricted T-cell receptor usage. For example, Chella David and colleagues have shown that collagen-reactive T cells in DBA/1 mice have a very strong preference for using $V_{\beta6}$. This observation will take on more significance when we discuss possible approaches to therapy in the last section of this chapter.

Another animal model is ADJUVANT ARTHRITIS, which is produced by injection of complete Freund's adjuvant into rats. This adjuvant contains killed *Mycobacterium tuberculosis*, and preparations that induce adjuvant arthritis contain somewhat higher doses of this bacterium than those conventionally used. Several investigators have demonstrated that animals with adjuvant arthritis make cellular immune responses to type II collagen, and T-cell lines from such animals react with collagen (and can transfer the disease). It looks, however, as though adjuvant arthritis may be a bit more interesting. Irun Cohen and his colleagues at the Weissman Institute purified a 65-kd protein from mycobacteria that was responsible for inducing arthritis. This protein was subsequently identified as hsp 60 (see above). This has opened the possibility that the autoantigen is also a stress protein. In any case, some (but not all) T-cell lines that react with this bacterial protein are capable of transferring the disease to normal animals.

Type I Diabetes

In the last 20 years it has become clear that type I diabetes (insulin-dependent diabetes, juvenile-onset diabetes mellitus) is an autoimmune disease in which the β cells that produce insulin in the pancreas are destroyed. Both autoantibodies and infiltrating T cells are detected, and this autoimmunity is specifically focused on the β cells, leaving the other cells of the pancreas alone. The autoantigen that is recognized, either in the human disease or in the animal models, is not known.

Since the advent of insulin therapy in the 1920s, the incidence of acute deaths in diabetes has been greatly reduced. Long-term consequences of this disease, however, can include blindness, kidney failure, and neurological problems. Some of the secondary effects of diabetes may be related to the autoimmune condition, as antibodies to neurons and cells of the adrenal cortex have been detected in some patients.

The genetics of type I diabetes and the phenomena identified in the animal models make this autoimmune disease of particular interest to immunologists.

Animal Models of Type I Diabetes

Until animal models for diabetes became available, the role of the immune system in the onset of this disease was controversial. This is because histologic analysis of pancreatic tissue involved in insulin production (the islets of Langerhans) showed destruction of these regions in diabetic patients but rarely showed evidence of an autoimmune reaction. It was possible, however, that autoimmune destruction of these pancreatic β islet cells occurs only at the onset of disease (which is much harder to observe in humans). Experiments with the animal models, however, established the autoimmune nature of diabetes and underscored the important role of T-cell-mediated responses. For example, it is possible to transfer the disease from a diabetic to a normal animal by transferring T cells or T-cell lines. Further, because the onset of diabetes in these animal models is predictable, it is possible to observe the autoimmune event leading to destruction of the pancreatic islet cells. This event involves lymphocyte infiltration of the pancreas (Figure 1). Later, the lymphocytes are gone, and as in humans, the evidence of the autoimmune assault is the destruction of the islet cells.

Two of the best animal models of diabetes are in rodent species in which some strains show a genetic predisposition to the disease. One such strain is the BB RAT (Biobreeding), in which approximately 60% of animals develop diabetes between 2 and 4 months of age. At this time, there is a massive infiltration of lymphocytes into the pancreatic islets, followed by β-islet-cell destruction. Bone marrow and thymus transplantation studies have shown that the defect that leads to diabetes resides in the stem cells, but that diabetes can be prevented when T cells mature in an allogeneic thymus. The susceptibility to diabetes in these animals is controlled by more than one genetic locus, but it is strongly associated with class II MHC haplotype.

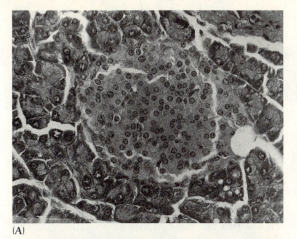

(A)

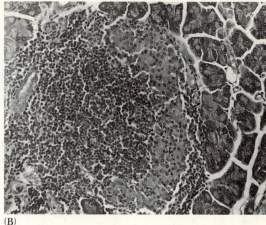

(B)

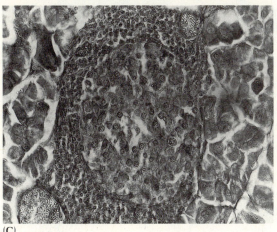

(C)

1   Cell-Mediated Immune Destruction of Pancreatic Islets in the Onset of Type I Diabetes. Histologic sections of pancreatic islets are shown from (A) nonobese diabetic (NOD) mouse pancreas before the onset of diabetes, (B) NOD pancreas during the onset of diabetes, and (C) NOD pancreas 2 months after the onset of diabetes. Note that the pancreatic islet cells in the center of the photograph appear healthy in (A) and damaged in (C), but that no evidence of cellular infiltration can be observed in (C). The autoimmune cell-mediated destruction is observed only in (B), during the onset of the disease. [Courtesy of B. Singh, University of Alberta]

More than one gene also contributes to development of disease in the NOD MOUSE (nonobese diabetic), and again, there is a strong association with class II MHC haplotype. Approximately 70 to 80% of female (but less than 20% of male) NOD mice develop diabetes by around 7 months of age, and this correlates with a marked infiltration of lymphocytes into the pancreas. Cloned T-cell lines from these mice have been generated that appear to recognize pancreatic islet cells, and these T cells are capable of transferring disease into young NOD mice.

An interesting (and, as yet, unexplained) finding regarding these two diabetic strains was made by Bhagirath Singh and his colleagues in Edmonton. They found that treatment of young NOD or BB animals with complete Freund's adjuvant results in a dramatic protection against developing the disease. Further, this resistance can be transferred with lymphoid cells that lack B- or T-cell markers. This finding presents a paradox: complete Freund's adjuvant is used in the *induction* of some experimental autoimmune diseases (immunization for EAE or collagen arthritis, and a larger dose for adjuvant arthritis). Why then, does it prevent this one? The answer to this question may give us new insights into the mechanisms of autoimmune diabetes (and perhaps some new approaches to therapy).

SYNTHESIS
The Limits of Tolerance

There is no doubt about it: the immune system is fully capable of making immune responses to self. We have discussed autoantibody responses and their consequences and considered the important role of autoreactive T cells in several autoimmune diseases. The critical problem then arises of how autoimmunity proceeds in the face of tolerance. When we discussed B-cell tolerance and autoimmunity in the last chapter, we weaseled out of the problem by suggesting that helper T cells, responding to foreign carriers, stimulate autoreactive B cells when the carrier is linked to an epitope cross-reactive with self. The astute reader will no doubt have seen the hand waving here. By brushing aside the question of why autoreactive B cells even exist, we deny the phenomenon of B-cell tolerance. We have seen, however, that B-cell tolerance is a real phenomenon (see Chapter 31). The problem of autoreactivity becomes even more profound when it is the T cell that reacts with autoantigens. As we know, autoantigens are processed and presented just like any other antigen (see Chapter 20), but the T cells that respond to autoantigens should be either functionally or actually deleted (see Chapters 24 and 31). At the core of the problems of autoreactive T and B cells is the fundamental question of autoimmunity: Why do the mechanisms of tolerance fail? The simple answer to this question is that there are limits on tolerance in the immune system.

Immunologic Privilege

If an autoantigen is normally SEQUESTERED from the immune system, then tolerance to this antigen seems unlikely. For example, in males, sperm antigens are not normally available to the immune system. If, for some reason, a male is systemically exposed to his own sperm, an immune response will ensue. This sometimes occurs following vasectomy or can be demonstrated in experimental animals.[2] Similarly, antigens found only in the eye are generally secure from immune exposure. If however, one eye is damaged, thus releasing these antigens into the system, the ensuing immune response can severely damage the other eye. Many other examples exist. Areas in the body that have this characteristic are collectively called IMMUNOLOGICALLY PRIVILEGED SITES.[3]

Immunologic "Ignorance"

Immunologically privileged antigens account for only a fraction of the specificities of autoreactive lymphocytes. What about autoreactivity to autoantigens that are not sequestered? Here again, we have to consider the limits to tolerance. N. Avrion Mitchison pointed out several years ago that some autoantigens seem to be normally present at too low a concentration to induce tolerance. This class of self-antigens, such as the F antigen of the liver, is simply "ignored" by the immune system. If, for some reason, however, the concentration of one of these antigens increases, immunity to the antigen can occur. The idea, then, is that the immune system is not tolerant but rather is simply ignorant of many antigens in the body.

Similarly, the immune system may be ignorant of certain *epitopes* on autoantigens. This has been demonstrated in cytotoxic T cells by Hans-Georg Ramensee and colleagues in Tübingen. They generated cytotoxic T-cell lines using peptides derived from a number of autologous proteins, such as β_2-microglobulin, hemoglobin, and liver proteins. These are autoantigens to which the animals are tolerant, but the peptides induced immune responses nevertheless. The CTL lines were specific for the peptides plus class I MHC, as expected, but did not kill autologous cells in the

---

[2] The experiment in which autoimmune testitis was induced by immunization with autologous sperm has a nickname, but decorum prevents specifically stating it. For the curious, a hint: it *could* be called the "Jerry Lee Lewis experiment" (goodness! gracious!...). We are indebted to Dr. Tom Wegmann for pointing this valuable piece of immunologic folklore out to us.

[3] Privileged sites are not as completely cut off from the immune system as we once believed, however. If foreign antigen is placed into such a site, for example, the anterior chamber of the eye, tolerance to the antigen is often generated. Tom Ferguson at Washington University has shown that such tolerance induction requires the presence of T cells in the privileged site. It may be, then, that this route of tolerance induction is a "backup system" designed to prevent autoreactivity if, for some reason, T cells enter a privileged site.

absence of the peptides. It appears, then, that normal processing of these autoantigens does not give rise to these particular peptides, and therefore, the T cells have not been tolerized to these particular combinations of peptide and MHC. This suggests that an alteration in the way that an autoantigen is processed and presented by the immune system could trigger autoimmune responses. Such an alteration might be produced by inappropriate expression of a protease not normally found in the cell that produces the autoantigen.

There are therefore several ways in which an autoantigen can evoke an immune response rather than tolerance. The antigen can be sequestered from the immune system, such that it is, for all intents and purposes, foreign to the system. It can be normally present at too low a concentration to be recognized for tolerance induction. Alternatively, the antigen may be normally processed in specific ways, such that a change in processing will produce a novel antigenic peptide.

Evasion of T-Cell Tolerance

At least three other mechanisms might also account for autoreactive T cells, and there may well be more. We saw in Chapter 24 that negative selection tests developing T cells for autoreactivity, and any autoreactive cells that are triggered at this point usually die. If, for some reason, cells avoid this suicide process, then autoreactive T cells can enter the system. This has been demonstrated in some experimental systems (see below), but the role of this process in naturally occurring autoimmunity is still unclear. Another mechanism might involve overcoming the state of anergy associated with peripheral T-cell tolerance (see Chapter 31). These anergic lymphocytes are normally unresponsive but are still present in the immune system. It is possible that there are signals that can override this anergy and thus activate autoreactivity. Recall from Chapters 26 and 31 that when antigen is presented to anergic T cells, the cells express IL-2R. If IL-2 were present at high enough concentrations, these cells might become activated.

Finally, some autoreactive T cells may be controlled by regulatory mechanisms, such as suppressor T cells (see Chapter 30). Several laboratories have shown that T cells reactive to autologous insulin are present in several species, including mice and humans. Judith Kapp and colleagues at Washington University have shown that removal of CD8$^+$ cells reveals the presence of CD4$^+$ T cells with reactivity to autologous insulin. Whether or not such regulatory T cells normally control the anti-insulin response in vivo is not yet known.

Autoreactive T Cells, MHC, and Autoimmunity

The idea that autoreactive T cells contribute to autoimmune disease has been proved in a number of systems. In this section and the next we will look at a few predictions based on this idea and see how our knowledge of T-cell function points to new approaches to therapy for autoimmunity. The first prediction is perhaps the most obvious: if autoreactive T cells are involved in autoimmunity, there should be a role for MHC. In many types of autoimmune disease, certain alleles of MHC genes are, indeed, linked to disease, but, so far, the reasons for this linkage are not really clear.

MHC and Relative Risk

In order to assess the contribution of a particular marker (say, an MHC allele) to a human disease, we can employ a measurement called RELATIVE RISK. A list of some autoimmune disease–HLA associations and their relative risks is given in Table 1. Relative risk is calculated by assessing the presence or absence of the marker in populations with or without the disease:[4]

$$\text{relative risk} = \frac{(\text{patients with marker}) \times (\text{controls without marker})}{(\text{patients without marker}) \times (\text{controls with marker})}$$

We can see from this that a relative risk of 1 indicates that the marker is no more frequent in the patient population than in the control population and therefore is not linked to the disease. A relative risk of >1, however, means that the marker is more frequent among those with the disease than among those without it, indicating an association between the marker and the disease. The allele might actually contribute to the disease state, but to demonstrate this requires a more complete analysis of the mechanisms of the disease. By itself, however, a relative risk of >1 does *not* necessarily mean that the allele *causes* the disease. The reason for this is the phenomenon of LINKAGE DISEQUILIBRIUM.

Linkage disequilibrium occurs when an allele at one locus is found together with an allele at a linked locus at a higher frequency

---

[4] Another way to calculate relative risk gives the same result but may be easier to follow: For each population, calculate the ratio $R = $ (number with marker)/(number without marker). Relative risk $= R_{\text{patient}}/R_{\text{control}}$.

Table 1 Some associations between HLA alleles and autoimmune diseases.[a]

Disease	HLA allele	Relative risk
Ankylosing spondylitis	B27	87.4
Rheumatoid arthritis	DR4	2.8-13.4
Juvenile rheumatoid arthritis	DR5	5.2-7.0
Graves' disease	DR3	3.3-5.5
Multiple sclerosis	DR2	4.1-4.8
Myasthenia gravis	DR3	2.5
Goodpasture's syndrome	DR2	13.1-15.9
Pernicious anemia	DR5	5.4
	DR2	2.0-3.7
Type I diabetes	DR3	2.9-15.3
	DR4	3.1-14.2
Celiac disease	DR3	10.8-54.0
Ulcerative colitis	DR2	5.1

Source: Data from Stastny et al., 1982. *Immunol. Rev.* 70: 113; and Svejgaard et al., 1982. *Immunol. Rev.* 70: 193.

[a] This table lists only a few HLA allele–autoimmune disease associations. Relative risk is defined in the text. Differences in relative risk depend on many factors, including race, disease definition, and the HLA typing reagents used in the study. Note that a significant relative risk (>1) does not prove that the specific HLA allele is, itself, involved in the disease—the allele may be closely linked with an allele that is involved (see discussion of linkage disequilibrium in text).

than expected. This may occur if the particular combination of alleles confers a selective advantage or may occur for any of a number of other reasons. Because of linkage disequilibrium, an association between an HLA allele and a disease cannot be taken as proof that the allele contributes to the disease. For example, the association between HLA-DR3 (and DR4) and diabetes (see Table 1) is not a demonstration that the DR locus plays a role in diabetes. As we'll see below, there is an interesting polymorphism in HLA-DQ that is also associated with diabetes, and for reasons we'll discuss, it seems somewhat more likely that this locus (rather than DR) may be important in the disease. Linkage disequilibrium is probably the reason that many autoimmune diseases were originally thought to be linked to class I MHC alleles. The availability of antibodies that detect class I polymorphisms previously made their identification easier than those of class II. Now that similar antibodies are available to identify class II polymorphism, we realize that class II alleles often (but not always) show a stronger association with autoimmunity than do class I alleles.

More recently, molecular biological approaches to identifying MHC polymorphisms are revealing even stronger associations between certain MHC alleles and autoimmunity. One such association is considered next.

MHC and Diabetes

As mentioned above, diabetes mellitus (or type I diabetes) is an autoimmune disease in which susceptibility is linked to the MHC, and one of the animal models of type I diabetes is the NOD mouse, a strain that has a high frequency of autoimmune diabetes among females. As in people, susceptibility to diabetes in NOD mice is linked to MHC haplotype.

Hugh McDevitt and his co-workers at Stanford studied human and mouse MHC genes that are associated with diabetes, and found that a polymorphism in the HLA-DQ$_\beta$ chain carries a relative risk of 107 (compare with Table 1 to see how high a risk factor this is). The polymorphism results in a change in a single amino acid (residue 57) in the HLA-DQ$_\beta$ protein from an aspartic acid to any of a number of other amino acids. They then examined the β chain of the I-A molecule, the homolog of HLA-DQ, in the NOD mouse. They found that this chain differs from that of all other mouse I-Aβ chains in that it lacks an aspartic acid in residue 57!

In the BB rat, the class II MHC allele associated with the disease also lacks an aspartic acid at residue 57. This polymorphism, however, is also seen in Lewis rats, which are not prone to diabetes. It is quite possible, though, that this allele nevertheless contributes to the disease in BB rats, while in Lewis rats other genetic elements that are also required for the development of disease are lacking.

If the structure of class II MHC molecules is similar to that of class I MHC molecules, then residue 57 lies within the antigen-binding groove of the molecule (see Chapter 20). Something about the role of residue 57 in antigen presentation (or, possibly, thymic selection, see Chapters 24 and 25) contributes to susceptibility to autoimmune diabetes.

Diabetes is not the only autoimmune disease linked to this polymorphism. An autoimmune skin condition, pemphigus vulgaris, is also linked to this change at residue 57 of HLA-DQ$_\beta$, and there may be others. These observations tell us that antigen presentation by class II MHC molecules is part of the process of some autoimmune diseases, but we don't yet know why an alteration in the MHC molecule can contribute to the disease. A possible clue may come from studies of the T-cell receptors that are used by autoreactive T cells. As we mentioned in our discussions of EAE and collagen autoimmune arthritis, there seems to be a very restricted usage of T-cell receptor V regions among autoreactive T cells. It may be that the reactivity (and perhaps, selection) of these T cells depends on the interactions of these T-cell receptors with the appropriate MHC molecule.

Inappropriate MHC Expression and Autoimmunity

We know from our previous discussions that class I MHC molecules are expressed on all the cells of the body. The levels of expression, however, can vary by orders of magnitude in different tissues. Class II MHC expression, on the other hand, is much more limited and in some cell types is only seen following some form of induction (see Chapter 20). Considerations of the distribution and levels of MHC have led to the idea that autoimmunity is either caused by or facilitated by an inappropriate expression of MHC molecules on the "wrong" tissues.

The idea, as originally suggested, seems somewhat unlikely. Several investigators had noted that extensive class II MHC expression can be observed in organs under attack by autoreactive lymphocyte infiltrates. They suggested that some inducing agent, a virus, for example, had caused cells in the tissue to begin to express high levels of class II MHC, and these cells then presented self-antigens in an unusual way that activated T cells. For some reason, these T cells would not be activated by the autoantigen presented on more conventional APCs. Thus, the inappropriate expression of class II MHC might serve as a "trigger" for autoimmunity.

Although most immunologists don't believe that this idea solves the problem of how autoimmunity occurs, it is very likely that changes in MHC expression contribute to the autoimmune process. Some autoreactive T cells, upon activation, will release lymphokines (such as γ-interferon) that elevate MHC expression. These T cells will then respond more efficiently because the APCs now bear increased levels of MHC molecules. The result is a feed-forward effect that, without appropriate control, leads to total destruction of the tissue.

Such destruction is very reminiscent of the rejection of foreign grafts (discussed in Chapter 37). In fact, the same changes in MHC expression occur in graft rejection and autoimmune attack on a tissue. This similarity has led many investigators to study graft-versus-host disease (GVHD, see Chapter 18) as a model for some types of autoimmunity. The major difference, of course, is that we know why antihost cells are present in GVHD, but not why they are present in autoimmunity.

Negative Selection and Autoimmunity

In Chapter 24, we discussed negative selection, one of the best understood mechanisms for the development of self–nonself discrimination in the immune system. Immature T cells that are stimulated by antigens presented in the thymus die, and the result of this is that autoreactive T cells should not mature. A defect in this process would result in autoreactive T cells entering the body, and clearly this could be a cause of autoimmunity.

Two experimental systems illustrate the potential of such a defect to produce autoimmune disease. In neither case, however, has it been formally proved that the autoimmunity that follows the experimental treatment is actually due to an escape from negative selection.

The immunosuppressive drug cyclosporin A interferes with activation-induced cell death in the thymus, and animals treated with this drug show an increase in T cells that are normally negatively selected (see Chapter 24). If a rat or mouse is treated with cyclosporin A from birth or following a bone marrow transplant, an autoimmune syndrome develops after the treatment stops. This syndrome is marked by lymphocyte infiltrates into many different organs, including thyroid, pancreas, and ovaries. In addition, autoantibodies are produced against a similar variety of tissues. When we consider the ability of cyclosporin A to interfere with negative selection, it seems very likely that the self-reactive T cells that escape this process are responsible for the autoimmune disease that develops.

Another system that may be related to defects in negative selection involves thymectomy of mice at an early age. Shimon and Noriko Sakaguchi, who have also studied the cyclosporin A model mentioned above, have shown that animals thymectomized between days 2 and 4 after birth develop a generalized autoimmune disorder with infiltrating T cells and autoantibodies. While it has not been shown that such thymectomy results in an escape from negative selection, this conclusion is fairly likely: several groups have shown that mature T cells that are normally absent from adult mice (due to negative selection) can sometimes be identified in mice shortly after birth. A likely interpretation of this finding is that some autoantigens are not expressed until some time after birth, and therefore there is no negative selection of the T cells that recognize such antigens.

How, then, are the responses of such T cells normally controlled? The Sakaguchis have shown that in both the thymectomy and cyclosporin A models, autoimmune disease can be prevented simply by injecting normal, syngeneic, CD4$^+$ T cells before the disease appears. Whatever these inhibitory T cells are doing (see Chapter 30), it seems very possible that they play an important, but as yet undefined, role in controlling autoimmunity.

It may not be surprising that defects in negative selection can cause problems for the control of self–nonself discrimination and lead to autoimmunity. What is frustrating, however, is that the search for such defects in animals genetically prone to autoimmune disease has not turned up much of interest. In general, such animals seem to show normal negative selection during T-cell development. This suggests either that there are other mechanisms for the generation of autoreactive T cells (e.g., escape from peripheral tolerance) or else we've missed the important defects in negative selection that lead to autoimmune disease in such animals. The latter is possible, since negative-selection studies have so far been restricted to assessment of T-cell-receptor V_β usage in mature T cells, or else maturation of T cells in T-cell-receptor–transgenic mice (using anti-nonself T-cell receptors). Undoubtedly, the maturation of T cells in animals made transgenic for autoreactive T-cell receptors will be studied, and these investigations may shed light on the role of negative selection in generating autoimmunity.

Immunologic Approaches to Therapy of Autoimmune Diseases

The role of autoreactive T cells in the generation of autoimmune diseases suggests several approaches to the immunotherapy of autoimmunity. As with our other discussions of therapy in this book, we will focus on those therapies that illustrate immunologic phenomena. Keep in mind, though, that there are other therapies (mostly pharmacologic) that have been used for many years to help to limit the consequences of autoimmunity and prolong the lives of such individuals.

Two of the three approaches we consider below employ antibodies to block or remove T cells involved in autoimmunity. The third approach is completely different and depends on immunization with T cells or T-cell receptors to generate a new regulatory environment in which autoimmunity cannot proceed. Each of these approaches has real potential as an immune therapy and will certainly be undergoing clinical trials in the next few years.

Antibodies That Block T-Cell Activation

We know that T cells are activated through interactions between the T-cell receptor complex and its ligand, MHC plus antigenic peptides, and there is no reason to suspect that the activation of autoreactive T cells is any different. Therefore, antibodies that prevent this interaction should be capable of interfering with autoimmunity. In many experimental models of autoimmune disease, the effects of treatment with such antibodies have been striking.

Antibodies that bind to class II MHC molecules and block T-cell recognition have been extensively used in this context, and their use has helped to underline the importance of T-cell activation in the generation of autoimmunity. Injection of anti-I-A antibodies into mice can prevent or even reverse EAE, experimental myasthenia gravis, and NZB autoimmune nephritis. Anti-I-A antibodies also prevent diabetes in NOD mice. In addition, anti–class II MHC antibodies have been shown to be effective in blocking and reversing EAE in rhesus monkeys. While it is likely that these antibodies work by blocking T-cell activation, in some cases they also appear to kill class II MHC$^+$ cells, especially B cells, and this effect may contribute to the immunosuppression.

Even more impressive results have been obtained using anti-CD4 antibodies. As we discussed in Chapter 26, such antibodies efficiently block the activation of CD4$^+$ T cells. Although some anti-CD4 antibodies kill T cells in vivo, other antibodies [or (Fab)$_2$ fragments] do not, and the latter also are effective in preventing or reversing autoimmunity. Rat and mouse EAE, collagen arthritis, experimental thyroiditis, NZB/NZW SLE, and diabetes in NOD mice have all been inhibited with anti-CD4 antibodies. Most interestingly, treatment with anti-CD4 can produce a state of specific tolerance, such that the animals are now resistant to induction of the autoimmune disease (and do not require further anti-CD4 treatments). This phenomenon, although not really understood, makes anti-CD4 therapy particularly attractive.

The ability of anti-CD4 to block NZB/NZW disease is evidence that T cells are involved in this autoimmunity, even though other evidence has suggested that they are not required [see discussion of (NZB × NZW)F$_1$ in Chapter 35]. We have also suggested that B-cell hyperactivity (even in the absence of T cells) helps to account for this disease. In light of the effects of anti-CD4 treatment, however, it is clear that there is still some work to do to understand the role of T cells in this disease.

The results with anti-CD4 also imply that if CD8$^+$ T cells are involved in autoimmune diseases, they are dependent upon CD4$^+$ cells (or else play only a very minor role). Some investigators have observed that treatment of animals prone to diabetes or experimental thyroiditis with *both* anti-CD4 and anti-CD8 antibody can be more effective than treatment with anti-CD4 alone.

Immunotoxins

In Chapter 33 we described the use of immunotoxins, antibodies to which a toxin or cytotoxic drug is attached, for the destruction of tumor cells. Similar strategies can be applied to autoimmunity, and some of these may turn out to be powerful new approaches to therapy.

One approach may be effective in autoimmune diseases in which autoantibodies play a major role in the disease process (see Chapter 35). If we know the antigen, we can convert it to a therapeutic agent by the attachment of toxin to the antigen. B cells that bind and internalize the agent will then be killed, thus removing the source of the autoantibodies. Erwin Deiner and others have demonstrated the potential of this approach to induce specific B-cell unresponsiveness in vivo. One problem with this approach, however, is that the effects will only last until the toxic conjugate is gone from the system and new B cells have a chance to mature. Nevertheless, it may turn out to be a useful therapy for acute conditions.

Another strategy is even more clever and targets activated T cells. As discussed in Chapter 27, when a T cell becomes activated it expresses the IL-2 receptor α molecule, also called CD25. In an individual under autoimmune attack, the activated autoreactive T cells will therefore express this marker. Immunotoxins composed of anti-CD25 and a toxin will kill these activated cells, sparing T cells that are not active at the time of the treatment (those that are antiforeign). As with the antigen–toxin conjugate, however, it is possible that autoimmunity will resume when the conjugate is clear and new T cells develop. Continuous treatment with this reagent would be unadvisable, since it will destroy T cells that are activated in response to pathogens. On the other hand, it is possible that the mechanisms of tolerance will reassert themselves given the chance. In any case, the therapy has some potential for extremely acute situations.

T-Cell "Vaccines"

One of the most exciting approaches to the therapy of autoimmune diseases has been developed mainly through the efforts of Irun Cohen and colleagues in Israel. Like others, they had observed that while some cloned T-cell lines that react to an autoantigen are capable of transferring disease to normal animals, others are not. They further observed that some of these non-disease-causing T cells are actually capable of *preventing* induction of (or even reversing) the disease. When these T cells are irradiated (so that they cannot proliferate) and injected into animals, a long-lasting state of resistance is generated. This method employing T-CELL VACCINES has been applied to EAE, experimental thyroiditis, and adjuvant arthritis. In every case, the protection is specific for the particular autoimmune disease, and responses to foreign antigens remain normal. The protection is effective against challenge with autoantigen or transfer of autoimmunity with autoreactive T cells.

Cohen and his colleagues have also shown that T cells taken directly from autoimmune animals can be used to vaccinate against induction of autoimmunity, especially if the cells are treated with hydrostatic pressure (which has been shown to increase the immunogenicity of some tumor cells). They found that the prolonged protection produced by either clones or treated T cells can be transferred to other animals with T cells from the treated animals. The T cells that transfer the resistance can be either $CD4^+$ or $CD8^+$, and the latter were found to be capable of specifically killing T-cell lines used to vaccinate. The ability of such $CD8^+$ T cells to suppress immune responses is reminiscent of the experiments of Binz and Wigzell discussed in Chapter 30.

It seemed possible that T-cell vaccination results in the generation of T cells that react against the T-cell receptors on the cells used to vaccinate. If this is true, then the fact that the induced T cells protect against the disease suggests that autoreactive T cells probably employ a limited number of different T-cell receptors. As we've seen, this is the case in several experimental models of autoimmune disease.

Although Cohen and his co-workers were unable to protect animals by vaccination with T-cell membranes, other investigators have taken this research an important step forward. Synthetic peptides have been designed that correspond to regions within the T-cell receptor V regions of autoreactive T cells in EAE. Immunization with these peptides produced a state of resistance to the induction of EAE. Again, T cells were found to be capable of transferring the protection. CD8$^+$ T cells from the immunized animals were capable of killing other T cells bearing the appropriate T-cell receptors.

Not only does this work point the way to a dynamic new approach to prevention and therapy of autoimmune diseases, but it also tells us some important things about the immune system. Based on this work, it is likely that idiotype–anti-idiotype reactions between T-cell receptors can occur, and that these may play an important role in maintaining tolerance.

Summary

1. Many autoimmune diseases are caused by autoreactive T cells that infiltrate a tissue and produce damage via delayed-type hypersensitivity. This has been demonstrated in animal models in which a particular autoimmune disease can be adoptively transferred to normal animals by injection of T cells or cloned T-cell lines from autoimmune animals.

2. One way in which autoreactive T cells can develop is if the antigen is normally present at very low concentrations or if it is normally sequestered from the immune system. Alternatively, autoimmunity can result from evasion of negative selection. While the latter has been suggested in some models employing manipulation of the developing immune system, it has not yet been demonstrated in any naturally occurring disease.

3. Many autoimmune diseases are associated, at least in part, with particular MHC alleles. Why some alleles but not others seem to increase the risk of autoimmunity is not fully understood, but this association further supports an important role for T cells in many autoimmune diseases.

4. Several new approaches to therapy depend on our knowledge of T-cell function in autoimmunity. Antibodies that block activation or kill activated cells are effective in blocking or reversing autoimmunity. Another strategy takes advantage of the fact that autoreactive T cells seem to employ a very limited number of T-cell receptors, and protective immunity against these receptors can be induced.

Additional Readings

Acha-Orbea, H., L. Steinman and H. O. McDevitt. 1989. T-cell receptors in murine autoimmune diseases. *Annu. Rev. Immunol.* 7: 371.

Cohen, I. R. 1986. Regulation of autoimmune disease, physiological and therapeutic. *Immunol. Rev.* 94: 5.

Zamvil, S. S. and L. Steinman. 1990. The T lymphocyte in experimental allergic encephalomyelitis. *Annu. Rev. Immunol.* 8: 579.

TRANSPLANTATION

Overview   The ability to respond to foreign antigen undoubtedly is important in the survival of the species (or else why would there be immunologists?). However, the response can be an impediment to surgical intervention when we wish to replace parts of the body. Surgeons have made the necessary technical advances that allow them to hook up the plumbing for kidneys, hearts, and livers. But these procedures would all be doomed to failure, because of the immune response of the host, if adequate immunosuppression were not possible. The combined use of cyclosporin A, azathioprine, and prednisone have made kidney and other organ transplantation possible.

It is amazing to think that within the lifetimes of some of the more mature readers of this book there was still a question about whether or not foreign tissue could be transplanted and what the nature of the rejection mechanism could be. We will see that the immunologic basis of rejection is now firmly established, and the success of clinical transplants has come about through our ability to control these phenomena.

Graft Rejection as an Immune Phenomenon

For many years surgeons had been faced with a dilemma when treating burn patients needing such large amounts of new skin that skin from the patient would not be sufficient to cover the area. They could either use "pinch grafts" to make one piece of skin do the job of two or three, or use skin from another individual. Although Flexner in 1911 had shown clearly that skin cannot be transferred from one individual to another, many surgeons continued the practice. As Peter Medawar pointed out in his 1957 Harvey lecture, "Holding their critical faculties in abeyance, [these surgeons] had convinced themselves that the skin of rabbits or dogs could flourish on human soil. The problem of whether or not skin grafts could survive transplantation from one person to another was still thought to be worth debating as recently as fifteen years ago [that is, 1942]."

In 1943, in fact, Medawar had done an experiment showing convincingly that foreign skin is rejected by "a mechanism of active immunization."

A 22-year-old burn patient was treated with 52 pinch autografts from her own thigh and 50 homografts from her brother's. A second set of 28 pinch homografts from her brother were transplanted 15 days after the first. The autografts grew and formed a continuous sheet. In contrast, the first set of homografts started growing, but by biopsy could be seen to be degenerating by 15 days and degeneration was complete by 23 days. The second set of homografts were in an advanced state of degeneration by day 8. [T. Gibson and P. B. Medawar, 1943. *J. Anat.* 77: 299]

It was clear to Medawar that the second set of grafts was being rejected at the same time as the original. He concluded that the patient had made an immune response to the first set of homografts and this caused the accelerated rejection of the second set of grafts. In other words, graft rejection is an immune phenomenon. In a classic paper in 1945 (Report to the War Wounds Committee of the Medical Research Council) Medawar summarized his experiments with the transplantation of skin of rabbits. "Resistance to homologous grafted skin therefore belongs to the general category of actively acquired immune reactions." [P. B. Medawar, 1945. *J. Anat.* 79: 157]

In 1954 Medawar's student, N. Avrion Mitchison, showed that immunity to a tumor can be transferred from one mouse to another with lymph node cells from an immunized animal, but not with serum. This was so similar to the transfer of DTH, which Chase had shown many years before, that the idea that tissue rejection is the result of an immune response became firmly established. It will be recalled from Chapter 15 on the MHC molecule that at about this same time Peter Gorer and George Snell were showing that tumor rejection and homograft rejection have the same mechanism. The stage was now set to understand graft rejection in terms of a cell-mediated immune response.

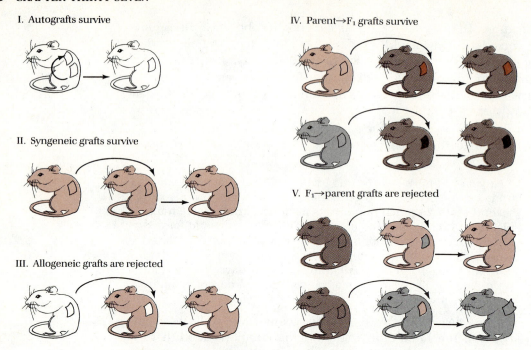

I. Autografts survive

II. Syngeneic grafts survive

III. Allogeneic grafts are rejected

IV. Parent→F₁ grafts survive

V. F₁→parent grafts are rejected

1 **The Laws of Transplantation.** (I and II) Autografts and grafts between syngeneic recipients survive because there are no T cells that are able to recognize the self-syngeneic antigens on the graft. (III) Allografts are rejected because the recipient has T cells that are reactive to the antigens on the graft. (IV and V) Parent-to-F_1 grafts survive because the F_1 host has antigens of the parent and therefore has no reactive T cells against these antigens. In contrast, F_1-to-parent grafts are rejected because the parent has reactive T cells to the other parent's antigens.

The Laws of Transplantation

Since the fate of a graft depends upon the ability of the host to respond to foreign antigens, the use of inbred mice was crucial for carrying out careful studies to determine the factors involved. From these studies, the LAWS OF TRANSPLANTATION were developed (Figure 1). In describing these laws we will be referring to tissue antigens that are recognized on the graft. Of course, we now know that MHC molecules are the most important of these, but the laws apply to all tissue antigens.

- *Law I. Autografts survive.* An AUTOGRAFT is the grafting of tissue from one area of the body to another area of the body on the same individual. There may be anatomical barriers to such a procedure, but there are no immunologic barriers because the recipient's immune system is seeing no new antigens.

- *Law II. Syngeneic grafts survive.* Since syngeneic animals are animals of the same inbred strain, this law is really a truism because in inbred strains of mice, each member is as genetically close to another member as an identical twin (the differences being in sex). Identical twins have the same set of antigens, and they can exchange grafts.
- *Law III. Allografts are rejected.* The grafting of tissue from one strain to another is called an ALLOGRAFT, just as members of the same species but with different genetic composition are ALLO-GENEIC. An allograft introduces genetic differences to which the recipient responds. Allografts are therefore rejected unless some means of preventing the host's immune system from responding to the foreign antigen is used.
- *Law IV. Parent-to-F_1 grafts survive.* Given two strains of mice, P and Q, the (P $\times$ Q)F_1 will express the antigens of both parental types. Thus when parental tissue is grafted to the F_1, which has both P and Q antigens, the F_1 host will not see any foreign antigens on the parental graft because it is tolerant to both P and Q. The graft will therefore succeed. In cases where the graft is immunologically competent (i.e., contains lymphocytes) the graft itself may respond to the foreign antigens of the recipients or host. This is a graft-versus-host reaction (GVH) and was discussed in Chapter 11. We will see below that this is a serious problem in bone marrow transplantation.
- *Law V. F_1-to-parent grafts are rejected.* In this case the F_1 has the antigens of both parental strains, P *and* Q. The recipient is one of the parental types, P *or* Q. The parental recipient P will therefore see the antigens of Q as foreign on the (P $\times$ Q)F_1 graft and will respond to it (just as Q will see the antigens of P as foreign). The graft will therefore be rejected.

Mechanism of Graft Rejection

Hyperacute Rejection

On rare occasions graft rejection can occur very rapidly (within days). This type of rejection is called HYPERACUTE REJECTION and is known to be mediated by preexisting antibodies to the donor antigens. The mechanism seems to be due to antibody's binding to antigen in the vasculature of the graft, causing thrombosis. In addition, the complement cascade, as well as the release of various vasoactive compounds, may be important.

Chronic Rejection

In some cases a slow rejection phase begins many months or even years after transplantation. This CHRONIC REJECTION appears to be due to the slow buildup of antibody directed against the antigens on the graft.

T-Cell-Mediated Rejection

The majority of rejection episodes to engrafted tissue are mediated by T cells. There is no clear-cut mechanism known, and we are not even sure which subset of T cells is involved. Studies in which CD4 or CD8 cells are eliminated from an animal by treatment with monoclonal anti-CD4 or anti-CD8 antibody have given equivocal results. These studies are always open to question because of the assay systems that must be used, that is, living animals in which it is impossible to rule out the reappearance of small numbers of the cell that has been eliminated. Nevertheless, the dominant body of immunological thought implicates both $CD4^+$ cells in a DTH-like reaction and $CD8^+$ cells in a cytotoxic response.

The Passenger Leukocyte Concept

In all the discussion above (and most of what follows) the reader has seen that the dominant idea in the barrier to successful tissue transplantation is that the host recognizes the antigens on the cells of the graft and mounts an immune response to them. There is a body of thought, however, that states that transplantation antigens are not the primary barrier to grafting. Rather, the argument goes, it is "PASSENGER" LEUKOCYTES that are carried along in the donor tissue that provide the major immunogenic stimulus for the host. If the idea is correct, then it would make good clinical sense to alter tissue immunogenicity as well as altering host responsiveness.

The idea that leukocytes in the graft are an important source of antigen goes back to observations made at the Jackson Laboratory by Nathen Kaliss and Andrew Kandutsch in 1956. These pioneers in transplantation noted that a recipient could be sensitized to a tumor allograft by injecting spleen or lymph node cells but not antigen extracts. George Snell suggested that these cells are responsible for the immunogenicity of the transplanted tissue, and the term *passenger leukocyte* was coined in 1968 by Elkins and Guttmann.

If the idea of the passenger leukocyte is correct, then it follows that ridding the graft of these cells should increase the survival time. Kevin Lafferty and his colleagues have reviewed the literature on this subject recently, and we will see in the section on pancreatic islet transplantation that this technique may have real potential in transplantation of β cells.[1]

Clinical Transplantation

Kidney Transplantation

There has been more clinical experience with the transplanting of the kidney than any other organ, and we will devote most of our attention to that organ. The history of modern transplantation began in 1954 when the first kidney was successfully transplanted between identical twins. At the time it was known that there would not be a problem with tissue incompatibility, and the procedure was viewed as showing that the surgical technique was adequate for human organ transplantation to be considered a viable treatment. But it was also realized that although the surgeons could transplant the kidney, there would have to be some way of getting around the immunologic rejection of the organ when donor and recipient were not identical twins. Two approaches were taken; one was the attempt to minimize the HLA differences between donor and recipient in the hope that the more similar the tissues the less chance of rejection. The second approach was to suppress the immune response of the recipient for a period of time so that the grafted organ could not be rejected and hope that a state of tolerance would be established.

Matching Donor and Recipients

At the beginning of the era of transplanting human kidneys between nonidentical twins (ca. 1968), it was assumed that HLA matching would be the critical determinant. The data in Figure 2 show the results of kidney transplantation at one transplantation

---

[1] The reader should be aware of the fact that one of the most amazing events in modern immunology centered around ridding grafts of passenger leukocytes. William Summerlin claimed that he was able to effect the complete allogeneic transplantation of skin in either mice or humans by culturing the skin for long periods of time. He was unable to reproduce his own early results and resorted to painting a black patch on the back of a white mouse. This desperate gesture was of course easily spotted, and the result was a great scandal. The story is beautifully told in a book by Joseph Hixon called *The Patchwork Mouse* (Anchor Press, 1976). A brilliant review of the book and the situation by Peter Medawar can be found in *The New York Review of Books* (April 15, 1976, page 6).

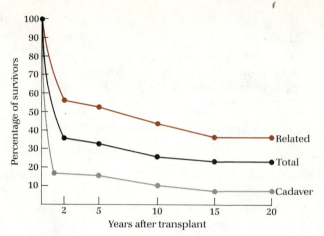

2 **Survival Rates for Kidney Transplantation from 1963 to 1968.** With tissue typing only ca. 50% survival rate was possible for kidneys from related donors. Cadaver kidneys had a very low survival rate. [Based on data from Sutherland et al., 1985. *Transpl. Proc.* 17: 110]

center in the era before adequate immunosuppression. From the results it is clear that while related recipients have a better chance of retaining the graft of the donor than do the recipients of unrelated cadaver kidneys, HLA compatibility does not by itself prevent rejection. This indicated that other factors, perhaps minor histocompatibility antigens, were responsible for rejection of the unrelated donor kidneys. It became obvious then that immunosuppression would be the crucial factor.

Immunosuppression in Transplantation

The first drugs used to suppress the immune response in kidney transplantation were the nucleic acid analog AZATHIOPRINE in 1961 and the corticosteroid PREDNISONE in 1963. The combined use of these two drugs has remained a mainstay of immunosuppression not only in kidney transplantation but in all other organ transplantation in humans. But the event that changed the practice of transplantation was the discovery of the drug CYCLOSPORIN A. This drug, which has revolutionized the practice of transplantation, was discovered during routine screening of culture broths of microbes for antibacterial and antifungal activity at the Sandoz pharmaceutical company in Switzerland. Antimicrobial drugs are discovered in the pharmaceutical industry by large-scale "screening" of sample microorganisms. At Sandoz in late 1971 a sample that had limited antibacterial activity was run through a larger battery of screening tests. Each week Sandoz ran about 20 candidate drugs through a battery of 50 tests. Included in these tests were cell culture assays to determine if the material would inhibit cell proliferation, and also tests of immune suppression. The sample gave a positive in only one of the tests: it inhibited the immune response of mice. It did not inhibit cell proliferation, and the only apparent side effect was slight nephrotoxicity.

> Thus, the results obtained in December 1971 and January 1972 in this screening programme already disclosed the three most important features of the biological effects of this preparation which was later found to consist mainly of cyclosporin A: effective immunosuppression with a well-tolerated dose, no general inhibition of cell proliferation (in contrast to azathioprine or cyclophosphamide) and impairment of kidney function at very high doses. [Stahelin, 1986. *Prog. Allergy* 38: 19]

The first report of the drug's success in kidney transplantation came in 1978. The data in Figure 3 show the result at a typical transplantation center from the precyclosporin era (1980–1983 in

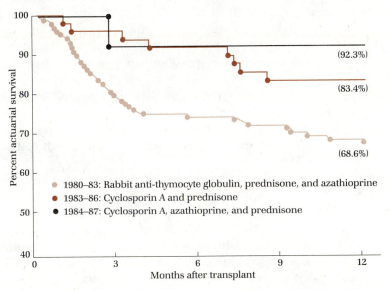

3 **The Effect of Immunosuppression on Kidney Grafts.** In the precyclosporin era immunosuppressive therapies included the use of rabbit anti-human thymocyte antiserum (rabbit anti-thymocyte globulin), glucocorticoids (prednisone) and nucleic acid analogs (azathioprine). The triple therapy of cyclosporin, azathioprine, and prednisone is now routine and over 90% graft survival is achieved. [Data from Posner et al., 1989. *Transpl. Proc.* 21: 1594]

figure) and the combined use of cyclosporin, azathioprine, and prednisone. It is clear that the use of this TRIPLE THERAPY has made kidney transplantation between unrelated donors a viable therapy.

Because of the potential toxicity for the kidney, the dose of cyclosporin and the length of time that it is administered are always kept to a minimum.

Cancer in Organ Transplant Recipients

There is an increase in cancer in organ transplant recipients. When the data are examined, it is found that the cancers that arise in transplant recipients are different from the ones that are seen in the general public. The most common forms of cancer in the general public are lung, prostate, colon and rectum, female breast, and invasive carcinoma of the uterine cervix. But these were not the forms of cancer seen in the transplant patients studied. In these patients the most common cancers were skin and lip. Even the type of skin and lip cancer was different. In the transplant patients squamous cell carcinomas were the most frequent, but in the general population basal cell carcinomas predominate.

In the age group of the transplant patients studied, Hodgkin's is the most common form of lymphoma, but in the transplant population, non-Hodgkin's was most common. Lymph node involvement is seen in 50 to 75% of patients in the general population, but extranodal disease predominated in the transplant recipients (70%).

There is a 400 to 500 increase in Kaposi's sarcoma in renal transplant recipients. In one study it accounted for 5.7% of the malignancies among transplant recipients. This is in comparison with 0.02 to 0.07% in the general population (before the AIDS epidemic).

One very important and perhaps instructive point with both the non-Hodgkin's lymphomas and the Kaposi's sarcoma is that many of them regressed when the immunosuppression was removed. Nontransplant patients who are undergoing immunosuppression (e.g., for autoimmune disease therapy) also show an increase in cancers, and these seem to be the same types that the transplant patients develop. The obvious conclusion from this is that certain kinds of tumors are held in check by the immune system, and that reducing the effectiveness of the immune system allows these tumors to grow. Observations of this type have led many immunologists to rethink aspects of immune surveillance (see Chapter 32). It will be seen later that AIDS patients exhibit similar patterns of tumors (see Chapter 39).

Monoclonal Antibodies in Acute Rejection

The data in the figures above show graft survival over a period of years. Even though cyclosporin has been extremely successful as a primary immunosuppressant as part of the triple therapy, some patients exhibit early signs of graft rejection. Most of these early episodes are handled by increasing the dose of steroid, but in some cases (about 20–30%) the rejection episode is not stopped by the steroid therapy and the patient must receive other treatment. One of the most successful of these is the murine monoclonal anti-human CD3 antibody called OKT3.

Figure 4 shows the use of OKT3 either as primary treatment of initial rejections or as treatment of those cases of acute rejection that were first treated with steroids but did not respond to that treatment. Results are shown for both related donor and cadaver kidneys. It is apparent from this figure that the monoclonal antibody therapy is very successful in reversing the course of acute kidney graft rejection.

OKT3 has been very useful, but as we discussed in Chapter 9,

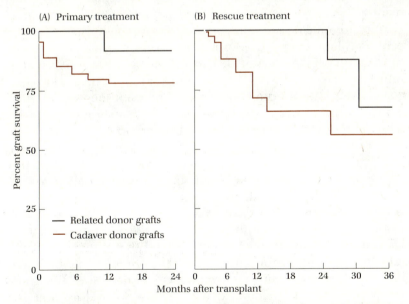

4   Graft Survival in Patients Undergoing Acute Kidney Graft Rejection and Treated with OKT3. Graft survival in (A) patients who showed symptoms of acute graft rejection and were treated with the monoclonal anti-CD3 OKT3 as primary treatment of initial rejection and (B) those who received OKT3 as rescue treatment after high-dose steroid therapy failed to reverse the rejection symptoms. [Redrawn from Norman et al., 1987. *Nephron* 46 (suppl. 1): 41]

murine monoclonal antibodies have the potential limitation of being immunogenic, that is, the recipient can make anti-monoclonal antibodies. This response has been called the HAMA (*human anti-monoclonal antibody*) response and is of importance if there is a recurrence of the rejection episode, that is, if the monoclonal antibody must be used for a second course of treatment. The use of humanized and human monoclonal antibodies will eliminate this problem for anti-isotype responses, but it remains to be seen if long-term treatment even with human monoclonal antibody will eliminate the anti-idiotype response. The presence of these antibodies in the serum of the recipient causes the injected monoclonal antibody to be neutralized or, even worse, may lead to antigen–antibody complexes in the kidney or to allergic reactions.

Transplantation of Pancreatic Islets

In insulin-dependent diabetes the insulin-producing cells (β cells) in the islets of Langerhans have been destroyed. While the reason for this remains unknown, the therapy for diabetes has long been the injection of insulin. As successful as this therapy has been, however, there are complications in the disease that develop over many years. These involve the eye (leading to blindness), kidney (leading to renal failure), and cardiovascular system (leading to the early development of arteriosclerosis). It is generally agreed that the complications are not due to the diabetic state per se, but rather to the inability of the present therapy to maintain blood sugar levels within normal limits at all times. It follows then that a most desired therapy would be the transplantation of islet cells.

Experimental studies in rodents are carried out by inducing a diabetic state by injecting either *streptozotocin* or *alloxan*. These agents have a specific cytotoxic action on the β cells, and this causes a consequent fall in blood sugar. Transplantation of syngeneic islet cells from rats into such treated animals results in a rise in blood sugar to normal levels. Not unexpectedly, the transplant of allogenic islet cells results in rapid rejections. But Paul Lacy and his colleagues in St. Louis found that if they incubated rat islet cells in vitro for 7 days at 24°C before injecting them into diabetic rats along with antilymphocyte serum (ALS), the grafts survived. In fact, they found that there was survival for over 100 days, even though they had crossed a major histocompatibility barrier. It is important to remember that in these studies neither incubation alone nor ALS alone was sufficient to allow graft survival. The combination of the two was needed. Various forms of preparing the tissue are now receiving great attention (treatment with monoclonal antibodies against various surface markers, for example).

Bone Marrow Transplantation

Bone marrow transplantation differs from the other forms of transplantation that we have been discussing because the bone marrow contains immunocompetent cells. So even if the host is rendered immunoincompetent, the cells in the graft are able to react to the antigens of the host. This will be familiar to the readers as a GVH response.

Two methods have been used with growing success to overcome the GVH response. One of these is to remove T cells by agglutinating them with soybean agglutinin, and the other, more promising, method is to treat either the recipient or the bone marrow with a monoclonal antibody against a T-cell marker. We mentioned in Chapter 9 that ricin-conjugated anti-CD5 has been used successfully to overcome acute GVH disease following bone marrow transplantation.

Other Tissues

The introduction of the triple therapy as immunosuppressant and the use of OKT3 as rescue therapy have been used in heart and liver transplantation and have allowed much greater survival of these organs. The patterns of rejection are different for each organ,

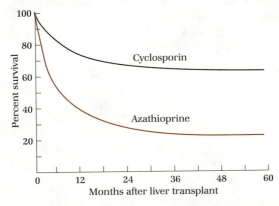

5   The Survival of Liver Recipients. Survival of liver transplant recipients in the precyclosporin era (1963–1979) and after introduction of cyclosporin–steroid therapy (1980–1987) at one transplant center. [Redrawn from Starzl et al., 1989. *Transpl. Proc.* 21: 2197]

and the proper regimens of immunosuppression must be correctly worked out, but it seems safe to say that the combination of immunosuppressive agents and monoclonal antibodies have removed the obvious immunologic barriers to transplantation of most tissue. This is seen dramatically for liver transplantation in Figure 5.

Summary

1.   Tissues from one individual cannot survive in a genetically non-identical recipient because the antigens are recognized as foreign and the host mounts a cell-mediated immune response against the graft.
2.   The "laws of transplantation" say that syngeneic grafts will survive but allogeneic grafts will be rejected. In inbred strains, parental grafts into F_1 are accepted because the F_1 has the same antigens as each of the parental types. F_1 grafts into parental inbred strains are rejected because each parent recognizes the antigens of the other on the graft.
3.   The advent of combined immunosuppression of cyclosporin, azathioprine, and prednisone has allowed tissue transplantation in humans to become a very real therapeutic alternative.

Additional Readings

Borel, J. F., ed. 1986. Ciclosporin. *Prog. Allergy* 38.

Lafferty, K. J., S. J. Prowse, C. J. Simeoniovic and H. S. Warren. 1983. Immunobiology of tissue transplantation: A return to the passenger leukocyte concept. *Annu. Rev. Immunol.* 1: 143.

Land, W. 1989. Kidney transplantation—State-of-the-art. *Transplant. Proc.* 31: 1425.

Luke, R. G., ed. 1988. Use of monoclonal antibodies in organ transplantation. *Am. J. Kidney Dis.* 11(2).

Penn, I. 1988. Tumors of the immunocompromised host. *Ann. Rev. Med.* 39: 63.

IMMUNODEFICIENCY AND IMMUNOPROLIFERATIVE DISEASES

Overview   Perhaps the most serious pathologic conditions involving the immune system are those that result in a loss of function of all or part of the system. These conditions are called imunodeficiency diseases. Imunodeficiency diseases are usually congenital, but some are acquired. In this chapter our emphasis on the congenital diseases will be an attempt to analyze the point in the differentiative pathway of lymphocytes at which the defect has occurred so that we can understand the cellular manifestations of the defect. In fact, these tragic "experiments of nature" are often important tools in defining the normal differentiative pathway.

   In immunodeficiency diseases the defect is manifest in all the cells of the type involved. The other malfunction that we will consider in this chapter presents the opposite problem. In immunoproliferative diseases, a single cell, in the course of differentiation, undergoes a malignant transformation and begins to proliferate rather than continuing along its differentiative pathway. This results in lymphoma or leukemia, diseases in which there is an accumulation of cells of the lymphoid or myeloid series. We will discuss these disorders in terms of the cells involved and the consequences to the patient.

Immunodeficiency Diseases

The immunodeficiency diseases that we will now describe all have in common the fact that all or some part of the immune system is not functioning. Patients affected by these deficiencies present a range of symptoms, but the underlying symptom is always inability to resist infection. These diseases were originally discovered because the patients had recurring infections. Over the years, as the defects became more clearly identified, it became clear that there are many forms of immunodeficiency diseases. Given the

671

complexity of the immune response, it is not surprising that things can go wrong at many sites. What follows is to some extent a catalog of immunodeficiency diseases, with an attempt to identify where in hemopoietic differentiation the congenital defects occur and to identify the cells affected.

Congenital Immunodeficiency Diseases

Immunodeficiency Diseases as Defects in Differentiation

In Chapter 12 we saw that the cells of the immune systems derive from the multipotent STEM CELL. From the practical point of view, if immunodeficiency disorders are to be corrected, it is imperative that we know where the defect has occurred. Table 1 is a list of immunodeficiency disorders classified according to the site of the defect.

Defects of Stem Cells and Progenitor Cells

These diseases, most of which are very severe, are due to a malfunction of the lymphoid system very early in differentiation. Because the defect occurs so early in the differentiative pathway, both the humoral and cell-mediated limbs of the response are affected.

Reticular dysgenesis   This is a rare and fatal disease in which there is no lymphoid or myeloid development. However, erythroid and thrombocyte development continues. Thus the defect must be at a very early stage in lineage establishment (but one at which erythroid and megakaryocyte progenitors have already been determined).

Severe Combined Immunodeficiency Diseases (SCIDs)   There is a fairly wide range of diseases that seem to have their basis in defects in early differentiation of cells along the lymphoid pathway. The term SEVERE COMBINED IMMUNODEFICIENCY is very descriptive, because in these diseases both the B-cell and T-cell lineages are affected (sometimes in varying degrees). SWISS-TYPE AGAMMAGLOBULINEMIA or AUTOSOMAL RECESSIVE ALYMPHOPENIC AGAMMAGLOBULINEMIA was first described by the Swiss physician W. H. Hitzig. It is an autosomal recessive disease (thus affecting both sexes) in which all classes of Ig are depressed, the clotting system malfunctions, and there is a severe decrease in the number of lymphocytes. Numbers of other blood cell types are normal. The thymus is atrophic, and the few circulating lymphocytes that the patient has are not reactive to T-

Table 1 Classification of immunodeficiency disorders according to function affected.

Classification	Diseases
Antibody (B cell) immunodeficiency diseases	X-linked (congenital) hypogammaglobulinemia
	Transient hypogammaglobulinemia of infancy
	Common, variable, unclassifiable immunodeficiency (acquired hypogamma-globulinemia)
	Immunodeficiency with hyper-IgM
	Selective IgA deficiency
	Selective IgM deficiency
	Selective deficiency of IgG subclasses
	Secondary B cell immunodeficiency associated with drugs, protein-losing states
	B cell immunodeficiency associated with 5′-nucleotidase deficiency
Cellular (T cell) immunodeficiency diseases	Congenital thymic aplasia (DiGeorge syndrome)
	Chronic mucocutaneous candidiasis (with or without endocrinopathy)
	T cell deficiency associated with purine nucleoside phosphorylase deficiency
Combined antibody-mediated (B cell) and cell-mediated (T cell) diseases	Severe combined immunodeficiency disease (autosomal recessive, X-linked, sporadic)
	Cellular immunodeficiency with abnormal immunoglobulin synthesis (Nezelof's syndrome)
	Immunodeficiency with ataxia-telangiectasia
	Immunodeficiency with eczema and thrombocytopenia (Wiskott-Aldrich syndrome)
	Immunodeficiency with thymoma
	Immunodeficiency with short-limbed dwarfism
	Immunodeficiency with adenosine deaminase deficiency
	Episodic lymphopenia with lymphotoxin
	GVH disease
Phagocytic dysfunction	Chronic granulomatous disease
	Glucose-6-phosphate dehydrogenase deficiency
	Myeloperoxidase deficiency
	Chédiak-Higashi syndrome
	Job's syndrome
	Tuftsin deficiency
	"Lazy leukocyte syndrome"
	Elevated IgE, defective chemotaxis, eczema, and recurrent infections
Complement abnormalities and immunodeficiency diseases	C1q, C1r, and C1s deficiency
	C2 deficiency
	C3 deficiency (type I, type II)
	C4 deficiency
	C5 dysfunction, C5 deficiency
	C6 deficiency
	C7 deficiency
	C8 deficiency
	C9 deficiency

Source: Data from Altman and Fudenberg, 1982. In Sites et al., eds., *Basic and Clinical Immunology,* 4th ed.; and Buckley, 1988. In Cecil, ed., *Textbook of Medicine.*

cell mitogens. The symptoms, which manifest themselves shortly after birth, are recurring severe infections. The only treatment is bone marrow transplantation. PRIMARY LYMPHOPENIC IMMUNOLOGIC DEFICIENCY is a disease whose symptoms are similar to those of Swiss-type agammaglobulinemia, but it is sex-linked, occurring only in males. SCID WITH ADA-DEFICIENCY patients also exhibit symptoms similar to those of Swiss-type agamaglobulinemia, but there is also an additional bone defect and a very unusual defect in the enzyme adenosine deaminase (ADA). The relationship between the ADA deficiency and the immunodeficiency is not clear, because members of the !Kung tribe in the Kalahari desert and some Arabian horses have the ADA defect without the immunodeficiency. ATAXIA-TELANGIECTASIA is an immunodeficiency disease that has its onset by 2 years of age. It results in abnormalities in both T and B cells. The defect is thought to be in the endoderm or endoderm–mesoderm interaction. The thymus is atrophic, and Ig levels are reduced. Aside from recurring infection, this disease also exhibits cerebral ataxia and oculocutaneous telangiectasia (loss of ability to control the muscles controlled by the cerebellum, and dilation of the vasculature of facial skin and eyeball).

Deficiencies of B-Cell Origin

A group of congenital immunodeficiencies is due to a defect in the differentiation of B cells. Patients with these diseases suffer from recurrent infections, but the infections are predominantly bacterial. Because much of viral immunity is due to T cells, these patients very often are able to defend themselves against virus infections.

X-Linked Infantile Hypogammaglobulinemia (Bruton) Description of Bruton-type hypogammaglobulinemia is thought to be the first clinical description of an immunodeficiency disorder. The symptoms, first described in 1952 in a male child, are recurrent pyogenic infections beginning at about 6 months, severely depressed IgG levels, and absence of IgM, IgA, IgD, and IgE, as well as an absence of peripheral B cells. The disease is X-linked, so only boys develop it. Because the disease is limited to B-cell function, injection of pooled IgG from normal individuals is effective in limiting infection in these children because normal IgG contains antibodies against most common bacteria. This treatment, of course, does not restore B-cell function, and survival into the second or third decade is rare.

Immunodeficiency with Thrombocytopenia and Eczema (Wiskott-Aldrich Syndrome)   This is another X-linked disease, affecting only boys. Levels of lymphocytes and thrombocytes are decreased, resulting in both recurring infections and bleeding.

Selective Ig Disorders   There are a variety of disorders showing selective decreased levels of one or more classes of Ig. Examples include selective IgG, IgM, and IgA deficiency. In these patients the levels of other Ig classes are normal, as is T-cell function.

Common Variable Immune Deficiencies   These are a group of immunodeficiencies that appear after 4–5 years of age that have different defects and cannot be associated with an identifiable cause. The defects are predominantly in antibody and may be associated with abnormalities in B-cell numbers or maturation. But some may be due to defects in helper T cells. Whatever the cause, the clinical manifestation is seen as a decrease in one or more Ig class.

Deficiencies of T-Cell Origin

Defects in T-cell development have far-reaching consequences because the T-cell population contains helper, effector, and regulatory cells. Because the thymus is the hemopoietic inducing microenvironment for T-cell development, it is possible in some cases to pinpoint the defect to the absence of the entire organ or to the reticular cells within it.

Thymic Aplasia (Di George)   Immediately following birth, children with Di George syndrome exhibit the symptoms: characteristic facial features, hypoparathyroidism, congenital heart disease, and immunologic defects. These children are born without a thymus. The syndrome reflects a defect that occurs in the twelfth week of intrauterine life. At that time the thymus and parathyroid have already developed from the third and fourth pharyngeal pouches, and the philtrum of the lip, the ear tubercule, and aortic arch structures are becoming differentiated. This developmental sequence accounts for the grouping of the symptoms. Di George patients have an absence of T cells and T-cell functions, with some impairment of B-cell function. Thymus transplantation is of value in correcting the immunologic disorder, but the patients often have such severe heart disease that survival is threatened.

Thymic Dysplasia (Nezelof) Unlike Di George, in which the thymus is absent, this is an autosomal disease in which the thymus is vestigial and devoid of lymphocytes. This deficiency probably indicates a defect in the reticular elements of the thymus, which are necessary for the organ to act as a hemopoietic inducing microenvironment.

PNP Deficiency This is a disease with a T-cell defect, but it is also characterized by a deficiency in the enzyme purine nucleoside phosphorylase (PNP). The connection between the enzyme and the immune malfunction is not known, and it appears that the disease may affect only some subsets of T cells. The point of origin of the defect is not known.

Trauma-Associated Immunodeficiency There is a transient immunodeficiency that is associated with traumatic injury (including multiple trauma, surgical trauma, and severe burns). The extent of the immunodeficiency is directly correlated with the severity of the trauma, and in such patients bacterial and some viral infections are a major cause of mortality. This immunodeficiency is associated with defects in myeloid and T-cell function. The complexity of the pathological effects of trauma has made the precise identification of the central causes of this immunodeficiency syndrome difficult.

Disorders of Granulocytes

There are a few diseases that affect the differentiation of granulocytes and are manifested by GRANULOPENIA or NEUTROPENIA. Infantile genetic agranulocytosis, familial neutropenia, and cyclic neutropenia are examples of these defects. In all these cases the lymphoid tissue is normal but the patients have decreased resistance to infection because of loss of granulocyte function.

Defects in the Complement System

Both the classical and alternative pathways mature with the gestational age of the fetus, and low complement activity is one of the predisposing factors for infection in premature infants. Genetic deficiencies in all the components have been described, but not all consistently predispose the individual to infections. This should not be too surprising, since we saw in Chapter 8 that the classical and alternative pathway function simultaneously and can be complementary. In addition, most genetic defects in complement components are autosomal recessive mutations, and the heterozygote has one-half the normal level of the relevant component, so that complete deficiencies are very rare. Only C2 deficiency occurs with significant frequency (1 in 10,000) and is an important cause of pneumococcal septicemia in children. Because of the central role of C3, patients with deficiencies in this component suffer life-threatening recurrent infections with encapsulated bacteria.

Figure 1 is a simplified diagram of the complement system and indicates the diseases associated with deficiencies.

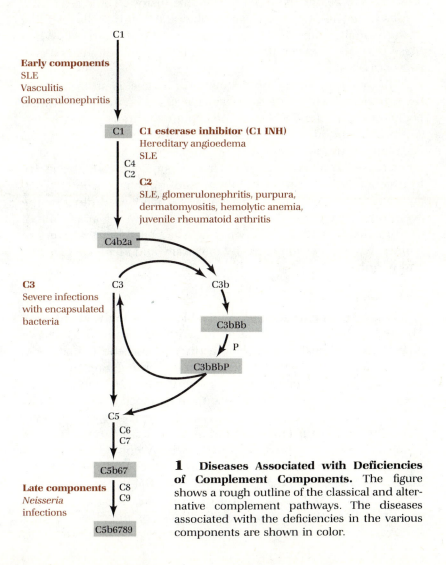

1   Diseases Associated with Deficiencies of Complement Components. The figure shows a rough outline of the classical and alternative complement pathways. The diseases associated with the deficiencies in the various components are shown in color.

Lymphoproliferative Diseases

Leukemias and Lymphomas

Earlier in this chapter we saw some of the consequences of defects in the differentiation pathways of hemopoietic cells, defects that lead to the failure of the stem cells to establish certain lineages and result in almost a complete absence of the end cells. These defects affect *all* the cells that differentiate along the affected pathway. Another pathologic form is the loss of regulatory control of an *individual cell* at some point in its life history. The disease that results from this is the excessive proliferation of the cells resulting in the clonal expansion of the progeny of the affected cell. When these diseases occur in the lymphoid system, they are called LYMPHOPROLIFERATE DISEASES.

The result of excess proliferation, of course, is an increase in the number of cells above the normal level. When this proliferation occurs, tumors can develop at the site. In lymphoid tissue, excessive proliferation in an organ such as a lymph node or the thymus is called a LYMPHOMA. When the proliferation of cells is manifest as an increase in the number of cells in the blood, it is called LEUKEMIA. In practice the two terms are often used interchangeably.

Leukemias and lymphomas are classified according to the symptoms they cause and the tissue in which they arise. One of the practical benefits of the work on the cell-surface markers of lymphocytes has been the ability to classify and identify leukemias and lymphomas.

Leukemias

LEUKEMIA is the accumulation of white blood cells in the circulation. The leukemias are classified as either acute or chronic on the basis of both the clinical course of the disease and the hematologic features, especially the maturation of the accumulating cells. Leukemia, either acute or chronic, can be of either the lymphoid or the myeloid cell lineages. The neoplasms associated with B cells are seen in Figure 2.

ACUTE LEUKEMIA is characterized by a block in maturation early in the differentiation process (in either the lymphoid or the myeloid cells). This defect causes the progeny of the cell with the defect to proliferate and accumulate first in the bone marrow and then in the peripheral blood. CHRONIC LEUKEMIA is similar, except that the cells that accumulate are farther along the differentiation pathway, and therefore partially functional.

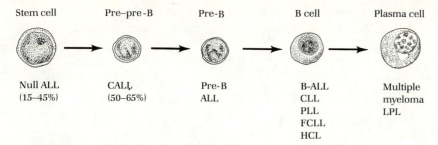

Stem cell	Pre–pre-B	Pre-B	B cell	Plasma cell
Null ALL (15–45%)	CALL (50–65%)	Pre-B ALL	B-ALL CLL PLL FCLL HCL	Multiple myeloma LPL

2   B-Cell Lymphoid Neoplasms. The differentiation steps in B-cell development are shown with the neoplasms that are associated with each step. The frequencies of the more common leukemias are shown. Abbreviations: Null ALL, null acute lymphoblastic leukemia; CALL, common ALL; Pre-B ALL, common ALL with intracytoplasmic Ig_μ H chain (C_μ); B-ALL, B-cell ALL (Burkitt's lymphoma); CLL, chronic lymphocyte leukemia; PLL, prolymphocytic leukemia; FCCL, follicular center cell lymphoma; HCL, hairy-cell leukemia; LPL, lymphoplasmacytoid leukemia (Waldenström's macroglobulinemia).

Because leukemias can involve cells of either lymphoid or myeloid cell lineages, there can be acute lymphoid leukemia, acute myelocytic leukemia, chronic lymphoid leukemia, chronic myelogenous leukemia, and a disease called hairy-cell leukemia that is a leukemic reticuloendotheliosis. Table 2 lists the leukemias as classified according to the cell type involved. This decision is most often made on the basis of cell-surface markers.

The symptoms of leukemia are fever, malaise, spontaneous bleeding in the skin and subcutaneous tissues, frequent infections, and enlargement of the lymph nodes and spleen. The diagnosis is made by observing increased numbers of leukocytes in the circulation. Very often there are large numbers of immature cells, and often there are anemia and thrombocytopenia due to a reduction in erythrocytes and platelets.

Acute Lymphoblastic Leukemia (ALL)   ALL is the most frequent neoplasm of children. Immature lymphocytes, called blast cells, are found in the blood. The disease is often rapidly progressive, and death can occur in a few months if the patient is not treated.

The disease is divided into four types, according to the pattern of markers expressed on the surface of the cells. COMMON-ALL cells have neither B-cell nor T-cell antigens but express a COMMON-ALL ANTIGEN (CALLA or CD10). NULL-ALL cells express neither B-cell, T-cell, nor CALLA antigens. This is the most common form of the disease, constituting close to two-thirds of all cases of ALL. About

Table 2 **Leukemias and lymphomas of the immune system.**

Cell of origin	Neoplasm
B CELL	
Medullary B cell	Chronic lymphocytic leukemia, diffuse small lymphocytic lymphoma
Follicular B cell	Follicular lymphomas, diffuse mixed lymphoma, diffuse large cell lymphoma, Burkitt's lymphoma
Immunoblastic B cell	Diffuse immunoblastic lymphoma
T CELL	
Thymic T cell	Lymphoblastic lymphoma
Mature T cell	Peripheral T-cell lymphomas, chronic lymphocytic leukemia (rare), HTLV-I-associated lymphoma, mycosis fungoides, Sézary's syndrome
Immunoblastic T cell	Diffuse immunoblastic lymphoma
HISTIOCYTIC	
Histiocyte	Malignant histiocytosis, true histiocytic lymphoma (rare)
UNKNOWN	Hodgkin's disease

Source: After Portlock, 1988. In Cecil, ed., *Textbook of Medicine.*

20% of ALL patients have cells that do not express B or CALLA markers but do express a T-cell marker.

At the time of diagnosis, the tumor mass in patients can consist of 10^{12} cells. With multiple drug therapy, the number of leukemic cells can be reduced by 99.9%. This results in a remission of all symptoms but still leaves a tumor load of ca. 10^9 cells. In recent years multiple drug therapy has resulted in primary remission in 95% of children with the disease. Because of the blood–brain barrier that impedes the entry of the drug into the brain, patients are then often treated with cranial irradiation as prophylaxis to eliminate more of the remaining tumor cells and are then given maintenance levels of the drugs for several years.

Chronic Lymphocytic Leukemia (CLL) Chronic lymphocytic leukemia is a disease of adults and is characterized by the progressive accumulation of small lymphocytes in blood, bone marrow, lymph nodes, and other organs. In over 95% of the patients the lymphocytes are B cells. Because the disease is monoclonal, that is, almost always arising from the transformation of a single cell, the serum of these patients very often displays a single "spike" of Ig when subjected to electrophoresis. This Ig is of one isotype, most usually IgM. This can often be a slowly progressive disease with an unusually high incidence of autoimmune hemolytic anemia and tumors (over 15% of the patients develop malignant solid tumors).

Myeloid Leukemias   There are several diseases of myeloid cells that are both chronic and acute. CHRONIC MYELOGENOUS LEUKEMIA (CML) results in the overproduction of granulocytes. This disease is of scientific interest because it is associated with the "Philadelphia chromosome." Chromosome 22 is shortened, and half of its longer arm is translocated to chromosome 9. The Philadelphia chromosome also is present in the erythroid and thrombocyte series of cells, as well as in the granuloid series, but it is not present in lymphoid cells.

There are two forms of ACUTE MYELOGENOUS LEUKEMIA (AML) called acute *monocytic* leukemia and acute *myelomonocytic* leukemia.

HAIRY-CELL LEUKEMIA is a rare but increasingly diagnosed disease affecting older adult males. The cells involved have a mixed series of markers on their surfaces, including some lymphoid, but they are glass-adherent and phagocytic.

Lymphomas

Transformed cells that continue to reside in the lymphoid organ in which they arose are called LYMPHOMAS. Lymphomas are divided into two classes, *Hodgkin's* and *non-Hodgkin's*.

Hodgkin's Disease   Hodgkin's disease (which is named after Thomas Hodgkin, who described it in 1822) is characterized by painless enlargement of the lymph nodes, fever, skin eruptions, and anemia. The enlarged nodes show HODGKIN CELLS—large (40μm) cells with a single nucleus and one large eosinophilic nucleolus. These cells give rise to REED–STERNBERG CELLS, which are cells with multiple nuclei and prominent nucleoli. Hodgkin's patients show impaired immune function, with reduced DTH and graft rejection ability and an increased susceptibility to infection. The origin of the Reed–Sternberg cells is not known, although

Table 3   **Rye Conference classification of Hodgkin's disease.**

Histologic classification	Frequency (%)
Lymphocyte predominance	10–15
Nodular sclerosis	40–70
Mixed cellularity	20–40
Lymphocyte depletion	5–10

current evidence seems to favor the monocyte–macrophage lineage. Because there is no immunologic classification, the standard classification is based on the histologic findings. The Rye Conference classification of Hodgkin's disease is shown in Table 3.

Non-Hodgkin's Lymphomas: T-Cell Tumors

Thymomas   These tumors of the thymus are rare and may be lymphoid or epithelial, or mixed.

Lymphoblastic Lymphoma   This lymphoma is a rare childhood disease in which the tumor cells spread from the thymus-dependent zones of the lymph nodes and spleen. Leukemia is often the terminal phase of this disease.

Mycosis Fungoides and Sézary's Syndrome   Mycosis fungoides begins in the skin and is characterized by a dermatitis that may last for years before giving rise to gross tumors. Sézary's syndrome is a leukemic form of the disease.

Non-Hodgkin's Lymphomas: B-Cell Tumors

Multiple Myeloma   This disease is characterized by the presence of tumor cells in the bone marrow and high levels of serum Ig. Bence–Jones proteins are L chains excreted in the urine. Waldenström's macroglobulinemia is characterized by monoclonal serum IgM.

Burkitts's Lymphoma   Found originally in Africa, this disease is associated with the Epstein-Barr virus (EBV). The American version of the disease seems to be more virulent than its African counterpart. The EBV is also associated with INFECTIOUS MONONUCLEOSIS, which, although not a form of cancer, does show a lymphocytosis of both T and B cells and lymphadenopathy. Antibodies to EBV are present in this disease and are used as a diagnostic tool.

Summary

1. Immunodeficiency diseases are syndromes in which all or part of the immune system does not function. Congenital immune deficiencies are a result of a defect at some stage in the differentiation of the B cell, T cell, or macrophage.
2. Congenital immunodeficiencies of the T-cell line can be due to the failure of the thymus to form, failure of the reticular cells to develop, or failure of lymphocytes to develop and function. B-cell defects are less well identified because of the lack of an identifiable hemopoietic inducing microenvironment.
3. Immunoproliferative diseases are the result of a single cell's losing its proliferative regulatory mechanisms. These cells are trapped at some early stage of differentiation, and the diseases that result from this accumulation of lymphoid or myeloid cells are called leukemias or lymphomas.
4. Leukemias are the accumulation of early forms of blood cells in the blood. Lymphomas are the accumulation of these cells at a single site. The leukemias can be of either lymphoid or myeloid origin and can take the form of an acute or chronic disease.
5. Lymphomas are divided into either Hodgkin's disease or non-Hodgkin's types.

Additional Reading

Altman, A. J. and H. H. Fudenberg. 1982. Immunodeficiency diseases. In D. P. Stites, J. D. Stobo, H. H. Fudenberg and J. V. Wells, *Basic and Clinical Immunology*, 4th ed. Lange Medical, Los Altos, Calif.

Cline, M. J., et al. 1979. Acute leukemia: Biology and treatment. *Ann. Intern. Med..* 91: 758

Holborow, E. J. and W. G. Reeves. 1983. *Immunology in Medicine: A Comprehensive Guide to Clinical Immunology*, 2nd ed. Grune & Stratton, London.

Kaplan, H. S. 1981. Review: Hodgkin's disease: Biology, treatment and prognosis. *Blood* 57: 813

Koeffler, H. P. and D. W. Golde. 1981. Chronic myelogenous leukemia: New concepts. *N. Engl. J. Med.* 304: 1201, 1296.

ACQUIRED IMMUNE DEFICIENCY SYNDROME

CHAPTER

39

Overview In the last decade a new and catastrophic disease affecting the immune system has become known. Acquired Immune Deficiency Syndrome, or AIDS, is before us every day in the newspapers, television, and scientific journals. Had this disease appeared a decade earlier, we would not have known enough about the workings of the immune system to understand it and to begin to apply the advances in basic science to clinical medicine to devise treatments.

We will see that this is a disease caused by a virus, the human immunodeficiency virus (HIV) that infects $CD4^+$ cells. The reader already knows the crucial role played by these cells in the immune response. Patients who develop AIDS become susceptible to opportunistic infections by rather ubiquitous agents that people with intact immune systems fight off regularly and with ease. There is also an effect on the nervous system that is attributable both to HIV infection of the brain and to opportunistic infections. The challenge facing the scientific community is how to reverse the effect of HIV infection before the decline in T cells begins and to develop means of preventing infection by immunization. The necessary public health measures will also be needed to prevent the further spread of this preventable disease.

This chapter is not intended to be a comprehensive analysis of the virus, the epidemiology, or the social significance of AIDS. Rather it is meant, like the rest of this book, to prepare the reader to understand the literature so that progress can be evaluated. This is probably more important in this area of research than in any other that is covered in the entire book. There is more interest in AIDS than any other disease in recent memory, and the supercharged social and political implications of the work make a solid understanding of the immunology essential.

The Immunology of AIDS

The First Appearances of AIDS

In 1981 three papers appeared in *The New England Journal of Medicine* describing immunodeficiency in previously healthy homosexual men. The disease was characterized by an increased incidence of *Pneumocytsis carinii* pneumonia and herpes simplex infection. Shortly after that it was noted that there was an unusually high incidence of disseminated Kaposi's sarcoma in male homosexuals. By the middle of 1982 it was clear to both the medical and the gay communities of New York and San Francisco that a disease of epidemic proportions was spreading through the gay community and that it was fatal. By the end of the year the entire world knew of ACQUIRED IMMUNE DEFICIENCY SYNDROME, or AIDS, and by 1985 AIDS was a feared, misunderstood, and controversial disease.

The number of AIDS cases has been increasing at an exponential rate since 1982 (Figure 1), and there is still no agreement among public health officials as to whether the numbers will level off or continue to rise at this rate. As a point of reference, the number of paralytic polio cases in 1952, the worst year, was 21,000.

Immune Defects in AIDS

AIDS, as the name describes, is an *acquired* failure of the immune system. Table 1 shows the CDC classification of human immunodeficiency virus (HIV) infection and AIDS. From this table it appears that the majority of the symptoms (fever, diarrhea, weight loss, various infections) can be traced to the failure of the immune system. There are also neurological symptoms (see below) that can be attributed to viral infection of the brain. The immunologic symptoms are all consistent with a loss of $CD4^+$ T cells.

The characteristic symptom (Table 1) is OPPORTUNISTIC INFECTIONS in AIDS patients. As the immune system declines, these individuals become infected with organisms that are probably present in the environment and never establish residence long enough to cause infection in people who can mount normal immune responses. The list of the most common opportunistic infections in AIDS is seen in Table 1. Note also from this table that there is an increase in neoplasms as well. This suggests that these tumors could be held in check by the immune system.

Table 2 describes some of the immunologic failures seen in

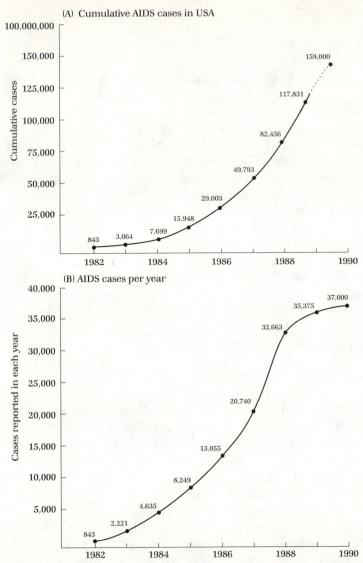

1   Cases of AIDS in the United States. (A) The cumulative cases reported to the CDC between 1982 and 1990. The 1990 total is projected from the March numbers. (B) The numbers of cases reported each year. The slight discrepancy between the top and bottom figures is due to a change in reporting in 1987. [Data from Centers for Disease Control]

AIDS. Lymphopenia, absence of DTH, reduced in vitro proliferative responses, and decreased antibody responses are, as seen in the table, exactly the list of defects we would expect from an absence of CD4$^+$ cells. The explanation for elevated IgG and IgA levels and

Table 1   Centers for Disease Control classification scheme for HIV infections.

Group	Description
I	**Acute HIV infection**
II	**Asymptomatic HIV infection**
III	**Persistent generalized lymphadenopathy (PGL)** Lymphadenopathy (>1 cm diameter) at two or more extrainguinal sites, lasting more than 3 months, and no other condition to explain the findings.
IV	**Other HIV disease**
IV-A	**Constitutional disease** One or more of the following: fever for more than 1 month; 10% weight loss; diarrhea lasting more than 1 month. No other condition to explain the findings.
IV-B	**Neurologic disease** One or more of the following: dementia; myelopathy; peripheral neuropathy. No other condition to explain the findings.
IV-C	**Secondary infectious diseases**
IV-C1	One of the 12 specified symptomatic or invasive diseases that define AIDS: *Pneumocystis carinii* pneumonia; chronic cryptosporidiosis; toxoplasmosis; extraintestinal strongyloidiasis; isoporiasis; candidiasis (esophogeal, bronchial, or pulmonary); cryptococcosis; histoplasmosis; *Mycobacterium artum* complex (or *M. kansasii*); cytomegalovirus; chronic mucocutaneous or disseminated herpes simplex viral infection; progressive multifocal leukoencephalopathy.
IV-C2	Symptomatic or invasive disease with one of the following: oral hairy leukoplakia; multidermatomal herpes zoster; recurrent *Salmonella* bacteremia; nocardiosis; tuberculosis; oral candidiasis.
IV-D	**Secondary cancers** Diagnosis of one of the following known to be associated with HIV infection: Kaposi's sarcoma; non-Hodgkin's lymphoma (small, noncleaved lymphoma or immunoblastic sarcoma); primary lymphoma of the brain.
IV-E	**Other conditions in HIV infection** Includes a variety of clinical headings that may be attributable to HIV disease, including chronic lymphoid interstitial pneumonitis; constitutional symptoms not meeting subgroup IV-A; patients with infectious diseases not meeting subgroup IV-C; and patients with neoplasms not meeting subgroup IV-D.

Source: Adapted from Centers for Disease Control, 1986. MMWR 35: 335.

increased spontaneous Ig secretion from B cells is not so obvious, and tells us that these B-cell functions may be under subtle control of T cells. However, we will see below that the immunology of the disease presents some very challenging problems whose solution will be important not only for the control of the disease but in understanding some aspects of T-cell control of normal function.

Table 2   Immunologic abnormalities in AIDS.

CHARACTERISTIC ABNORMALITIES

Lymphopenia

Quantitative reduction of CD4$^+$ cells

Decrease or absence of DTH

Elevated serum IgG and IgA levels

Increased spontaneous Ig secretion by B cells

CONSISTENTLY OBSERVED ABNORMALITIES

Decreased in vitro proliferative response to mitogens, antigen, and alloantigen

Decreased cytotoxic activity of cytotoxic T cells and NK cells

Decreased antibody response to new antigens

Altered macrophage function

Elevated serum levels of immune complexes

Source: Modified from Seligmann et al., 1984. *N. Engl. J. Med.* 311: 1286.

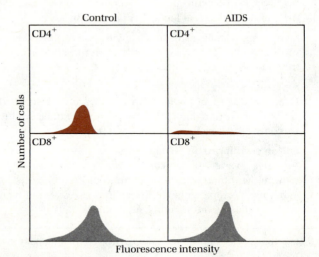

2   FACS Analysis of CD4$^+$ and CD8$^+$ Cells in AIDS. FACS analysis of peripheral blood lymphocytes from a patient with AIDS and a normal control subject, showing the concentrations of CD4$^+$ and CD8$^+$ cells. Cells were incubated with monoclonal anti-CD4 or anti-CD8 and then with fluorescence-labeled goat anti-mouse Ig. Values on the x axis represent fluorescence intensity; values on the y axis represent the number of cells with that intensity. It is clear that the CD4$^+$ cells have been dramatically reduced in the AIDS patient. [Redrawn with background fluorescence subtracted from Fauci et al., 1984. *Ann. Int. Med.* 100: 92]

The dramatic loss of CD4$^+$ cells is seen in Figure 2. This reduction in the absolute number of CD4$^+$ cells results in the increased percentage of CD8$^+$ cells, thus altering the CD4/CD8 ratio. In normal persons this ratio is approximately 1.2 to 1.5. It can be seen in Table 3 that AIDS patients have a ratio of 0.34. Moreover, AIDS PRODROME patients (those who did not have the symptoms of the disease when the study began but who developed them during the course of the study) have a severely reduced CD4/CD8 ratio. Those patients with what is called the AIDS-RELATED COMPLEX or ARC (CDC group III), which is characterized by lymphadenopathy, also have a significantly reduced ratio. From the point of view of distinguishing between AIDS and congenital immune deficiency, patients with common variable immune deficiency (see Chapter 38) have a normal *ratio* of T-cell types, even though the absolute number of their lymphocytes may be decreased.

Risk Groups and Modes of Transmission

Since the discovery of AIDS in the male homosexual population, two other groups have been identified as high-risk groups. These are intravenous drug users and hemophiliacs who receive either blood or blood fractions.

The common denominator of these groups was the opportu-

Table 3   CD4$^+$/CD8$^+$ ratios and anti-HIV antibodies.

Patient category	CD4$^+$/CD8$^+$	HIV$^+$ (%)[a]
AIDS	0.34	68
Risk group		
Prodrome	0.58	100
Lymphadenopathy	0.77	100
Controls		
Healthy; AIDS risk	1.20	0
Sexual contact with AIDS patient	1.09	40
Common variable immune deficiency	1.52	0

Source: Based on Laurence et al., 1984. *N. Engl. J. Med.* 311: 1296.

[a]Note that anti–AIDS virus antibody is found in all the groups associated with AIDS except the healthy at-risk group. Other studies have begun to show that the incidence of antibody may be significant in this group. The group with congenital immunodeficiency has neither the antibody nor a reduced CD4$^+$/CD8$^+$ ratio.

nity for an infectious agent to be transmitted via blood. The intravenous drug users were at risk because of the possibility of using a contaminated needle, and the hemophiliac patients because they relied on intravenous injection of blood and blood products, either of which could be contaminated with the agent. Among male homosexuals, the disease could be spread during anal intercourse, during which blood vessels may be torn, thereby allowing the agent to be transmitted. So, based on the risk groups involved, it seemed that the etiological agent would be blood-borne. Because hemophiliac patients receive blood products that are filtered and free of bacteria and fungi, a virus was the most likely candidate.

Human Immunodeficiency Virus (HIV)

By early 1984 the virus that causes the disease was independently isolated by the groups headed by Luc Montagnier and his colleagues at the Institut Pasteur in France and by Robert Gallo and his colleagues at NIH. There is almost universal agreement that the disease is caused by a retrovirus of the lentivirus subfamily that is called HIV (*h*uman *i*mmunodeficiency *v*irus).

Lentiviruses produce "slow" diseases (*lentus* in Latin means "slow"; *lento* and *lentissimo* indicate a slow tempo in music). Other members of this subfamily include visna, maedi, and progressive pneumonia (PPV) viruses in sheep, caprine arthritis–encephalitis virus (CAEV) of goats, and equine infectious anemia virus (EIAV) of horses. HIV is the first member known to infect humans. A similar virus infects primates (simian immunodeficiency virus, or SIV) and cats (feline immunodeficiency virus, FIV).

There are two *subtypes* of the human virus, called HIV-1 and HIV-2. HIV-1, the initial isolate, is epidemic in the United States and Western Europe as well as Haiti and Central Africa. HIV-2 is found in West Africa and sporadically in Europe and parts of South America.[1]

There is very great heterogeneity among the isolates of HIV, a fact that has allowed virologists to gain insight into the mechanisms of the virus but also something that must be considered in thinking about a vaccine or a drug that will be active against the virus. In addition to heterogeneity in genetic structure, cell tropism, and replication kinetics, there are differences between isolates in cytopathic effect and plaque and syncytium formation. The fact

---

[1] We will discuss primarily HIV-1 in the rest of this chapter and so will refer to it as HIV.

that there is probably heterogeneity in latency and inducibility as well as antigenic composition must also be kept in mind.

The life cycle of HIV is seen in Figure 3. The crucial feature here is that the virus attaches to cells through the interaction of the cell-surface receptor CD4 and the viral envelope glycoprotein gp120.

The primary HIV infection is probably accompanied by a viremia (presence of virus in the blood) that until very recently was thought to be transient. We now know that many (if not all) patients in all CDC classifications have circulating infectious HIV that can be isolated by current improved methods of viral cultivation. This is seen dramatically in Figure 4, which shows that none of the normal control subjects had detectable virus in either their plasma or peripheral blood mononuclear cells but all the HIV$^+$ subjects did. HIV positivity refers to seropositivity, that is, the presence of anti-HIV antibodies in the serum indicating that the persons, who were asymptomatic, had been exposed to the virus.

CD4 as Viral Receptor

HIV infects cells through the high-affinity binding of the HIV envelope glycoprotein gp120 to the CD4 molecule on the surface of T cells and some macrophage–monocytes. In an elegant series of experiments, it was shown that transfection of a variety of human cells with the gene encoding human CD4, but not CD8, rendered these cells susceptible to infection with HIV. This included T cells, B cells, and epithelial cells, and indicates that the kind of cell is not important, only that it express CD4. Mouse cells transfected with the human CD4 gene could not be infected with HIV. This was shown not to be due to some intracellular block, since AIDS virus DNA introduced into these cells was able to replicate. But the virus could also be shown to bind to the surface CD4 with the same affinity as in human cells, arguing that the block was in the ability of the virus–CD4 complex to be internalized. These data seem to indicate that while CD4 is necessary, it may not be sufficient for infection and another, perhaps ubiquitous molecule that is present on human cells but absent from mouse cells is also involved.

To determine where on the CD4 molecule the gp120 of the virus binds, a series of truncated and substituted soluble derivatives of CD4 was produced. It was found by studying the truncated molecules that the gp120-binding site is solely within the first 106 amino acids (the V_1 domain) of CD4. This is a region with great

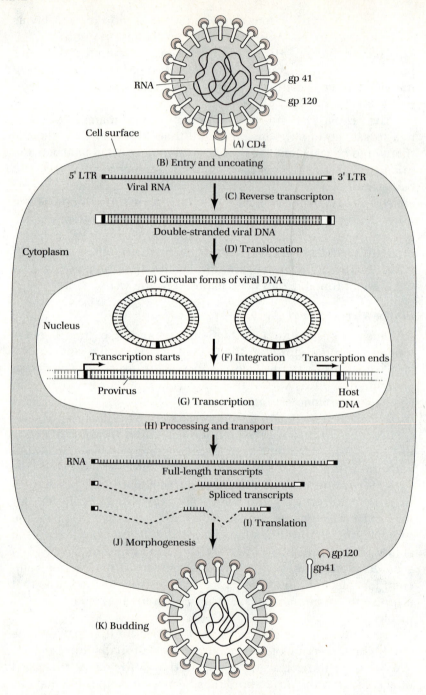

RNA

gp 41

gp 120

Cell surface

(A) CD4

(B) Entry and uncoating

5' LTR   3' LTR
Viral RNA

(C) Reverse transcripton

Double-stranded viral DNA

Cytoplasm   (D) Translocation

(E) Circular forms of viral DNA

Nucleus

Transcription starts   (F) Integration   Transcription ends

Provirus   (G) Transcription   Host DNA

(H) Processing and transport

RNA

Full-length transcripts

Spliced transcripts

(I) Translation

(J) Morphogenesis

gp120
gp41

(K) Budding

◄**3**   **Life Cycle of HIV.** (A) HIV attaches to cells by interaction between gp120 and cell-surface CD4. (B) After the virus enters the cell and is uncoated, (C) virion-associated reverse transcriptase converts the viral RNA into double-stranded DNA, which is (D) translocated from the cytoplasm to the nucleus and (E) converted to supercoiled molecules containing one or two copies of the long terminal repeat (LTR), which (F) is then integrated. (G) HIV gene expression and (H) processing occur, and the full-length transcripts are spliced and transposed to the cytoplasm. The full-length transcripts are messenger RNAs for *gag* and *gag-pol* precursors and genomes for assembly of virions. The spliced transcripts are (I) translated into viral protein (only gp120 and gp41 are shown). (J) Morphogenesis involves formation of a ribo-nucleoprotein core that consists of two molecules of HIV genomic RNA complexed with *gag* and *pol* gene products. (K) This core buds through the cellular membrane and acquires a coat containing *env* glycoproteins. [From Peterlin and Luc, 1988. *AIDS* 2(Suppl. 1): S29. With permission]

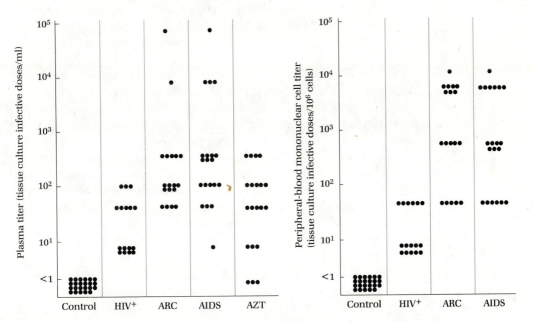

4   **HIV in Plasma and Peripheral Blood Cells.** Titers of infectious HIV in plasma and peripheral blood mononuclear cells (PBMCs) in 22 controls and 54 patients. ARC, patients with AIDS-related complex. AZT, patients receiving long-term AZT treatment. HIV[+], asymptomatic seropositive patients. [From Ho et al., 1989. *New Engl. J. Med.* 321: 1621. With permission]

sequence homology to Ig V regions. Analysis of the substitution mutants defined a discrete binding site within this domain. This site is structurally homologous to the second CDR of the Ig domain.

The binding of the virus gp120 to a domain that has homology to Ig V domains is of interest because CD4 can also be shown to associate with class II MHC molecules that have homology to Ig. Recently Maurizio Zanetti and his colleagues in San Diego showed that there is definite binding of recombinant CD4 to the V region of Ig H chains. This appears to be a domain–domain interaction and may be of importance in the infection process in HIV. If the virus has reacted with an anti-HIV antibody that then associates with CD4 through domain–domain interaction, the antibody may be acting to focus the virus onto its receptor. This must be given serious consideration in thinking about vaccines against HIV.

Depletion of CD4$^+$ T cells

So far we have seen that HIV causes the immunosuppression of AIDS by infecting CD4$^+$ cells, which leads to a selective depletion of CD4$^+$ T cells. The question is: How does the infection cause the depletion?

Since CD4$^+$ T cells are infected, one mechanism for their decline and disappearance could certainly be a *direct cytopathic effect* in which the virus destroys the cell. But the picture is obviously more complicated than this since there is a long latency period (or at least a period of low virus replication) during which the number of CD4$^+$ T cells may be stable or only slowly declining. In contrast, the development of AIDS follows activation of HIV expression and a rapid fall in the number of CD4$^+$ T cells.

There are other mechanisms that might be at work. One can visualize CD4$^+$ cell destruction due to massive budding of the virus at the cell surface, an accumulation of viral products inside the cell, or the formation of gp120–CD4 complexes intracellularly. In vitro infected cells can form syncytia of large, multinucleated cells by fusion, which could occur in vivo as well. It has been suggested that uninfected cells could then be brought into these syncytia.

It has also been argued that the immune system itself may play a crucial role in the destruction of infected cells. For example, antibodies or cytotoxic T cells directed against infected cells may eliminate CD4$^+$ T cells. In fact, the sera of HIV-infected patients have been shown to contain a wide array of anti-viral and anti-cell-surface antibodies. One of the more intriguing observations is that a subset of cytotoxic $CD4^+$ T cells that are specific for gp120 can lyse *uninfected* autologous $CD4^+$ T cells in the presence of gp120. The process is dependent upon the uptake of gp120 by T cells. It will be recalled that most CTLs are $CD8^+$, and this exceptional system may be critical in destroying uninfected $CD4^+$ T cells.

The normal function of the immune system could be responsible in part for the activation of virus in HIV-infected cells. Daniel Zagury and his colleagues in 1986 worked out culture conditions in which it was possible to maintain normal T cells that had been infected with HIV in culture. When these cells were activated with the mitogen PHA, it was found that the virus was activated and the cells died. This is of course in contrast to uninfected cells, which are induced to proliferate by PHA. In fact, activation of HIV-infected T cells increases virus expression by up to 50-fold.

Gary Nabel and David Baltimore examined the products of activated T cells and identified a transcription factor (NF–κB) that binds to the viral enhancer. The implication of this study is that if infection of $CD4^+$ T cells by HIV is random, then activation of the T cells during the course of a normal immune response would pose a risk of activating the virus because the infected cell may be specific for the antigen to which the response is being made.

SYNTHESIS
AIDS and the Immune System

Up to now we have seen that AIDS is a disease in which there is a depletion of $CD4^+$ T cells. This loss of helper T cells results in a susceptibility to infection. The disease is caused by a virus, HIV, that gains entry to the cells by using the CD4 surface molecule of cells through an interaction of cell-surface CD4 with a viral envelope glycoprotein gp120. Unfortunately, HIV is highly variable. The problem facing immunologists is to design a strategy for immunizing against the virus based on the known interactions but in the face of antigenic variability.

Immunization against AIDS

From what we discussed above it is clear that if a vaccine can be developed against HIV one must be both careful and clever in choosing the immunization strategy. There is no doubt that the initial infection with HIV induces a vigorous antibody response to the virus and that seroconversion to HIV^+ is a valid test for infection. But the fact that significant numbers of people with antibody directed against HIV go on to develop AIDS indicates that these antibodies are not always protective (and may even have contributed to the activation of the virus). In one study in which sera from HIV^+ donors were pooled and injected into chimpanzees to determine if the antibody could prevent infection, it was found that the treated animal became infected within the same time period as did the control (no anti-HIV antibodies injected) animal. Chimpanzees do not develop the symptoms of AIDS, but these data indicate that the antibodies that result from infection are not enough to be protective, and we must attempt to devise more efficient immunization procedures.

If the natural infection appears not to routinely give protective antibody, what approach should be taken to attempt to get protection? Table 4 describes the envelope domains of HIV. From in vitro studies it has been established that most neutralizing antibodies are directed toward targets in either the viral gp41 or gp120. A glance at the viral structure (Figure 3) shows that antibodies against these structures will inhibit the early stages of infection, that is, binding to the CD4 receptor, fusion of T-cell membranes, or penetration of the viral elements into the cell. Most HIV-infected individuals have antibodies directed against these regions, and yet they are not protected. This can be because the antibodies are in fact not neutralizing in vivo or because of the heterogeneity of the antigenic sites on HIV.

This heterogeneity has been well documented over the last few years. Different isolates of virus from individuals, and indeed, from the same individual over a period of time, have shown that many serotypes of HIV exist. If the very epitopes that are potentially protective are highly changeable, then the immune system may constantly be fighting the last war, that is, making antibodies against the wrong epitopes.

Another limitation on developing an AIDS vaccine is that it is almost imperative that the immunogen be a recombinant molecule because of the danger of infectious virus in killed or attenuated viral preparations. Knowing the functions of the domains of the virus is an important start toward this end.

Recently a group at NIH has shown that it is possible to develop $CD8^+$ CTLs in mice to recombinant gp160 of HIV. The animals were immunized with the protein in IMMUNOSTIMULATING COMPLEXES (ISCOMs). These are stable molecular structures with a diameter

Table 4   **HIV envelope domains.**[a]

gp120		gp41	
SELECTED FUNCTIONAL DOMAINS			
105–117	gp41 complementarity (?)	518–527	Fusogenic sequence
269	Postbinding, viral entry	579–601	gp120 complementarity (?)
303–337	Postbinding, fusion	691–712	Membrane span
420–463	CD4 binding	840–862	Viral infectivity, cytopathicity
VIRUS NEUTRALIZATION EPITOPES			
254–274		582	Neutralization-resistant mutation
303–337	Variable	584–609	
458–484		616–633	
491–523		735–752	Conserved
T-CELL EPITOPES			
112–124		584–609	
315–329	CTL variable		
410–429	$CD4^+$ CTL		
428–443			
ADCC TARGETS			
315–329	Variable		
474–518	Conserved		
651–670	(Not precisely mapped)		
REGIONS OF HOMOLOGY WITH KNOWN MOLECULAR STRUCTURES			
254–274	6-glucophosphoisomerase	518–527	Fusogenic domain
	HLA-DR	583–599	Immunosuppressive sequence
		831–837	HLA-DR
		840–862	Interleukin-2
IMMUNODOMINANT EPITOPES			
504–518		579–601	

Source: From Bolognesi, 1989. *AIDS* 3[Suppl. 1]: S112. Used with permission.

[a]Selected amino acid sites of the HIV envelope grouped into various categories. Other epitopes that have been mapped on gp120 and gp41 include binding sites of monoclonal antibodies.

of 35 nm in which protein or peptide antigens are incorporated into a matrix of the adjuvant glycoside Quil A. The spleen cells of the immunized mice were then restimulated in vitro with fibroblasts that were expressing a transfected gp160 gene. They produced CTLs that killed target cells expressing gp160 or cells that were pulsed with a 15-residue peptide of gp160. More immunologists will be turning their attention toward CTLs now that it can be shown that cytotoxic cells can be generated to defined gene products. The hope obviously is that if antibodies continue to prove to be less than satisfactory in developing protection, perhaps cytotoxic cells will be more promising.

SYNTHESIS
A Strategy for Immunizing against HIV?

The problem of gearing up the immune response in defense against AIDS is twofold. One would want to intervene in the natural history of the virus to prevent the establishment of infection. If this fails, then one would want to prevent infection from turning into disease. It is clear that AIDS is a communicable disease of viral origin, and as such it seems reasonable that we should be able to immunize against it. Therefore, the research in the coming months and years must be to determine how to get either neutralizing antibodies or cytotoxic cells, or how to augment NK cells or ADCC. We are fortunate that we know enough about the virus and the receptors that it uses to have made a good start. The problem is made more difficult because the infection is in the cells of the immune system and failure to prevent infection from turning to disease results in a decline of the very system that we want to use as defense.

AIDS and the Nervous System

It is clear now that infection with HIV is very often associated with a neurological syndrome called AIDS DEMENTIA COMPLEX (ADC). This is characterized by cognitive, motor, and behavioral disturbances. A recent statement by the American Academy of Neurology provides a succinct recapitulation of the consensus view of the clinical picture as of the end of 1989:

> Different neurologic manifestations occur during different stages of HIV-1 infection. With seroconversion to HIV-1 or shortly after the time of primary infection (CDC group I), some individuals

develop acute aseptic meningitis with headache, fever, and stiff neck and pleocytosis and antibody to HIV-1 in the CSF. In the asymptomatic stages of HIV-1 infection (CDC groups II and III), HIV-1 seropositive individuals may have silent pleocytosis in the CSF or may develop acute (Guillain-Barré syndrome) or chronic inflammatory demyelinating polyneuropathy, myopathy, or herpes zoster radiculitis.

However, most neurologic problems do not become manifest until constitutional symptoms develop such as weight loss, fever, night sweats or chronic diarrhea, or opportunistic infections such as oral thrush (CDC groups IV-A and IV-C2). The neurologic complications that occur during the asymptomatic stages of HIV-1 infection may also occur in patients with (so-called) AIDS-related complex (ARC), who in addition may develop mild cognitive impairment, mononeuritis multiplex or distal symmetric polyneuropathy.

Although (some) patients will develop dementia as their initial AIDS-defining disease, dementia in the absence of HIV-related constitutional symptoms or immunocompromise is thought to be rare. Once AIDS has developed, a wide variety of neurologic problems may occur, which include dementia (AIDS dementia complex (ADC), HIV-1 encephalopathy (HIVE), sub-acute encephalitis, vacuolar myelopathy, mild cognitive abnormalities, distal symmetric polyneuropathy, and CNS opportunistic infections and neoplasms such as toxoplasmosis, cryptococcal meningitis, progressive multifocal leukoencephalopathy, or primary lymphoma of the brain. In children, primary lymphoma of the brain has been reported and a progressive encephalopathy probably caused by HIV-1 has been described. [Janssen et al., 1988. *Ann. Neurol.* 23(suppl): S27]

It is clear from this account that there are many neurological manifestations of AIDS and HIV infection, but they all seem to arise either from direct infection of nervous tissue with HIV or with opportunistic infections of the nervous system as a result of the failure of the immune system in AIDS. Figure 5 shows the time scales of HIV-related systemic and central nervous system disease.

HIV Infection of the Brain

In 1985 a group at NIH through a large collaborative effort found DNA of the AIDS virus in the brains of five AIDS patients at autopsy. A year later another group at NIH and one in La Jolla were able to show that the virus was not localized in neurons but rather was found in mononucleated and multinucleated macrophages and capillary endothelial cells. It became clear that ADC and other neurological symptoms in AIDS could be attributed to viral infec-

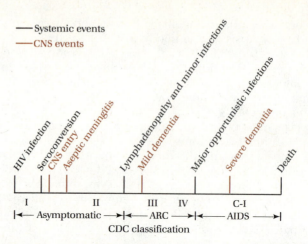

— Systemic events
— CNS events

HIV infection
Seroconversion
CNS entry
Aseptic meningitis
Lymphadenopathy and minor infections
Mild dementia
Major opportunistic infections
Severe dementia
Death

I   II   III   IV   C-I
|← Asymptomatic →|← ARC →|← AIDS →|
CDC classification

5   Time Scale of HIV-Related Systemic and CNS Events. The figure shows the rough relationship between the systemic and CNS events after HIV infection leading to AIDS. The time course varies between individuals, and any individual may have varying degrees of symptoms (including none) after seroconversion. [Redrawn from Price et al., 1988. *Ann. Neurol.* 23(Suppl.): S27]

tion in the brain, but not of the neurons. Therefore, the symptoms were secondary to infection of supporting cells rather than nerve cells. In addition to this, there is also infection of the brain by opportunistic viral and nonviral agents that one sees in the systemic infections (Table 5).

The frequency of virus-infected cells in the *brain macrophages* is thought to be between 10,000- and 100,000-fold higher than in blood cells. Since the macrophage is usually a $CD4^-$ cell, there must be some other mechanism of entry that HIV uses. HIV could enter the macrophage by direct phagocytosis or through *receptor-mediated endocytosis* (see Chapter 32). This latter mechanism would use either the Fc receptor (FcR) or the complement receptor (CR1).

Entry into established cell lines of macrophages in vitro has been shown to occur via the FcR. In these experiments HIV was reacted with serum from seropositive individuals, and it could be shown that at low concentration these antisera *enhanced* HIV infection. The enhancement could be either blocked with heat-aggregated IgG or eliminated if $(Fab)_2$ fragments of the antibody were used. In another study, it was shown that neither anti-CD4 antibody nor soluble CD4 prevented this enhancement of infection. In contrast, antibody to the FcR did.

Table **5**   Diseases associated with AIDS.

Category	Carrier or condition
Bacterial	*Salmonella* spp.
	Nocardia asteroides
	Listeria monocytogenes
	Mycobacterium avium
	Mycobacterium tuberculosis
Viral	Cytomegalovirus
	Adenovirus
	Varicella zoster
	Epstein-Barr virus
	Papovirus-JC
Fungal	*Candida* spp.
	Aspergillus spp.
	Cryptococcus neoformans
	Histoplasma capsulatum
Protozoan	*Cryptosporidium* spp.
	Toxoplasma gondii
	Pneumocystis carinii
	Isospora belli
Neoplasms	Kaposi's sarcoma
	Non-Hodgkin lymphoma
	Cloacogenic carcinoma of the rectum
	Squamous carcinoma of the tongue

SYNTHESIS
AIDS and the Nervous System

It is clear that the brain is a major site of HIV infection and may in fact be the major reservoir of virus in the body. The neurological symptoms of ADC made it seem logical that the neurons would be infected, but as we have seen, it is the macrophages that are the infected cells in the brain. The neurological aspects of AIDS become important not only because of the neurological symptoms but also because these cells can act as a major reservoir of virus. Any therapy must take this into account. Clearly, the interaction of HIV with both the immune and nervous systems is a problem of overwhelming complexity and monumental importance. We fervently hope that among the readers of this book there will be some who will be moved to try to make inroads into this problem.

Summary

1. Acquired immune deficiency syndrome (AIDS) is caused by a retrovirus called HIV (human immunodeficiency virus). The disease is characterized by failure of the immune system, resulting in fever, diarrhea, weight loss, and susceptibility to infection.
2. These symptoms are the result of a decline of CD4$^+$ T cells. The number of CD8$^+$ T cells remains constant; however, the ratio of CD4$^+$ to CD8$^+$ cells changes.
3. The virus uses the CD4 molecule on T cells as a receptor. The viral envelope protein gp120 binds to CD4 to facilitate entry into the cell. Entry into macrophages is probably by receptor-mediated endocytosis with the complex of anti-HIV–HIV reacting with an Fc receptor.
4. The virus is very heterogeneous, and this poses a problem in developing an effective vaccine.
5. Infection of brain macrophages with HIV results in neurological symptoms collectively termed AIDS dementia complex (ADC).

Additional Reading

Arthos, J., K. C. Deen, M. A. Chaikin, J. A. Fornwald, G. Sathe, Q. J. Sattentau, P. R. Clapham, R. A. Weiss, J. S. McDougal, C. Pietropaolo, R. Axel, A. Truneh, P. J. Maddon and R. W. Sweet. 1989. Identification of the residues in human CD4 critical for the binding of HIV. *Cell* 57: 469.

Castro, B. A., C. Cheng-Mayer, L. A. Evans and J. A. Levy. 1988. HIV heterogeneity and viral pathogenesis. *AIDS* 2(Suppl. 1): S17.

Cease, K. B. and J. A. Berzofsky. 1988. Antigenic structures recognized by T cells: Towards the rational design of an AIDS vaccine. *AIDS* 2(suppl 1): S95.

Centers for Disease Control. 1990. *HIV/AIDS Surveillance Report*. April: 1.

Homsy, J., M. Meyer, M. Tateno, S. Clarkson and J. A. Levy. 1989. The Fc and not CD4 receptor mediates antibody enhancement of HIV infection in human cells. *Science* 244: 1377.

Lifson, A. R., G. W. Rutherford and H. W. Jaffe. 1988. The natural history of human immunodeficiency virus infection. *J. Infect. Dis.* 158: 1360.

Peterlin, B. M. and P. A. Luc. 1988. Molecular biology of HIV. *AIDS* 2(Suppl. 1): S29.

Afterword

No textbook of immunology can cover the entire field, up to the minute. But since it was our intention *not* to do that, we think we have succeeded. We hope that those of you who are learning about immunology have gained some insights not only into the immune system but into how that system is studied. We also hope that we've communicated some of the excitement we feel about this field. Those of you who knew immunology before reading this book (and didn't take our advice not to read it) will certainly have found some holes in our view of the immune system. You are invited to communicate any suggestions to us.

In 1988, when we decided to collaborate on this Second Edition of *Immunology: A Synthesis*, we thought it would be an easy job. After all, the first edition had just been published, and because the book focused on experiments rather than interpretations, we assumed it would lay all the foundations for a few recent updates. We weren't even close.

A number of important findings required that much of modern immunology be reframed. These included (but were not restricted to) the elucidation of the ligand for the T-cell receptor; the structure of MHC molecules; the processes of negative and positive selection in T-cell development; and the molecular and cellular bases of lymphocyte activation. Some areas of immunology had been redrawn in broad strokes. In the past year, other important findings have altered some of our views, and we were forced to make the decision to either publish this edition or continue to rewrite it indefinitely. In the next edition we will fill some of these unavoidable holes, though undoubtedly new ones will form. It's a losing battle, but an enjoyable one nonetheless.

Some Immunologic Abbreviations

ADCC Antibody-dependent cell-mediated cytotoxicity
AFC Antibody-forming cell
Ag–Ab Antigen–antibody
APC Antigen-presenting cell
BSA Bovine serum albumin
C Constant (region); Complement
CD Cluster of differentiation
CDR Complementarity-determining region
CEA Carcinoembryonic antigen
CFA Complete Freund's adjuvant
CMI Cell-mediated immunity
CML Cell-mediated lympholysis
ConA Concanavalin A
CSF Colony-stimulating factor
DTH Delayed-type hypersensitivity
EBV Epstein–Barr virus
ELISA Enzyme-linked immunosorbent assay
FcR Fc receptor
FITC Fluorescein isothiocyanate
GALT Gut-associated lymphoid tissue
GVHD Graft-versus-host disease
H Heavy (chain)
H-2 Mouse MHC
HEV High endothelial venule
HGG Human gamma globulin
HLA Human leukocyte antigen (human MHC)
HSA Human serum albumin
ICAM Intercellular adhesion molecule
Id Idiotype
IEF Isoelectric focusing
IFA Incomplete Freund's adjuvant
IFN Interferon
Ig Immunoglobulin
IL Interleukin
IR Immune response

K cell Killer cell
KLH Keyhole limpet hemocyanin
L Light (chain)
LFA Leukocyte functional antigen
LGL Large granular lymphocyte
LK Lymphokine
LPS Lipopolysaccharide
MAC Membrane attack complex
MALT Mucosa-associated lymphoid tissue
MHC Major histocompatibility complex
MLR Mixed lymphocyte reaction
NIP 4-Hydroxy,5-iodo,3-nitrophenylacetyl
NK Natural killer
NP 4-Hydroxy,3-nitrophenylacetyl
OVA Ovalbumin
PAGE Polyacrylamide gel electrophoresis
PBL Peripheral blood lymphocytes
PC Phosphorylcholine
PCA Passive cutaneous anaphylaxis
PFC Plaque-forming cell
PHA Phytohemagglutinin
PMN Polymorphonuclear neutrophil
PPD Purified protein derivative
PWM Pokeweed mitogen
RAST Radioallergosorbent test
RBC Red blood cells
RIA Radioimmunoassay
SLE Systemic lupus erythematosus
SRBC Sheep red blood cells
T$_C$ Cytotoxic T cell
T$_H$ Helper T cell
T$_S$ Suppressor T cell
TCR T-cell receptor
TNF Tumor necrosis factor
TNP Trinitrophenyl
V Variable (region)

Glossary

Accessory cell A cell required for immune responses (in addition to helper and effector cells). Generally describes a macrophage or other antigen-presenting cell.

Acquired immunity Immune resistance that develops following initial exposure to antigen. Generally antigen-specific.

Active immunization Production of immunity by the administration of a specific antigen leading to the induction of an immune response.

Acute-phase proteins A set of proteins that are induced rapidly during inflammatory reactions and many infections.

Adaptive immunity (See Acquired immunity.)

ADCC (See Antibody-dependent cell-mediated cytotoxicity.)

Adenopathy Swelling or enlargement of glands. (See Lymphadenopathy.)

Adherent cell Often refers to macrophages or dendritic cells, both of which stick to glass or plastic.

Adjuvant Material that nonspecifically increases the specific immune response to an antigen. Examples include complete Freund's adjuvant (CFA), incomplete Freund's adjuvant (IFA), alum, and killed *Bordetella pertussis.*

Adoptive transfer The transfer of an immunologic effect to a recipient by the administration of lymphocytes from an antigen-treated donor.

Affinity The binding strength between a receptor (e.g., one binding site on an antibody) and a monovalent ligand (e.g., an epitope on an antigen). Equal to the association constant.

Affinity maturation The increase in the average affinity of antibodies produced during secondary (or subsequent) immune responses to an antigen.

Agglutination The aggregation or clumping of insoluble antigen caused by reaction with multivalent antibody.

Agretope The region of an antigenic peptide responsible for binding to an MHC molecule for effective antigen presentation to T cells.

Allele One variant form of a gene at a particular locus. There is only one allele for any locus per haploid genome.

Allelic exclusion The restriction of a lymphoid cell to the production of an antigen-receptor molecule encoded by only one haploid chromosome (rather than both). Controlled at the level of gene rearrangement.

Allergen An antigen responsible for inducing an allergic reaction (usually type I hypersensitivity).

Allergic reaction A hypersensitive response to an antigen resulting in inflammation and host tissue damage. Usually refers to type I (immediate) or type IV (delayed) hypersensitivity reactions.

Alloantiserum Antiserum produced in an individual against allelic antigens of another individual of the same species.

Allogeneic Genetically different, but of the same species.

Allogeneic effect The activation of antigen-specific B cells by nonimmune, allogeneic helper T cells.

Allograft A tissue transplant between two genetically different members of the same species.

Allotype Protein encoded by an allelic gene. Generally refers to an allelic form of an immunoglobulin isotype.

Altered self Theory suggesting that T-cell receptors recognize conformational changes in MHC induced when the latter binds antigen.

Alternative pathway Complement activation independent of antigen–antibody interaction. Involves C3 and factors B, D, P, H, and I, which form a C3 convertase under the influence of an activator.

Anamnestic response Used to describe immunologic memory. An anamnestic response is an increased immune response following previous exposure to antigen. Literally, "does not forget."

Anaphylatoxins Complement peptides C3a and C5a, which cause mast cell degranulation and smooth muscle contraction.

Anaphylaxis Immediate-type hypersensitive response to antigen mediated by IgE and mast cell degranulation that results in life-threatening vasodilation and smooth muscle contraction (especially of the bronchus).

Antibody A set of related proteins capable of binding specifically to antigen. Produced by B cells in response to immune challenge. Synonymous with *immunoglobulin.*

Antibody-dependent cell-mediated cytotoxicity (ADCC) Cytotoxicity mediated by effector cells (often myeloid "K cells") that recognize targets via passively acquired antibody bound to Fc receptors on their surface.

Antibody-forming cell (AFC) B cell producing antibody, as determined in experimental assays. (See Plaque-forming cell.)

Anergy A state in which a cell and/or individual is incapable of responding to an antigen. When referring to a cell or clonal populations this implies that the cells are present but nonresponsive.

Antigen Any substance that reacts specifically with antibodies and/or T cells.

Antigen-binding site The part of an immunoglobulin molecule that specifically binds antigen. In immunoglobulins this site is formed by the V_H and V_L regions, but it could refer to such a site on any antigen-binding molecule (e.g., MHC, some T-cell receptors).

Antigen presentation Display on the surface of an antigen-presenting cell of a ligand (composed of antigenic fragments associated with an MHC molecule) which is recognized by the T-cell receptor.

Antigen-presenting cell (APC) Usually refers to cells bearing class II MHC molecules that can process and present antigen to $CD4^+$ helper cells. (Rarely used to describe cells that present antigen to $CD8^+$ T cells.)

Antigen processing The degradation of antigen into fragments and the association of these fragments with MHC molecules for presentation by antigen-presenting cells to specific T cells.

Antigen receptor The molecule on B or T lymphocytes responsible for conferring antigen specificity. Refers to surface immunoglobulin on B cells, or to T-cell receptors on T cells.

Antigenic determinant One site on an antigen which is recognized by an individual antibody or T-cell receptor. Synonymous with *epitope.*

Antiserum Serum containing specific antibodies from an immunized animal.

Apoptosis Developmental or "programmed" cell death characterized by membrane blebs, extensive chromatin condensation, and DNA fragmentation. Plays a role in many developmental and other processes, including negative selection of developing T cells and the killing of targets by cytotoxic T lymphocytes.

Arthus reaction An example of type III hypersensitivity produced by localized formation of antigen–antibody complexes.

Ascites Fluids accumulating in a body cavity (e.g., the peritoneum) as a result of the growth of a non-solid tumor. When produced by B-cell hybridomas, these fluids are rich in monoclonal antibodies.

Atopy Clinical manifestation of type I hypersensitivity (IgE-mediated allergy).

Autoantibody An antibody which reacts against antigens of the host in which it was generated (i.e., against "self" or autoantigens).

Autoantigen A "self"-antigen. Usually refers to antigens normally present and not those appearing as a result of infection, drugs, or tumors.

Autochthonous Coming from self. (Greek *autokhthon,* "one sprung from the land itself," hence, indigenous.)

Autograft Tissue graft from one part to another of the same individual.

Autoimmunity An immune response directed against "self" antigens.

Autologous Derived from the same individual.

Autosomes Those chromosomes which are not sex-determining (in mammals, all chromosomes except X and Y).

Avidity The functional binding strength between two molecules, such as between an antigen and an antibody. Avidity is a function of affinity and valency.

B lymphocytes (B cells) Cells that rearrange and express immunoglobulin genes. Cell-surface immunoglobulin acts as an antigen receptor on these cells.

Bence–Jones protein Immunoglobulin light chains (usually dimeric) present in monoclonal form in the urine of some multiple myeloma patients. These proteins were the first source of pure, uniform immunoglobulin for characterization and protein sequencing.

Blast cell A cell stage displaying a higher cytoplasm-to-nucleus ratio than does a resting cell. In lymphocytes, this stage appears shortly after activation and before cell division.

Blastogenesis Formation of blast cells. Usually refers to activation of lymphocytes by antigen or mitogens.

Bursa of Fabricius The primary lymphoid organ of B-cell development in birds; found at the junction of the hindgut and cloaca.

Bystander lysis Lysis of cells in the vicinity of specific targets. These "innocent bystanders" cannot, by themselves, activate the cytolytic effector pathway.

C domains Constant domains of antibodies and T-cell receptor molecules. C domains show relatively little variability between molecules. They do not participate in antigen recognition but may function in effector functions of antibody.

C genes The gene regions encoding the C domains of immunoglobulins and T-cell receptor molecules.

Capping Extensive aggregation of cell-surface molecules to form a "cap." Often requires metabolic and cytoskeletal activity by the cell.

Carcinoembryonic antigen (CEA) An antigen shared by embryonic and malignant tissues, absent from (or found in very low amounts on) normal adult tissues.

Carcinoma An epithelial cancer.

Carrier A molecule to which a hapten can be conjugated, allowing the hapten to be immunogenic. The carrier generally contains determinants recognized by T cells.

Carrier effect The experimental observation that a mixture of two lymphocyte populations, one immunized against a hapten and one immunized against a carrier, will generate a secondary immune response if challenged with the linked hapten–carrier. The carrier effect is produced by the recognition of hapten by B cells and carrier by T cells, which interact in the presence of the hapten–carrier conjugate.

CD markers Cell-surface molecules. These markers are designated by international convention (see Appendix 2), recognized by monoclonal antibodies, and often used to differentiate cell populations.

CD2 A molecule present on the surface of T cells. CD2 interacts with LFA-3 on antigen-presenting cells to facilitate antigen presentation via adhesion. This molecule can also transduce an activation signal (distinct from that of the CD3–TCR complex), although the normal function of this activation pathway is not known.

CD3 A set of molecules (γ, δ, ϵ, ζ, η) associated with the T-cell receptor and involved in its function. Also called T3.

CD4 A molecule present on the surface of a population of T cells that recognize antigenic peptides presented by class II MHC molecules. CD4 is often, but not always, associated with helper function. It is also the receptor for HIV.

CD8 A molecule present on the surface of a population of T cells that recognize antigenic peptides presented by class I MHC molecules. Often, but not always, associated with cytotoxic effector function.

CD25 The low-affinity IL-2 receptor, IL-2Rα. Also called Tac.

CDRs (complementarity-determining regions) Sequences in the variable region of an antibody (or T-cell receptor) responsible for antigen recognition. In antibodies these correspond to the hypervariable regions.

Cell cycle The four phases of cell division: G_1, S, G_2, and M. DNA replication occurs during S and mitosis during M. Cells enter the cell cycle from the resting G_0 stage.

Cell-mediated immunity (CMI) Historically, immune responses mediated by cells as opposed to by humoral factors (antibody). Presently used to describe delayed-type hypersensitivity and CTL reactions (e.g., tuberculin response, graft rejection, contact sensitivity).

Cell-mediated lympholysis (CML) The process of destruction of one cell by another. Usually refers to cytotoxic T-cell–mediated lysis.

Central tolerance Antigen-specific nonresponsiveness induced in lymphocytes during their development. (See Tolerance; Peripheral tolerance.)

Chemotaxis Directed movement of cells in response to the concentration gradient of an attractant.

Chimera A mythological animal with the head of a lion, the body of a goat, and the tail of a snake. Refers to an individual containing tissues derived from another, genetically distinct, individual. For example, a *bone marrow chimera* is an individual transplanted with bone marrow from a genetically distinct animal.

Class I MHC Major histocompatibility molecule consisting of a polymorphic, integral membrane polypeptide noncovalently associated with β_2-microglobulin. Encoded by HLA-A, B, and C in humans; H-2K, D, and L in mice. Expressed on nearly all cells. These molecules present peptide antigen fragments to CD8$^+$ T cells.

Class II MHC Major histocompatibility molecules composed of two integral membrane polypeptides (α and β). Encoded by HLA-DR, DQ, and DP in humans; I-A and I-E in mice. Expressed on antigen-presenting cells, including B cells, dendritic cells, and some macrophages. Also called *Ia*. These molecules present peptide antigen fragments to CD4$^+$ T cells.

Class III MHC Molecules, encoded by genes within the MHC, that are not involved in presenting peptide antigen fragments to T cells. Include some complement components.

Class switch The process by which a single B cell produces a new immunoglobulin isotype (class) without altering the specificity of the antibody produced. Occurs by gene rearrangement of a new heavy-chain C gene to the VDJ, deleting the previous C gene in the process.

Classical pathway Classical complement pathway; the activation of the complement cascade by antigen–antibody complexes. Involves components C1, C4, and C2, leading to the formation of a C3 convertase distinct from that of the alternative pathway. (See Alternative pathway.)

Clonal deletion The theory that immune tolerance is due to the removal of lymphocytes which react with "self"-antigens. In T-cell development, the negative selection that occurs in the thymus to eliminate cells reactive to self-MHC.

Clonal selection The central paradigm of modern immunology. Cells bearing a single antigen-receptor specificity are stimulated to proliferate and differentiate by interaction with specific antigen.

Clone Cells derived from a single progenitor cell.

Clonotype A unique marker on members of a single clone. In T cells, the clonotype (or clonotypic marker) is the variable region(s) of the T-cell receptor.

Cluster of differentiation markers (See CD markers.)

Colony-stimulating factors (CSFs) A group of factors that control the growth and differentiation of hemopoietic and other cells.

Combinatorial diversity The diversity generated in lymphocyte receptors by the choice of a unique heavy chain and a unique light chain (in B cells) or two T-cell receptor chains (in T cells). Can also refer to the diversity generated by choice of V, D, and J gene segments. (See Recombinational diversity.)

Complement The set of serum proteins that, when activated, form a cascade of interactions leading to lytic attack of cell membranes, chemotaxis, and phagocyte activation. (See Alternative pathway; Classical pathway; Membrane attack complex.)

Complete Freund's adjuvant (CFA) A potent adjuvant consisting of mineral oil and mycobacteria. Antigen in aqueous solution is emulsified in CFA for primary immunization. Named after its inventor, Jules Freund (1890–1960). (See Incomplete Freund's adjuvant.)

ConA (Concanavalin A) A lectin, extracted from jack beans, that binds mannose and glucose residues. ConA binds most cells, but is a potent mitogen for T cells in many species.

Concomitant immunity Immunity in which infectious agents or tumors are not eradicated, but in which new inocula are resisted.

Congenic Individuals that differ genetically at only one locus or genetic region. Synonymous with *coisogenic*.

Constant region (C region) The relatively invariant carboxyl terminal portion of immunoglobulin heavy and light chains, and the α, β, γ, and δ chains of the T-cell receptor.

Contrasuppression An immunoregulatory T-cell activity in which target cells are rendered resistant to the effects of suppression.

Conventional antigen Usually refers to defined, soluble protein antigens or xenogeneic red cells, added to a system to induce an immune response. Synonymous with *nominal antigen*.

Coombs' test A test for the detection of antibodies bound to red cells by the addition of anti-immunoglobulin antibody. One diagnostic test of systemic autoimmunity (e.g., systemic lupus erythematosus). Named for Robin Coombs, who devised the test.

Cross-reactivity The ability of an antibody or T-cell receptor, specific for one antigen, to recognize another.

Cyclophosphamide A drug that is differentially cytotoxic for lymphocyte subpopulations at different doses. May either augment or suppress immune responses, depending on its use. Frequently used in immunosuppression for transplantation.

Cyclosporin A (CsA) A potent immunosuppressive drug widely used in prevention of graft rejection.

Cytokines Growth and differentiation factors. Often (but not always) refers to those *not* produced by lymphocytes. (See Lymphokines; Monokines.)

Cytophilic Having a propensity to bind to cells. (Literally, cell-loving.)

Cytostatic Having the property of inhibiting cell growth without killing.

Cytotoxic Having the property of killing cells.

D genes Diversity genes. In immunoglobulin heavy chain genes, D genes are situated between V and J genes. Also found in the T-cell receptor β and δ gene complexes. D rearranges to J, then V to DJ, during B- and T-cell ontogeny.

Degranulation Exocytosis of cytoplasmic granules upon activation in mast cells, or lysis of cytoplasmic granules in granulocytes after phagocytosis.

Delayed-type hypersensitivity (DTH) Type IV hypersensitivity. A cell-mediated immune response in which T cells, in response to antigen, release growth and differentiation factors for the recruitment and activation of macrophages. These responses take 24 hours to several weeks to develop (in contrast to immediate hypersensitivity). Examples of DTH are tuberculin reaction, contact hypersensitivity, and granuloma formation.

Dendritic cells A particularly active type of antigen-presenting cell with long, branching processes found in lymph node (follicular), spleen (splenic), thymus (thymic), and other tissues. The term is also used to refer to a CD3$^+$ cell present in skin, but this cell is a T cell and not an APC.

Desetope The part of an MHC molecule responsible for binding to peptides for presentation to T cells.

Determinant The part of an antigen that is recognized by an antibody or T-cell receptor. (See Epitope.)

Differentiation antigen A cell-surface structure found only on cells of a particular lineage or at a particular developmental stage. Identified by the use of specific antibodies (hence the term "antigen.").

Domain A region of a protein having a coherent tertiary structure. In immunoglobulins the structural unit is approximately 110 amino acids and has an internal disulfide loop. This same domain structure is found in all members of the immunoglobulin superfamily.

Dominant idiotype An idiotype found on a major fraction of the antibodies generated in response to a specific antigen.

DR antigens One type of class II MHC molecules in humans (the others are DQ and DP). Sometimes loosely and incorrectly used to describe all human class II MHC.

Edema Swelling due to accumulation of fluid in tissue spaces.

Epstein-Barr virus (EBV) A virus with the ability to transform human B cells. The causative agent of infectious mononucleosis, Burkitt's lymphoma, and nasopharyngeal carcinoma.

Effector cells Refers to cells responsible for mediating an immune function, as opposed to helper and regulatory cells.

Endocytosis Active internalization of extracellular matter.

Endogenous Originating internally (i.e., within an individual or a cell).

Endosome The intracytoplasmic vesicle produced when a molecule is bound to membrane receptors and carried into the cell.

Endothelium Cells lining the blood vessels and lymphatics.

Endotoxin Gram-negative bacteria contain these lipopolysaccharides in their cell walls. Endotoxins are responsible for most pathogenic effects of these organisms. Some are B-cell mitogens (e.g., *E. coli* LPS).

Enzyme-linked immunosorbent assay (ELISA) A solid-phase antibody quantitation assay employing enzyme-linked antibody and a colored substrate to measure the activity of the bound enzyme.

Epitope The site on an antigen that interacts with an antibody or T-cell receptor.

Erythema Redness caused by the movement of erythrocytes into tissue spaces. One of the "Four Cardinal Signs of Inflammation" (redness, swelling, heat, and pain).

Etiology The origin of a disease.

Exon Region of a gene that, when transcribed, is retained in mRNA.

Exotoxin A class of proteins secreted by both Gram-negative and Gram-positive bacteria, responsible for many pathogenic effects. Some exotoxins are superantigens, interacting with a large percentage of T cells.

Fab The antigen-binding fragment of an antibody, consisting of a light chain and part of a heavy chain, that is produced by digestion of immunoglobulin with the enzyme papain. The cleavage occurs at the hinge region above the inter-H chain disulfide bonds.

Fc The "crystalizable," non-antigen–binding part of an immunoglobulin generated by cleavage with pepsin. It contains the C-terminal domains of the H chains along with the binding sites for C1q complement components and for Fc receptors on cells.

Fc receptor (FcR) Receptor on the surface of some lymphocytes, mast cells, macrophages, and other cells that binds the Fc portion of an Ig molecule.

Flare The erythema (reddening) of the skin caused by local vasodilation.

Fluorescein isothiocyanate (FITC) A fluorescent green dye that can be conjugated to proteins, including antibodies.

Framework regions Portions of antibody (or possibly T-cell receptor) V regions that occur between the CDRs (hypervariable regions) and may be relatively constant among V regions.

Freund's adjuvant (See Complete Freund's adjuvant; Incomplete Freund's adjuvant.)

Gamma globulins A major fraction of serum proteins. Appears closest to the cathode following electrophoresis and includes the antibodies.

Genetic restriction Phenomenon in which cooperation between cells is most effective when they share particular alleles.

Germinal center A region within antigen-stimulated peripheral lymphoid tissue (e.g., lymph nodes, spleen), populated mostly by proliferating B cells.

Germ line The genetic material transmitted to offspring via the gametes. It is unmodified by the genetic rearrangements found in some somatic cells (e.g., T and B cells).

Giant cells Large, multinucleate cells found in granulomatous reactions. In vitro, giant cells can result from the fusion of macrophages.

Graft-versus-host reaction (GVH) Effect caused by transplanted T cells that respond to the host but to which the host does not respond.

Graft-versus-host disease (GVHD) The pathological consequences of GVH. Can be either acute or chronic.

Granulocyte Any of the granular myeloid cells (neutrophils, eosinophils, or basophils).

Gut-associated lymphoid tissue (GALT) Those parts of the immune system associated with the gastrointestinal tract. Properties of GALT are shared by the lymphoid tissue of all mucosal surfaces (e.g., lung, mouth), hence the alternative term MALT (mucosal associated lymphoid tissue).

H-2 The murine major histocompatibility complex.

Haplotype A combination of alleles at linked loci found on one chromosome. Often used with reference to MHC.

Hapten A compound, usually of low molecular weight, that can act as an epitope but not an immunogen—that is, it cannot itself induce an immune response (unless coupled to a carrier molecule).

Heavy chain (H chain) The larger of the two types of polypeptides from which immunoglobulins are constructed. The heavy chains carry the constant regions that determine isotype of the antibody.

Helper T cells (T_H) Functional class of T cells that induces effector cell function by releasing growth and differentiation factors upon induction. Helper T cells are usually CD4$^+$ and restricted to class II MHC.

Hemagglutinin A molecule able to cause agglutination of red blood cells, e.g., antibodies to red cells.

Hemolysis Lysis of red blood cells.

Hemopoiesis The development of blood cells. Synonymous with *Hematopoiesis*.

Heterologous From a different source.

High endothelial venule (HEV) Area of the capillary venule through which lymphocytes move from the blood to the lymph node.

Hinge region The flexible region of an antibody molecule that allows the two combining sites to operate independently. Usually encoded by a separate exon.

Histamine A vasoactive amine present in granules of mast cells and basophils, released upon degranulation.

Histocompatibility Acceptance of grafts between individuals; controlled by histocompatibility molecules.

HLA (human leukocyte antigen) The human major histocompatibility complex.

Humoral Pertains to serum and lymph.

Humoral immunity Immune responses mediated by antibody and complement (in contrast to cell-mediated immunity).

Hybridoma A cell line produced by fusing a lymphocyte (B or T) and a tumor cell. The resulting hybridoma retains some properties of the lymphocyte (e.g., production of antibody) and some of the tumor (e.g., ability to grow in vitro). Used in producing monoclonal antibodies.

Hypersensitivity An immune response that causes damage to the individual (e.g., allergic reaction). May be mediated by antibodies (type I, II, III) or T cells (type IV).

Hypervariable regions The most variable parts of the V regions of immunoglobulin and T-cell receptor chains. Contribute to the antigen binding site. Synonymous with CDRs.

Ia "Immune-response associated" class II MHC molecules.

ICAM-1 (Intercellular adhesion molecule-1) A cell-surface molecule found on a variety of cells (including white cells) that interacts with LFA-1 on lymphocytes and other cells.

Idiotope A single antigenic determinant on a V region of an antibody or a T-cell receptor. The idiotopes make up the idiotype. (See Idiotype; Paratope.)

Idiotype (Id) The set of antigenic determinants (idiotopes) on an antibody which make that antibody unique. The idiotype is associated with the V regions, often at the antigen-combining site.

Immune complex Antigen bound to specific antibody. Immune complexes precipitate more readily than either component alone, which can result in immune complex disease (type III hypersensitivity).

Immune response gene (Ir gene) A gene that determines T-cell responsiveness to a particular antigen. Ir genes commonly map to the class II genes.

Immunofluorescence A method for identification of antigens on cells or tissues. Uses a conjugate of specific antibody and fluorescent dye.

Immunogen A substance that can elicit an immune response. Note that although all immunogens are antigens, some antigens (e.g., haptens) are not immunogens.

Immunogenic Having the property of an immunogen.

Immunoglobulin (Ig) Antibody.

Incomplete Freund's adjuvant (IFA) An adjuvant composed of mineral oil. Antigen in aqueous solution is emulsified in IFA for secondary and subsequent immunization. (See Complete Freund's adjuvant.)

Induration Hardening of tissue, for example in the area of a delayed-type (type IV) hypersensitivity response.

Innate immunity Host defenses that are present even before initial exposure to a specific antigen (in contrast to acquired immunity).

Interferon (IFN) A class of factors that increase resistance of cells to viral infection and act as differentiation factors. IFNγ mediates some T-cell functions.

Interleukins (IL) A group of growth and differentiation factors with immunological and other functions. See Chapter 27 for a complete list.

Internal image From network theory, a site on some anti-idiotype antibodies (Ab2) that mimics the original antigen, that is, it stimulates immune responses reactive with the antigen to which the idiotype (Ab1) binds.

Intron Noncoding region of a gene; separates the coding regions (exons). Introns are removed during formation of mRNA by RNA splicing.

In vitro Refers to experiments with tissue, cells, or cell components performed outside the body. (Literally, "in glass.")

In vivo Refers to experiments performed in a living individual.

Isoelectric focusing (IEF) Separation of molecules on the basis of charge in a pH gradient.

Isotype Generally refers to antibody class (e.g., IgM versus IgG). Encoded by immunoglobulin constant-region genes.

Isotype switch Conversion of antibody production by a B cell or its progeny from one class (isotype) to another, while expressing the same V regions. Produced by genetic rearrangement of the heavy-chain constant-region genes.

J chain A polypeptide that "joins" monomeric IgA or IgM into their polymeric forms.

J genes Joining gene segments. These gene segments are recombined during lymphocyte ontogeny and form part of immunoglobulin light and heavy chains and all T-cell receptor chains.

Junctional diversity Diversity generated by imperfect joining during immunoglobulin gene rearrangement.

Kappa (κ) chain One of the types of immunoglobulin light chains. (See Lambda chain.)

Killer cell (K cell) A lymphoid cell (non-T, non-B) that bears Fc receptors allowing it to bind and kill antibody-coated targets.

Killer T cell Cytotoxic T cell.

Kupffer cells Macrophage-like cells that line the liver sinusoids and may act as antigen-presenting cells.

Lambda (λ) chain One of the two types of immunoglobulin light chains. (See Kappa chain.)

Langerhans cell A very active antigen-presenting cell found in the skin.

Large granular lymphocytes (LGLs) Lymphoid cells, defined by morphological criteria, that include NK (natural killer) cells and K (killer) cells.

Leader (See Signal peptide.)

Lectin Glycoproteins that specifically bind sugar residues. Some lectins are also mitogens.

Leukocyte (or leucocyte) "White cell"; i.e., any blood cell that is not an erythrocyte.

Leukocyte functional antigens (LFAs) Three molecules (LFA-1, 2, and 3) that mediate intercellular adhesion. (See ICAM-1.)

Leukotrienes Family of mediators produced from arachidonic acid via the lipoxygenase pathway.

Ligand The molecule (or molecular complex) bound by a receptor.

Light chain (L chain) The smaller of the two polypeptides that constitute an immunoglobulin molecule. Two different light chains are found in most mammalian species: kappa (κ) and lambda (λ).

Linkage disequilibrium The situation in which two genes are found together at a higher frequency than predicted by the product of their individual frequencies. This can result in an observed trait being mapped to the wrong gene.

Linked recognition The observation that T–B interaction requires hapten and carrier determinants on the same molecule.

Lipopolysaccharide (LPS) A common bacterial endotoxin that nonspecifically activates B cells and macrophages.

Locus Genetically mapped chromosomal location of a gene.

Ly markers A group of cell-surface markers on murine cells. These have been assigned CD designations, which are now more widely used than the Ly designations.

Lymph The fluid that circulates through the lymphatics. Lymph is a serum exudate from capillaries.

Lymphadenopathy Enlargement of the lymph nodes.

Lymphocyte A small cell with little cytoplasm. T and B lymphocytes are responsible for all specific recognition of antigen.

Lymphoid Pertaining to lymphocytes.

Lymphokines Biologically active substances produced by lymphocytes, especially by T cells. Other cells may produce lymphokines as well, but then the substances are often called *cytokines*; thus the term is often used loosely. (See also Monokines.)

Lymphoma A cancer of lymphoid tissue.

Lymphopoiesis The differentiation of lymphocytes from hemopoietic stem cells.

Lymphoproliferation gene (*lpr*) A gene that is defective in MRL mice, leading to massive enlargement of lymph nodes and spleen (caused by lymphocyte proliferation) and autoimmune disorders.

Lymphotoxin One of the tumor necrosis factors (TNFβ).

Lytic pathway The complement pathway leading to formation of the membrane attack complex (C5–C9)

Macrophage Large, myeloid phagocytic cell derived from monocytes. In tissues they were sometimes called *histiocytes*.

Major histocompatibility complex (MHC) A complex of highly polymorphic genes that encode the cell-surface molecules responsible for rapid graft rejection and needed for antigen presentation to T cells. Other molecules (with other functions) are also encoded by genes in the MHC. Currently only described in vertebrates.

Mast cell A bone marrow-derived cell found in tissues; resemble basophils. Mast cells degranulate to release a number of stored mediators (e.g., histamine) and also synthesize mediators upon activation. Degranulation may be induced by a number of stimuli, including cross-linking of IgE bound to cell-surface Fcε receptors.

Megakaryocyte Myeloid cell responsible for platelet production.

Membrane attack complex (MAC) Formed from complement components C5–C9 via the lytic pathway. Leads to a membrane pore in the target cell.

Memory (immunologic) The ability of the immune system to alter (usually heighten) its response to a specific, previously encountered antigen.

Metastasis The spreading of a malignant tumor by the release and growth of transformed cells. May also refer to the secondary tumor.

MHC (See Major histocompatibility complex.)

MHC restriction The observation that T cells and antigen-presenting cells interact most effectively when they share MHC haplotypes. MHC restriction is due to the specific recognition of antigenic peptides *plus* MHC molecules by the T-cell receptor.

β$_2$-Microglobulin Polypeptide that is noncovalently associated with class I MHC molecules. β$_2$-Microglobulin is a member of the immunoglobulin superfamily, but has little or no polymorphism and is encoded outside the MHC.

Migration inhibition factor (MIF) A lymphokine capable of inhibiting the migration of macrophages. Believed to play a role in delayed-type hypersensitivity.

Minor histocompatibility antigens Polymorphic antigens, encoded outside of the MHC, that can contribute to graft rejections. They are recognized, together with MHC molecules, by T cells.

Mitogen A substance that nonspecifically induces cell proliferation.

Mixed lymphocyte reaction (MLR) Proliferation of T cells induced by cells bearing allogeneic MHC molecules.

Monoclonal Derived from the progeny of a single cell.

Monokines Biologically active factors secreted by monocytes and macrophages. Some of these are produced by other cells as well, but as such are referred to as *lymphokines* or *cytokines*.

Mucosa-associated lymphoid tissue (MALT) Lymphoid tissue associated with the gastrointestinal tract (GALT), bronchi, and other mucosa.

Multiple myeloma An oncologic disorder of the bone marrow characterized by plasma cell tumors, high levels of immunoglobulin, and bone lesions.

Myeloma Tumor of plasma cells that often secretes a monoclonal antibody, suggesting that it arose from a single cell.

Natural killer cell (NK cell) A large, granular lymphocyte lacking immunoglobulin or T-cell receptors that has the ability to recognize and destroy some types of tumor cells. NK cells do not undergo clonal selection.

Necrosis Cell death due to injury. Necrotic cells show swelling and disruption of cytoplasmic organelles before observable effects on the nucleus.

Neoplastic Cancerous.

Network theory Proposed regulation of the immune system via the direct interactions of immunoglobulin V regions.

Nominal antigen (See Conventional antigen.)

Nude mouse A mouse carrying a homozygous genetic defect (*nu/nu*) that results in the absence of a thymus. This or a closely linked gene also causes a lack of hair (hence the term "nude").

Null cells Lymphocytes lacking T or B markers (especially surface Ig and T-cell receptor).

NZB/NZW Related mouse strains displaying autoimmune defects. The F_1 is a model for systemic lupus erythematosus.

Oncogene Genes identified from their roles in the development of different types of tumors. If derived from viruses they are designated "v-" (e.g., v-myc). Counterparts in normal cells are proto-oncogenes and are designated "c-" (e.g., c-myc).

Oncogenic Causing cancer.

Opsonin A substance that enhances phagocytosis by binding to both the particle and receptors on the phagocytic cell. Examples are antibodies and C3b.

Opsonization The enhancement of phagocytosis by an opsonin.

Paratope An idiotope (antigenic site on an antibody) involved in binding to the antigenic determinant (epitope). Term used mostly in network theory.

Passive cutaneous anaphylaxis (PCA) Technique used to detect antigen-specific IgE. A test animal is injected intravenously with antigen and dye, and serum (containing IgE) is injected intradermally. The resulting antigen-IgE interaction allows the dye to leave the blood and enter the extravascular space. The diameter of the leaked dye is then used as a measure of the amount of IgE in the intradermally injected serum.

Pathogen An organism capable of causing disease.

Peripheral tolerance Antigen-specific nonresponsiveness induced in lymphoid cells that are fully differentiated. Appears not to involve negative selection but rather cellular paralysis or active suppression. (See Tolerance; Central tolerance.)

Phagocytosis The process by which cells (e.g., macrophages or neutrophils) ingest cellular and particulate matter and enclose it within a vacuole (called a phagosome) in the cytoplasm.

Phagolysosome Vacuole in phagocytic cells produced upon fusion of phagosomes (containing engulfed material) and lysosomes (containing degradative enzymes). The ingested material is digested in the resulting phagolysosome.

Phagosome Vacuoles in phagocytic cells that contain ingested (phagocytosed) materials.

Pinocytosis Process by which soluble molecules or very small particles are taken up by cells into endosomes.

Plaque-forming cell Antibody-forming cell identified in the Jerne plaque assay or related assays.

Plasma Blood after the removal of cells. Contains all clotting factors. (See Serum.)

Plasma cell An antibody-producing cell that is terminally differentiated from an activated B cell.

Plasmacytoma A transformed plasma cell that causes multiple myeloma in humans. Used as fusion partner in producing monoclonal antibodies.

Platelet A small, anuclear cellular structure that ruptures to release thrombin, leading to blood clotting. Produced by megakaryocyte differentiation.

Pokeweed mitogen (PWM) A mitogen that induces human B-cell proliferation and, in the presence of T cells, B-cell secretion of antibody.

Polyclonal Products of a number of different clones of lymphocytes. (See Monoclonal.)

Polymorphism Existence of multiple alleles at a particular gene locus.

Polymorphonuclear neutrophil (PMN) A granulocyte that is morphologically characterized by a multilobed nucleus and neutrophilic granules. Eosinophils and basophils have multilobed nuclei (polymorphous) but have either eosinophilic or basophilic granules.

Primary lymphoid tissue Those tissues and organs in which lymphocytes differentiate from stem cells. These tissues include bone marrow, thymus, fetal liver, and (in birds) the bursa of Fabricius.

Primary response The cellular and humoral immune response to an initial exposure to antigen. This response has a longer lag phase, shorter duration, and smaller effects (e.g., antibody titer) than the secondary response.

Prime To expose to antigen for the first time.

Private specificity An antibody-defined epitope on an MHC molecule that distinguishes it from other haplotypes. (See Public specificity.)

Prophylaxis A protective treatment such as vaccination.

Prostaglandins Derivatives of arachidonic acid via the cyclooxygenase pathway that have a wide range of effects, including roles in inflammation and immunity.

Prozone Antibody concentrations that are too high to allow immune precipitation (high antibody excess).

Pseudogenes Genes that have close sequence homology to other genes but are incapable of being expressed.

Public specificity An antibody-defined epitope on an MHC molecule that is found on MHC molecules of other haplotypes. (See Private specificity.)

Purified protein derivative (PPD) An antigen prepared by ammonium sulfate precipitation of supernatants of *Mycobacterium tuberculosis* cultures.

Quiescent Inactive.

Radioallergosorbent test (RAST) A solid-phase radioimmunoassay used for the detection of IgE antibody to a specific allergen.

Radioimmunoassay (RIA) A technique for the measurement of antigen–antibody interactions. Employs radiolabeled antibodies.

Reagin Antibody that mediates immediate (type I) hypersensitivity. IgE is the major reagin in most mammals and binds to basophils or mast cells via its heavy-chain constant regions.

Reaginic antibody (See Reagin.)

Recombinational diversity Joining of DNA segments chosen from two sets of genes to generate diversity. For example, the selection of a V region and a J region during immunoglobulin gene rearrangement in B-cell development.

Respiratory burst Rapid increase in oxidative metabolism in granulocytes or macrophages following phagocytosis and/or exposure to some growth factors.

Reticuloendothelial system Bone marrow-derived phagocytic cells associated with connective tissue throughout most of the body. Responsible for the uptake and clearance of particulate material.

Rheumatoid factor An antibody (usually IgM) found in individuals with rheumatoid arthritis and many other autoimmune diseases. Rheumatoid factor is an autoantibody specific for IgG.

Rosette A cell surrounded by bound cells or particles. Rosetting can be used to identify and/or isolate cell populations. For example, human T cells form rosettes with sheep red blood cells.

Sarcoma A cancer of supporting tissue (e.g., bone or muscle).

Secondary response The heightened, more rapid immune response that follows a second or subsequent exposure to antigen.

Second-set rejection Secondary response to an allograft in a recipient immunized by a previous graft.

Secretory component Protein produced by some epithelial cells in the mucosa. Binds to dimeric IgA and transports it through the cell and into the mucosal secretions.

Serological Involving methods that employ antibodies.

Serum Fluid portion of blood that remains after the cells and clotting factors have been removed. (See Plasma.)

Serum sickness Type III hypersensitivity reaction (immune complex disease) produced when antigen is administered intravenously into an individual with high levels of circulating antibody. This injection results in large amounts of circulating immune complexes, which precipitate at many sites. Serum sickness was originally described in patients treated with multiple injections of antibody from another species (antisera).

Signal peptide The leader (amino terminal portion) of a newly synthesized secreted or membrane protein that "signals" the polyribosome to associate with the membrane of the endoplasmic reticulum (ER). Once the protein enters the ER, the signal peptide is cleaved off.

Somatic mutation A single base mutation in non-germ-line DNA. In immunology, point mutations that occur in rearranged antibody genes, probably following activation of the B cell. These mutations play a role in the refinement of the antibody response (affinity maturation) through clonal selection.

Specificity Ability of a lymphocyte antigen receptor (or antibody) to discriminate between antigenic determinants. Also refers to the precise determinants recognized by a particular receptor or antibody.

Stem cell Cell from which differentiated cells derive. Most stem cells are regenerating (i.e., they produce more stem cells).

Superantigen An antigen capable of stimulating any T cell bearing a particular T-cell receptor $V\beta$.

Suppressor T cell (T_S) Functionally defined T-cell population that can specifically or nonspecifically inhibit immune responses. The existence of T_S as a unique T-cell lineage is controversial, although the existence of this T-cell function is not.

Synergism Cooperative interaction in which the result is greater than the sum of the parts.

Syngeneic Genetically identical (except for sex).

Systemic lupus erythematosus (SLE) A human autoimmune disease, characterized by antibodies to red blood cells, nuclei, double-stranded DNA, and other intracellular molecules. The name derives from the characteristic "wolf mask" (*lupus*, wolf) on the face, caused by the deposition of immune complexes in the skin.

T cells Lymphocyte population defined by the presence of a rearranged T-cell receptor. Most T cells require a thymus for their maturation from hemopoietic precursors.

T-cell receptor (TCR) The heterodimeric protein on the surface of T cells responsible for antigen/ MHC specificity of the cell. May consist of either γδ dimer (called TCR 1) or αβ (TCR 2). TCR is assembled with CD3 molecules for cell-surface expression. Sometimes referred to as Ti, as in "Ti-T3 complex" (the complex of TCR and CD3 molecules).

T-dependent antigen An antigen that elicits an antibody response only in the presence of helper T cells.

T-independent antigen An antigen that can elicit an antibody response in the absence of helper T cells (although T cells can affect this response).

Thy-1 A glycoprotein (previously called *theta*). Present on T cells, it can be used to distinguish them from B cells. Also found in brain, some fibroblasts, and some hemopoietic stem cells. Human Thy-1 is not present on mature T cells but is found in brain and kidney. A member of the immunoglobulin superfamily, its function is unknown.

Thymocyte A developing T cell present in the thymus.

Titer The relative strength of an antiserum or antibody preparation. Equal to the reciprocal of the highest dilution giving a measurable effect.

Tolerance A state of induced immunological unresponsiveness to a specific antigen.

Tolerogen Refers to antigen that is being employed to induce immunologic tolerance. (Contrast with Immunogen.)

Toxoid Bacterial toxin that has been treated so that it retains its immunogenicity and antigenicity but has lost its toxicity.

Tuberculin Protein fraction from supernatants of *Mycobacterium tuberculosis* cultures.

Tumor necrosis factor (TNF) Biologically active factors produced by macrophages and some T cells; have multiple functions. TNFα is responsible for many pathophysiologic effects (such as those observed in endotoxic shock). TNFβ is also called lymphotoxin.

V genes Genes that combine with J genes (or DJ) of immunoglobulin or T-cell receptors during lymphocyte ontogeny to encode V regions.

V region Variable amino acid terminal domains of immunoglobulin light and heavy chains and T-cell receptor chains. Responsible for antigenic specificity of the molecule. (See CDRs; Hypervariable regions.)

Vaccination Immunization against a pathogen.

Vasoactive amines Molecules released from mast cells, basophils, and platelets that induce contraction of endothelium and smooth muscle. Examples are histamine and 5-hydroxytryptamine.

Wheal-and-flare A transient, sharply delineated swelling of the skin due to edema (wheal) with surrounding redness (flare). Characteristic of type I (immediate) hypersensitivity reactions on the skin.

White pulp The periarteriolar sheaths of lymphocytes and myeloid cells in the spleen.

Xenogeneic From a different source.

Xenograft A tissue or organ graft from a different species.

Amino Acid Abbreviations

ABBREVIATION		Amino Acid	Mnemonic
1-letter	**3-letter**		
G	Gly	Glycine	Glycine
M	Met	Methionine	Methionine
A	Ala	Alanine	Alanine
S	Ser	Serine	Serine
I	Ile	Isoleucine	Isoleucine
L	Leu	Leucine	Leucine
T	Thr	Threonine	Threonine
V	Val	Valine	Valine
P	Pro	Proline	Proline
H	His	Histidine	Histidine
C	Cys	Cysteine	Cysteine
Y	Tyr	Tyrosine	tYrosine
F	Phe	Phenylalanine	Fenylalanine
E	Glu	Glutamic acid	gluEtamic
W	Trp	Tryptophan	tWyptophan
R	Arg	Arginine	Rginine
D	Asp	Aspartic acid	asparDic
N	Asn	Asparagine	Not aspartic
K	Lys	Lysine	liKe sine
Q	Gln	Glutamine	CUEtamine

Human CD Designations

Designation	Main cellular distribution[a]	Recognized membrane component
CD1a	Thy, DC, B subset	gp49
CD1b	Thy, DC, B subset	gp45
CD1c	Thy, DC, B subset	gp43
CD2	T	CD58(LFA-3) receptor, gp50
CD2R	Activated T	CD2 epitopes restr. to activ. T
CD3	T	CD3-complex (5 chains), gp/p 26, 20, 16
CD4	T subset	ClassII/HIV receptor, gp59
CD5	T, B subset	gp67
CD6	T, B subset	gp100
CD7	T	gp40
CD8	T subset	Class 1 receptor, gp32, $\alpha\alpha$ or $\alpha\beta$ dimer
CD9	Pre-B M, Plt	p24
CD10	Lymph. Prog., cALL, Germ Ctr. B, G	Neutral endopeptidase, gp100,CALLA
CD11a	Leukocytes	LFA-1, gp180/95
CD11b	M, G, NK	C3bi receptor, gp155/95
CD11c	M, G, NK, B subset	gp150/95
CDw12	M, G, Plt	(p90–120)
CD13	M, G	Aminopeptidase N, gp150
CD14	M, (G), LHC	gp55
CD15	G, (M)	3-FAL, X-hapten
CD16	NK, G, Mac.	FcRIII, gp50–65
CDw17	G, M, Plt	Lactosylceramide
CD18	Leukocytes broad	β chain to CD11a, b, c
CD19	B	gp95
CD20	B	p37/32, ion channel?
CD21	B subset	C3d/EBV-Rec. (CR2), p140
CD22	Cytopl. B/surface B subset	gp135, homology to myelin assoc. gp (MAG)
CD23	B subset, act. M, Eo	FcεRII, gp45–50
CD24	B, G	gp41/38?
CD25	Activated T, B, M	IL-2R βchain, gp55
CD26	Activated T	Dipeptidylpeptidase IV, gp120
CD27	T subset	p55 (dimer)
CD28	T subset	gp44
CD29	Broad	VLA β-, integrin β1-chain, Plt GPIIa

Appendix 2 (continued)

Designation	Main cellular distribution[a]	Recognized membrane component
CD30	Activated T, B; Reed–Sternberg	gp120, Ki-1
CD31	Plt, M, G, B, (T)	gp140, Plt, GPIIa
CDw32	M, G, B	FcRII, gp40
CD33	M, Prog., AML	gp67
CD34	Prog.	gp105–120
CD35	G, M, B	CR1
CD36	M, Plt, (B)	gp90, Plt GPIV
CD37	B, (T, M)	gp40–52
CD38	Lymph. Prog., PC, act. T	p45
CD39	B subset, (M)	gp70–100
CD40	B, carcinomas	gp50, homology to NGF receptor
CD41	Plt	Plt GPIIb–IIIa complex and GPIIb
CD42a	Plt	Plt GPIX, gp23
CD42b	Plt	Plt GPIb, gp135/25
CD43	T, G, M, brain	Leukosialin, gp95
CD44	Leukocytes, brain, RBC	Pgp-1, gp80–95
CD45	Leukocytes	LCA, T200
CD45RA	T subset, B, G, M	restricted T200, gp220
CD45RB	T subset, B, G, M	restricted T200
CD45RO	T subset, B, G, M	restricted T200, gp180
CD46	Leukocytes	Membrane cofactor protein (MCP), gp66/56
CD47	Broad	gp47–52, *N*-linked glycan
CD48	Leukocytes	gp41, PI-linked
CDw49b	Plt, cultured T	VLA-α2 chain, Plt GPIa
CDw49d	M, T, B, (LHC), Thy	VLA-α4 chain, gp150
CDw49f	Plt, (T)	VLA-α6 chain, Plt GPIc
CDw50	Leukocytes	gp148/108
CDw51	(Plt)	VNR-α chain
CDw52	Leukocytes	Campath-1, gp21–28
CD53	Leukocytes	gp32–40
CD54	Broad, activated	ICAM-1
CD55	Broad	DAF (decay-accelerating factor)
CD56	NK, act. lymphocytes	gp220/135, NKH1, isoform of N-CAM
CD57	NK, T, B sub, brain	gp110, HNK1
CD58	Leukocytes, epithel.	LFA-3, gp40–65
CD59	Broad	gp18–20
CDw60	T subset	NeuAc-NeuAc-Gal-
CD61	Plt	Integrin β3-, VNR-β chain, Plt GPIIIa
CD62	Plt act.	GMP-140 (PADGEM), gp140
CD63	Plt act., M, (G, T, B)	gp53
CD64	M	FcRI, gp75
CDw65	G, M	Ceramide-dodecasaccharide 4c
CD66	G	Phosphoprotein gp180–200
CD67	G	p100, PI-linked

Appendix 2 (continued)

Designation	Main cellular distribution[a]	Recognized membrane component
CD68	Macrophages	gp110
CD69	Activated B, T	gp32/28, AIM
CDw70	Activated B,-T, Reed–Sternberg	Ki-24
CD71	Proliferating cells, Mac.	Transferrin receptor
CD72	B	gp43/39
CD73	B subset, T subset	ecto-5′-nucleotidase, p69
CD74	B, M	Class II assoc. invariant chain, gp41/35/33
CDw75	Mature B, (T subset)	p53?
CD76	Mature B, T subset	gp85/67
CD77	Resting B	Globotriaosylceramide (Gb3)
CDw78	B, (M)	?

Source: Adapted from *Immunology Today*, 1989. 10:8, p. 253.

[a]Thy, thymocytes; DC, dendritic cells; B, B cells; T, T cells; M, monocytes; G, granulocytes; Plt, platelets; Prog, progenitor cells; Germ Ctr. B, germinal center B cells; NK, natural killer cells; Mac, Macrophages; cytopl, cytoplasmic; LHC, epidermal Langerhans cells; Reed–Sternberg, Reed–Sternberg cells; lymph. prog., lymphocyte progenitor cells; epithel., epithelial cells; act., activated; Eo, eosinophil; PC, plasma cell; RBC, red blood cell.

A Last-Minute Update on Mls and MMTV

We were just finishing this book when the following information became available and, while we have not generally made a special effort to keep the contents "up to the minute," we thought that these observations give an important new slant to some of the experiments presented in the text. The observations concern the identities of the *Mls* (minor lymphocyte stimulatory) loci and the nature of their products. (See Box 1 in Chapter 24 for a quick overview of Mls.)

Recently the laboratories of Brigitte Huber, Elizabeth Simpson, Ed Palmer, Philippa Marrack, and others have determined that the Mls determinants and other self-"superantigens" are in fact encoded by retroviruses—specifically, mouse mammary tumor viruses (MMTV, or *mtv* when we refer to the virus as a locus), distributed throughout the murine genome.

Mls loci are defined by their ability to induce proliferation in T cells bearing particular Vβ's. These are listed with the *Mls* loci, their chromosomal locations, and the endogenous *mtv* that maps to the site.

Mls locus	Chromosome	Vβ	*mtv* locus
Mls-1	1	6,7,8,1,9	*mtv-7*
Mls-2	4	3	*mtv-13*
Mls-3	16	3	*mtv-6*
Mls-4 (*Mls-2*-like)	7	3	*mtv-1*

Each *Mls* locus has two alleles: "*a*" indicates that cells from the individual induce proliferation in T cells from a "*b*," or negative, strain. The alleles correlate with the presence or absence (*a* or *b*, respectively) of the particular endogenous *mtv*.

The definitions of *Mls-2* and *Mls-4* differ between labs, and all of this will take at least a few months to get sorted out. Other *mtv* (8, 9, and others) can also cause deletion of T cells within particular Vβ, and these probably account for other "self-superantigens" (discussed in Chapter 24).

MMTV is composed of a 5' long terminal repeat (ltr), *gag, pol,* and *env* genes, and a 3' ltr. The 3' ltr contains an open reading frame (ORF) encoding an Mr 37-Kd protein of unknown function. Different endogenous *mtv* show a high degree of homology, except in this ORF. Transfection of the LBB.1 cell line with a construct containing the ORF from one *mtv* causes the cell to be capable of stimulating a population of T cells expressing a dominant Vβ. Although it isn't formal proof, this suggests that the protein that acts as Mls is encoded by this gene.

Conclusions from these and similar studies are that the Mls loci are in fact different endogenous *mtv*, and that the 3′ ltr ORF encodes a variety of superantigens reactive with T cells bearing particular TCR Vβ. Although these observations do not dramatically change the conclusions that are based on studies of Mls (e.g., studies on negative selection and tolerance such as those discussed in Chapters 24 and 31), it does place these studies in an interesting new light. Among other things, it forces us to consider why viruses and the immune system coevolved such that some viral antigens are recognized by one or a few Vβ's. It will also be very interesting to determine if an analogous relationship exists between viruses and the human immune system.

Additional Reading

Dyson, P. J., A. M. Knight, S. Fairchild, E. Simpson and K. Tomonari. 1991. Genes encoding ligands for deletion of Vβ11 T cells cosegregate with mammary tumor virus genomes. *Nature* 349: 531.

Frankel, W. N., C. Rudy, J. M. Coffin and B. T. Huber. 1991. Linkage of Mls genes to endogenous mammary tumour viruses of inbred mice. *Nature* 349: 526.

Janeway, C. 1991. MLS: Makes a little sense. *Nature* 349: 459.

Marrack, P., E. Kushnir and J. Kappler. 1991. A maternally inherited superantigen encoded by a mammary tumour virus. *Nature* 349: 524.

Woodland, D. L., M. P. Happ, K. J. Gollob and E. Palmer. 1991. An endogenous retrovirus mediating deletion of αβ T cells? *Nature* 349: 529.

Index